Modern System of Ophthalmology (MSO) Series

Disorders of Lens and Cataract Surgery

Second Edition

Modern System of Ophthalmology (MSO) Series

Disorders of Lens and Cataract Surgery

Second Edition

AK Khurana MS FAICO CTO (London)
Professor and Head
Department of Ophthlmology
SGT Medical College, Hospital and Research Institute
Gurugram, Haryana, India

Former Senior Professor and Head
Regional Institute of Ophthalmology
Postgraduate Institute of Medical Sciences
Rohtak, Haryana

Assisted by

Aruj K Khurana DNB FICO FVRS
Assistant Professor
Department of Ophthalmology
Vitreo-Retinal Services
SGT Medical College, Hospital and Research Institute
Gurugram, Haryana, India

Bhawna P Khurana MS DNB FICO FNN FRCS
Associate Professor
Squint, Paediatric Ophthalmology
Orbit and Oculoplasty Services
Department of Ophthalmology
SGT Medical College, Hospital and Research Institute
Gurugram, Haryana, India

CBSPD

CBS Publishers & Distributors Pvt Ltd

New Delhi • Bengaluru • Chennai • Kochi • Kolkata • Lucknow • Mumbai
Gujarat • Hyderabad • Jharkhand • Nagpur • Patna • Pune • Uttarakhand

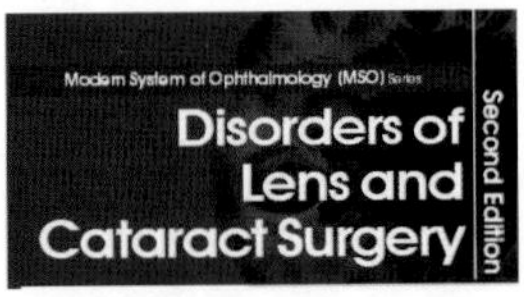

ISBN: 978-93-5466-566-0

Second Edition 2024
Reprint **2026**
First Edition 2014
Reprint 2018, 2020, 2021

Published by Satish Kumar Jain and produced by Varun Jain for

CBS Publishers & Distributors Pvt Ltd

4819/XI Prahlad Street, 24 Ansari Road, Daryaganj, New Delhi 110 002, India

Ph: 011-23289259, 23266838 Website: www.cbspd.com e-mail: delhi@cbspd.com

Corporate Office: 204 FIE, Industrial Area, Patparganj, Delhi 110 092, India

Ph: 011-49344934 Fax: 011-49344935
e-mail: publishing@cbspd.com; publicity@cbspd.com

Branches

- Bengaluru: Seema House 2975, 17th Cross, KR Road, Banasankari 2nd Stage, Bengaluru 560 070, Karnataka, India
  Ph: +91-80-26771678/79 Fax: +91-80-26771680 e-mail: bangalore@cbspd.com
- Chennai: No.18/8B, Subbarayan Street, Shenoy Nagar, Chennai 600 030, Tamil Nadu, India
  Ph: +91-44-42032115, 26681266 e-mail: chennai@cbspd.com
- Kochi: 42/1325, 1326, Power House Road, Opposite KSEB, Power House, Ernakulum 682018, Kochi, Kerala, India
  Ph: +91-484-4059061–67 Fax: +91-484-4059065 e-mail: kochi@cbspd.com
- Kolkata: 147, Hind Ceramics Compound, 1st Floor, Nilgunj Road, Belghoria, Kolkata 700056, West Bengal, India
  Ph: +91-33-25330055/56 e-mail: kolkata@cbspd.com
- Lucknow: Basement, Khushuma Complex, 7 Meerabai Marg (behind Jawahar Bhawan), Lucknow 226001, UP, India
  Ph: +91-522-4000032 e-mail: tiwari.lucknow@cbspd.com
- Mumbai: PWD Shed, Gala No. 25/26, Ramchandra Bhatt Marg, Next JJ Hospital Gate No. 2, Opp. Union Bank of India, Noorbaug, Mumbai 400009, Maharashtra, India
  Ph: +91-22-66661880/89 e-mail: mumbai@cbspd.com

Representatives

- Gujarat 0-9879558667
- Nagpur 0-8692091830
- Uttarakhand 0-9716462459
- Hyderabad 0-9885175004
- Patna 0-9334159340
- Jharkhand 0-9811541605
- Pune 0-9664372571

Printed at Goyal Offset Works Pvt. Ltd., Haryana (INDIA)

Foreword

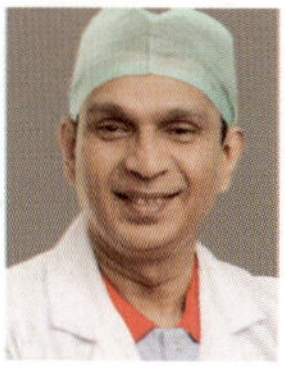

Disorders of lens, especially cataract and its surgical management, has always fascinated ophthalmologists. It gives me immense pleasure to mention that the evolution in cataract surgery from the times of Jacques Daviel and Sushruta to the current date has changed the lives of many. India has made incredible advancements in cataract surgery, probably unparalleled worldwide. Dr Khurana in his book, '*Disorders of Lens and Cataract Surgery*' has crystallized his experience into a beautiful set of clear and succinct guidelines

It gives me immense pleasure to write Foreword for second edition of this remarkable book, a part of Modern System of Ophthalmology (MSO) Series, of which Dr AK Khurana is the Chief Editor. This book builds on a systemic approach with a clear statement of the fundamental issues relating to the disorders of lens and the details that are important in the initial assessment, diagnosis and management.

This book is concise yet a complete textbook on disorders of lens and their management. The book comprises 20 chapters divided into two sections. Section I "Disorders of Lens" covers the basic aspects including anatomy, embryology, physiology and biochemistry of lens, along with clinical profile of the lenticular disorders. Section Il includes the essential aspects of surgical techniques of cataract surgery.

Dr AK Khurana has done all a real service in compiling so much insight and experience into this easy-to-follow text. The book is an enthusiastic celebration of various disorders of the lens and cataract intricately woven with surgical management. I highly recommend this book to everyone.

Dr Khurana, Prof and Head, Department of Ophthalmology, SGT Medical College, Hospital and research institute, Budhera, Gurugram and former Senior Professor and Head, Regional Institute of Ophthalmology, PGIMS, Rohtak, a humble teacher, as I have known him, is an established and well-read author in ophthalmology. Comprehensive Ophthalmology, a textbook for undergraduate students, authored by him, is an indispensable text today. His other books have also been well-received by residents in ophthalmology. I am more than sure that the second edition of the book *Disorders of Lens and Cataract Surgery* will be useful to residents and practicing general ophthalmologists. I appreciate Prof Khurana's efforts and extend him my best wishes.

Prof Amar Agarwal
MS, FRCS, FRCOphth
Chairman and Managing Director
Dr Agarwal's Group of Eye Hospitals
and Eye Research Centers
Chennai, Tamil Nadu, India

Acknowledgements

Second edition of the book has been possible as a result of active criticism, suggestions and generous help of many teachers and students. Surely, I owe sincere thanks to them all. Those who need special mention are Prof RC Nagpal (Former Head, RIO, PGIMS, Rohtak); Prof Jagat Ram (Ex-Dean, PGIMER, Chandigarh); Prof and Head, Swapan Samanta, Govt. Medical College Raigarh; Prof Atul Kumar, Prof JS Titiyal, Prof Namarata sharma and Prof Tanuj Dada from Dr RP Centre for Ophthalmic Sciences, AIIMS, New Delhi; Prof SP Singh, Faridkot; Prof CS Dhull, WCMSR, Jhajjar; Prof Sanjiv Mittal, AIIMS, Rishikesh, Uttarakhand; Prof Kirti Singh, Prof Subhash Dadeya, and Prof Ruchi Goel, MAMC, New Delhi; Prof Harsh Bahadur and Prof Renu Dhasmana from HIMS, Jolly Grant, Dehradun; Prof Manisha Gupta, SGRRIHMS, Dehradun; Prof SP Singh and Prof Kamaljeet Singh from Prayagraj; Prof Rupali Chopra and Prof Nitin Batra, CMC, Ludhiana; Prof Gursatinder Singh, Head, Department of Ophthalmology, Adesh Medical College and Hospital, Shahbad, Kurukshethra; Prof Anand Aggarwl, Head, Department of Ophthalmology, Government Medical College, Patiala; Prof Prempal Kaur, Head, Department of Ophthalmology, Government Medical College, Amritsar; Prof Manjeet Kaur from SHKM, Government Medical College, Mewat; Dr Sumeet Khanduja from Karnal; and Dr Mahipal S Sachdev, Medical Director, Centre for Sight, New Delhi. I acknowledge the special help rendered by Dr Supriya, Dr Harmanjot Singh, Dr Divya Rana, and Dr Amandeep Arora, Residents from SGT Medical College, in updating this edition. I acknowledge with thanks, the respect, affection and cooperation of faculty members of Department of Ophthalmology, SGT Medical College, Hospital and Research Institute, Gurugram namely Prof JP Chugh, Prof Neeraj Sharma, Dr Tulika Gupta, and Faculty of Regional Institute of Ophthalmology (RIO), PGIMS, Rohtak namely, Dr RS Chauhan, Senior Professor and Head, Dr Manisha Rathi, Dr Neebha Anand, Dr Manisha Nada, Dr Urmil Chawla, Dr Ashok Rathi, Dr Sumit Sachdeva, Dr Reena Gupta, Dr Jitender Phogat, Dr Jyoti Deswal, and Dr Ruchi Dabas. The contribution made by Dr Aruj K Khurana and Dr Bhawna P Khurana in completion of this edition is duly acknowledged. The love and moral support, in addition to the editorial help, rendered by my daughter Dr Arushi and Son-in-Law Dr Gurukripa, Asst. Professors of Medicine, Mayo Clinic College of Medicine and Science Rochester, Minnesota, USA, and my wife Dr Indu Khurana, Professor Emeritus, SGT University, and Former Professor of Physiology and Dean-cum Principal, World College of Medical Sciences and Research, Gurawar, Jhajjar, and Former Professor and Head, Department of Physiology, PGIMS, Rohtak, made my task untiring.

I also thank Shri Manmohan Singh Chawla (Managing Trustee); Ms Madhupreet Chawla (Chairperson); Shri Ram Bahadur Rai (Chancellor); Prof Sham Lal Singla (Advisor); Prof OP Kalra (Vice-Chancellor); Prof Gen. SPS Kochar (Dean, FMHS); GL Khanna (Head, HR Department), SGT University, for providing atmosphere conducive to such academic activities.

The enthusiastic cooperation received from Mr SK Jain (Managing Director); Mr YN Arjuna (Senior Vice President—Publishing, Editorial and Publicity), and Mrs Ritu Chawla (AGM, Production) CBS Publishers & Distributors, New Delhi, needs special acknowledgement. Mr Dinesh Chandra Gupta (Senior Editor), Mr Sanju (Graphic Artist), Mr Sunil Dutt, who initially made hand drawings and Mrs Jyoti Kaur (DTP Operator), need special mention because of their efforts to provide considerable beauty to this volume.

AK Khurana

Chief Editor

Contents

DISORDERS OF LENS: BASIC AND CLINICAL ASPECTS

SECTION I

ANATOMY AND PHYSIOLOGY OF LENS

CHAPTER 1

ANATOMY OF THE LENS

The lens is a transparent, biconvex, crystalline structure placed between iris and the vitreous in a saucer-shaped depression, the *patellar fossa.* The posterior surface of the lens capsule is in intimate contact with the vitreous in this fossa and is attached to it in a circular area with ligamentum hyaloidocapsulare (Weigert's ligament). Inside this circle, between hyaloid face and the lens capsule is a small cavity or potential space called retrolental or *Berger's space.* The *equatorial diameter* of the lens, about 6.5 mm at birth, increases to 9–10 mm in the second decade and then remains almost constant. Its *thickness* (axial or anteroposterior diameter) varies with age between 3.5 mm (at birth) and 5 mm (at extreme of age). Its *weight* varies from 135 mg (0–9 years) to 255 mg (40–50 years of age). It has two surfaces. The *anterior surface,* less convex than the posterior, is the segment of a sphere whose radius averages 10 mm (8–14 mm). The *posterior surface,* more curved than the anterior, presents a radius of about 6 mm (4.5–7.5 mm). These two surfaces meet at the *equator,* which is almost circular and has a rippled or undulated appearance. The centres of the anterior and posterior surfaces are called the anterior pole and posterior pole, respectively. The anterior pole is about 3 mm from the back of cornea.

The *refractive index* of the lens is 1.39 (nucleus 1.42, cortex 1.38). Its refractive power is about 16–17 dioptres. Its accommodative power varies with age, being 14–16 D at birth; 7–8 D at 25 years of age and 1–2 D at 50 years of age.

The *colour* of the lens also changes with age. A transparent lens in infants and young adults is colourless, acquires a definite yellow tinge after about 30 years of age and appears amber-coloured in old age. The *consistency* of the lens cortex differs from the nucleus; the former being softer than the latter.

STRUCTURE OF THE LENS

1. LENS CAPSULE

The lens capsule is a thin, transparent, hyaline collagenous membrane which surrounds the

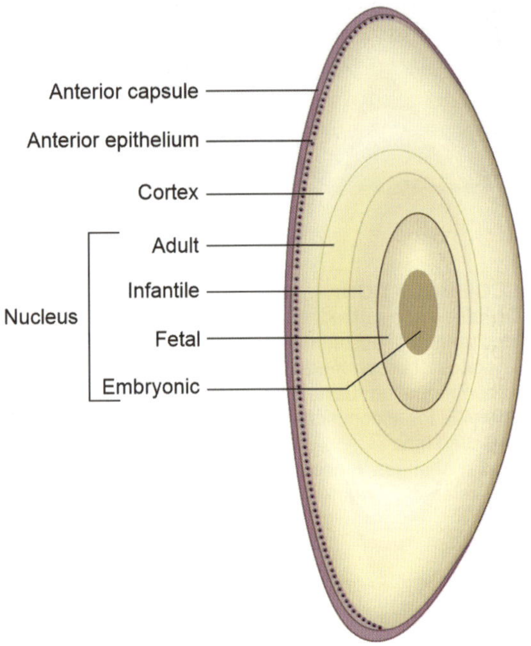

Fig. 1.1. *Structure of crystalline lens.*

lens completely (Fig. 1.1). The lens capsule is highly elastic but does not contain any elastic tissue. It is secreted by the basal cell area of the lens epithelium anteriorly and by the basal area of the elongating fibres posteriorly. Produced continuously throughout life, the lens capsule is the thickest base in membrane in the body. Capsule thickness varies according to the age and is not consistent through its extent.

It is thicker anteriorly than posteriorly and at the equator than at the poles, being thinnest at posterior pole (Fig. 1.2). The Salzman's data for capsular thickness are shown in Table 1.1.

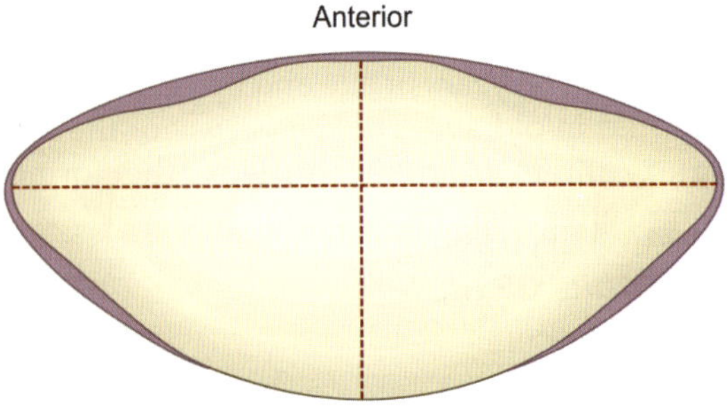

Fig. 1.2. *Variable thickness of lens capsule.*

Table 1.1 *Salzman's data for capsule thickness*

Age (yrs)	*Capsule thickness (mm)*		
	Anterior pole	*Posterior pole*	*Equator*
25	8	2	7
35	14	4	17
71	14	23	9

On light microscopy, the capsule appears as a homogenous structure and stains with PAS. However, on ultramicroscopic examination, it shows a lamellar appearance.

Each lamella contains fine filaments. In true exfoliation of the lens capsule, superficial zonular lamella of the capsule splits off from the deeper layer. The lens capsule is composed principally of type IV collagen and 10% glycosaminoglycans. It contains enzyme, ATP and glycolytic intermediates but cannot be considered to have an independent metabolism. There are chemical and antigenic similarities between the lens capsule and basement membrane of kidney and glomeruli, blood vessels, spleen and lungs.

2. ANTERIOR LENS EPITHELIUM

It is a single layer of cuboidal nucleated epithelial cells which lies deep to the anterior capsule (Fig. 1.1). These cells contain all the organelles found in a typical epithelial cell. Almost all the metabolic, synthetic and transport processes of the lens occur in this layer. In the equatorial region, these cells become columnar, are actively dividing and elongating to form new lens fibres throughout life. There is no posterior epithelium, as these cells are used up in filling the central cavity of the lens vesicle during development of the lens.

Zones of lens epithelium. The anterior lens epithelium can be divided into three zones:

a. *Central zone.* It consists of cuboidal cells which are polygonal in flat section. Their nuclei are round and located slightly apically. These cells are stable and their number, like those of corneal endothelium, slowly reduces with age. Under normal circumstances, these cells do not mitose, but can do so in response to a wide variety of injurious insults including uveitis. During injury repair, epithelial cells are elongated; resembling fibroblasts and can pile up to 10 layers thick under the capsule. Metaplasia of these central zone lens epithelial cells into spindle-shaped myofibroblast-like cells can lead to anterior subcapsular cataract like the shield cataract in atopic dermatitis and glaukomflecken seen after an attack of acute congestive close angle glaucoma.

b. *Intermediate zone.* It consists of comparatively smaller and more cylindrical cells located peripheral to the central zone. Their nuclei are round and central. These cells mitose occasionally.

c. *Germinative zone.* It consists of columnar cells which are most peripheral and located just pre-equatorial. Nuclei of these cells are flattened and lie in the plane of cell axis. Cells of the germinative zone are actively dividing to form new cells which migrate posteriorly to become lens fibres. This process continues throughout life. These cells are extremely susceptible to irradiation. Dysplasia of these transitional zone cells can lead on to posterior subcapsular cataracts (PSCs) as seen in radiation cataract, myotonic dystrophy and neurofibromatosis-II.

Features of lens epithelium

- The anterior lens epithelium has the highest metabolic rate (content of ATP and enzymes is highest in this area of lens).
- The lens epithelial cells are remarkable in that they have a prominent, well-characterized cytoskeletal network consisting of actin, vimentin, spectrin, microtubules, alpha actinin and myosin. The cytoskeletal network is in the form of a polygonal array of geodomes located subjacent and attached to their apical membrane.
- The lateral membrane of the lens epithelial cells is markedly inflamed and has small number of gap junctions—hydrophilic passage between neighbouring cells. Uncommon feature of the lens epithelial cells' lateral membrane is that it lacks tight/occluding junctions.
- The apical membrane of the lens epithelial cells is planar and interfaces with the apical membrane of elongating fibre cells as they migrate to their sutural location. The unique apico-apical interface is known as epithelial fibre cell interface (EFI). The EFI is characterized by transcytotic events and plays a key role in the lens physiology.
- Na-K ATPases and acid phosphatases are localized on the apicolateral membrane.

3. LENS FIBRES

Formation

The epithelial cells elongate to form the lens fibres. At first, the lens fibres are formed from the posterior epithelium which runs from posterior to anterior to fill the lens vesicle. But later on, the lens fibres are derived from the cells of the equatorial region of the anterior epithelium. These cells divide, elongate and differentiate to produce long, thin, regularly arranged lens fibres that constitute the bulk of the lens. Successively, the new lens fibres are laid on the older deeper fibres. The superficial (new) fibres are nucleated with elongation of the cell; the nuclei assume a relatively more anterior position. As the new fibres are laid down, the anterior shifted nucleus forms a line convex forward at the equator, known as *lens* or *nuclear bow* (Fig. 1.3).

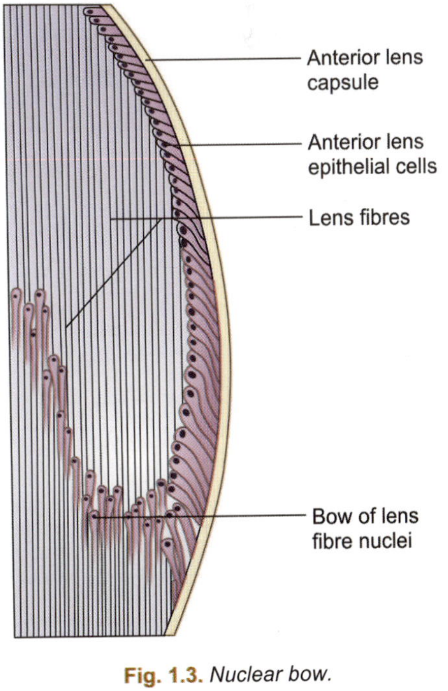

Fig. 1.3. *Nuclear bow.*

Structure of the lens fibres

On cross-section, the lens fibres are almost hexagonal in shape and are bound together by the ground substance (Fig. 1.4A). The cytoplasm of the cells of the superficial bow region and the newly formed lens fibres contain a nucleus, mitochondria, Golgi apparatus, rough endoplasmic reticulum, and polysomes. The ribosomal content of the newly formed lens fibres is more than the epithelial cells indicating an elevated protein synthesis. The nuclei of the lens fibres are present temporarily and disappear later on. Thus the cytoplasm of the older lens fibres is devoid of nuclei, is homogenous and granular with very few organelles. There are interlocking processes between cells (ball-and-socket and tongue-and-groove interdigitations) with zonulae occludentes present (Fig. 1.4B). It is interesting to note that the interdigitations are less complicated in the superficial zone of the lens; and this may permit moulding of the lens shape during accommodation.

Structural arrangement of the lens fibres

The initial fibres forming the fetal nucleus just surrounding the embryonic nucleus are arranged in such a way that they terminate with two Y-shaped sutures on the anterior (upright Y) and the posterior (inverted Y) surfaces of the lens (Fig. 1.5). Later in gestation and following birth, the growth of the lens sutures is much more irregular. Instead of simple Y-sutures, more complicated dendritic patterns (Fig. 1.6) are observed due to asymmetrical fibre growth.

Zonal arrangement of the lens fibres

The lens fibres are formed throughout life and are arranged in zones that delineate the various periods of development of the lens (Fig. 1.1). This stratification is due to optical differences between the older, more sclerotic regions of the central lens and the newer, more transparent peripheral areas. In an adult, the lens fibres are arranged compactly as nucleus and cortex of the lens.

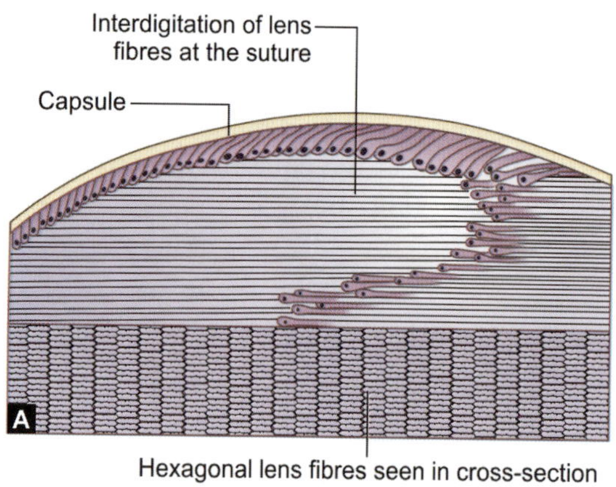

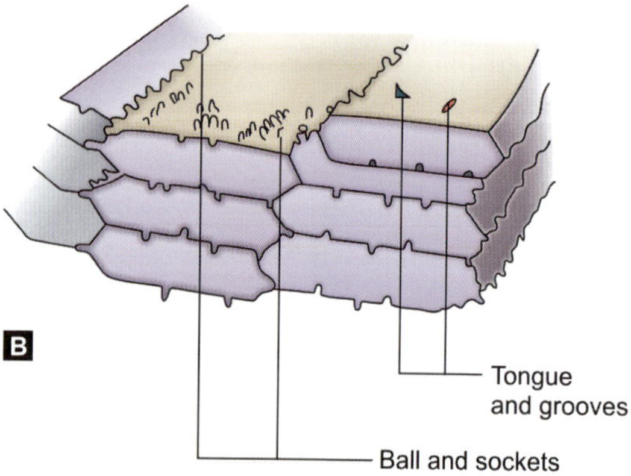

Fig. 1.4. *Structure of lens fibres: **(A)** Hexagonal arrangement of lens fibres in cross-section; **(B)** Interlocking processes in between the lens fibres.*

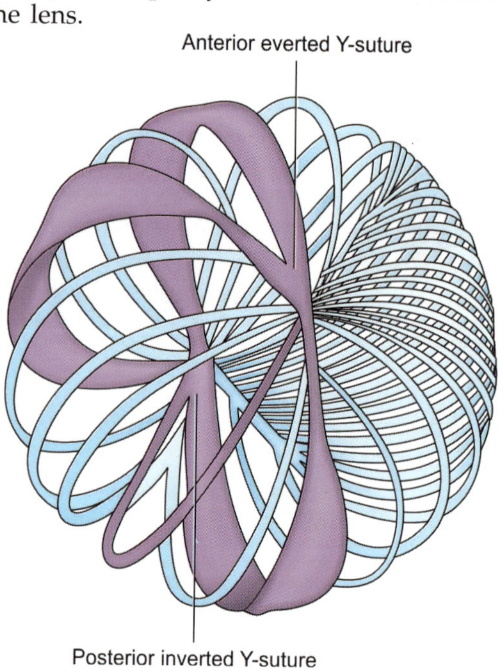

Fig. 1.5. *Y-shaped arrangement of lens fibres around embryonic nucleus.*

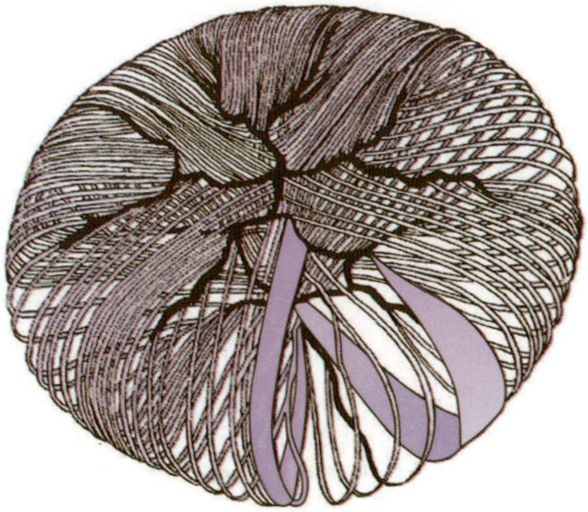

Fig. 1.6. *Dendritic pattern of lens fibres.*

a. ***Nucleus.*** It is the central part containing the oldest fibres. It consists of different zones, *embryonic nucleus* is its innermost part (formed at 1–3 months of gestation). Outside the embryonic nucleus, successive nuclear zones are laid down as the development proceeds and depending upon the period of formation, are called *fetal nucleus* (corresponding to lens from 3 months of gestation till birth), the *infantile nucleus* (corresponding to lens from birth to puberty) and the *adult nucleus* (corresponding to lens in adult life). The size of the embryonic and fetal nuclei remains constant while that of adult nucleus is always increasing.

b. ***Cortex.*** It is the peripheral part of the lens which lies just outside the adult nucleus. It comprises the youngest (most recently formed) lens fibres.

APPLIED ANATOMY OF THE LENS

BIOMICROSCOPIC STRATIFICATION OF THE LENS

Biomicroscopic examination of the lens with the pupil dilated reveals stratification of the lens into concentric layers from front to backwards which are as follows (Fig. 1.7A):

1. ***Capsule*** **(Ca).** The outermost layer, formed by capsule (Ca), is seen as a fine stratum.

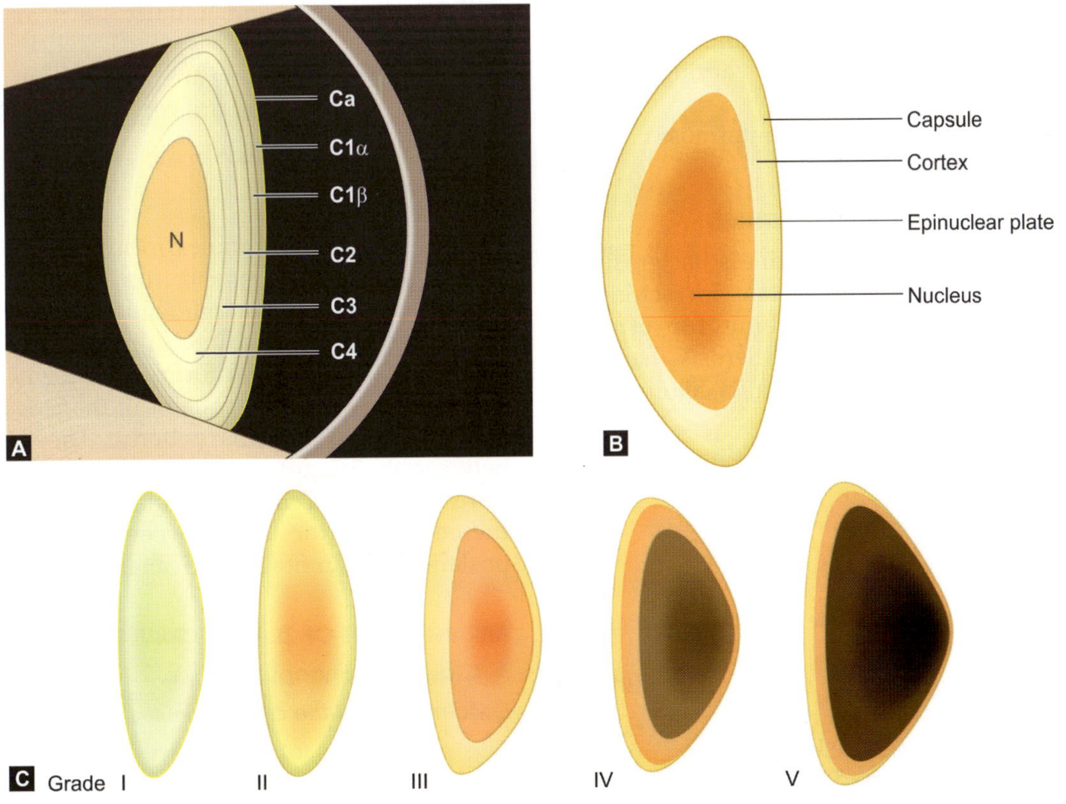

Fig. 1.7. *Applied anatomy of the crystalline lens:* ***(A)*** *Biomicroscopic stratification;* ***(B)*** *Surgical anatomy depicting capsule, cortex, epinuclear plate and nucleus;* ***(C)*** *Grading of the nucleus hardness in the cataractous lens.*

2. ***Superficial cortex.*** It is further stratified into three layers in the beam of slit-lamp:
- C1a. First cortical clear zone or the sub-capsular clear zone.
- Cl b. First zone of disjunction, seen as a bright narrow, scattering zone of discontinuity.
- C2. Second cortical clear zone or the subclear zone of cortex.

3. ***Deep cortex*** is stratified into the following two perinuclear zones which autofluoresce a brilliant green under blue exciting light:
- C3. It is the bright light scattering zone of deep cortex.
- C4. It is the relatively clear zone of deep cortex.

4. ***Nucleus*** **(N)** represents the prenatal part of the lens. It shows following further stratifications:
- Central part of nucleus, which lacks scattering of light, represents the embryonic nucleus.
- Anterior and posterior peripheral light scattering zones of nucleus.

SURGICAL ANATOMY OF THE LENS

From the surgical viewpoint, the lens can be divided into four parts (Fig. 1.7B):
- A *central hard nucleus* surrounded by
- An *epinuclear plate* (EN) of varying thickness surrounded by
- A *layer of cortex*, and the outermost
- *Capsule*

GRADING OF NUCLEUS HARDNESS

Grading of nucleus hardness (sclerosis) in cataractous lens is important for setting the parameters of the machine for effective phacoemulsification. The sclerosis (hardness) of nucleus, depending upon its colour, can be graded as below (Fig. 1.7C):
- Grade I: Whitish/green yellow
- Grade II: Yellow
- Grade III: Amber
- Grade IV: Brown
- Grade V: Black.

The hardness of the lens nucleus can also be classified into:
- Ultra-soft (grade I)
- Soft (grade I+)
- Soft-medium (grade II)
- Medium-hard (grade III)
- Hard (grade IV)
- Ultra-hard (grade V).

CILIARY ZONULES

The ciliary zonules (zonules of Zinn or suspensory ligaments of lens) consist essentially of a series of fibres which run from the ciliary body and fuse into the outer layer of the lens capsule around the equatorial zone. Thus, they hold the lens in position and enable the ciliary muscle to act on it.

STRUCTURE

The zonular fibres are transparent, stiff and not elastic. Each zonular fibre has a diameter of about 0.35–1.0 μ. It is composed of microfibrils with a diameter varying from 8–40 nm. Zonular fibres are composed of glycoproteins and muco-polysaccharides and are similar in structure to the microfibrils of the elastic fibres. Their susceptibility to hydrolysis by α-chymotrypsin has been *used to advantage in intracapsular cataract surgery.* Structurally, three different types of zonular fibres have been described.
- *First type fibres.* These are thick, about 1 μ in diameter, wavy and usually lie near the vitreous.
- *Second type fibres.* These are thin and flat.
- *Third type fibres.* These are very fine and run a circular course.

Gross Appearance

Grossly, the ciliary zonules form a complete ring of fibres, which extend from ciliary body to the lens equator circumferentially (Fig. 1.8). On cut section, the ciliary zonules appear to be arranged in a triangular form. The base of the triangle is towards the equator of the lens and apex towards the ciliary body. The space between the triangle is filled with the zonular fibres except for a circumferential space around the equator of the lens between anterior and posterior zonular fibres—the canal of Hannover.

ARRANGEMENT OF ZONULAR FIBRES

A. Classical concept

I. *Main fibres of the ciliary zonules*

The main fibres of the ciliary armies which bind the lens with the ciliary body, depending upon their arrangement can be classified into the following four groups (Fig. 1.9A):

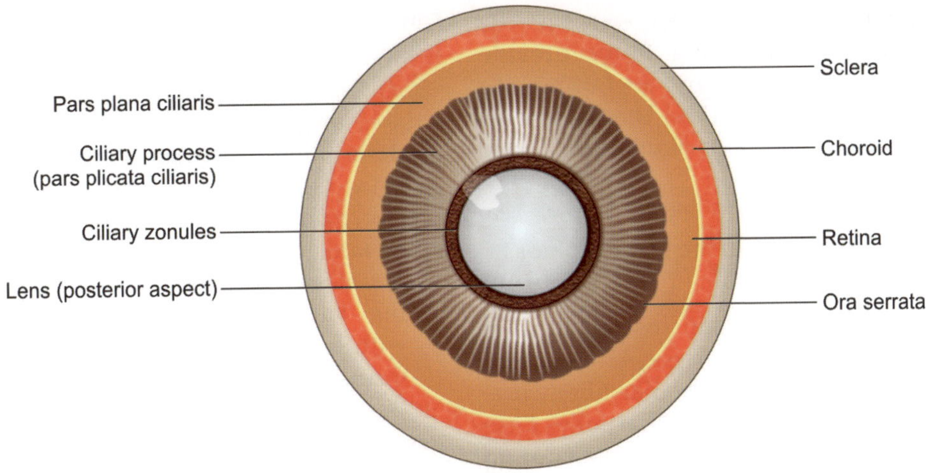

Fig. 1.8. *Gross appearance of ciliary zonules as seen from interior of the eyeball in relation to posterior surface of the lens.*

1. ***Orbiculoposterior capsular fibres.*** These are the most posterior and innermost zonular fibres. These take origin from the ora serrata, pass anteriorly in close contact with the anterior limiting layer of the vitreous and are inserted together with *hyaloidocapsular ligament* in the posterior capsule of the lens. Structurally, they are secona type fibres.

2. ***Orbiculoanterior capsular fibres.*** These are the thickest and strongest (structurally of first type) zonular fibres. They arise from the pars plana of ciliary body (orbicularis ciliaris), pass anteriorly to get inserted anterior to the equator. By the supporting (auxiliary) fibres, they are attached to the valleys and sides of the ciliary processes.

3. ***Ciliposterior capsular fibres.*** These are the most numerous zonular fibres. They arise mainly from the valleys and a few from the sides of the ciliary processes, pass posteriorly and get inserted on the posterior capsule anterior to the insertion of the orbiculoposterior capsular fibres.

4. ***Cilioequatorial fibres.*** These fibres arise from the valleys of the ciliary processes and pass almost directly inward to be inserted at the equator. They occupy the whole of the interval between the anterior and posterior group of fibres. These are third type of fibres. These are present in abundance in youthful eyes and tend to disappear and become sparse with advancing age.

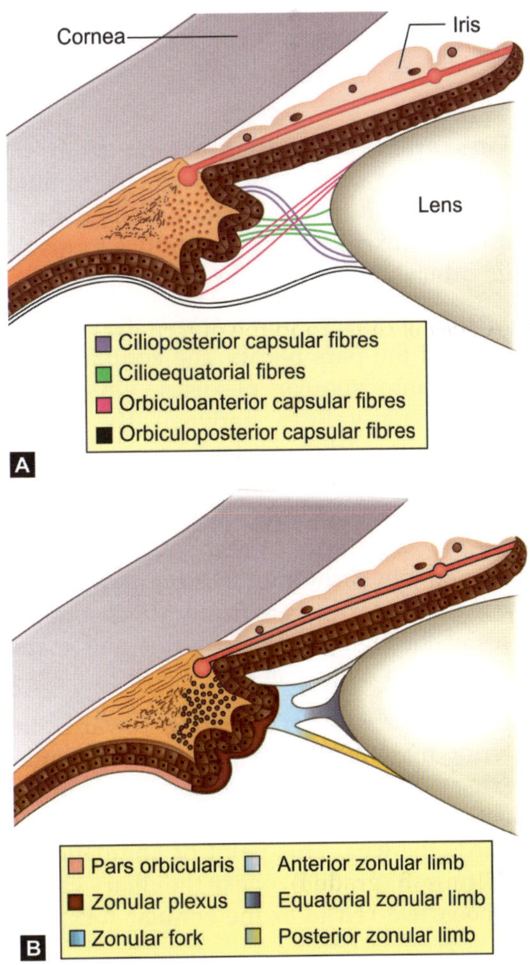

Fig. 1.9. *Arrangement of main zonular fibres:* ***(A)*** *Old concept;* ***(B)*** *New concept.*

II. Auxiliary fibres

The auxiliary or supporting fibres provide strength to main fibres by anchoring the individual portions of zonules. These also help to hold the various portions of the ciliary body together.

B. Recent concepts about the zonular fibres

I. Main zonular fibres

Recent scanning electron microscopy studies do not approve the above classical description of the arrangement of the zonular fibres. It is reported that vast majority of the zonules arise from the posterior end of the pars plana up to 1.5 mm from the ora serrata. They run a more or less complex but continuous course from ora serrata to the edge of lens. However, for description purposes, the suspensory zonular complex can be divided into four zones (Fig. 1.9B):

1. ***Pars orbicularis.*** After arising from the posterior end of the pars plana, the zonular fibres pass forward over the pars plana as a feltwork. This portion of the zonules forms the pars orbicularis.

2. ***Zonular plexuses.*** After reaching the posterior margin of the pars plicata, the zonular fibres segment into zonular plexuses, which pass through the valleys between the ciliary processes. Thus the zonular plexuses are that part of the zonules which lie between the ciliary processes in the region of the pars plicata. Each zonular plexus consists of fibres which cross and join each other in a regular pattern. The zonular plexuses are firmly attached to the bases of the ciliary valleys by fine and coarse fibrils known as *tension fibres.*

3. ***Zonular fork.*** After reaching towards the anterior margin of pars plicata, the zonular plexuses consolidate into zonular bundles which bend almost at right angle to proceed towards the lens. This point of angulation of the zonules at the mid-zone of the ciliary valleys has been referred to as the zonular fork.

4. ***Zonular limbs.*** At the level of the zonular fork, the zonular fibres divide into three zonular limbs—the anterior, equatorial and posterior—running to the anterior, equatorial and posterior lens capsule, respectively.

   i. *Anterior zonular limb.* It is analogous to the *orbiculoanterior capsular fibres* of old classical description. The anterior zonular fibres are relatively dense and all insert at approximately the same distance from the equator (about 1.5 mm), as an irregular double row of bundles. It has been reported that anterior zonules decrease in number with age and that the site of the anterior insertion becomes displaced more centrally.

   ii. *Equatorial zonular limb.* It replaces the term *cilioequatorial fibres* of old classical description. The equatorial fibres are sparse and poorly developed but fan out in a brush-like manner to get inserted into the capsule of the equatorial region.

   iii. *Posterior zonular limb.* It can be considered a substitute for the orbiculoposterior capsular fibres and cilioposterior capsular fibres of old classical description. Posterior fibres fan out more and show less interconnections than the anterior zonules. They are inserted into the posterior capsule in two or three layers in a zone starting from the posterior edge of the equator to about 1.25 mm.

II. Hyaloid zonule

The hyaloid zonule comprises a single layer of zonules connecting the anterior hyaloid at the border of the patellar fossa with the pars plana and pars plicata. This layer is indistinguished in the untouched eyes because its fibres are closely apposed to those of the posterior zonules. The space between the hyaloid zonule and the posterior zonule is the *canal of Petit.*

III. Hyalocapsular zonule

It is a circular band of zonular fibres which is at the site where the anterior hyaloid membrane is attached to the posterior lens capsule at the rim patellar fossa. It probably corresponds to the ligament of Wiegert.

IV. Circumferential zonular girdles

Anterior ciliary girdle. It is a circular band of fibres which binds the ciliary processes with the anterior hyaloid membrane of the vitreous.

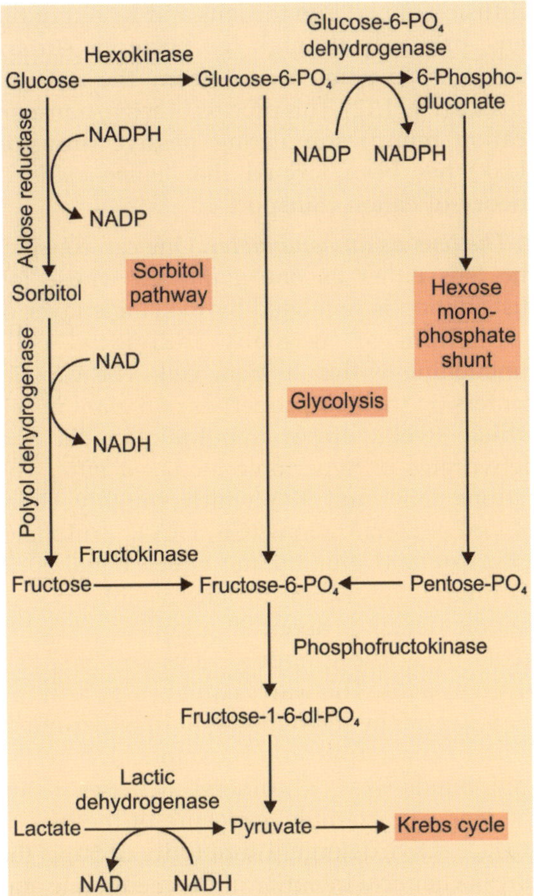

Fig. 1.10. *Pathways of glucose metabolism in the crystalline lens.*

In this pathway, glucose is converted into sorbitol (by the enzyme aldose reductase) which in turn is converted into fructose by the enzyme polyol dehydrogenase. The fructose is converted into fructose-6-phosphate (by the enzyme fructokinase) which enters into the glycolytic pathway (Fig. 1.10).

PROTEIN METABOLISM

Protein synthesis. Mechanisms occurring in the lens are similar to those occurring in all other tissues of the body. Proteins are synthesized from free amino acids which are actively transported into the lens from the aqueous. The formation of peptides from amino acids requires ATP and the appropriate RNA template. The ATP is acquired from glucose metabolism. Incorporation of amino acids into the RNA to form lens proteins occurs at a rather slow rate. It has been reported that glycine and serine are incorporated at no more than 5% per day. Further, rate of protein synthesis varies in different parts of the lens, nucleus being the slowest.

Protein breakdown in the lens is catalyzed by the enzyme peptidases and proteases. *In vitro* under sterile conditions, the lens undergoes autolysis. However, normally *in vivo*, the process of autolysis is inhibited.

PERMEABILITY AND TRANSPORT MECHANISMS OF THE LENS

Active and passive (permeability dependent) transport mechanisms of the lens are essential to provide nutrients for metabolism, to dispose of waste products of metabolism and to regulate water and cation balance in the lens. The salient features of biochemical composition of the lens vis-a-vis aqueous humour and the chemical exchange between the two is depicted in Fig. 1.11.

Active transport mechanisms are concerned with the transport of amino acid, potassium, taurine, inositol and extrusion of sodium. As discussed earlier, about 90% of the energy in

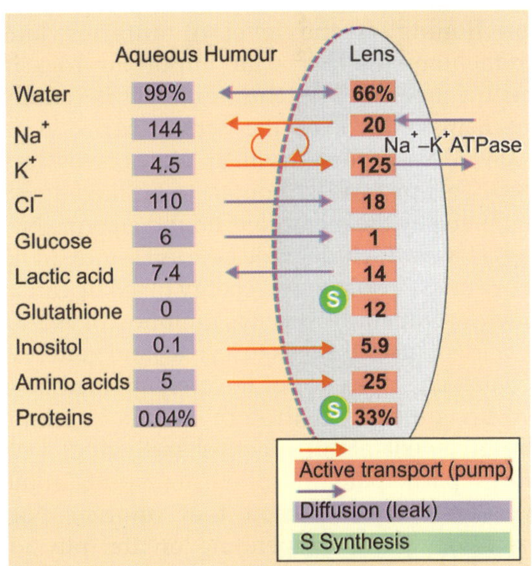

Fig. 1.11. *Chemical composition of the lens vis-à-vis aqueous humour and chemical exchange (pump-leak mechanism) between them. Values are in mmol/kg of lens water unless otherwise stated.*

the form of ATP generated from the glucose metabolism in the lens is utilized for these active transport mechanisms. ***Passive exchange (transport)*** across the lens capsule occurs for water, ions and waste products of metabolism, such as lactic acid and carbon dioxide. Exchange of these substances between the lens and aqueous humour meets with a little resistance from the capsule. It has been confirmed in laboratory studies that the isolated capsule is permeable to all low molecular weight compounds but restricts the movement of the larger colloidal material.

Following transport mechanisms of the lens need special description:

- Water and electrolyte transport
- Transport of amino acid and inositol
- Glucose transport

WATER AND ELECTROLYTE TRANSPORT

The electrolyte and water content of the lens resemble that of an intact cell, whereas Na^+, Cl^-, and K^+ ions and water content of the aqueous and vitreous are similar to that in plasma or extracellular fluids. The lens maintains its electrolyte and water gradient against the surrounding fluid by following mechanisms:

1. ***An energy-dependent cation pump.*** It is functioning at the level of anterior lens epithelium and plays an important role in cation balance in the lens. This pump mechanism involves the active extrusion of sodium (Na^+) coupled with uptake of potassium (K^+). This process is thought to be linked and mediated by the membrane bound enzyme Na-K-ATPase which degrades the ATP into ADP, inorganic phosphate and energy (used by cation pump). Oubain, a specific inhibitor of Na-K-ATPase, causes the lens to lose K^+ and gain Na^+ (confirming presence of the enzyme-mediated cation pump). Although there is some disagreement about whether individual lens fibres participate in cation transport, some workers have reported that another Na^+ extrusion 'pump' depending on the physiochemical integrity of lens fibres also exists.

As a result of the active extrusion of Na^+ and uptake of K^+ at the anterior surface of the lens generates a chemical gradient which stimulates diffusion of Na^+ into the lens and K^+ out of the lens, primarily through the posterior surface and also to some extent from the anterior surface (Fig. 1.12). This process of active transport (cation pump) stimulating passive diffusion (leak) has been termed the *"pump-and-leak"* theory of cation transport.

2. ***The lens as an osmometer.*** One can consider the lens either as one giant cell whose ion distribution is regulated by the single layer of epithelium or as many individual cells functioning within a giant cell. The capsule confers on the lens properties of a giant in cell which swells up in hypotonic media and dehydrates in hypertonic media *in vitro*. The cations (Na^+ and K^+) which roughly equal 145 mEq/l, and anions (Cl^-, HCO_3^-, sulphate, ascorbate and glutathione) which equal 50 to 60 mEq/l, contribute to lens osmolarity. An anionic deficit of about 90 mEq/l is probably made by acidic groups of lens proteins and glycoproteins. The water equilibrium between the lens and the surrounding fluid is disrupted, if the concentration of osmotically active compounds (Na^+, K^+, others) increases inside the lens. For example, exposure of the lens to surface active detergent antibiotics disrupts the physiochemical integrity of the membrane and

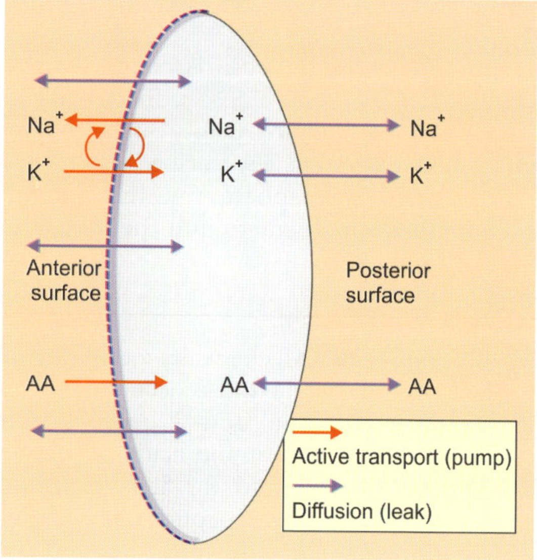

Fig. 1.12. *The 'pump-and-leak' mechanism of cation balance in the lens.*

the Na^+ extrusion pump which subsequent gain of Na^+ ions and water by the lens. Lens swelling, and eventually, complete loss of lens transparency follows.

TRANSPORT OF AMINO ACIDS AND INOSITOL

Amino acids are actively transported into the lens at the anterior epithelial surface and are, therefore, included in the "pump-and-leak" concept (Fig. 1.12). Three different pumps—one each for acidic, basic and neutral amino acids—have been reported. The transport of amino acids is in some way linked to the transport of cations. Inside the lens, amino acids are incorporated into the proteins, metabolized and used for energy or diffuse back into the aqueous by "leak" mechanism (Fig. 1.13).

Inositol is also actively transported into the lens, but its exact mechanism is not known.

GLUCOSE TRANSPORT

Simple diffusion and facilitated diffusion (mediated transfer) are the two mechanisms involved in the transport of sugars across the lens. Unlike the active transport of cations and amino acids which occur only at the anterior epithelial surface, the transfer of glucose occurs across both anterior and posterior surfaces of the lens.

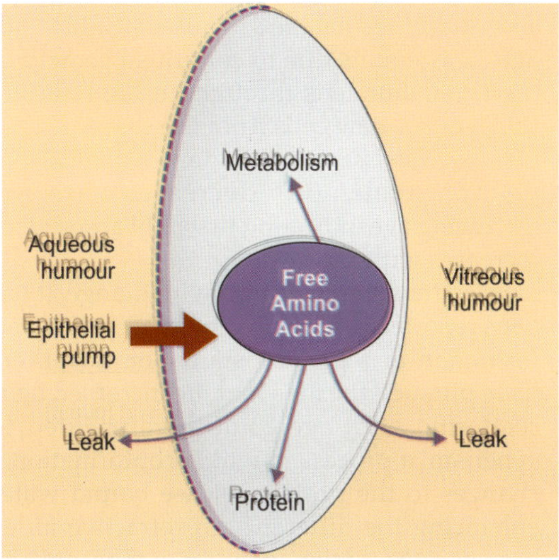

Fig. 1.13. *Fate of amino acids in the lens.*

ELECTRICAL PHENOMENA OF THE LENS

As a result of distribution of the ions inside the lens and its bathing medium (aqueous and vitreous), there exists a resting potential or an electrical potential difference in the lens. The inside of the lens is electronegative with respect to the bathing medium. Potential of about –70 mV is recorded across the intact lens capsule and of –23 mV in the lens fibres. Further, there exists a difference of –23 mV between the anterior and posterior surfaces of the lens. Thus, the flow of electrolytes into the lens is directed by an electrical gradient.

It is hoped that elucidation of electrophysiologic finding in the lens might eventually provide an ideal tool for detecting early membrane changes during cataractogenesis.

LENS CULTURE

The lens is an excellent tissue for *in vitro* incubation owing to its avascularity and simple structure. Thus, most of the physiologic and biochemical investigations on the lens are carried out *in vitro*. Various methods have been employed to incubate the lens in artificial culture media.

The most commonly employed method is '*closed* system' in which the carefully excised animal lens is placed in a culture flask containing an isotonic oxygenated balanced solution with glucose such as Tyrode's or Krebs-Ringer's solution. Under such conditions, a lens can be readily maintained for at least 24 hours. TC 199, a tissue culture medium containing salts, glucose, amino acids, and vitamins is used for long-term lens culture for days or weeks. The *in vitro* studies which are frequently carried out while the lens is in culture include: Glucose utilization, cation and amino acid transport and lens transparency. Chemicals or drugs harmful or beneficial to the lens in culture can be tested by comparing the treated lens with the control contralateral lens of the same animal. Several criteria for the viability of a cultured lens have been used, including mitotic activity and cation balance.

LENS TRANSPARENCY

Normal lens is a transparent structure transmitting almost 80% of light energy. It consists of a composite system of fibre-cells with their own individual membranes separating their contents from the interstitial fluid or cement substance which is itself separated by the lens capsule and epithelium from the surrounding aqueous and vitreous humours. The transparency of this system must presumably depend upon the avoidance of large transitions of refractive index between cells and surrounding cement substance. In other words, the transparency of lens must simply be a consequence of the low number of scattering centres. Moreover, the lens cell is composed largely of protein molecules about 10 nm in diameter which are present in a non-opalescent colloidal solution. The particle size is sufficiently small and the concentration is sufficiently low so much that scattering, although present, reduces the transmission of white light only by a few percentage units. Torkel has proposed that the lens transparency is due to the regular arrangement of lens fibres and the uniform distribution and paracrystalline state of proteins within the cell. Jones and Lerman reported that the lamellar conformation of lens proteins rather than helical structure may also contribute to transparency. Benedek, however, has suggested that if the protein molecules are not too large, then their precise arrangement is of lesser importance.

In general, the factors that play significant role in maintaining the outstanding clarity of the normal lens are:

- Single layer of epithelial cells which is not thick.
- Semipermeable character of the lens capsule.
- Sparsity and highly packed nature of lens cells. The lens extracapsular space is less than 5% of its total volume, so the zones of discontinuity are very small compared to wavelength of light.
- Characteristic arrangement of lens proteins.
- Pump mechanism of the lens fibre, which regulates the electrolyte and water balance in the lens and thus maintains relative dehydration of the lens.
- Avascularity of the lens
- *Auto-oxidation.* High concentration of reduced glutathione in the lens maintains the lens proteins in a reduced state and ensures the integrity of the cell membrane pump.

Thus, appearance of vacuoles (both intracellular and extracellular), local precipitation of proteins resulting in larger aggregates and distortion of lens structure, probably all lead to increased light scatter and clinically the changes are described as cataract. Changes in transparency are certainly associated with changes in electrolyte and water content.

The layers of normal lens have different refractive indices. This change is not gradual, there is stepwise increase towards the interior. The refractive index of the nucleus is higher (1.40) than the cortex (1.38) owing to the comparative hardness of the nucleus.

CHANGES IN AGEING LENS

There are three stages of age-related changes in the crystalline lens: Development, growth and ageing. Many changes occur to the clear lens with increasing age. These are not to be confused with the changes occurring in the cataractous lens, though many of these changes are seen in a more extreme form in cataract and some are the forerunners of the cataractous changes. Changes in the ageing lens can be grouped as: Physical changes, metabolic changes, changes to crystallins and changes to plasma membranes and cytoskeleton.

1. *PHYSICAL CHANGES*

- *Lens weight and thickness* increase steadily with age. This results due to continued growth of the crystalline lens throughout life building up layers of new cells from the equator.
- *Light transmission* by the lens especially at lower wavelengths decreases with the increasing age indicating that light absorbance increases with the age.
- *Light scattering* is increased with the age. It has been reported to be caused by aggregation and formation of a gel-like state. Some workers have pursued the idea that the increased light scattering with age could be attributed to synerism, a process in which conformational changes to the protein release bound water enhancing the difference in refractive index between the 'drier' protein region and its surroundings.

- *Fluorescence* property of lens has been confirmed to increase with the age.
- *Refractive index* in the nucleus of bovine lens is reported to increase with age. However, no such change was found in human lens.

2. METABOLIC CHANGES

Most of the metabolic activities of the lens decrease with age. A few important ones are as follows:

- The proliferative capacity of human lens epithelial cells declines during adult life.
- Many enzyme activities decline in the whole lens with age.
- There occurs an increase in the urea-soluble proteins, at the expense of soluble proteins, on going from cortex to nucleus.
- Three enzymes of glutathione metabolism, viz. glutathione peroxidase, glutathione reductase and glutathione S-transferase do not significantly decline with age. However, both glutathione and ascorbate levels decrease in lens with age.
- Both superoxide dismutase and glucose-6-phosphate dehydrogenase activity are lost with age but the denatured enzyme protein remains.

3. CHANGES IN CRYSTALLINS

Various studies have been carried out to study the changes in crystallins with age. The reported changes are as below:

- The earlier claim that high-molecular weight aggregates accumulate in bovine and human lens nucleus with age has not been supported by recent experiments using fast high performance gel chromatography. However, α-crystallins have been reported to almost disappear from soluble extracts of the nucleus and β-crystallins become more polydisperse.
- There occurs an age-related loss of γ-crystallins.
- The γ-crystallin fraction in particular shows an increase in disulphide bonds with age.
- There occurs a limited unfolding of bovine crystallins with age.
- It has been reported that all crystallin fractions of human lens contain fluorophor other than tryptophan. The non-tryptophan fluorescence increases with age (greater in nucleus than the cortex).

4. CHANGES OF PLASMA MEMBRANE AND CYTOSKELETON

- The loss of hexagonal cross-section of fibre cells and of their interlocking devices, and the lack of cytoskeleton in the lens nucleus have been reported to occur as age changes.
- There occur age-related losses of membrane proteins and lipids and of cytoskeletal proteins.
- A loss of membrane potential and an increase in lens sodium and calcium occur with age.
- All the large membrane polypeptides are reported to decrease in parallel with age.
- Main junctional polypeptide (MP-26) is converted into smaller variants with age.
- Changes in membrane rigidity also occur with ageing.

ACCOMMODATION

DEFINITION AND RELATED TERMS

As we know that in an emmetropic eye, parallel rays of light coming from infinity are brought to focus on the retina, with accommodation at rest. Our eyes have been provided with a unique mechanism by which we can even focus the diverging rays coming from a near object on the retina in a bid to see clearly (Fig. 1.14). This mechanism is called accommodation. In it, there occurs increase in the power of the crystalline lens.

Far point, near point, range and amplitude of accommodation

The nearest point at which small objects can be seen clearly is called near point or *punctum proximum* and the distant (farthest) point is

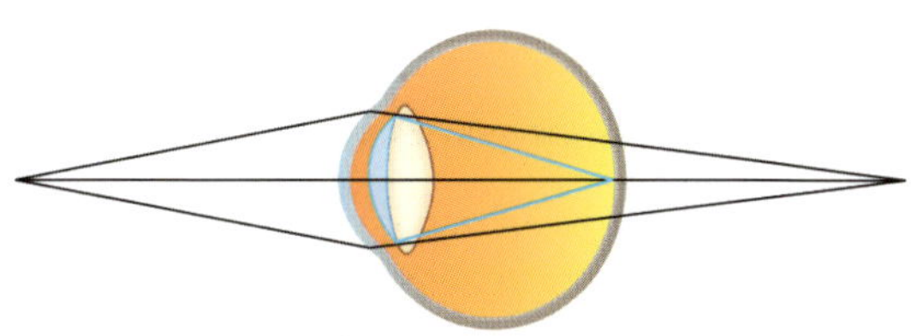

Fig. 1.14. *Effect of accommodation on divergent ray entering the eye.*

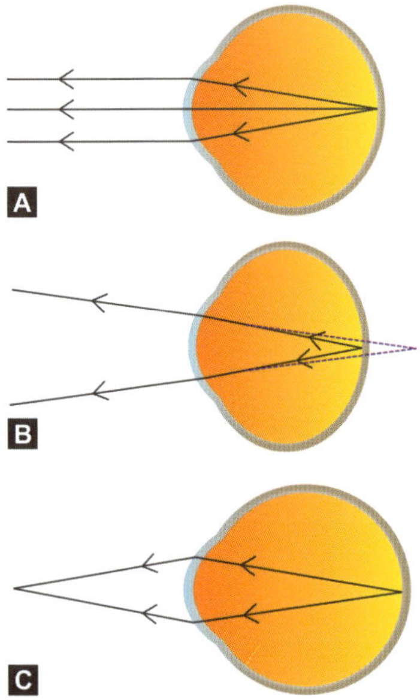

Fig. 1.15. *Showing far point in:* ***(A)*** *emmetropic eye;* ***(B)*** *hypermetropic eye;* ***(C)*** *myopic eye.*

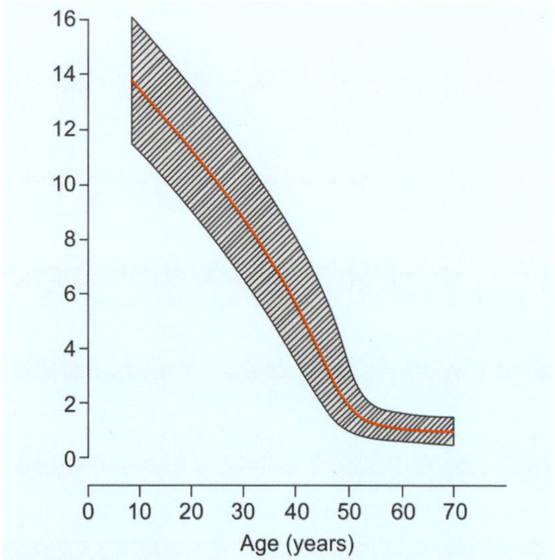

Fig. 1.16. *Showing decrease in the amplitude of accommodation with age in human (From Duane, A. Arch Ophthalmol 54; 568, 1925).*

called far point or *punctum remotum.* The distance between the near point and the far point is called *range of accommodation.* The difference between the dioptric power needed to focus at near point (P) and to focus at far point (R) is called *amplitude of accommodation* (A). Thus, A = P–R.

Far point and near point of the eye vary with the static refraction of the eye. In hypermetropic eye, far point is virtual and lies behind the eye, while in myopic eye, it is real and lies in front of the eye (Fig. 1.15). In an emmetropic eye, far point is at infinity and near point varies with age; being about 7 cm at age of 10 years, 25 cm at the age of 40 years and 33 cm at the age of 45 years. Thus the amount that the eye can alter its refraction is greatest in childhood and slowly decreases until it is lost in middle age. Amplitude of accommodation in dioptres as function of the age, as studied by Duane, is depicted in Fig. 1.16.

Depth of field and depth of focus

When an object is accurately focused monocularly, often the objects somewhat near and somewhat farther away are also seen clearly without any change in accommodation. This range of distance from the eye in which an object appears clear without change of accommodation is termed depth of field. Depth of field reduces the necessity for precise accommodation.

The range at the retina in which an optical image may move without impairment of clarity is termed depth of focus. The depth of field and depth of focus are markedly influenced by the diameter of the pupil (Fig. 1.17). Depth of field is inversely proportional to pupil size. Size of the blur circle produced on retina is proportional to pupil size.

Depth of field should not be mistaken for accommodation. The apparent range of accommodation also includes depth of field and tolerance of blur (i.e. depth of focus).

MECHANISM OF ACCOMMODATION

Accommodation is the result of a change in the form of the lens brought about by contraction of the ciliary muscle. Therefore, a review of the anatomy of ciliary body and ciliary muscle and lens with its capsule and the zonules will be useful to understand the mechanism of accommodation.

As we know, accommodation is a process by which one can focus the objects at different distances in a bid to have a clear vision. Its

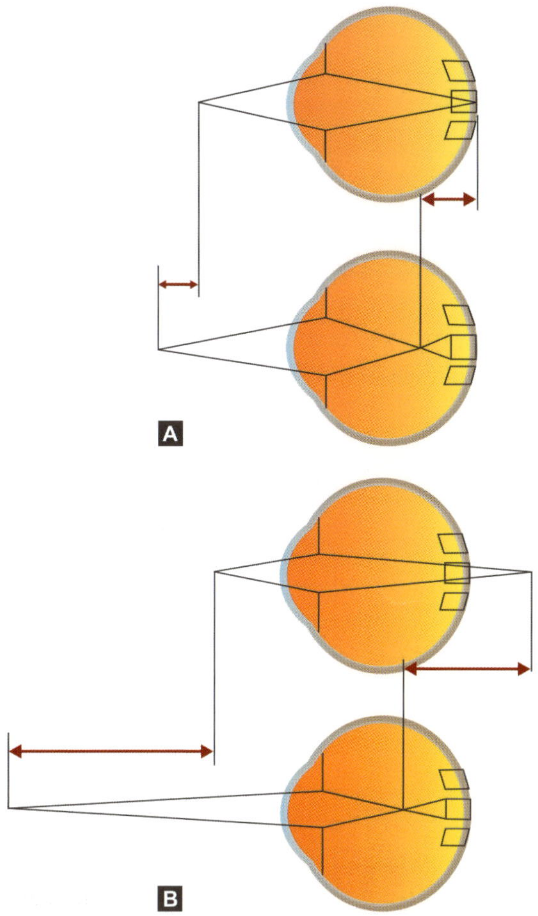

Fig. 1.17. *Effect of pupil diameter on depth of field and field of focus:* ***(A)*** *Large pupil;* ***(B)*** *Small pupil.*

mechanism varies from species to species. Just for interest, examples of a few species are given below.

- Some fish retract their lenses to focus on distant objects.
- Snakes and frogs have a mechanism to move the lens forward for near vision.
- Horses, by moving their heads, tilt the retina so that different regions lie at appropriate distances behind the lens.
- In man, the process of accommodation is achieved by a change in the shape of the lens.

THEORIES OF ACCOMMODATION IN HUMAN

The mechanism of human accommodation and disaccommodation, i.e. the ability of the focus from far to near and near to far, respectively, has been debated with surprising passion, since 1801 when Young reported that lens is responsible for accommodative properties of the human eye. In a bid to account for the changes taking place in the lens during accommodation, numerous theories have been proposed, a few of which warrant serious consideration are discussed below.

1. The relaxation theory (Helmholtz theory)

The relaxation theory also known as *capsular theory* is probably, most widely accepted, although it is not necessarily supported by experimental evidence. This theory was first proposed by Thomas Young and elaborated by Helmholtz in 1885, by whose name it is known generally. The importance given to the lens capsule was emphasized by Fincham in 1937. The main points of the relaxation theory are as follows:

- When the eye is at rest (unaccommodated) the malleable substance of young lens is compressed in its capsule (which is an elastic structure) by tension of the zonules. The surfaces of the compressed lens are less curved and these change the dioptric power in lens.
- Zonules are kept under tension by a pull executed on them by the elastic choroid (Helmholtz original assumption). However, recently it is being assumed by many workers that the zonules are kept under tension by the relaxation of fibres of the ciliary muscle.
- Contraction of the ciliary muscle causes the ciliary to shorten and move forward the equator of the lens. It also pulls the choroid forward. As a result, the zonules are relaxed *(basic mechanism of relaxation theory)*, the tension on the capsule is relieved and the lens attains a more spherical shape. As the refractive index of lens (1.39) is more than refractive index of aqueous and vitreous, increase in convexity of the lens increases its dioptic power and thus allows the near objects to be focused clearly on the retina.

Points in favour of relaxation theory

Glasser and Kaufman developed experiments to confirm the classical description of the mechanism of accommodation in primates. Many latest techniques also support this theory.

The imaging techniques show that the apex of the ciliary muscle moves antero-inward and the equatorial edge of the lens moves away from the sclera during accommodation (about 250 μm for 10 D of accommodation). Goniovideography shows that the zonular fibres extending from the ciliary processes to the lens equator are relaxed during accommodation. UBM imaging shows the posterior zonular fibre extending between the posterior attachment of the ciliary muscle, and the ciliary processes are stretched during accommodation by the forward and axial movement of the apex of ciliary muscle.

Points against relaxation theory

There are some points against this theory. According to Helmholtz hypothesis, since the equatorial diameter increases with age (i.e. since the crystalline lens equator is getting closer to the ciliary muscle), the zonules should relax. As one ages, the power of the crystalline lens should increase while viewing distant objects in the accommodated state. One should become more myopic and the crystalline lens should become unstable, but in fact, one becomes slightly hyperopic and the crystalline lens remains stable. Helmholtz theory also is not consistent with the decrease in spherical aberration that occurs during accommodation.

Helmholtz attributes the universal linear decrease in the amplitude of accommodation with age to hardening of the crystalline lens. No tissue in the body hardens in a linear fashion with age.

Role of lens capsule

Although, at first, Helmholtz regarded the lens to be an elastic body as a whole which would assume the spherical shape of its own when made free from the tension of zonules. However, he soon realized his fallacy that being a semisolid mass the lens may be deformed by the external force but being inelastic cannot return to its original shape when the deforming force is removed. Helmholtz found it necessary, therefore, to attribute elastic properties to the lens capsule to account for the change in the shape of lens when it was free from the tension of zonules. It was seen that the lens surfaces were not perfectly spherical in contour; the anterior surface, in particular, is more convex centrally during accommodation. Fincham suggested that variations in thickness of lens capsule (Fig. 1.2) account for the local variations in curvature. He proposed that during accommodation the thicker ring of anterior capsule surrounding the central region contracts under the lessened zonular traction, while the thinner central capsule bulges forward in a more pronounced fashion. The physiological anterior lenticonus thus formed has a short radius of curvature and high refraction.

Gullstrand mechanical model of accommodation

Based on the Helmholtz hypothesis, Gullstrand devised a mechanical model to explain the mechanism of accommodation. Description of Gullstrand's model (as shown in Fig. 1.18) is as below: The cord between the two springs represents the zonules. The upper spring represents the lens, and its contraction represents change of the shape of the lens during accommodation. The lower spring represents the elasticity of choroid. In the eye, at rest this spring is sufficiently strong to overcome the pull of the upper string, which must always be slightly on the stretch and, therefore, must be the weaker of the two (presently now the lower spring is thought to be represented by relaxation of the fibres of the ciliary muscle and not the choroid). A cord passed over the pulley supporting the weight represents the pull of the circular fibres of the ciliary muscle. In the unaccommodated eye (Fig. 1.18A), the weight is at rest and exerts no pull. When accommodation at place (Fig. 1.18B) due to pull exerted by the contraction of ciliary muscle, the lower spring pulled, and the zonules are slackened; this allows the upper spring to contract (i.e. change in the shape of lens).

2. Theory of increased tension (Tscherning theory)

This theory attributes to the increased curvature of the capsule increasing tension on the zonules. It states that contraction of the ciliary muscle pulls on the zonules directly and increases the

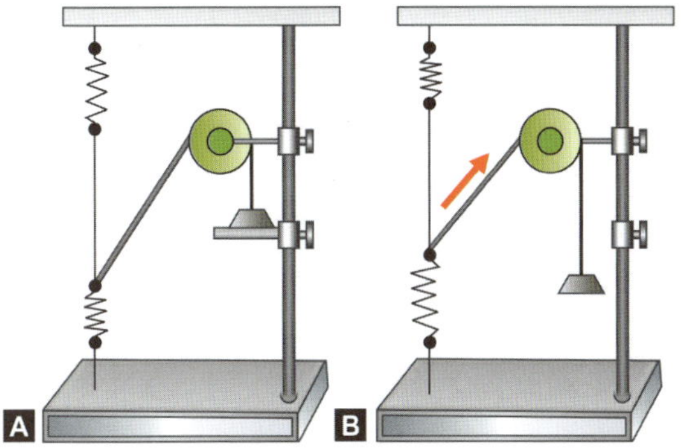

Fig. 1.18. *Gullstrand's mechanical model showing the forces which produce accommodation according to the Young-Helmholtz theory:* ***(A)*** *Unaccommodated stage;* ***(B)*** *Accommodated stage.*

tension on the capsule. This results in a compression of the capsule at the equator of the lens so that the poles bulge. Accommodation is brought about, therefore, by increasing the tension of the zonules.

However, now all the evidences (anatomical and physiological) are against this view and so this theory is no longer accepted.

3. Schachar's theory

Recently, media attention focused on a new theory of accommodation and presbyopia and its resulting surgical treatment, which Schachar suggested, may restore accommodation. This theory seems to be a modification of Tscherning's theory of increased tension and states that accommodation occurs when ciliary muscle contraction tenses rather than relaxes, the equatorial zonules. The lens would then be stretched equatorially or coronally (i.e. the lens edge moves toward the sclera) but the biomechanical properties of the lens are such that the central part of the lens rounds up and moves anteriorly, increasing its refracting power.

In Schachar's theory, the anterior and posterior zonules act like supportive ligaments of skeletal joints and are stabilizing components, which are tense during distance vision and relax during accommodation. The equatorial displacement of the crystalline lens occurs as a result of increased tension on the equatorial zonules produced by contraction of the anterior radial muscle fibres of the ciliary muscle. Since an active force is involved in accommodation, the amount of force that the ciliary muscle can apply is dependent on how much the ciliary muscle is stretched.

The Schachar's theory thus contradicts the classical Helmholtz mechanism, in which ciliary muscle contraction is thought to relax the zonules, allowing centripetal elasticity of the lens capsule to spherisize the lens (i.e. the equatorial or coronal diameter of the lens decreases, the equatorial edge of the lens recedes from the sclera, and the lens as a whole round up).

According to Schachar's theory, presbyopia results from growth in the equatorial diameter of the lens, such that the perilenticular space is reduced and ciliary muscle contraction can no longer tense the zonules and expand the lens coronally. Based on his theory, Schachar introduced a new surgery for presbyopia, i.e. the use of scleral expansion bands (SEB). The aim of these segments is to increase the working distance between the ciliary muscle and the lens equator, which should theoretically, as suggested by Schachar, allows the muscle to work again. However, recently conflicting reports regarding the effectiveness of SEB surgery have appeared in the literature and have challenged the validity of the Schachar's theory.

4. Cotenary (hydraulic suspension) theory of accommodation

Recently, Coleman et al. have stated that many observations during accommodation can neither be explained by 'capsular theory' of Helmholtz nor by Schachar's theory. The most difficult objection to these theories is to overcome the precise, rapid and anatomical reproducible shape of the lens in accommodated state. In addition, the ciliary muscle does not have the necessary anatomic rigidity or the attachments to support an equatorial fraction force to flatten the lens as proposed by Schachar theory. The capsule itself does not have the elastic properties to round up the lens mass reproducibly and rapidly. Coleman et al have demonstrated the observable feature of accommodation by a mechanical model of Cotenary theory of accommodation. The Cotenary theory of accommodation was proposed by Coleman in 1970 and demonstrated by a simple Cotenary model to support his concept in 1986. The Cotenary (hydraulic suspension) theory propounds that the lens zonules and anterior vitreous comprise a diaphragm between the anterior and vitreous chambers of the eye. It has been proposed that contraction of ciliary muscle generates a pressure gradient between the aqueous and vitreous, causing anterior movement of the lens zonule diaphragm and steepening of anterior central lens curvature and slight flattening of the anterior peripheral lens curvature. Coleman and Fish in their mechanical model of Cotenary theory have demonstrated that the anterior capsule and zonules form a trampoline shape or hammock-shaped surface that is totally reproducible depending on the circular dimensions, i.e. the circumference of the ciliary body. Thus, he stated that the ciliary body directs the shape like the pylons of a suspension bridge, but does not need to support an equatorial fraction force to flatten the lens as required by a capsular theory.

According to the cotenary system of Coleman and Fish, presbyopia occurs due to increasing lens volume with age that results in a reduced response of anterior radius of curvature to the vitreous pressure gradient created by ciliary body contraction.

Conclusion

Despite a wealth of contradictory observations, the von Helmholtz capsular theory is probably most widely accepted. In light of the abundant evidence provided by experimental physiology throughout the last century, it is remarkable that fundamental elements of the mechanism of accommodation remain contentious. Nevertheless, using ultrasound biomicroscopy and goniovideography, Glasser and Kaufman have provided strong support for the classical Helmholtz theory, namely that upon accommodative effort, contraction of ciliary muscle releases zonular tension on the equatorial crystalline lens, allowing the lens to assume more spherical geometry. However, still there are elements of the mechanism that await further elucidation; for example, the role of the iris as suggested by Crawford et al. and role of the vitreous pressure as suggested by Cramer in 19th century and Coleman and Fish recently in 2001.

ACCOMMODATION: CERTAIN PHYSIOLOGICAL ASPECTS

STIMULUS FOR ACCOMMODATION

There is not only a single important stimulus to accommodation. All of the following factors must be responsible in eliciting the appropriate accommodative response:

- Image blur
- Apparent size and distance of object
- Chromatic aberrations
- Oscillation of accommodation
- Scanning movements of the eye

It has been reported that the initial accommodative adjustment is based on 'trial and error'.

REACTION TIME

Reaction time refers to the time lapse between the presentation of an accommodative stimulus and occurrence of the accommodative response. Some of the observations made regarding reaction time are as follows:

- Average reaction time for 'far-to-near' ac accommodation is 0.64 seconds.
- Average reaction time for 'near-to-far' accommodation is 0.56 seconds.
- Reaction time for accommodation is considerably larger than that for the contraction of the pupil to light (0.26–0.30 seconds). Reaction time of convergence response is about 0.20 seconds.

OCULAR CHANGES IN ACCOMMODATION

The changes which take place in the eye during accommodation can be summarized as below:

1. ***Slackening of the zonules.*** Zonules are normally tense and keep the lens flat. They slacken during accommodation due to contraction of ciliary muscle.

2. ***Changes in the curvature of lens surface.*** The principal change in the lens during accommodation is seen in the anterior surface of the lens. At rest, the radius of curvature of the anterior surface of the lens is 11 mm and that of posterior surface is 6 mm. In accommodation, the curvature of posterior surface remains almost the same, but the anterior surface changes, so

that in strong accommodation its radius of curvature becomes about 6 mm in the periphery and 3 mm in the central part which bulges more. The central part of the anterior surface bulges more because the anterior capsule is thinner here (Fig. 1.19) as compared to the peripheral part. The posterior capsule is the thinnest region and so the posterior surface has a greater curvature even in the unaccommodated lens.

3. *Anterior pole* of the lens moves forward carrying the iris with it, resulting in shallowing of the anterior chamber in the centre.

4. *Axial thickness* of the lens is increased owing to forward movement of the anterior pole (posterior pole remaining fixed).

5. *Changes in the tension of lens capsule* have also been studied. During accommodation, the anterior capsule becomes slack.

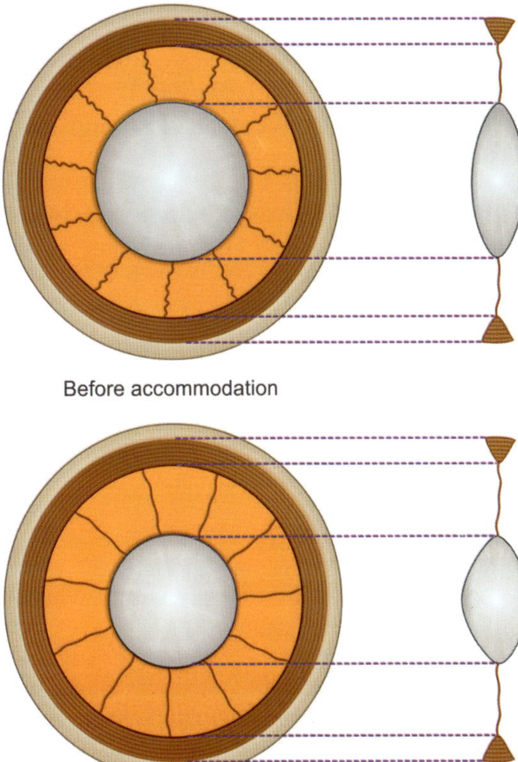

Fig. 1.19. *Changes in the ciliary body ring, zonules and shape of lens during accommodation.*

6. *Lens sinks down* because the accommodated lens is held less firmly by its zonular attachment, it is influenced by the force of gravity and tends to sink within the globe.

7. *Changes within the lens substance.* In addition to the changes in curvature of the lens, the changes in the lens substance also create a change in the refractive power of the lens. The internal changes are brought about by changes in curvature of the various portions of lens having different indices of refraction.

8. *Pupillary constriction and convergence of eyes.* In addition to the changes in the lens and zonular system, the pupil constricts and the eyes converge, almost simultaneously. These changes occur in a bid to achieve clear vision for near objects. The pupillary constriction is a synkinesis and not a true reflex, it does not depend on either accommodation or convergence alone for its appearance.

9. *The choroid* is stretched forward by the ciliary muscle contraction.

10. *The ora serrata* moves forward about 0.05 mm with each dioptre of accommodation.

AGE-RELATED CHANGES IN ACCOMMODATION

As discussed earlier, in an emmetropic eye, far point is infinity and near point changes with age, being about 17 cm at the age of 10 years, 25 cm at the age of 40 years, 33 cm at the age of 45 years and about 50 cm at the age of 50 years. Therefore, at the age of 10 years, amplitude of accommodation (A) = 100/7 (dioptric power needed to see clearly at near point)—I/a (dioptric power needed to see clearly at far point); i.e. A (at age 10) = 14 dioptres. Similarly 'A' at age 40 years = (100/25 – I/a) = 4 dioptres; at age 45 years A = 3 dioptres and at 50 years = 2 dioptres. Since, we usually keep the book at about 25 cm, so we can read comfortably up to the age of 40 years and after that the near point recedes beyond the normal reading or working range. This condition of failing near vision due to related decrease in the amplitude of accommodation or increase in the near point (punctum proximum) is called presbyopia.

Pathophysiology of presbyopia

Theories proposed to explain the development of presbyopia include:

1. Changes in the elastic properties of lens capsule
2. Hardness or sclerosis of the lens, and
3. Weakening of the ciliary muscle.

Changes in the elastic property of lens capsule

Lens capsule has a definite role in the occurrence of presbyopia. But many workers have reported that the elasticity of the lens capsule does not change markedly with age.

Sclerosis or hardening of the lens

It is generally believed that the principal cause of presbyopia is the result of sclerosis or hardening of the nucleus of the lens so that the forces (capsule's elasticity) which normally deform the soft lens during youth, are now no longer effective. For many years, it was thought that the hardening of the ageing lens correlated with a decrease in water content, particularly in the nuclear region. However, now it is clear that there is no significant loss of water in the aging human lens, although this is a frequent observation in other mammalian species. The age-related hardening of the lens must, therefore, be due to an alteration in the structural proteins of the lens or to increased adhesions between lens fibres.

Weakening of the ciliary muscle

Although, age-related morphologic changes are known to occur in the ciliary muscle, however, there is little evidence to support the concept of a weakened ciliary muscle. In presbyopes also, the ciliary muscle contracts vigorously under the influence of pilocarpine. Thus, from the above, it can be concluded that the principal factor for causing presbyopia is age-related hardening of the lens nucleus. But change in the elasticity of the lens and weakening of the ciliary muscle also might be playing some role.

BIBLIOGRAPHY

1. Adler, FH. Quoted from Adler's physiology of the eye ed by Moses, RA 342 The CV Mosby Company, 1970.
2. Arkin W, Madalinaki W, Trzcincka Z. Acta XVIIIth Int Cong ophthal Brussels, 1:693 In Duke Elder, 5(ed): System of ophthalmology, Vol IV, 375, Henry Kimpton, London, 1968.
3. Augusteyn RC, and Spector A: Biochem J, 124: 345–355;1971.
4. Barbar, GW. Invest Ophthalmol, 7:564–583;1968.
5. Bassems, GJH, Keizer, E, Wollen Sak, J Hoenders, HJ. Age-related variations in distribution of crystallins within the bovine lens. Exp Eye Res, 43, 1019–1030;1988.
6. Bates, CJ, Cowen, TD. Effects of age and dietary vitamin C on the contents of ascorbic acid and acid-soluble thiol in lens and aqueous humor of guinea pigs. Exp Eye Res, 46, 937–945; 1988.
7. Bellows, JG. Cited in Biochemistry of Eye ed by Graymore, CN Pub by Academic Press London, 194:236,320;1971.
8. Benedek GB. Theory of transparency of the eye Applied Optics 10:456–473;1971.
9. Berzelius. Lib D Chemie, Reutingen, 4 (1832): Quoted by Duke-Elder, S: System of Ophthalmology, Vol IV, 149, Henry Kimpton, London, 1968.
10. Bittar, EE (ed). Membranes and Ion Transport, Vol 1, New York, Wiley-Interscience, 1970.
11. Bjork, I. Exp Eye Res, 1:145–154;1961.
12. Bjork, I. Exp Eye Res, 3:254;1964.
13. Brassil, D and Kern, HL: Invest Ophthalmol, 7:441;1968.
14. Burger (1963). Vision Res, 3: 227 Quoted by Duke Elder, S: System of Ophthalmology Henry-Kirnpton London, Vol IV, 372, 1968.
15. Carta, Santori Maraini (1960). Ann Ottal, 92:23 Quoted by Duke-Elder, S: System of ophthalmology Henry Kimptom London, Vol IV, 377, 1968.
16. Clark, R, Zigman, S, Lerman, S. Exp Eye Res, 8:172–182;1969.
17. Clayton RM. Comparative aspects of lens proteins. In Davson H, Graham LT Jr (Eds): The Eye Vol 5 New York, Academic Press, 400–494; 1974.
18. Cotlier, E. Rb transport, water, and cation concentrations in lenses exposed to polymyxin B sulfate Exp Eye Res 15:711;1973.
19. Dark, AJ. The distribution of lipids in the bovine lens and cornea Arch Ophthal, 59:676;1958.
20. Duke-Elder's System of ophthalmology, Vol IV, 365, ed by Duke-Elder, S Henry Kimpton, London, 1969.
21. Elbrink, J, Bihler, I. Characteristics of the membrane transport of sugars in the lens of the eye, Biochem Biophys Acta 282:337–351,1972.

22. Feldman, GL. Lipids a of human lens Biochemistry of the Eye, Symp Tutzing Castle, 348;1966.
23. Feldman, GL and Feldman, L. New concepts of human lenticular lipids and their possible role in cataracts Invest Ophthal, 4:162;1965.
24. Fischer, FP (1938). Documents Ophthal, 1: 79 Cited in Biochemistry of eye, 185, ed by Graymore, C N, Published by Academic Press, London, New York, 1970.
25. Hans, W, Hockwin, O, Kleifeld, O. Die Bestimmung des Sauerstoffverbrauches der Linse auf polaro graphischem Wege Albrecht von Graefes Arch Klin Ophthalmol 157:72–84; 1956.
26. Hanson, H. Proteolytische Enzyme der Augenlinse In Dardenne MU (ed): Biochemistry of the Eye, Symposium, 1966, Basel, Karger, 325–343; 1968.
27. Harding, JJ, Crabbe, MJC. The lens: Development, proteins, metabolism and cataract in the eye, Vol IB (Ed H Davson) Academic Press, London, 207–492;1984.
28. Harding, JJ. Free and protein-bound glutathione in normal and cataractous human lenses Biochem 117,957–960;1970.
29. Heath H. The distribution and possible functions of ascorbic acid in the eye Exp Eye Res 1:362–367;1962.
30. Hockwin, O, Slum, G, Korte I, Murata, T, Radetzki, W, Rast, F. Studies on the citric acid cycle and its portion of glucose breakdown by calf and bovine lenses vitro, Ophthalmic Res 2: 143–148;1971.
31. Jones HA, Lerman S. Optical rotatory dispersion and circular dichroism studies on ocular lens proteins Can J Biochem 49:426–430;1971.
32. Kern, HL, Ho, CK. Localization and specificity of the transport system for sugars in the calf lens, Exp Eye Res 15:751–765;1973.
33. Kern, HL, Roosa, P, Murray, S. Evidence for active transport of alkali metal cations by calf lens Exp Eye Res 1:385–395;1962.
34. Kinoshita, JH, et al. Factors affecting the formation of sugar alcohols in the ocular lens, Biochem Biophys Acta 74:340;1963.
35. Kinoshita, JH. Pathways of glucose metabolism in the lens, Invest Ophthalmol 72:554;1964.
36. Krause, AC. Chemistry of lens V relation of the anatomic distribution of the lenticular proteins to their chemical composition Arch Ophthal, 10:788;1933.
37. Kuck, JFR. Carbohydrates of the lens in normal and precataractous states Invest Ophthal, 4:638; 1965.
38. Latina, M, Chylack, LT, Fagerholm, P et al. Dynamic light scattering in the intact rabbit lens: Its relation to protein concentration Invest Ophthalmol Vis Sci, 28,175–83;1987.
39. Mehta, PD, Maisel, H. Biochemistry of the Eye, Symp Tutzing Castle, 271,1966.
40. Morner, Hoppe-Seyl (1893–94). Z Physiol Chem, 18:60:213 Quoted by Duke-Elder, S: System of Ophthalmology Vol IV Henry Kimpton London, 366,1968.
41. Nishida. S Scanning electron microscopy of the zonular fibres in human and monkey eyes ARVO Suppl: Invest Ophthalmol Vis Sci, 1:357; 1982.
42. Nordman and Mandel (1952). Ann Oculist (Paris), 185:929 Quoted from system of Ophthalmology ed by Duke Elder,S Henry Kimpton London 377;1968.
43. Paterson, CA, Neville, MC, Jenkins, RM II, Cullen, JP. An electrogenic component of the potential difference in the rabbit lens Biochem Biophys Acta 375:316,1975.
44. Patterson, JW. A review of glucose transport in the lens, Invest Ophthalmol 4: 667–679;1965.
45. Paulus, Hockwin, and Kleifeld: V Graefes Arch Ophthal, 163:309;1961.
46. Peterson, CA. Distribution and movement of ions in the ocular lens, Docum Ophthalmol 31:1–28;1972.
47. Pierscionek, BK, Chan, DYC, Ennis, JP et al. Non-destructive method of constructing three-dimensional gradient Index Models for crystalline lenses I Theory and experiment Am J Optom Physiol Opt 65, 481–491;1988.
48. Rabaey, M. Nature, London, 198:206;1963.
49. Reddy, DVN and Kinsay, VE. Studies on the crystalline lens IX Quantitative analysis of free amino acids and related compounds Invest Ophthal, 1:635;1962.
50. Reddy, DVN. Transport of organic molecules in the lens Exp Eye Res 15:731–750;1973.
51. Rohen, JW. Scanning electron microscopic studies of the zonular apparatus in human and monkey eyes Invest Ophthalmol Vis Sci, 18:33; 1979.
52. Shapiro, AL. Invest Ophthalmol, 7: 544–550;1968.
53. Sippel, TO. Measurement of oxygen consumption in the rat lens with a flow respirometer Invest Ophthal, 1:377;1962.

CHAPTER 2

EMBRYOLOGY AND CONGENITAL ANOMALIES OF LENS

EMBRYOLOGY OF LENS

The first evidence of primitive eye formation occurs during the third week of gestation. The region of neural plate (Fig. 2.1A), which is destined to form the prosencephalon, shows a linear thickened area on either side (Fig. 2.1B), which soon becomes depressed to form the optic sulcus (Fig. 2.1C). Meanwhile the neural plate becomes converted into prosencephalic vesicle. As the optic sulcus deepens, the walls of the prosencephalon overlying the sulcus bulge out to form the *optic vesicle* (Fig. 2.1D and E). The proximal part of the optic vesicle becomes constricted and elongated to form the *optic stalk* (Fig. 2.1F to H).

FORMATION OF THE LENS PLACODE AND LENS VESICLE

As the optic vesicle grows laterally (during the third week of gestation), it comes in relation to the surface ectoderm. At about 27 days of gestation (embryo 4.0–4.5 mm), the area of the surface ectoderm overlying the optic vesicle becomes thickened to form the *lens placode* (Fig. 2.2A). The lens placode invaginates the sinus below the surface ectoderm to form a lens vesicle, which consists of a single layer of cells covered by a basal lamina (Figs 2.2B and C; and 2.3). It is soon separated from the surface ectoderm at 33rd day of gestation.

DEVELOPMENT OF LENS STRUCTURES

Formation of primary lens fibres

The cells of the posterior wall of the lens vesicle rapidly elongate and get filled with proteins called crystallines, which make them transparent. The bases of these densely packed cells remain anchored to the basal laminae posteriorly and their apices grow towards the anterior lens epithelium obliterating the lumen of lens vesicle (Fig. 2.3). These elongated transparent cells are known as primary lens fibres. The nuclei of the lens fibres are present more anteriorly within the cells to form a line convex forward called the nuclear bow. The primary lens fibres now become attached to the apical surface of anterior lens epithelium and

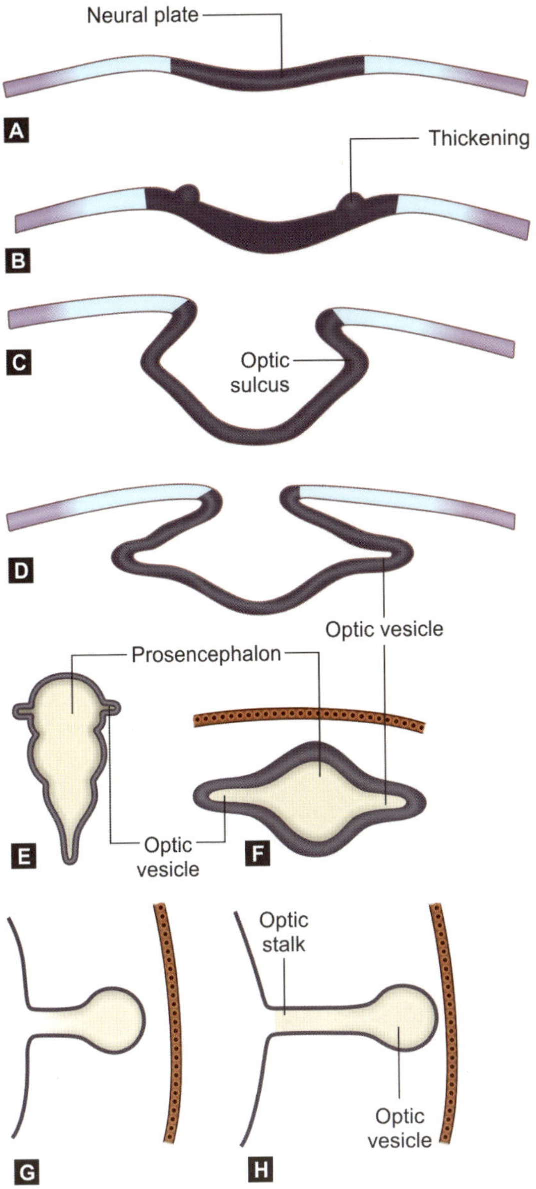

Fig. 2.1. *Formation of the optic vesicle and optic stalk.*

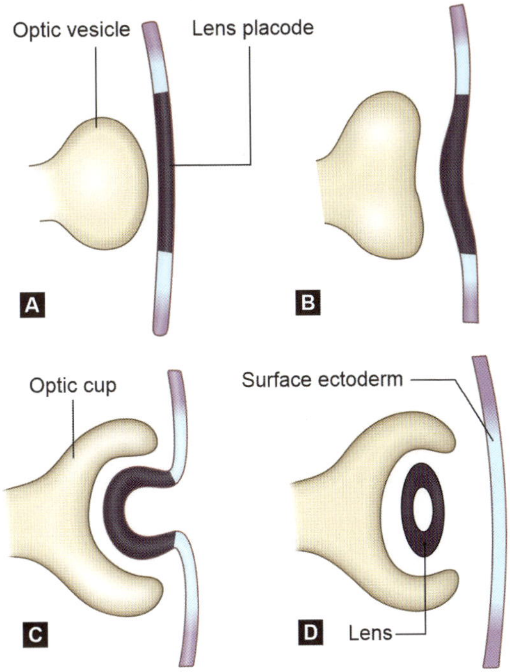

Fig. 2.2. *Formation of lens vesicle and optic cup.*

their nuclei disappear. The primary lens fibres are formed up to the 3rd month of gestation and are preserved as the compact core of the lens, known as embryonic nucleus. The posterior aspect of the lens, therefore, becomes devoid of epithelium.

Formation of secondary lens fibres

The equatorial cells of the anterior epithelium remain active throughout the life and form the so-called secondary lens fibres (Fig. 2.4). Since the secondary lens fibres are laid down concentrically, the lens on section has a laminated appearance. Depending upon the period of development, the secondary lens fibres are named below (*see* Fig. 1.1).

Fetal nucleus refers to the secondary lens fibres formed from 3rd to 8th month of gestation. The initial lens fibres of fetal nucleus reach both the anterior and posterior poles and they surround the embryonic nucleus. This process mandates that the primary lens fibres (embryonic nucleus) lose their original attachments with the lens epithelium anteriorly and their basal laminae posteriorly. The subsequently formed fibres of fetal nucleus can no longer extend from one pole to the other. Instead they meet at radiating lines or sutures that appear as an erect Y anteriorly and an inverted Y posteriorly (*see* Figs 1.5 and 2.5). Later in gestation and following birth, the growth of the lens fibres is asymmetric. Therefore, instead of simple Y sutures, a more complicated dendritic pattern is observed in infantile and adult nucleus (*see* Fig. 1.6).

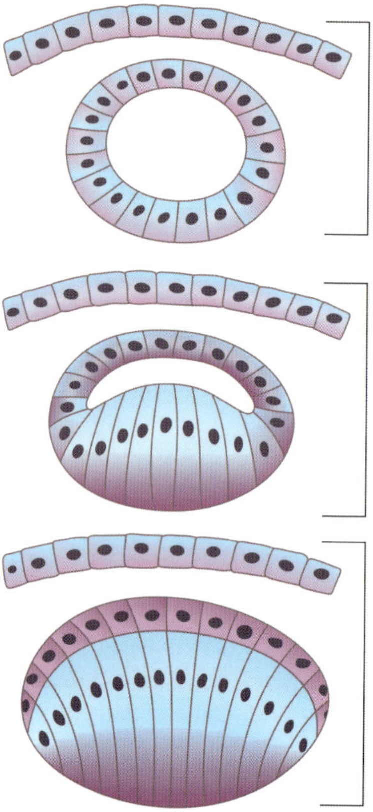

Fig. 2.3. *Development of the crystalline lens.*

Infantile nucleus refers to the secondary lens fibres formed during the last weeks of fetal life to puberty.

Adult nucleus is formed by the secondary lens fibres formed after the puberty.

Cortex consists of the recently formed superficial secondary lens fibres.

Tunica vasculosa lentis

During embryonic and fetal development, the lens receives nourishment via an intricate vascular capsule, the tunica vasculosa lentis, that completely encompasses the lens by approximately 9 weeks. It is formed from the mesenchyme that surrounds the lens. Three components of tunica vasculosa are anterior pupillary membrane, capsulo-pupillary membrane and posterior pupillary membrane (Fig. 2.6). In the earliest stages of development, tunica vasculosa lentis receives an abundant arterial supply from the hyaloid artery. Later, this blood supply regresses, and the vascular capsule disappears before birth. For its nutrition, the lens now depends on diffusion from the aqueous and vitreous.

Formation of lens capsule

The true lens capsule is a membranous non-cellular envelope that surrounds the lens. It is a true basement membrane produced as a result of basal laminae material deposited by the lens epithelium on its external aspect.

Formation of lens zonules

Lens zonules develop from the neuroectoderm in the ciliary region. The earliest fibres of the zonular apparatus are a continuation of the internal limiting membrane that thickens over the nonpigmented epithelium of the developing ciliary processes. They begin to develop at about the 10th week of gestation (45 mm stage). Later, zonular fibres are synthesized by the ciliary epithelial cells, and the zonules increase in number, strength and coarseness. By the 5th

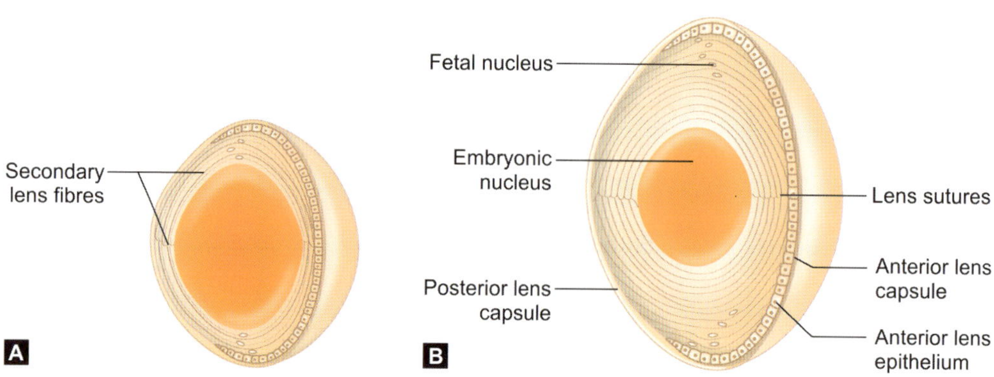

Fig. 2.4. *Formation of:* ***(A)*** *Secondary lens fibres 7 weeks;* ***(B)*** *Fetal nucleus.*

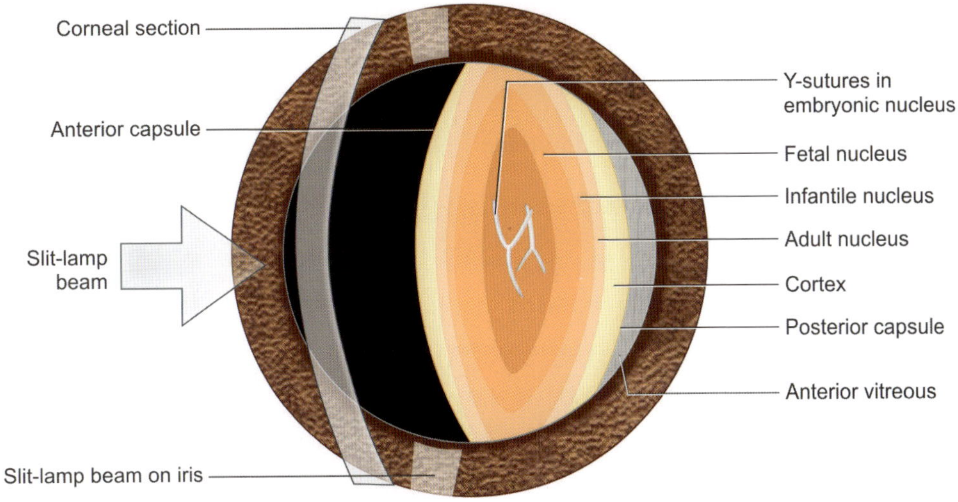

Fig. 2.5. *Y-shaped sutures around the embryonic nucleus can be seen on slit-lamp examination.*

month of gestation, the zonules have reached the lens and merge with both the anterior and posterior capsules.

Changes in the developing lens shape

The lens undergoes the following changes in shape during development:

- During initial development, the lens is elongated anteroposteriorly.
- It is nearly spherical, soft and reddish in tint at the 18–24 mm stage.
- As more and more secondary lens fibres are added to the equator, the lens becomes ellipsoid, a trend that continues till birth.
- At birth, the lens is almost spheroidal, being slightly wider in the equatorial plane. The anteroposterior diameter of lens at birth is nearly that of an adult, but its equatorial diameter is about two-thirds of that reached in the adult.

CONGENITAL ANOMALIES OF THE LENS

COLOBOMA OF LENS

- *Coloboma of lens* refers to focal inferior flattening or truncation of the lens in the lower

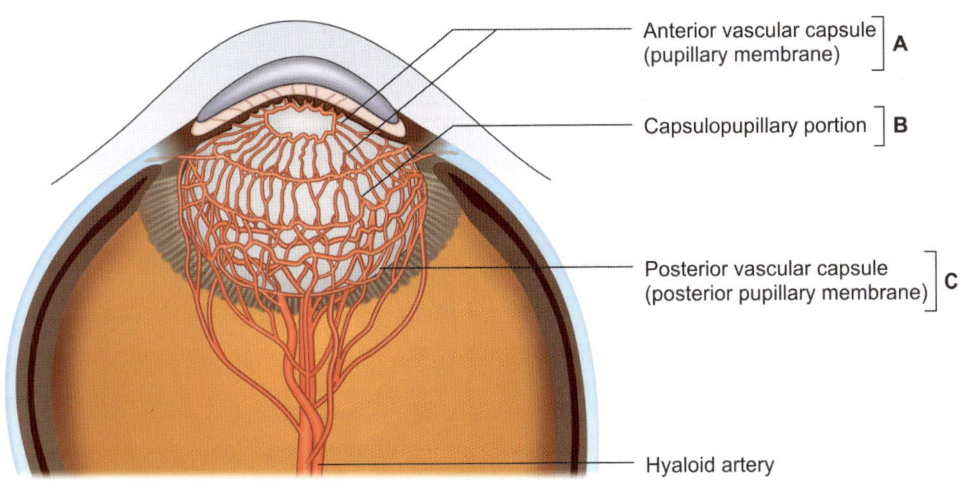

Fig. 2.6. *Three components of tunica vasculosa:* ***(A)*** *Anterior pupillary membrane;* ***(B)*** *Capsular pupillary membrane;* ***(C)*** *Posterior pupillary membrane.*

quadrant of equator resulting due to absence of zonular support (Fig. 2.7).

- Often *unilateral and hereditary*; can rarely be bilateral.
- *Double coloboma* of lens is also reported in the literature.
- *Coloboma* of the uveal tract may or may not be associated.
- *Visual acuity* may be decreased due to myopia, amblyopia and associated lenticular opacity.
- *Accommodation* may be decreased.
- *Slit-lamp examination* with dilated pupil confirms the diagnosis.

Treatment includes:

- Correction of refractive error and management of amblyopia.
- *Denticular opacity* may require cataract surgery.

LENTICONUS AND LENTIGLOBUS

Lenticonus

Lenticonus refers to cone-shaped projection of anterior pole (lenticonus anterior) or posterior pole (lenticonus posterior); or rarely both poles of the lens.

Characteristic features are as follows:

- *Lenticonus anterior* is a rare bilateral condition characterized by cone-shaped anterior pole (Fig. 2.8), often associated with Alport's syndrome.
- *Lenticonus posterior* is a cone-shaped bulge of posterior pole (Fig. 2.9). It may be associated with Lowe's syndrome.
- *Visual acuity* may be decreased due to myopia, and amblyopia.
- *Strabismus and nystagmus* may be present.

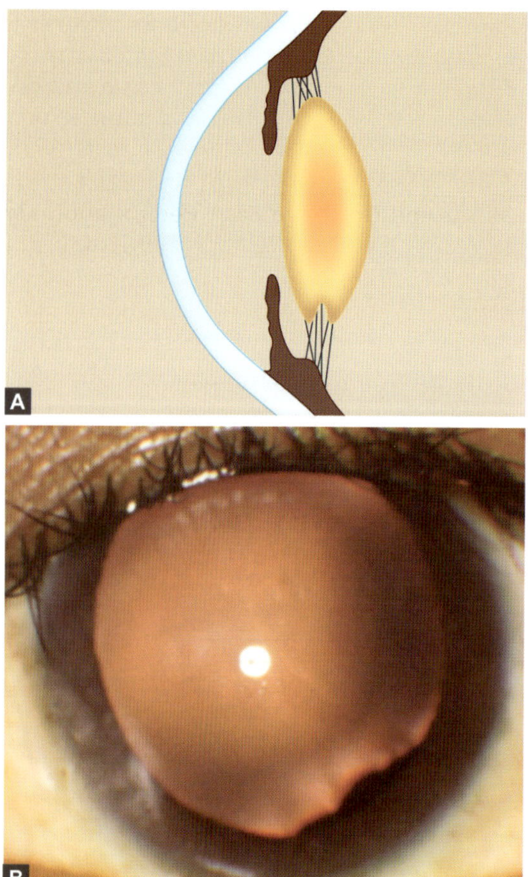

Fig. 2.7. Coloboma of the lens: **(A)** Diagrammatic; **(B)** Slit-lamp photograph of a patient.

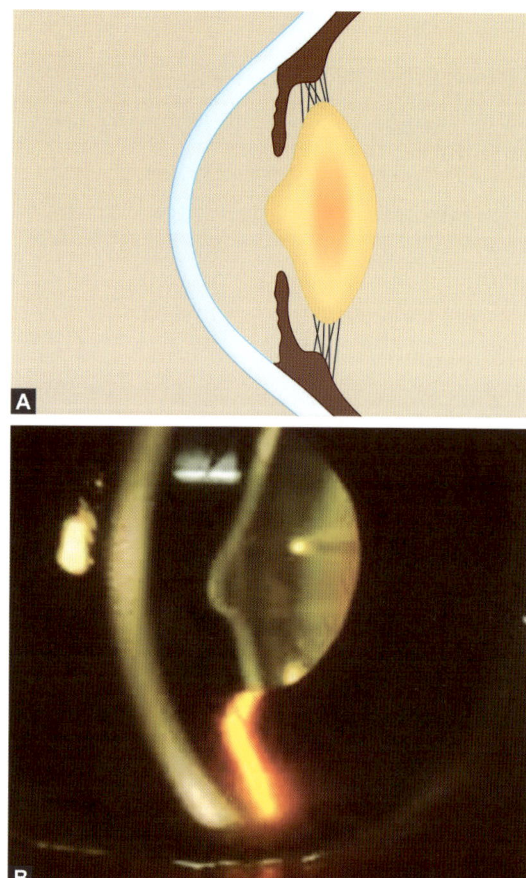

Fig. 2.8. Lenticonus anterior: **(A)** Diagrammatic; **(B)** Slit-lamp photograph of a patient.

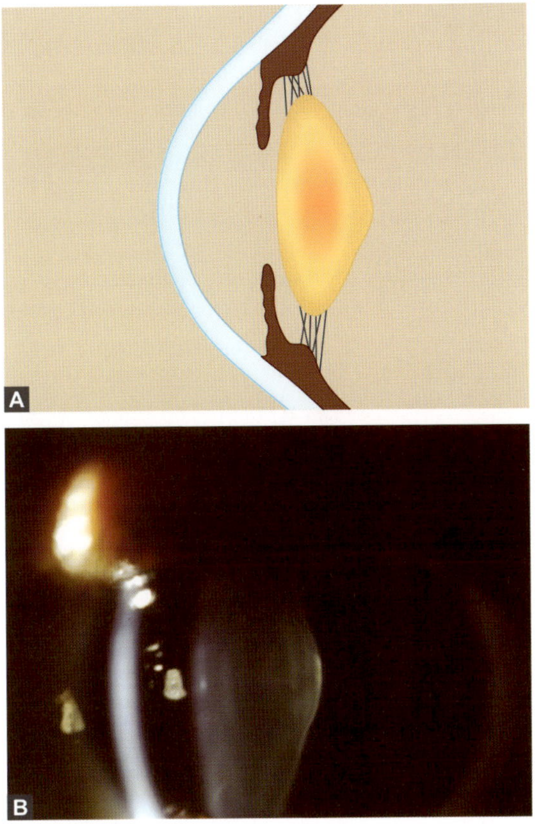

Fig. 2.9. *Lenticonus posterior:* ***(A)*** *Diagrammatic;* ***(B)*** *Slit-lamp photograph of a patient.*

- *Oil droplet sign* is positive, i.e. on distant direct ophthalmoscopy both anterior as well as posterior lenticonus present as oil globule lying in the centre of red reflex.
- *Slit-lamp examination* confirms the diagnosis (Figs 2.8B and 2.9B).
- *Lenticular opacification* may be present in both, lenticonus anterior as well as posterior.

Treatment includes:

- *Correction of refractive error* and occlusion therapy for amblyopia.
- *Phacoaspiration with IOL implantation* may be required for associated lens opacification and high lenticular astigmatism. Posterior capsulorrhexis should be performed in patients with lenticonus posterior.

Lentiglobus

Lentiglobus refers to the globe-shaped bulge at the anterior pole or posterior pole or both poles of the crystalline lens. In fact lentiglobus is the extreme form of lenticonus.

- *Anterior lentiglobus* is rare (accounts for 10% cases) and is often bilateral.
- *Posterior lentiglobus* accounts for 90% cases and is typically unilateral.
- *Glaucoma* may be associated with lentiglobus.
- *Lenticular opacity* may be associated.
- *Ultrasound A-scan* shows increased lens thickness.

Symptoms, signs and treatment are largely similar to advanced lenticonus.

MICROSPHEROPHAKIA AND MICROPHAKIA

- *Microspherophakia*. In this condition, the lens is spherical in shape (instead of normal biconvex) and is small in size (Fig. 2.10).
- *Microphakia* lens is small in size but normal in shape, i.e. biconvex.

Associations are as follows:

- *Microphakia* is usually associated with Lowe's syndrome.
- *Microspherophakia* may occur as an isolated familial condition (autosomal dominant) or as a feature of other syndromes such as Weill-Marchesani syndrome (*see* page 87), Marfan's syndrome (*see* page 84), Peter's anomaly, hyperlysinemia, Alport's syndrome and congenital rubella.

Clinical presentations of microspherophakia include:

- *Refrative error* may be present.
- *Amblyopia* may be associated.
- *Subluxation of lens* is a common presentation.

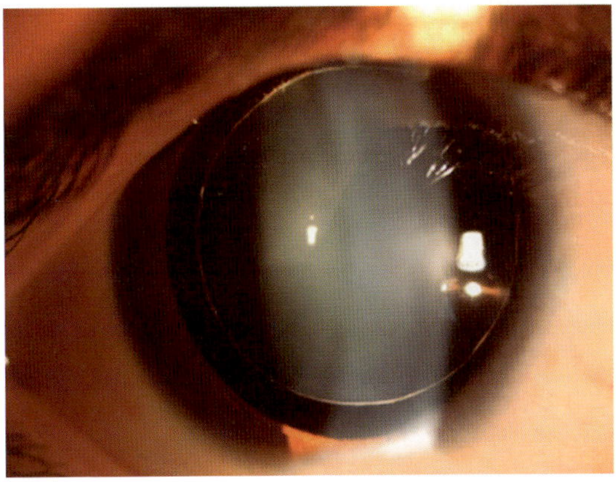

Fig. 2.10. *Microspherophakia.*

- *Pupil block glaucoma* may be a complication. The glaucoma is aggravated by miosis and relieved by mydriasis (that is why, it is called *inverse glaucoma*).

Management of microspherophakia includes:

- *Correction of refractive error* and treatment of associated amblyopia.
- *Subluxation of lens* may or may not need treatment.
- *Pupil block glaucoma* is relieved by cycloplegics. May require laser iridotomy or even lens extraction.

MITTENDORF DOT

- Mittendorf dot refers to a small white spot on the posterior lens capsule that represents the remnant of the posterior tunica vasculosa where the former hyaloid artery is attached (Fig. 2.11).
- Usually asymptomatic.
- May be associated with posterior polar cataract.
- Hyaloid artery (usually blood less remnant) may be seen in 10% cases. On ophthalmoscopy, it appears as a single vessel extending from the optic disc anteriorly through Cloquet's canal.

CONGENITAL ECTOPIA LENTIS

See Lens displacements (page 83)

CONGENITAL CATARACT

See page 50.

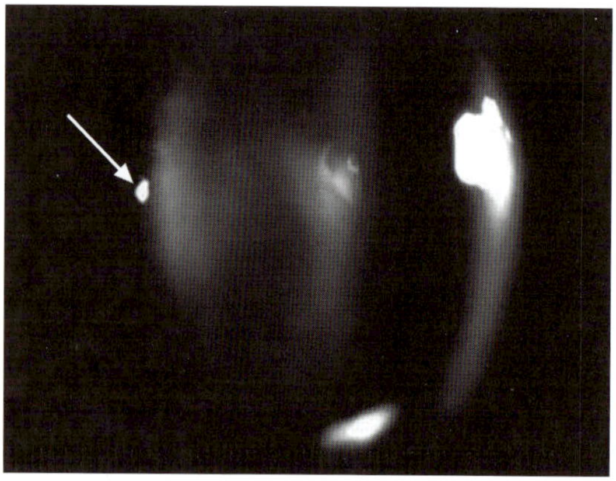

Fig. 2.11. *Mittendorf dot.*

BIBLIOGRAPHY

1. Barber AN. Embryology of Human Eye, The C.V. Mosby St. Louis 1955.
2. Buffam FV. Lacrimal diseases in Textbook of ophthalmology, Vol-4, Edited by Podos S.M. p7.1 to 7.3, Gower Medical Publication, London 1993.
3. Duke Elder S. System of Ophthalmology, Vol-III, Part-I, First edition, Henry Kimpton, London, 1964.
4. Dutta LC. Uveal effusion syndrome in Ophthalmology, First Edition pp 122–123 Current Books International, Kolkota 1995.
5. Hamming Nancy Apple D. Anatomy and embryology of the eye in Principles and Practice of Ophthalmology, Vol-I, 3–20, First Indian edition. Edited by Peyman GA, Sander DR. and Goldberg MF Jaypee Brothers, New Delhi, 1987.
6. Kozart DM. Embryology of the human Eye in Textbook of Ophthalmology, Ninth Edition p 79–92, Edited by Schcie HG, and Albert DM, WB Saunders Company, London, 1977.
7. Mann Ida; Development of Human Eye, Third Edition, British Medical Association, London, 1964.
8. Nema HV, Singh VD, Nema N. Congenital anomalies of the eye and its adnexa in Anatomy of the Eye and its Adnexa. Second edition. 162–165, Jaypee Brothers, New Delhi, 1991.
9. Review of medical embryology book by Ben Pansky, PhD, MD; chapter 169 – congenital malformations of the eye.
10. Schaffer DB. Abnormalities of the eye as a whole in Textbook of Ophthalmology, Ninth Edition, pp 209–293, Edited by Scheie H.G. and Albert DM, WB Saunders Company, Philadelphia, 1977.
11. Shields MB. Nanophthalmos in Textbook of Glaucoma, Fourth Edition, p 280, William and Wilkins Philadelphia, 1999.
12. Tayfun Bavbek, Mehdi S. Ogut, Haluk Kazokoglu. Congenital lens coloboma and associated pathologies. Documenta Ophthalmologica 1993, Volume 83, Issue 4, pp 313–322.
13. Vaughan D, Asbury T. General ophthalmology, Ninth Edition, 9–13, Lange Medical Publication, California, 1980.

CATARACT: DEFINITION, CLASSIFICATION, AND EPIDEMIOLOGY

3 CHAPTER

DEFINITION OF CATARACT

The term 'cataract' dates to the middle ages and has been derived from the Latin word *catarcta* and from the Greek word *katarraktes* meaning something that falls from above such as waterfall or a port cullis. This term was coined assuming that an abnormal humour developed and flowed in front of the lens and decreased the vision.

The term cataract was also introduced by Constantinus Africanus, an Arab ophthalmologist in 1018 AD, as a translation of the Arabic word '*suffusion*' meaning 'something deposited over something else'.

The present day definition of cataract came much later after the understanding of the lens anatomy and of the fact that the normal lens is a transparent structure. In the year 1 AD, Celsius, Ruffles and Galen, all described the structure of the lens with its anterior capsule and zonules. As of today, the term cataract refers to any opacification in the lens or capsule. Rolfinack (1650) is credited for this definition of cataract. However, clinically, cataract refers to an opacification of sufficient severity, on or in the human lens or its capsule to impair the vision (Dorland's Illustrated Medical Dictionary, WB Saunders, Philadelphia).

The lens opacification may occur by any of the two mechanisms:

- *Formation of opaque lens fibres*, i.e. instead of transparent, opaque lens fibres are being formed. This may occur due to abnormal development of the lens. When the disturbance occurs before birth, the lens opacity is called *congenital cataract* and when the disturbance occurs from infancy to adolescent, the resultant lens opacity is called *developmental cataract.*
- *Opacification of normally formed transparent lens fibres* may occur due to degenerative process. Biochemically, the lens fibre proteins get irreversibly denatured and coagulated. As a matter of fact, any factor physical, chemical or biological which disturbs the critical intra- and extracellular equilibrium of water and

electrolytes or deranges the colloid system within the lens fibres, tends to bring about lens opacification. Such an opacification of the previously clear lens fibres is called *acquired cataract.*

CLASSIFICATION OF CATARACT

The cataract can be variously classified.

A. ETIOLOGICAL CLASSIFICATION

I. ***Congenital and developmental cataract***

A. *Congenital capsular cataracts*
  1. Anterior capsular cataract
  2. Posterior capsular cataract

B. *Congenital polar cataracts*
  1. Anterior polar cataract
  2. Posterior polar cataract

C. *Congenital nuclear cataracts*
  I. Cataract involving embryonic nucleus
    1. Cataracta centralis pulverulenta.
  II. Cataracts involving fetal nucleus
    1. Lamellar cataract
    2. Sutural and axial cataracts
      - Floriform cataract
      - Coralliform cataract
      - Spear-shaped cataract
      - Anterior axial embryonic cataract
      - Dendritic suture cataract
  III. Cataract involving whole nucleus (embryonic, fetal and infantile)
    1. Total congenital cataract
    2. Congenital membranous cataract

D. *Cataracts involving adult nucleus and cortex*
  1. Coronary cataract
  2. Blue dot cataract

II. ***Acquired cataract***
  1. Age-related cataract
  2. Traumatic cataract
  3. Complicated cataract
  4. Metabolic cataract
  5. Electric cataract
  6. Radiational cataract
  7. Toxic cataract, e.g.
     - Corticosteroid-induced cataract
     - Miotics-induced cataract
     - Copper (in chalcosis) and iron (in siderosis) induced cataract.
  8. Dermatogenic cataract (cataract associated with skin diseases).
  9. Cataract associated with osseous diseases.
  10. Cataract with miscellaneous syndromes, e.g.
     - Dystrophica myotonica
     - Down's syndrome.
     - Lowe's syndrome
     - Treacher-Collins syndrome

B. MORPHOLOGICAL CLASSIFICATION (Fig. 3.1)

1. *Capsular cataract.* It involves the capsule and may be:
   - Anterior capsular cataract
   - Posterior capsular cataract

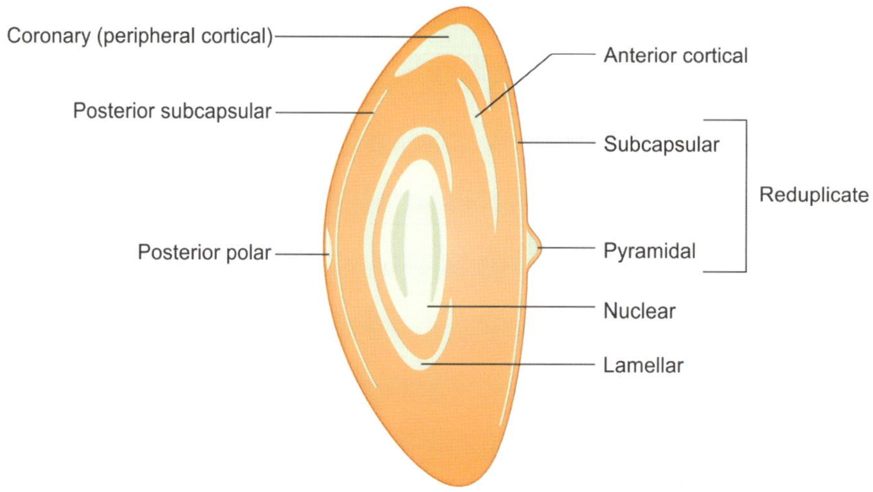

Fig. 3.1. *Morphological shapes of cataract.*

2. *Subcapsular cataract.* It involves the superficial most part of the cortex (just below the capsule) and includes:
   - Anterior subcapsular cataract
   - Posterior subcapsular cataract
3. *Cortical cataract.* It involves the major part of the cortex.
4. *Supranuclear cataract.* It involves only the deeper parts of cortex (just outside the nucleus).
5. *Nuclear cataract.* It involves the nucleus of the crystalline lens.
6. *Polar cataract.* It involves the capsule and superficial part of the cortex in the polar region only and may be:
   - Anterior polar cataract
   - Posterior polar cataract.

C. CLASSIFICATION BASED ON STAGE OF MATURITY

1. *Stage of lamellar separation*, i.e. earliest change characterized by demarcation of the lens fibres owing to their separation by fluid.
2. *Stage of incipient cataract*, i.e. early or very mild changes of lens opacification.
3. *Immature cataract.* It is characterized by presence of scattered opacities with areas of clear lens in between. When such a cataractous lens become swollen due to imbibation of fluid, the term *intumescent cataract* is used. Intumescence may persist even in the next stage of maturation.
4. *Mature cataract*, also termed *'riped cataract'*, is characterized by complete (total) opacification of the lens fibres.
5. *Hypermature cataract*, also termed *'over-riped cataract'* may present in two forms:
   - *Morgagnian hypermature cataract* which is characterized by total liquefaction of the cataractous cortex, and
   - *Sclerotic type of hypermature cataract* which is characterized by shrinkage of the opaque lens (due to leakage of water) associated with wrinkling and thickening of anterior lens capsule.

D. BIOMICROSCOPIC-PHOTOGRAPHIC CATARACT CLASSIFICATION SYSTEMS

The above described morphological and cataract maturity classifications are based on coarse and subjective scales. However, the need for more accurate and consistent system of cataract classification was felt for the studies being conducted on:

- Identification and quantification of mechanism of cataract formation,
- Cataractogenic toxicity of certain drugs, and
- Epidemiological studies on the risk factors for the human cataract formation.

A few of the cataract classification systems developed are as follows:

I. *In vitro classification systems*, e.g.
   - American cataract classification and research group (CCRG) classification system

II. *In vivo classification systems*, e.g.
   - Lens opacities classification system (LOCS), version I, II and III.
   - Oxford clinical cataract classification and grading system (OCCCGS).
   - Wilmer classification system.
   - Wisconsin classification system.
   - Japanese cooperative cataract epidemiology study group classification system.
   - WHO classification system.
   - Pentacam-Scheimpflug based cataract classification system.

I. *IN VITRO CLASSIFICATION SYSTEMS*

In early days, when the whole lenses were readily available from intracapsular cataract extraction (ICCE), a few in vitro classification systems were developed with isolated lenses. Of these, the popular comprehensive classification is the 'American CCRG classification system'.

AMERICAN CCRG CLASSIFICATION SYSTEM

This system divides the lens into two distinct zones: The cortex and the nucleus.

Cortex is further subdivided into six anatomic zones:

- Subcapsular anterior (SCA)
- Subcapsular posterior (SCP)
- Anterior cortical (CXA)
- Equatorial cortical (CXE)
- Posterior cortical (CXP)
- Supranuclear (SN), a zone found between the cortical and the nuclear zones.

Nuclear (N) region is not further subdivided.

Subscripts are added to the classification terms to indicate the extent or intensity of involvement in that particular region of the lens:

- *For CXA, CXE, CXP, and SN*, each zone is subdivided into four quadrants, and the total extent of opacification, even if scattered throughout the zone, is expressed in terms of the number of quadrants that are totally opacified; these are denoted by subscripts 1 to 4.
- *For SCA and SCP*, the extent of opacification is estimated by comparing the opaque zone with the area within each of a series of concentric circles, representing opacification of 3, 4, 25, 44, 69, and 100% of the area of the equatorial circle of the lens. The percentage of the total area involved is denoted as a subscript.

Although the CCRG classification system was designed primarily for use on extracted lenses; it proved useful to some ophthalmologists for in vivo classification.

II. *IN VIVO CLASSIFICATION SYSTEMS*

After the advent of extracapsular cataract extraction (ECCE), several in vivo classification systems have been developed based on the biomicroscopic and photographic techniques. Each system uses standard photographs that represent boundaries between different degrees of opacity. By comparing the patient's lens under defined lighting conditions with the standard photographs, a trained observer can define the type and extent of opacity in each lens zone. Systems differ not only in the number of photographs in each class of standards but also in the features that are emphasized as defining age-related cataract.

Essential features of some of the in vivo cataract classification systems are described below.

1. LENS OPACITIES CLASSIFICATION SYSTEMS (LOCS) I, II AND III

The most widely used classification system in the United States is the Lens Opacities Classification Systems I to III, which has been used in several national and international collaborative projects. LOCS uses a reference set of standard photographs that defines the *extent* of opacification in the cortical (C) and posterior subcapsular (P) zones, and the *intensity* of nuclear opalescence (NO) in the nuclear zone. Also in LOCS, nuclear colour (NC) is graded separately from opalescence.

LOCS I

It was originally designed for use in a case-control study of risk factors for age-related cataract sponsored by the National Eye Institute. In LOCS I, an ordinal scaling ranging from zero (no opacification) to 2 (definite opacification) for each class defines the severity of opacification or intensity of brunescence (Fig. 3.2).

Grade 0 implies the absence of lens opacities.

Grade 1 implies the presence of early opacification. It is subdivided into 1a and 1b classes.

- *Category 1a* includes minor, clinically insignificant opacification; and
- *Category 1b* includes early cortical cataract.

Grade 2 implies definite cataract.

The boundaries between the gradings are defined by a set of standard photographs, consisting of:

- *One slit-lamp colour photograph* used to grade nuclear opalescence and nuclear colour, and
- *Three black-and-white retroillumination photographs* used for posterior subcapsular and cortical classifications.

The standard photographs are reproduced on an 8½ by 11 inch transparency and placed on a light box located at eye level behind the patient's right shoulder when the patient is seated at the slit-lamp. The classifier can easily refer to the standards during the examination, which is done with the patient's pupils maximally dilated.

LOCS II

It is an expanded version of LOCS I, designed to further differentiate among the various degrees of cortical, subcapsular, and nuclear opacification. It was also designed for use in longitudinal studies. Coloured standards are used, and the number of reference standards is increased. LOCS II uses (Fig. 3.2):

- *Four nuclear standards* for grading nuclear opalescence,

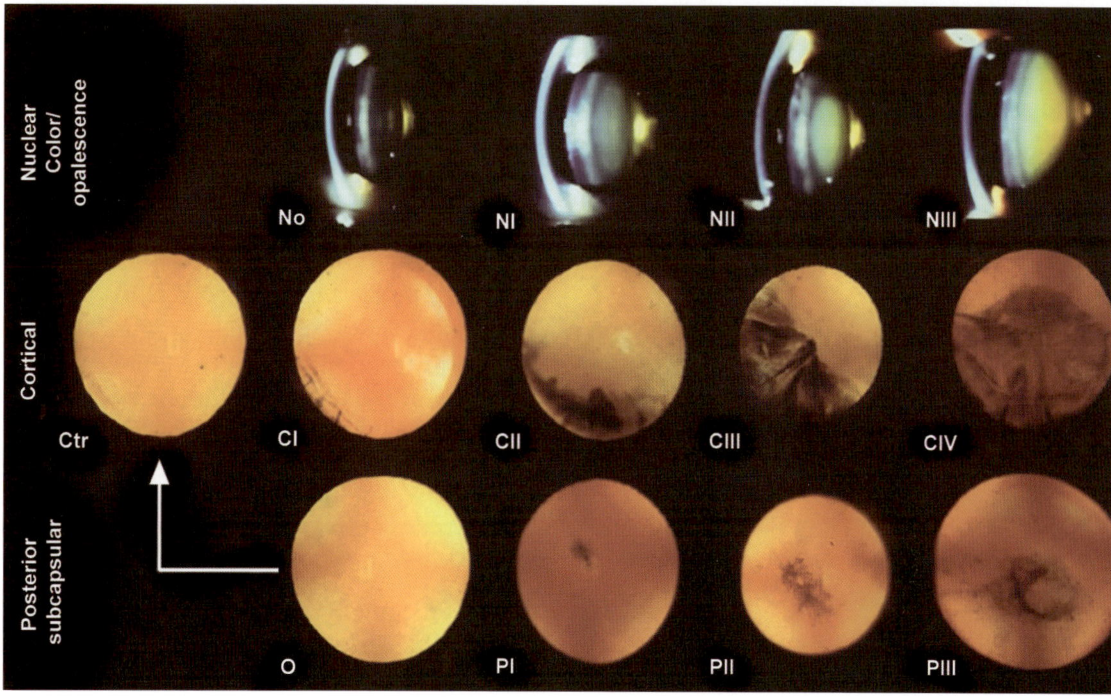

Fig. 3.2. *The Lens Opacity Classification System II (LOCS II) photographic grading standards. N = Nuclear photographs. Stage 0 = normal; I–III = various stages of nuclear cataract. For nuclear opalescence, the average opalescence across the entire nuclear region is used. An opalescence that is less than or equal to Photographic Standard 0 = grade 0; if the opalescence is less than or equal to Standard I, the grade is 1, and so on. For Colour Grading of the nucleus, only the N2 standard is used. (<N2 for colour = 0, equal to N2 in colour = 1, and N2 for colour = 2) C = Cortical photographs. 0-Trace (Tr) = normal; I–IV = various steps of cortical cataract (roughly CII ¼, CIII ½, CIV ¾. CV > ¾). P = Posterior subcapsular photographs. 0 = normal; I–III = various stages of posterior subcapsular cataracts (Chylack LT, Leske MC, McCarthy D, et al: Lens opacities classification system II [LOCS II]. Arch Ophthalmol 107:991, 1989)*

- *Five cortical standards*, and
- *Four subcapsular standards*.

The standards demarcate boundaries between various grades.

Grading of nuclear colour (NC). The nuclear colour (NC) is graded by comparing the colour of the posterior cortical–posterior subcapsular reflex to the nuclear I (NI) standard, which is the same standard as in LOCS I. The biomicroscopist uses the low-magnification view of the slit-lamp with the slit-beam oriented approximately 45° to the patient's visual axis, and the slit-height and brightness are set to equal those in the standard photograph. If the colour is less yellow than the standard, the nuclear colour is graded zero; if it is similar, it is graded 1; and if it is darker yellow, it is graded 2.

Grading of nuclear opalescence (NO). In grading nuclear opalescence (NO), the classifier estimates the average opalescence of the nucleus (the overall density of the entire lens enclosed within the zones of supranuclear scattering) and determines whether it is equal to or less than a specific nuclear standard. For example, if the average NO is more than the N0 but less than or equal to the N1 standard, the grade is N1.

Grading a cortical (C) or posterior subcapsular (P) opacity. The grader estimates whether the aggregate area of such an opacity is less than or equal to the aggregate area of the opacity in a particular standard. The classifier envisions an aggregate opacity by clumping all contiguous and non-contiguous opacities into one zone. The size of the opaque zone relative to the size of the opaque zone in the standards determines which class is chosen to grade the cataract. In the LOCS classification scheme, the cortical and posterior subcapsular zones are graded individually as C and P:

- *C zone* includes the subcapsular anterior, cortical anterior, cortical equatorial, cortical posterior, and supranuclear zones of the original American CCRG *in vitro* classification scheme.
- *P zone* includes the subcapsular posterior zone. The classification data are recorded on a form that contains guidelines for classifying each type of opacification.

LOCS III

The LOCS III system evaluates four features (Fig. 3.3):

- Nuclear opalescence (NO)
- Nuclear colour (NC)
- Cortical cataract (C)
- Posterior subcapsular cataract (PSC).

Nuclear opalescence and colour are graded on a decimal scale, based on a set of six standardized photographs, (NO1 to NO6 and NC1 to NC6).

Cortical and posterior subcapsular cataracts are graded based on five standardized photographs. (C1 to C5 and P1 to P5).

2. WILMER CATARACT CLASSIFICATION SYSTEM

In Wilmer system, the gradings are based on three criteria: visual acuity, density, and extent of the opacity.

Grading of nuclear opalescence (NO)

The nucleus is examined with a thin slit-beam that passes through the centre of the lens, and the clarity of the optical section of the nucleus is compared with the standard photograph and graded accordingly. The Wilmer system uses four nuclear standard photographs for grading nuclear opacity (NO1 to NO4), but does not grade nuclear colour (NC).

Grading of cortical (C) and posterior subcapsular (P) opacities

The cortical and posterior subcapsular opacities are examined using retroillumination. Only opacities that could be seen in retroillumination are graded by estimating the proportion of the total circumference of the lens occupied by the

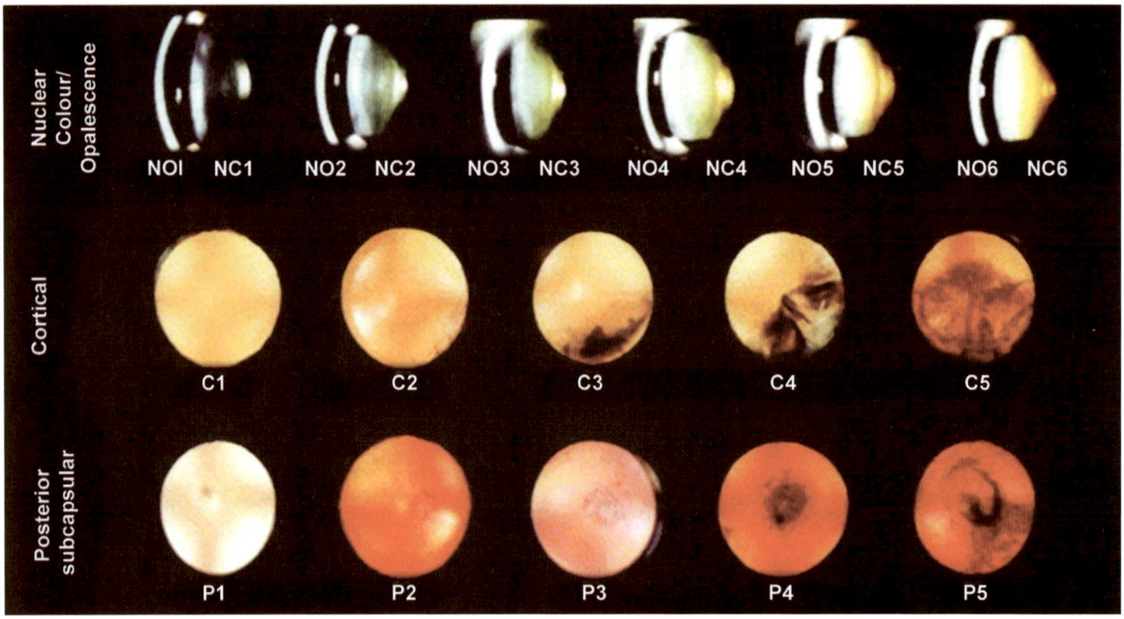

Fig. 3.3. *The LOCS III standard images in an 8.5-inch × 11-inch colour transparency as used in the office at the slit-lamp. The top row contains the standards for NO and NC. The second row contains the standards for grading cortical cataract (C) and the bottom row, for grading posterior subcapsular cataract (P). (Reproduced from Chylack et al. Arch Ophthalmol. 1993;105:1244–1250).*

combined cortical opacities as if they are adjacent, gives the cortical opacity grading definitions. The posterior subcapsular opacities are assessed by determining the overall vertical and horizontal dimensions measured using the calibration of the slit-beam height. These dimensions are then multiplied to give an approximation of area.

3. OXFORD CLINICAL CATARACT CLASSIFICATION AND GRADING SYSTEM (OCCGS)

Oxford system is a very comprehensive system of classifying and grading cataracts. It includes quantitation on a scale of 0 to 5 of such features as anterior clear zone thickness, anterior subcapsular opacity, posterior subcapsular opacity, cortical spoke opacity, waterclefts, vacuoles, retrodots, focal dots, nuclear brunescence, and white nuclear scatter.

Grading of cortical opacities

The system gives:
- *Anterior clear zone thickness* reference standards,
- *Diameter scale* reference standards for grading anterior and posterior subcapsular opacities
- *Pie segment* reference standards for grading spoke opacities and waterclefts
- *Vacuole* reference standards
- *Retrodot* reference standards
- *Focal dot* reference standards.

Grading of nuclear opacities

Nuclear brunescence is graded by comparing the posterior region of the nucleus just anterior to the posterior nuclear shell with a set of Munsell colour chips. The grade is selected according to the closest available match between the nucleus and the colour chips. White nuclear scatter is assessed as the amount of white light being scattered back to the observer by the lens nucleus and is compared with Munsell neutral-density gray-scale samples.

4. JAPANESE COOPERATIVE CATARACT EPIDEMIOLOGY STUDY GROUP CLASSIFICATION SYSTEM

The Japanese Cooperative Cataract Epidemiology Study Group system also uses a set of standard photographs in grading cortical, nuclear, and subcapsular opacities. These cataracts are graded on the basis of standard photographs of cortical and nuclear cataracts as follows.

Grading of cortical opacities

The subcapsular opacities are graded in reference to the pupil size as below:
- *Early (grade I).* An opacified area corresponding to the normal pupil size is graded I.
- *Moderate (grade II).* An area larger than a normal pupil but smaller than a moderately dilated pupil as II.
- *Advanced (grade III).* An area larger than a moderately dilated pupil as grade III.

Grading of nuclear opacities

Nuclear colouration is classified into four gradings:
- *Grade* I, pale yellow
- *Grade* II, yellow
- *Grade* III, brownish-yellow
- *Grade* IV, brown (including reddish-brown and black-brown).

5. WORLD HEALTH ORGANIZATION'S SIMPLIFIED CATARACT GRADING SYSTEM

There had been so many classification systems with their own merits and demerits so in an attempt to unify the methods of grading age-related cataract, WHO (2002) with the help of cataract classification experts have proposed a new simplified classification.

The WHO/PBD (prevention of blindness and deafness) simplified cataract grading system has been developed to encourage more clinical and epidemiological studies of cataract by ophthalmologists, otherwise not particularly involved in such research. It is based on slit-lamp examination only and is easy to use in field surveys as well as to teach any personnel with experience of slit-lamp examinations. It has been developed to:
- Facilitate epidemiological studies of the main forms of cataract and their possible risk factors.
- To give an estimate of cases that are likely to be in need of surgery.
- It can be easily combined with national blindness prevalence of surveys.

Essential features of WHO cataract grading system

The WHO cataract grading system described here has been summarized from the article by panel of experts who developed this system (B. Thylefors et al., Ophthalmic epidemiology-2002, Vol 9, no. 2, pg 83-95). This system involves slit-lamp examination of lens with dilated pupils (at least 6.5 mm diameter). It grades the three most common forms of cataract:

- Nuclear cataract (NUC)
- Cortical cataract (COR)
- Posterior subcapsular cataract (PSC).

Grading of nuclear cataract

Age-related nuclear change involves two related processes: Opacification (clouding) and colouration (browning). In the WHO/PBD classification system, nuclear cataract (NUC) is defined only in terms of the opacification of nucleus. For the purpose of grading the severity of the nuclear cataract, only a specified region of the nucleus (the 'grading region') should be examined. It includes the anterior shell, the anterior embryonal nucleus, the posterior embryonal nucleus, and the posterior shell. Between the component parts are three clearer zones called ground or background (Fig. 3.4).

The WHO/PBD NUC standards represent increasing opacification from standards 1 to 3 (Figs 3.5 to 3.7). The examiner assigns a severity grade by comparing the degree of opacification in the slit-lamp appearance of the grading region with the standard photographs. Grades are assigned as follows:

i. *Grade NUC-0:* Less than the NUC-STD 1
ii. *Grade NUC-1:* Equal to or greater than the NUC-STD 1 but less than the NUC-STD 2
iii. *Grade NUC-2:* Equal to or greater than the NUC-STD 2 but less than the NUC-STD 3
iv. *Grade NUC-3:* Equal to or greater than the NUC-STD 3
v. *Grade NUC-9:* Cannot grade

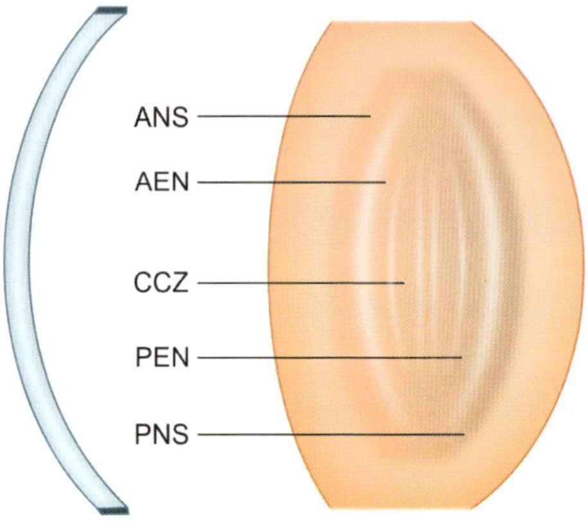

ANS : Anterior nuclear shell
AEN : Anterior embryonal nucleus
CCZ : Central clear zone
PEN : Posterior embryonal nucleus
PNS : Posterior nuclear shell

Fig. 3.4. *Image of lens with the 'grading region', as shown for early nuclear cataract, including the anterior and posterior nuclear shells, the embryonal nuclei and the central clear zone.*

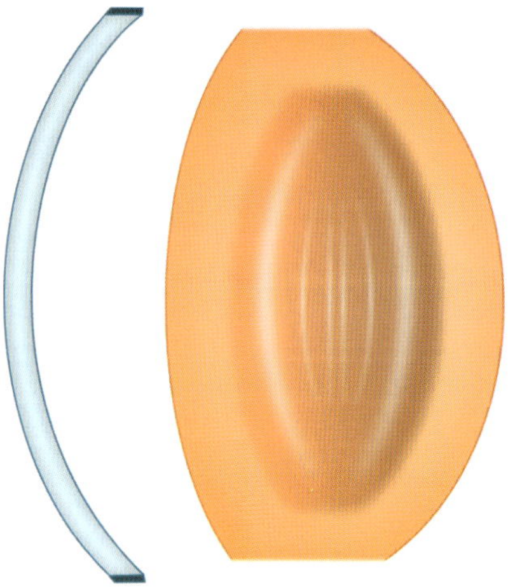

Fig. 3.5. *WHO PBD NUC standard I showing significant nuclear cataract formation.*

Note.

- Situations in which a grade of NUC-9 may occur include the presence of advanced corneal opacity or extensive corneal opacity, which obscures the lens nucleus, or if there is a Morgagnian cataract.
- In cases of very advanced nuclear cataract, it will not be possible to obtain sufficiently good retroillumination for grading of cortical and/or PSC cataract: Code 9 should apply in those instances.

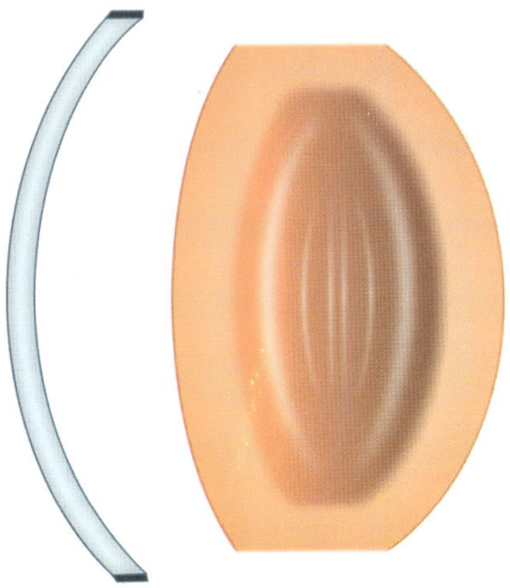

Fig. 3.6. *WHO/PBD NUC standard 2 showing moderately advanced nuclear cataract formation.*

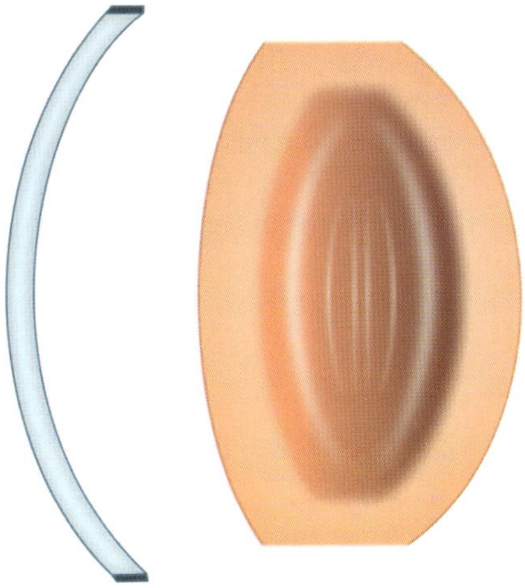

Fig. 3.7. *WHO/PBD NUC standard 3 showing very advanced nuclear cataract formation.*

Grading of cortical cataract

Only sharply and well-defined anterior and posterior cortical opacities seen on retroillumination at the slit-lamp should be graded as COR. A relatively short and broadly focused beam, positioned within the 3 or 9 o'clock border of the pupil should be used. In cases of a dispersed cortical cataract (with several non-contiguous spoke- or ring-like opacities), all of the opacities should be aggregated for the purposes of grading circumferential extent (Fig. 3.8):

i. *Grade COR-0:* Cataract involves less than one-eighth of the circumference.
ii. *Grade COR-1:* If cataract involves one-eighth, but less than a quarter of the circumference.
iii. *Grade COR-2:* If cataract involves a quarter but less than half of the circumference.
iv. *Grade COR-3:* If cataract involves half or more of the circumference.
v. *Grade COR-9:* Cannot grade.
vi. *Grade CEN:* Involvement of central optical zone of 3 mm diameter (yes/no).

Note.

- *Cortical opacities that do not extend to the circumference* should also be graded by extending straight radial lines from the papillary centre through the edges of the opacity to the pupillary margin and estimate the circumferential involvement between the radial lines (Fig 3.8).
- *Central optical zone involvement.* It is also of interest to measure the progression of cortical cataract towards the central optical zone. Therefore, the following should also be graded as central (CEN) involvement.

Grading of posterior subcapsular cataract

A posterior subcapsular opacity (PSC) is located just in front of the posterior lens capsule. Typical PSC is centred near the posterior pole of the lens and extends from varying distances

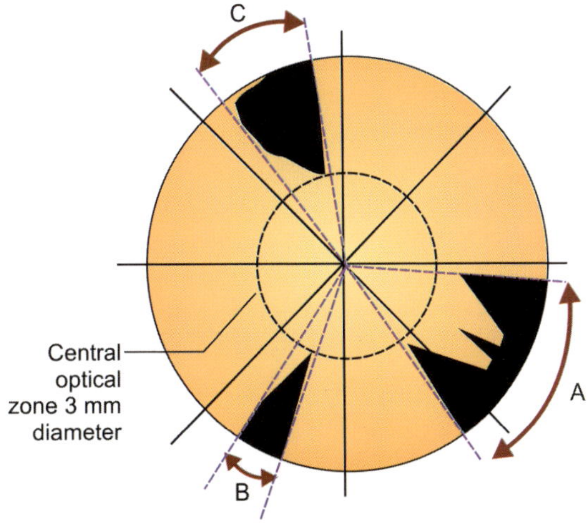

Fig. 3.8. *For case of grading, the circumference can be divided into octants (eights) by first dividing the pupillary aperture into quadrants with the imaginary lines between 6 and 12, and between 3 and 9 o'clock. A quadrant can then be halved to create one-eighth segments.*

towards the equator. PSC typically has a feathered appearance in contrast to the sharp, spoke-like cortical opacities. PSC is graded according to the vertical diameter (in mm). For measurement, the observer should adjust the height of the slit-beam to the maximum overall height of the PSC. The measurements are read of the gradicule scale that adjusts the beam height. If peripheral or several PSC opacities exist, only the most central, clearly defined entity should be graded, if it is at least partially within the 3 mm central optical zone. Furthermore, only clearly visible opacities with distant borders should be taken into account.

PSC definitions, measured in the vertical dimension are as follows:

i. *Grade 0:* Less than 1 mm
ii. *Grade PSC-1:* Equal to or greater than 1.0 mm, but less than 2.0 mm ('case')
iii. *Grade PSC-2:* Equal to or greater than 2.0 mm, but less than 3.0 mm ('progression which may require surgery')
iv. *Grade PSC-3:* Equal to or greater than 3.0 mm ('usually requires surgery')
v. *Grade 9:* Cannot grade

Note.

If the posterior capsule cannot be visualized because of advanced NUC or COR preventing visualization against the red reflex, a designation of 'cannot grade' should be made.

WHO/PBD simplified cataract assessment proforma

The proforma used to document the observations by the panel of experts of WHO/PBD simplified cataract grading system is depicted in Table 3.1.

6. PENTACAM SCHEIMPFLUG BASED CATARACT CLASSIFICATION SYSTEM

Recently attempts have been made to correlate the lens density measured using the Pentacam Scheimpflug system with LOCS III grading score.

- A linear increasing relationship between the lens density values and LOCS III grading score has been reported in patients with nuclear cataracts.
- Lens density value had a stronger significant correlation with **LOCS** III NO score than that with NC score. The correlation between the nuclear lens density value and log MAR visual acuity was stronger than that between NO score and log MAR visual acuity or between NC score and log MAR visual acuity.
- Certain areas of nucleus are reported to be more representative of the lens density on Scheimpflug imaging (region of interest) and that these areas correlated with the LOCS III, whereas the average lens density measurement on Pentacam did not correlate with the LOCS standards.

7. OPTICAL BIOMETRY BASED CATARACT GRADING SYSTEM (OBBCGS)

Gede Pardianto (2009) introduced the new Optical Biometry Based Cataract Grading System (OBBCGS) for phacoemulsification planning.

Cataract can be classified to Lens Opacity Classification System III (LOCS III) and Maturity Based Cataract Grading System (MBCGS), and then being converted to Optical Biometry Based Cataract Grading System (OBBCGS) using IOL Master Optical Biometry into following grades:

- No cataract (NC)
- Optical biometry examinable cataract (OBEC)
- Optical biometry un-examinable cataract (OBUC).

Criteria for conversion to OBBCGS

- LOCS III's NC0, C0 and P0 and MBCGS' no cataract can be converted to OBBCGS' NC.
- LOCS III's NC1-3, C1-3, P1-3 and MBCGS' insipiens or immature cataract can be converted to OBBCGS' OBEC.
- LOCS III's NC4-5, C4-5, P4-5 and MBCGS' nearly mature or mature cataract can be converted to OBBCGS' OBUC; and need to be examined using applanation ultrasonography biometry.

Implications of OBBCGS

- *OBBCGS' NC:* There is no cataract. No need of any cataract surgery. But if refractive lens extraction (RLE) is to be done, one can prepare a phacoemulsification for soft cataract with less vacuum, less until no power and less manipulation.
- *OBBCGS' OBEC:* One can prepare a phacoemulsification for soft to medium cataract

Table 3.1 *WHO/PBD simplified cataract assessment proforma*

	OD		*OS*	
1. **Mature or Morgagnian cataract present**	Yes	No	Yes	No
Gradable cataract present				
2. If 'Yes', proceed to (9)	Yes	No	Yes	No
If 'No'				
3. Phthisis	Yes	No	Yes	No
4. Corneal opacification	Yes	No	Yes	No
5. Aphakia	Yes	No	Yes	No
6. PCIOL present	Yes	No	Yes	No
7. ACIOL present	Yes	No	Yes	No
8. Other findings (specify)				
a.	Yes		Yes	
b.	Yes		Yes	
9. **Dilated pupil size ≥6.5 mm**	Yes	No	Yes	No
10. **WHO/PBD cataract severity grade** (please circle):				
	OD		*OS*	
a. **NUC**	0 1 2 3 9		0 1 2 3 9	
b. **COR**	0 1 2 3 9		0 1 2 3 9	
CEN	Yes	No	Yes	No
c. **PSC**	0 1 2 3 9		0 1 2 3 9	

with less vacuum, less power and less manipulation.

- *OBBCGS' OBUC:* One can prepare a phacoemulsification for medium to hard cataract with more vacuum, more power and may be more manipulation.
- *OBBCGS' OBUC grade tends to be medium to hard cataract except in cases with:*
  - Presenile cataracts (congenital and juvenile)
  - Traumatic or any secondary cataract
  - Posterior polar cataract (PPC)
  - Dense posterior subcapsular cataract

Advantages of OBBCGS

- OBBCGS is very useful in grading of cataract for phacoemulsification planning, especially for *beginner* and phaco surgeons who learn sub 2 mm Micro Incision Cataract Surgery (MICS). We suggest them to choose and select patient with OBBCGS' **OBEC** for better safety and result. OBBCGS' **OBEC** is the preferred criterion for ophthalmologists to perform any *research* of everything between phacoemulsification and posterior segment of the eyeball by using OCT, SLP, SLO, ERG, etc.
- OBBCGS is very useful in planning to consider vacuum, power and manipulation.
- OBBCGS is very useful to give some predictive information for patients and better informed consent.

EPIDEMIOLOGY OF CATARACT

Cataract poses a substantial economic and public health burden and is the leading cause of blindness worldwide, accounting for nearly 48% of all blindness.

THE BURDEN OF DISEASE

GLOBAL BURDEN

The World Health Organization estimates that the current global prevalence of blindness is 0.57% (range: 0.2–1%), with more than 82% of all blindness occurring in individuals aged 50 and older. Worldwide there are about 20 million bilateral blind due to cataract. By the year 2020, the projected numbers of persons with blinding cataract will exceed 40 million worldwide. Cataract accounts for 47.8% of the world's roughly 37 million blind individuals. 90% of the contribution of cataract to blindness is seen in developing countries.

Aim under 'Vision 2020' is to eliminate avoidable blindness due to cataract by the year

2020 by performing cataract extraction with intraocular lens (IOL) implantation. Strategy to achieve the aim to measure the increase in the cataract surgery rate (CSR), i.e. number of cataract surgeries per million population per year is given in Table 3.2.

Table 3.2 *Strategy to increase in the cataract surgery rate*

Year	*Global cataract surgery rate targets*	*Global number of cataract operation targets (million)*
2000	2000	12
2010	3000	20
2020	4000	32

Emphasis is to be placed on achieving:

- High success rates in terms of restored vision and quality-of-life outcome.
- Affordable and accessible services
- Measures to overcome barriers and increased use of services.

INDIAN SCENARIO

Cataract continues to be the single largest cause of blindness. According to latest National Survey in India (1999–2001), 62.6% of blindness in 50+ population of India was found to be cataract related. During 'Rapid Assessment of Avoidable Blindness (RAAB) conducted in 2006–07, the cataract is reported to be responsible for 72.2% of blindness in 50+ population.

OBJECTIVES AND TARGETS

Objective under vision 2020: Indian perspective is to improve the quantity and quality of cataract surgery and the targets include:

- The targets fixed for the cataract surgery rate (CSR) in the vision 2020 strategy were 4500 per million per the year by 2005, 5000 by 2010, 5500 by 2015 and 6000 by 2020.
- To improve the visual outcome of surgery to match the standards set by WHO (i.e. 80% to have visual outcome 6/18 or >6/18 after surgery).
- IOL surgery for >80% by the year 2005 and for all by the year 2010.
- YAG capsulotomy services at all district hospitals by 2010.

Strategic activities suggested to clear the backlog of cataract include:

- *Primary screening* by community health worker to identify persons with visual impairment (finger counting <6 m in any eye).
- *Case selections* by eye surgeons at screening camps and at base level (district hospital).
- *Cataract extraction with IOL implantation* to be done free of cost for bilateral cases, underserved poor people, especially women.
- *Reduction in disparities* based on geographical, socioeconomic and gender bases.

IMPACT OF DISEASE

Although 90% of cataract cases are found in developing countries, the disease has a substantial impact in developed world countries as well from social, physical, and financial perspectives. The burden of cataract extends beyond the financial costs to society. Patients with prevalent cataract are likely to have significantly reduced quality of life resulting from low vision. Cataract is primarily a disease of older age groups. Often, decreases in functional abilities are attributed to other age-related processes and not recognized as the onset of cataract. That is why cataract represents an important contributor to disability in older populations in developed countries also despite treatment availability.

In developing countries, the economic impact of vision loss from cataract is huge, including loss of jobs and increase in custodial care. It is estimated that 1500% of the cost of cataract surgery could be generated in 1 year through increased economic productivity. In fact, cataract surgery is ranked as one of the most cost-effective public health interventions for the developing world. Worldwide, the evidence for superior visual outcome and high patient satisfaction, coupled with the decline in cost of intraocular lenses (IOLs), has increased the demand for IOL surgery and acceptance of pseudophakia as the standard of care.

OUTCOME OF CATARACT SURGERY AND EFFECT ON QUALITY OF LIFE

Quality cataract surgery has been shown to enhance visual function and quality of life. The

National Study of Cataract Outcomes reported that severe complications of surgery were rare in the United States, and achievement of 20/40 or better vision in the operated eye occurred in greater than 90% of patients. In other countries, however, some evaluations have suggested that desirable outcomes were not as large as expected because of surgical complications, concurrent diseases, loss of aphakic spectacles, and development of posterior capsular opacification.

Clearly, lens opacification and associated visual loss influences the quality of life for patients. Research has documented the improvement in performance of tasks involving vision and improvement in psychological well-being following cataract surgery. Some data indicate that the improvement in depressive symptoms following cataract surgery may be a major pathway for the improvement in quality of life in other domains.

RISK FACTORS

Well-established risk factors for the development of age-related cataract that have been consistently reported are:

- Age
- Smoking
- Ultraviolet B radiation
- Diabetes

Risk factors where current understanding is evolving or reports conflicting results

- Race—nuclear cataract is seen more commonly in whites, whereas cortical is seen more commonly in African Americans; however, PSC cataract is prevalent at roughly the same, much lower, rate in both groups.
- Myopia
- Nutrition and supplement usage
- Weight status and fat consumption
- Corticosteroids
- Exogenous oestrogens
- Genetics
- Markers of inflammation

Note. Various risk factors for development of age-related cataract have been described in detail on page 60.

CATARACT AND MORTALITY

Nuclear cataract, particularly nuclear cataract mixed with other types, appears to be an independent predictor of early mortality. The association is present in Caucasians, African Americans, and African Caribbeans. Other predictors of mortality, such as frailty, smoking, diabetes, and other chronic conditions, do not explain this association. Thus the lens may provide an interesting window into the aging process, and there is considerable research interest in finding a common pathway between lens opacification and premortal events at the cellular or subcellular level.

CATARACT: OBSERVATIONS OF SOME IMPORTANT EPIDEMIOLOGICAL STUDIES

Although a lot of epidemiological studies have been carried out from time to time in relation to cataract, but due to lack of a widely accepted, standardized classifications system for lens opacities make it different to evaluate precisely the prevalence and incidence of cataract. Some of the important studies which had some impact are mentioned briefly:

Age-related eye disease study (AREDs report no 4 Am J Ophthalmol 2001; 131:167–75), has demonstrated a high degree of reliability in grading evenly of the lens opacities (AREDs system for classifying cataract from photography).

Beaver Dam eye study (ophthalmology, 1992;99: 546–552) reported that:

- *Visually significant cataract was present* in 38.8% of men and 45.9% of women above the age of 74 years.
- *Incidence of nuclear cataract, cortical cataract* and posterior subcapsular cataract reported was 13.1%, 8.2% and 3.4%, respectively.
- *Sex distribution.* In general, women were reported to have higher incidence of nuclear cataract vis-a-vis men.

Baltimore eye study (N Eng J Med, 1991;325: 1412–1417) reported that:

- *Leading cause of blindness* in the population above 40 years was cataract.
- *Racial difference* was reported in the incidence of blindness due to untreated cataract (Africans American, 27% and Caucasians, 13%)

Longitudinal study of cataract (LSC) (Arch Ophthalmol 1993;111:831–836) reported that:

- *Lens opacities classification system III* (LOCS III), was described by LSC group in 1993.
- *Risk factors* for nuclear cataract reported by LSC group (Am J Epidemiol 1998;147:36–41) include with increasing age, white race, lower education, gout medication, current smoking, family history of cataract, pre-existing PSC, and early end of eyeglasses.

Barbados eye study (Arch Ophthalmol 1997;115: 105–111) provided prevalence data of lens opacities in a predominant black population:

- *Cortical opacities* were the most frequent type of cataract; and
- *Women* had higher frequency of opacification.

BIBLIOGRAPHY

1. Barker FM. "Dietary supplementation: effects on visual performance and occurrence of AMD and cataracts". Curr Med Res Opin 26 (8): 2011–23; August 2010. doi:10.1185/03007995. 2010. 494549. PMID 20590393.
2. Buchberger W, Winkler R, Moser M, Rieger G. "Influence of iodide on cataractogenesis in Emory mice". Ophthalmic Res 23(6):303–308; 1991. doi:10.1159/000267127. PMID 1803312.
3. Christen WG, Manson JE, Seddon JM, *et al.* "A prospective study of cigarette smoking and risk of cataract in men". JAMA 268(8):989–993; August 1992. PMID 1501324.
4. Courtney P. "The National Cataract Surgery Survey: I. Method and descriptive features". Eye (Lond) 6 (Pt 5):487–92;1992. doi:10.1038/ eye. 1992.103. PMID 1286712.
5. "Death and DALY estimates for 2004 by cause for WHO Member States" (xls). World Health Organization. who.int. 2004.
6. Dobson, R. "Ozone depletion will bring big rise in number of cataracts". *BMJ* 331 (7528): 1292–1295;2005. doi:10.1136/bmj.331.7528.1292-d. PMC 1298891. edit
7. Duker, Jay S; Myron Yanoff MD; Yanoff, Myron; Jay S. Duker MD. Ophthalmology. St. Louis, Mo: Mosby/Elsevier, 2009. ISBN 0-323-04332-1.
8. Emmett T. Cunningham, Paul Riordan-Eva. Vaughan & Asbury's general ophthalmology. (18th ed. ed.). McGraw-Hill Medical. ISBN 978-0071634205.
9. Greiner J, Chylack L. "Posterior subcapsular cataracts: histopathologic study of steroid-associated cataracts". Arch Ophthalmol 97 (1): 135–144,1979. PMID 758890.
10. Guo Y, Yan H. "Preventive effect of carnosine on cataract development". Yan Ke Xue Bao 22 (2):85–8;2006. PMID 17162883.
11. Javitt, JC; Wang, F; West, SK. "Blindness Due to Cataract: Epidemiology and Prevention". Annual review of public health 17:159–177;1996. doi : 10.1146/annurev.pu.17.050196.001111. PMID 8724222. Cited in Five-Year Agenda for the National Eye Health Education Program *(NEHEP)*, p. B-2; National Eye Institute, US National Institutes of Health.
12. Kahn HA, Leibowitz HM, Ganley JP, Kini MM, Colton T, Nickerson RS, Dawber TR. "The Framingham Eye Study. I. Outline and major prevalence findings". Am J Epidemiol 106 (1): 17–32;Jul 1977. PMID 879158.
13. Klein, Barbara; Ronald Klein, Kristine Lee, and Lisa Grady. "Statin Use and Incident Nuclear Cataract". Journal of the American Medical Association 295 (23):2752–2758; 2006. doi:10. 1001/jama. 295.23.2752. PMID 16788130.
14. Lipman RM, Tripathi BJ, Tripathi RC. "Cataracts induced by microwave and ionizing radiation". Surv Ophthalmol 33(3):200–10;1988. PMID 3068822.
15. Matthew, Milan C, Ann-Margret Ervin, Jeremiah Tao, Richard M Davis (2012 Jun 13). "Antioxidant vitamin supplementation for preventing and slowing the progression of age-related cataract.". Cochrane Database Syst Rev. 6: CD004567. doi:10. 1002/14651858. CD004567. pub2. PMID 22696344.
16. Neale, RE; JL Purdie, LW Hirst, and AC Green. "Sun exposure as a risk factor for nuclear cataract". Epidemiology 14 (6):707–712;(2003–11). doi:10.1097/01.ede.0000086881.84657.98. PMID 14569187.
17. Organization, World Health. The global burden of disease: *2004* update. Geneva, Switzerland: World Health Organization, 2008. p. 35. ISBN 9789241563710.
18. "Posterior Supcapsular Cataract". Digital Reference of Ophthalmology. Edward S. Harkness Eye Institute, Department of Ophthalmology of Columbia University. 2003. Retrieved 2 April 2013.
19. "Priority eye diseases: Cataract". Prevention of Blindness and Visual Impairment. World Health Organization. WHO.int.
20. Rafnsson, V; Olafsdottir E, Hrafnkelsson J, Sasaki H, Arnarsson A, Jonasson F. "Cosmic radiation increases the risk of nuclear cataract in airline pilots: a population-based case-control study". Arch Ophthalmol 123(8):1102–1105; 2005. doi:10. 1001/archopht.123.8.1102. PMID 16087845.
21. Richa S, Yazbek JC. "Ocular adverse effects of common psychotropic agents: a review". *CNS*

Drugs 24(6):501–26;2010 Jun. doi:10.2165/ 11533180-000000000-00000. PMID 20443647.

22. Sliney DH (1994). "UV radiation ocular exposure dosimetry". Doc Ophthalmol 88 (3–4): 243–254. PMID 7634993.
23. Spencer R, Andelman S. "Steroid cataracts. Posterior subcapsular cataract formation in rheumatoid arthritis patients on long term steroid therapy". Arch Ophthalmol 74:38–41; 1965. PMID 14303339.
24. Sperduto RD, Seigel D, Seigel D. Sperduto RD. "Senile lens and senile macular changes in a population-based sample". Am J Ophthalmol 90 (1):86–91;Jul 1980. PMID 7395962.
25. van den Brûle J, Degueldre F, Galand A. "Cataractes incitées de médicament" [Drug-induced cataracts]. Revue médicale de Liège (in French) 53(12):766–769;1998 Dec. PMID 9927876.
26. Wang S, Wang JJ, Wong TY. "Alcohol and eye diseases". Surv Ophthalmol 53(5):512–525;2008. doi:10.1016/j.survophthal.2008.06.003. PMID 18929762.
27. Williams DL, Munday P. "The effect of a topical antioxidant formulation including N-acetyl carnosine on canine cataract: a preliminary study". Vet Ophthalmol 9 (5): 311–316, 2006. doi:10. 1111/j.1463-5224.2006. 00492.x. PMID 16939459.

CHAPTER 4

CONGENITAL AND DEVELOPMENTAL CATARACTS

DEFINITION, PREVALENCE AND ETIOLOGY
- Definition
- Prevalence
- Etiology

CLINICAL TYPES
- Congenital capsular cataracts
- Polar cataracts
- Nuclear cataracts
- Lamellar cataract
- Sutural and axial cataracts
- Generalized cataracts

DIFFERENTIAL DIAGNOSIS
- Other causes of leukocoria

MANAGEMENT
- Clinico-investigative work-up
- Prognostic factors
- Indications and timing of paediatric cataract surgery
- Contraindications to cataract surgery
- Preoperative counselling
- Surgical procedures
- Correction of paediatric aphakia
- Correction of amblyopia
- Visual prognosis
- Prophylaxis

DEFINITION, PREVALENCE, AND ETIOLOGY

DEFINITION

Congenital and developmental cataracts occur due to some disturbance in the normal growth of the lens. When the disturbance occurs before birth, the child is born with a *congenital cataract.* Therefore, in congenital cataract, the opacity is limited to either embryonic or fetal nucleus. *Developmental cataract* may occur from infancy to adolescence. Therefore, such opacities may involve infantile or adult nucleus, deeper parts of cortex or capsule. Developmental cataract typically affects the particular zone which is being formed when this process is disturbed. The fibres laid down previously and subsequently are often normally formed and remain clear. Congenital and developmental opacities assume most variegated appearance and minute opacities (without visual disturbance) are very common in normal population. These are detected with the beam of slit-lamp under full mydriasis.

PREVALENCE

- The prevalence of childhood cataract has been reported to be 1–15 cases in 10,000 children.
- It is estimated that globally, there are 2,00,000 children blind from bilateral cataract and about 20–40 thousand children are born with developmental cataract each year.
- Approximately 3/4th of world's blind children live in poorest regions of Africa and Asia.
- In India, about 60,000 childern are blind due to cataract.

ETIOLOGY

About 50% cases are idiopathic and one-third are hereditary and the rest due to other causes.

I. Idiopathic

About 50% cases are sporadic and of unknown etiology. Many of these occur due to new mutations and familial nature of these cataracts will be discovered in subsequent generations.

II. Heredity

About one-third of all congenital cataracts are hereditary.

Inherited cases without systemic disorders

In these cases, the mode of inheritance is usually autosomal dominant but rarely it may be autosomal recessive or X-linked also.

Inherited cases with systemic disorders include:

- *Chromosomal disorders,* e.g. trisomy 21, trisomy 13–15, trisomy 16–18, Turner's syndrome and Cri-du-chat syndrome.
- *Skeletal disorders,* e.g. Conradi-Hunermann syndrome, Stickler syndrome.
- *Central nervous system disorders,* e.g. Marinesco-Sjögren syndrome, Noorie's disease and cerebro-oculofacial syndrome.
- *Renal system disorders,* e.g. Lowe's syndrome.
- *Dermatological disorders,* e.g. congenital icthyosis, incontinentia pigmenti, Schafer syndrome, Siemens syndrome, syndrome of alopecia, cataract and syndactyly.
- *Muscle disorders,* e.g. myotonic dystrophy; cataract, lactic acidosis and cardiomyopathy.
- *Digital disorders,* e.g. Rubenstein-Taybi syndrome (syndactyly/polydactyly), Ellis-van Creveld syndrome.

Common familial cataracts include:

- Cataracta pulverulenta,
- Zonular cataract (also occurs as non-familial),
- Coronary cataract, and
- Total soft cataract (may also occur due to rubella).

III. Maternal factors

1. *Malnutrition* during pregnancy has been associated with non-familial zonular cataract.
2. *Infections.* Maternal infections like rubella are associated with cataract in 50% of cases. Other maternal infections associated with congenital cataract include toxoplasmosis and *cytomegalo-inclusion* disease.
3. *Drugs ingestion.* Congenital cataracts have also been reported in the children of mothers who have taken certain drugs during pregnancy (e.g. *thalidomide, corticosteroids).*
4. *Radiation.* Maternal exposure to radiation during pregnancy may cause congenital cataracts.

IV. Foetal or infantile factors

1. *Deficient oxygenation* (anoxia) owing to placental haemorrhage.
2. *Birth trauma,* may cause cataract.
3. *Metabolic disorders* of the foetus or infant, e.g. galactosaemia, galactokinase deficiency and neonatal hypoglycaemia.
4. *Cataracts associated with other congenital anomalies,* e.g. as seen in Lowe's syndrome, myotonia dystrophica and congenital ichthyosis.
5. *Ocular diseases* associated with developmental cataracts include persistent hyperplastic primary vitreous (PHPV), aniridia, anterior chamber cleavage syndrome, retinopathy of prematurity (ROP), lenticonus posterior, microphthalmos, congenital glaucoma, pigmentary retinopathy and subluxation of lens.
6. *Malnutrition* in early infancy may also cause developmental cataract.

CLINICAL TYPES OF CONGENITAL CATARACT

Congenital and developmental cataracts have been variously classified.

A simple morphological classification of congenital and developmental cataracts is as under:

A. *Congenital capsular cataracts*
   1. Anterior capsular cataract
   2. Posterior capsular cataract

B. *Congenital polar cataracts*
   1. Anterior polar cataract
   2. Posterior polar cataract

C. *Congenital nuclear cataracts*
   - I. Cataract involving embryonic nucleus
     1. Cataracta centralis pulverulenta.
   - II. Cataracts involving fetal nucleus
     1. Lamellar cataract
     2. Sutural and axial cataracts
        - Floriform cataract
        - Coralliform cataract
        - Spear-shaped cataract

- Anterior axial embryonic cataract
- Dendritic suture cataract

III. Cataract involving whole nucleus (embryonic, fetal and infantile)
1. Total congenital cataract
2. Congenital membranous cataract

D. *Cataracts involving adult nucleus and cortex*
1. Coronary cataract
2. Blue dot cataract

A. CONGENITAL CAPSULAR CATARACTS

1. ***Anterior capsular cataracts*** are non-axial, stationary and visually insignificant.
2. ***Posterior capsular cataracts*** are rare and can be associated with persistent hyaloid artery remnants and also as part of posterior polar cataract.

B. CONGENITAL POLAR CATARACTS

1. ***Anterior polar cataract*** The cataract involves the central part of the anterior capsule and the adjoining superficial most cortex. It may arise in the following ways:

- *Due to delayed development of anterior chamber.* In this case, the opacity is congenital usually bilateral, stationary and visually insignificant.
- *Due to corneal perforation.* Such cataracts may also be acquired in infantile stage and follow contact of the lens capsule with the back of cornea, usually after perforation due to ophthalmia neonatorum or any other cause.

Morphological types. Anterior polar cataracts may occur as any of the following morphological patterns:

- *Thickened white plaque* in the centre of anterior capsule, i.e. anterior pyramidal cataract. In it, the thickened capsular opacity is coneshaped with its apex towards cornea.
- *Reduplicated cataract* (double cataract). Sometimes along with thickening of central point of anterior capsule, lens fibres lying immediately beneath it also become opaque and are subsequently separated from the capsule by laying of transparent fibres in between. The burried opacity is called 'imprint' and the two together constitute reduplicated cataract (Fig. 4.1).

2. ***Posterior polar cataract:***
Posterior polar cataract is a common lens anomaly that consists of a small circular circumscribed opacity involving the posterior pole.

Associations. Posterior polar cataract may be associated with:

- Persistent hyaloid artery remnants (Mittendorf dot)
- Posterior lenticonus, lentiglobus
- Persistent hyperplastic primary vitreous (PHPV).

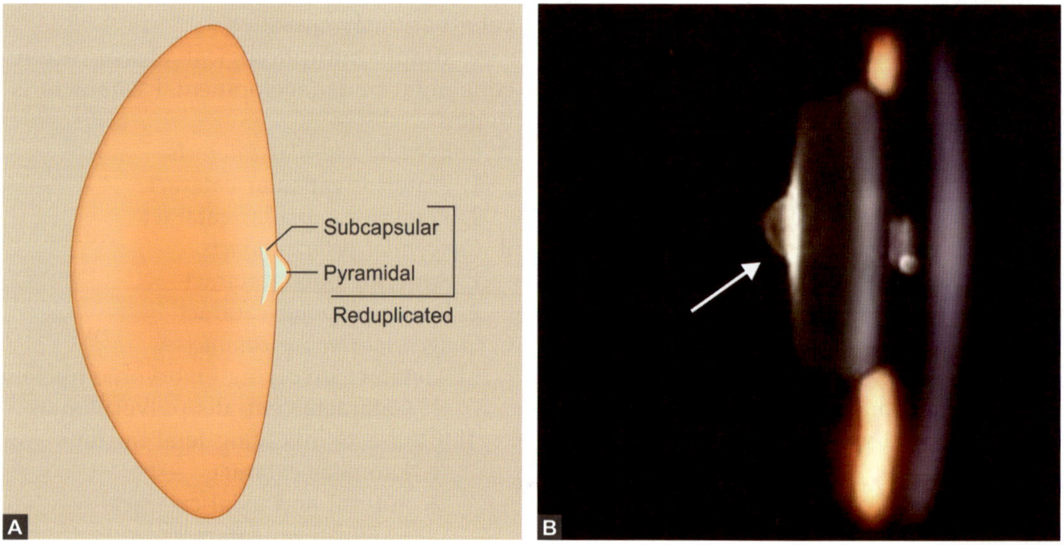

Fig. 4.1. *Reduplicated cataract: **(A)** Diagrammatic optical section; **(B)** Diffuse illumination photograph. Congenital and developmental cataracts.*

Types. Posterior polar cataract occurs in two forms:

- Stationary form
- Progressive form which progresses after birth. It typically has an 'onion whorl appearance' (Fig. 4.2).

C. CONGENITAL NUCLEAR CATARACTS

I. Cataract involving embryonic nucleus

Cataracta centralis pulverulenta (Embryonic nuclear cataract) It has dominant genetic trait and occurs due to inhibition of the lens development at a very early stage and thus, involves the embryonic nucleus. The condition is bilateral and is characterized by a small rounded opacity lying exactly in the centre of the lens. The opacity has a powdery appearance (pulverulenta) and usually does not affect the vision (Fig. 4.3).

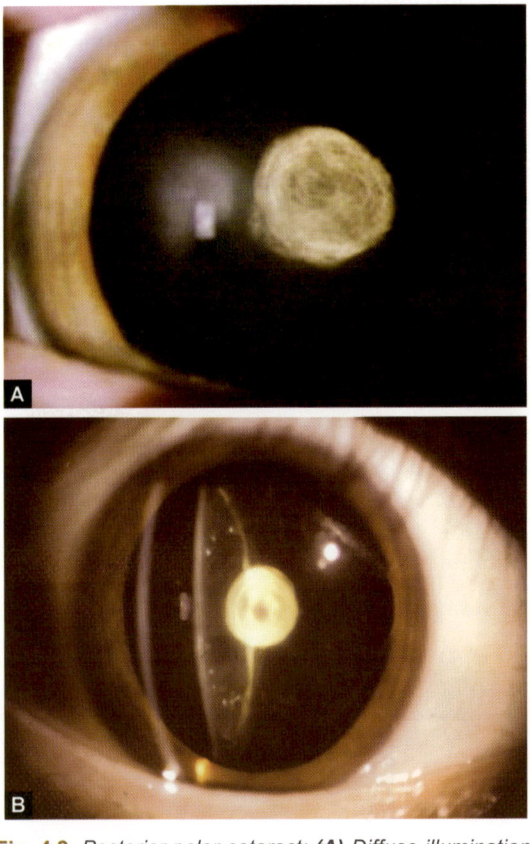

Fig. 4.2. *Posterior polar cataract: **(A)** Diffuse illumination; **(B)** Slit-lamp optical section.*

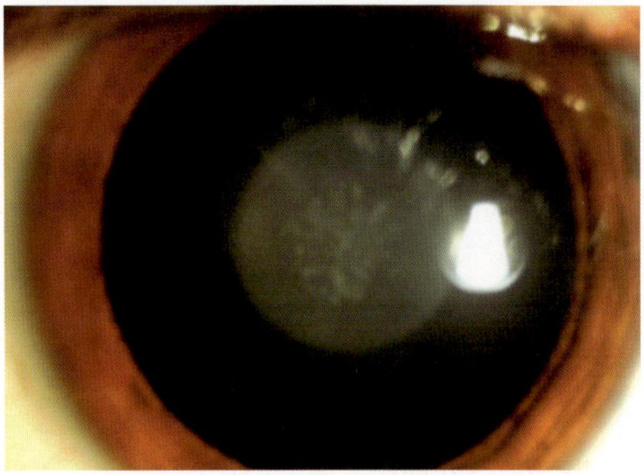

Fig. 4.3. *Cataracta centralis pulverulenta.*

II. Cataracts involving fetal nucleus

1. Lamellar (zonular) cataract. Lamellar or zonular cataract refers to the developmental cataract in which the opacity occupies a discrete zone in the lens. It is the most common type of congenital cataract presenting with visual impairment. It accounts for about 40% of the cases.

Etiology. It may be either genetic or environmental in origin.

- *Genetic pattern* is usually of familial autosomal dominant variety.
- *Environmental form* is associated with–Vitamin D deficiency – Hypocalcaemia – Sometimes maternal rubella infection contracted between 7th and 8th week of gestation may also cause lamellar cataract.

Characteristic features. Typically, this cataract occurs in a zone of fetal nucleus surrounding the embryonic nucleus (Fig. 4.4).

- Occasionally two such rings of opacity are seen.
- The main mass of the lens internal and external to the zone of cataract is clear, except for small linear opacities like spokes of a wheel (riders) which may be seen towards the equator.
- It is usually bilateral and frequently causes severe visual defects.

2. Sutural and axial cataracts. Sutural cataracts are comparatively of common occurrence and consist of a series of punctate opacities scattered around the anterior and posterior Y-sutures. Such cataracts are usually static, bilateral and

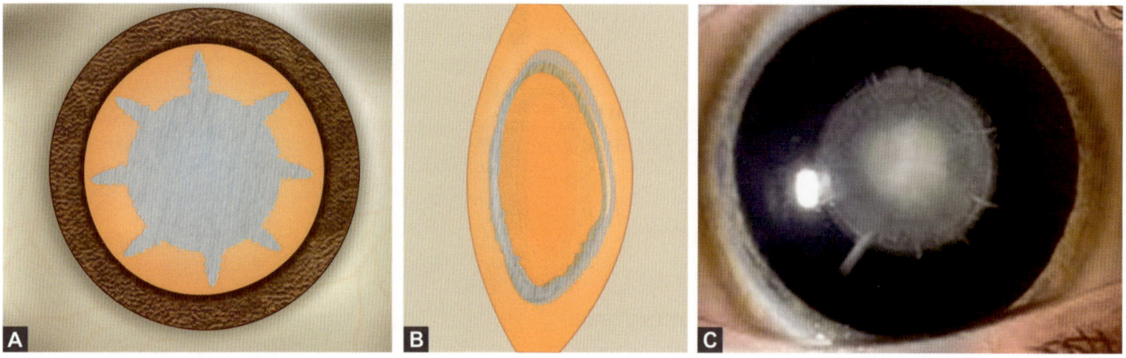

Fig. 4.4. *Lamellar cataract: **(A and B)** Diagrammatic depiction as seen on oblique illumination and in optical section with the beam of the slit-lamp, respectively; **(C)** Clinical photograph.*

do not have much effect on the vision. The individual opacities vary in size and shape and have different patterns and thus are named accordingly as under:

- *Anterior axial embryonic cataract* occurs as fine dots near the anterior Y-suture of foetal nucleus (Fig. 4.5). Sometimes opacities may form chalky bands around Y- sutures and may interfere with the vision. Almost bilateral and has autosomal dominant inheritance.
- *Floriform cataract*. Here the opacities are arranged like the petals of a flower.
- *Coralliform cataract*. Here the opacities are arranged in the form of a coral. It is also known as fusiform spindle shaped axial cataract and is characterized by an anterior posterior spindle shaped opacity with off shoots giving a resemblance a coral.
- *Spear-shaped cataract*. The lenticular opacities are in the form of scattered heaps of shining crystalline needles.
- *Dendritic suture cataract* occurs as fine dots along the dendritic sutures.

III. Cataract involving whole (embryonic, fetal and infantile) nucleus

1. Total congenital cataract. Total congenital cataract is a common variety and usually bilateral (Fig. 4.6). In many cases, there may be hereditary character. Its other important cause is maternal rubella. Total nuclear cataract usually involves the embryonic and fetal nucleus and sometimes infantile nucleus as well. It is characterized by a dense chalky white central opacity seriously impairing vision. The opacities are usually non-progressive

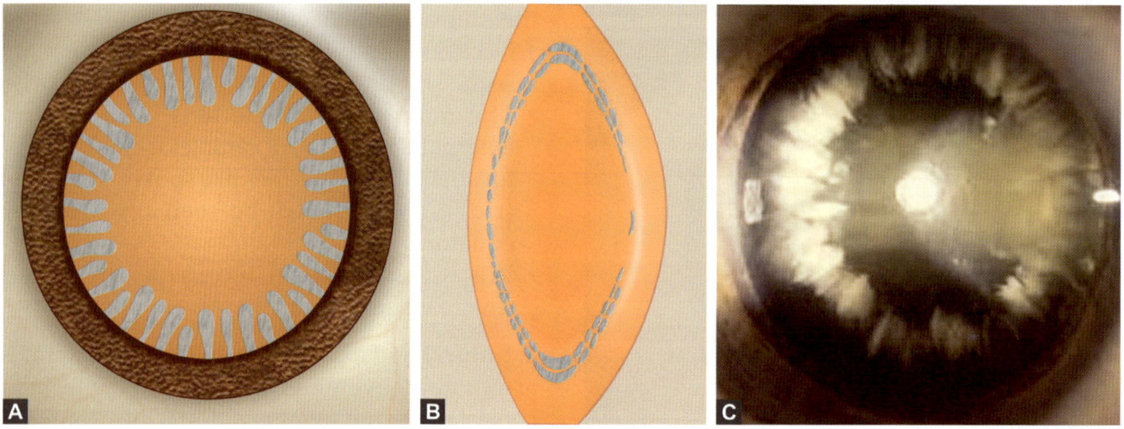

Fig. 4.5. *Coronary cataract: **(A and B)** Diagrammatic depiction as seen on oblique illumination and in optical section with the beam of the slit-lamp, respectively; (C) Clinical photograph.*

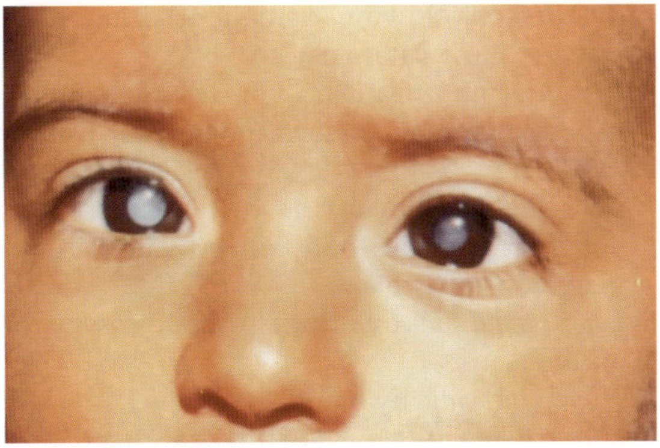

Fig. 4.6. *Total congenital cataract.*

Rubella cataract

- *Maternal rubella* infection acquired during first trimester (second or third month) may cause rubella cataract.
- *Rubella cataract* typically, the child is born with a 'pearly white' nuclear cataract. It is a progressive type of cataract.
- *Congenital Morgagnian cataract*, i.e. Lens matter may remain soft or may even liquefy
- *Cataractous nucleus* may harbour the virus up to two years of age. Therefore, removal of such a cataract is usually followed by a severe inflammatory reaction (uveitis or even endophthalmitis) probably due to liberation of retained viruses.

Note: Congenital rubella can be prevented by vaccination of the mother. Since, the rubella vaccine is toxic to fetus, it must, therefore, be administered at least three months before the pregnancy.

Rubella syndrome. Congenital rubella cataract may occur alone or as part of the classical rubella syndrome which consists of:

i. *Ocular defects*, e.g. congenital cataract, salt and pepper chorioretinopathy, microphthalmos, cloudy cornea and poorly dilating pupil.
ii. *Ear defects*, e.g. deafness due to destruction of organ of Corti.
iii. *Heart defects*, e.g. patent ductus arteriosus, pulmonary stenosis and ventricular septal defects.

2. Congenital membranous cataract. Sometimes there may occur total or partial absorption of congenital cataract, leaving behind thin membranous cataract. Rarely there is complete disappearance of all the lens fibres and only a fine transparent lens capsule remains behind. Such a patient may be misdiagnosed as having congenital aphakia. This is associated with Hallermann-Streiff-Francois syndrome.

D. CATARACTS INVOLVING ADULT NUCLEUS AND CORTEX

1. Coronary cataract

Coronary cataract (Fig. 4.7) is an extremely common form of developmental cataract occurring about puberty; thus involving either the adolescent nucleus or deeper layer of the cortex. The opacities are often many hundreds in number and have a regular radial distribution in the periphery of lens (corona of club-shaped opacities) encircling the central axis. Since the opacities are situated peripherally, vision is usually unaffected. Sometimes the associated large punctate opacities may marginally reduce the vision.

2. Blue dot cataract

Blue dot cataract, also called cataracta-punctatacaerulea, is perhaps the most common type of congenital cataract. It usually forms in the first two decades of life. The characteristic punctate opacities are in the form of rounded bluish dots situated in the peripheral part of adolescent nucleus and deeper layer of the cortex. Opacities are usually stationary and do not affect vision. However, large punctate opacities associated with coronary cataract may marginally reduce the vision.

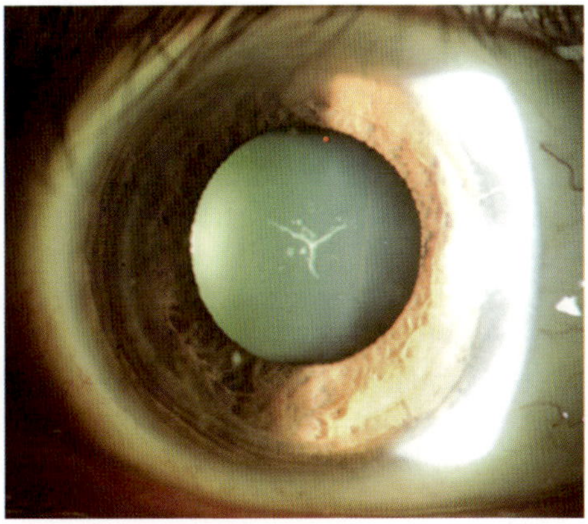

Fig. 4.7. *Anterior axial embryonic suture cataract.*

DIFFERENTIAL DIAGNOSIS OF CONGENITAL CATARACT

Other cause of leukocoria

Congenital cataracts presenting with leukocoria need to be differentiated from various other conditions presenting with leukocoria such as:

- Retinoblastoma, retinopathy of prematurity
- Persistent hyperplastic primary vitreous (PHPV). New term for PHPV is persistent fetal vasculature syndrome (PFVs)
- Inflammatory deposits in vitreous following a plastic cyclitis or choroiditis
- Coloboma of the choroid
- Toxocara endophthalmitis
- Exudative retinopathy of Coats.

MANAGEMENT OF CONGENITAL AND DEVELOPMENTAL CATARACTS

A. CLINICO-INVESTIGATIVE WORK-UP

A detailed clinico-investigative work-up is most essential in the management of paediatric cataract. It should aim at knowing the prognostic factors and indications and timing of surgery.

1. ***Ocular examination*** should be carried out with special reference to:

- *Density and morphology of cataract*. Density is indicated by quality of red reflex seen on distant direct ophthalmoscopy before and after dilation of pupil. Cataract morphology may suggest underlying cause.
- *Assessment of visual function* is difficult in infants and small children. An idea may be made from the density and morphology of the cataract by oblique illumination examination and fundus examination. Special tests like fixation reflex, forced choice preferential looking test, visually evoked potential (VEP), optic–kinetic nystagmus (OKN), etc. also provide useful information.
- *Associated ocular defects* which need to be noted include microphthalmos, glaucoma, PHPV, foveal hypoplasia, optic nerve hypoplasia, and rubella retinopathy, etc.

2. ***Laboratory investigations*** should be carried out to detect following systemic associations in non-hereditary cataracts:

- *Intrauterine infections*, viz. toxoplasmosis, rubella, cytomegalovirus and herpes virus by TORCH test.
- *Galactosaemia* by urine test for reducing substances, red blood cell transferase and glactokinase levels.
- *Lowe's syndrome* by urine chromatography for amino acids.
- *Hyperglycaemia* by blood sugar level.
- *Hypocalcaemia* by serum calcium and phosphate levels and X-ray skull.

B. PROGNOSTIC FACTORS

Prognostic factors which need to be noted are:

- Density of cataract,
- Unilateral or bilateral cataract,
- Time of presentation,
- Associated ocular defects, and
- Associated systemic defects.

C. INDICATIONS AND TIMING OF PAEDIATRIC CATARACT SURGERY

1. ***Partial cataracts and small central cataracts*** which are visually insignificant can safely be ignored and observed or may need non-surgical treatment with pupillary dilatation while visually significant cases need to be managed on priority. Visually significant cataracts include those that occupy 3 mm or more of the embryonal and foetal nucleus and those that obscure the view of retinal vessels with direct ophthalmoscope through an undilated pupil.

2. ***Bilateral dense cataracts*** should be removed early (within 6 weeks of birth) to prevent stimulus deprivation amblyopia. Second eye should be operated within a few days of the first eye.

3. ***Unilateral dense cataract*** should preferably be removed as early as possible (within days) after birth with optical correction in the first few weeks. However, it must be born in mind that visual prognosis in most of the unilateral cases is very poor even after timely operation, because correction of aphakia and prevention of amblyopia in infants is an uphill task.

D. CONTRAINDICATIONS TO CATARACT SURGERY

- Severe life-limiting disease such as Lowe's disease.

- Severe microphthalmia (cornea diameter <5 mm).
- Disorganised posterior segment.
- Presence of untreated retinoblastoma.

E. PREOPERATIVE COUNSELLING

It is most important. Parents must understand that surgery is only the first step of management. The child needs follow-up for a long period for repeated correction of residual and changing refractive error and occlusion therapy. Possibility of postoperative complications and need of secondary intervention must be emphasized.

F. SURGICAL PROCEDURES

Childhood cataracts (congenital, developmental as well as acquired) can be dealt with anterior capsulorrhexis and irrigation aspiration of the lens matter or lensectomy.

Surgical techniques of these procedures are described in Chapter 17, pages 306–311.

Note. The *needling operation* (which was performed in the past) is now obsolete because of high rates of complications and better available techniques.

G. CORRECTION OF PAEDIATRIC APHAKIA

It is still an unsolved query. Common views are as follows:

- *Children above the age of 2 years* can be corrected by implantation of posterior chamber intraocular lens during surgery.
- *Children below the age of 2 years* should preferably be treated by extended wear contact lens. Spectacles can be prescribed in bilateral cases. Later on, secondary IOL implantation may be considered.
- *Present trend* is to do primary implantation at the earliest possible specially in unilateral cataract, i.e. in all cases because most surgeons have reported negative experience in the compliance with glasses and contact lenses.

Paediatric IOL: Size, design, and power

The main concerns regarding the use of IOL in children are the growth of the eye, IOL power considerations, increased uveal reaction and long-term safety. Present recommendations are:

Size of IOL above the age of 2 years may be standard 12–12.75 mm diameter for in the bag implantation. In infants, IOL diameter should be between 10.5 and 12 mm. However, these IOLs are not easily available.

Design and material of IOL recommended previously has been one-piece PMMA with modified C-shaped haptics (preferably heparin coated). However, the capsular and inflammatory responses and large-sized incision remain the major problems with PMMA lenses. Therefore presently, most surgeons are preferring foldable IOLs made of hydrophobic acrylic material (e.g. Acrys of IOL manufactured by Alcon lab, USA).

Power of IOL. Most surgeons follow the following protocol:

- *In older children (>8 years),* emmetropia is the target.
- *In children between 2 and 8 years of age,* 10% under correction from the calculated biometric power is recommended to counter the myopic shift.
- *Below 2 years,* an undercorrection by 20% is recommended from the biometric reading. However, most surgeons follow Dahan et al's simplified approach based on the axial length only, which is depicted in Table 4.1.

Table 4.1 *Power of IOL–simplified approach (Dahan, et al.)*

Axial length	*IOL power*
17 mm	28D
18 mm	27D
19 mm	26D
20 mm	24D
21 mm	
22 mm	23D
23 mm	23D
>24 mm	Axial length –1D

H. CORRECTION OF AMBLYOPIA

It is the central theme around which management of childhood cataract and aphakia revolves. In spite of best efforts, it continues to be the main cause of ultimate low vision in these children. The management includes:

Spectacles may be prescribed as soon as inflammation has subsided and the media has cleared. The child is initially prescribed near correction in the pre-verbal age. As the child grows older and starts going to school, shift to bifocals for 2 pairs of spectacles (one for distance and one for near). The power of spectacles needs to be checked on every follow-up visit and any change of 0.5D or more needs to be incorporated. The parents should be told that the spectacle power will gradually decrease with the growth of the eye. Full time occlusion is a better option than part time occlusion in the initial phase of treatment. Parents need to be made to understand that compliance is of utmost importance for better visual outcome.

I. VISUAL PROGNOSIS

Visual prognosis is guarded and affected by many factors. A few common poor prognostic factors are:

- Associated PHPV.
- Presence of strabismus and/or nystagmus.
- Delayed surgery, especially in unilateral cataracts (beyond 4–6 months).
- Complications related to surgery especially severe inflammatory response and capsular opacification.
- Poor compliance to correction of residual refractive error and/or amblyopia.

J. PROPHYLAXIS FOR CONGENITAL CATARACT

Some measures which could bring down the incidence of congenital cataract include:

- Compulsory rubella vaccination for all girls after the age of 12 years or all children younger than one year can be considered.
- Discouragement for consanguineous marriages.
- Genetic counselling in the event of congenital cataract in the family.
- Avoidance of drugs (like thalidomide and corticosteroids) and radiation during pregnancy.

BIBLIOGRAPHY

1. Ashwin Reddy M, et al. Molecular Genetic Basis of Inherited Cataract and Associated Phenotypes. Survey of Ophthalmology 2004, May-June
2. Gimbel HV, DeBroff BM. Posterior capsulorhexis with optic capture: maintaining a clear visual axis after pediatric cataract surgery. J Cataract Refract Surg. 20:658–664;1994 Nov.
3. Holmes JM, Leske DA, Burke JP, Hodge DO. Birth prevalence of visually significant infantile cataract in a defined US population. Ophthalmic Epidemiol 10:67–74;2003 Apr.
4. J Mwende, A Bronsard, M Mosha, R Bowman, R Geneau, P Courtright. Delay in presentation to hospital for surgery for congenital and developmental cataract. Br J Ophthalmol 2005;89:1478–1482 doi:10.1136/bjo.2005.074146.
5. Lambert SR, Buckley EG, Drews-Botsch C, Dubois L, Hartmann EE, Lynn MJ, Plager DA, Wilson ME, Infant Aphakia Treatment Study Group. A randomized clinical trial comparing contact lens with intraocular lens correction of monocular aphakia during infancy: grating acuity and adverse events at age 1 year. Arch Ophthalmol 128:810–818;2010. Jul.
6. Mutations in the founder of the *MIP* gene family underlie cataract development in the mouse. Alan Shiels & Steven Bassnett. Nature Genetics 12:212–215;1996.
7. Outcome and complications of intraocular lenses in children with cataract. Journal of Cataract and Refractive Surgery. Volume 22, Issue 6, 730–736;1996 July-August.
8. Pandey SK, Wilson ME, Trivedi RH, et al. Pediatric cataract surgery and intraocular lens implantation: current techniques, complications and management. Int Ophthalmol Clin. 41(3):175–196;2001 Summer.
9. Rahi JS, Dezateux C. British Congenital Cataract Interest Group. Measuring and interpreting the incidence of congenital ocular anomalies: lessons from a national study of congenital cataract in the UK. Invest Ophthalmol Vis Sci 42:1444–1448; 2001 June.
10. RHC Markham, P A Bloom, A Chandna and EH Newcomb. Results of intraocular lens implantation in paediatric aphakia. *Eye* (1992) 6, 493–498; doi:10.1038/eye.1992.104
11. Vishwanath M, Cheong-Leen R, Taylor D, et al. Is early surgery for congenital cataract a risk factor for glaucoma? Br J Ophthalmol 88;905–910;2004.

ACQUIRED CATARACTS

5 CHAPTER

DEFINITION AND TYPES

We have studied that congenital and developmental cataracts occur due to disturbance in the formation of the lens fibres, i.e. instead of clear, opaque lens fibres are produced. While, in acquired cataract, opacification occurs due to degeneration of the already formed normal fibres.

Common types of acquired cataract

A few common varieties of the acquired cataract are:

1. Age-related (senile) cataract
2. Traumatic cataract
3. Metabolic cataracts
4. Complicated cataract
5. Drug-induced cataract, e.g.
   i. Corticosteroid-induced cataract
   ii. Miotics-induced cataract
6. Radiational cataract
7. Electric cataract
8. Syndermatotic cataract associated with skin diseases.
9. Cataract associated with osseous diseases.
10. Cataract with miscellaneous syndromes, e.g.
    i. Dystrophica myotonica
    ii. Down's syndrome.
    iii. Lowe's syndrome
    iv. Treacher-Collins syndrome

CLINICAL PROFILE OF ACQUIRED CATARACTS

AGE-RELATED CATARACT

'Age-related cataract', also called senile cataract is the commonest type of acquired cataract affecting equally persons of either sex usually above the age of 50 years. The condition is usually bilateral, but almost always one eye is affected earlier than the other.

Morphologically, the senile cataract occurs in two forms, the cortical (soft cataract) and the nuclear (hard cataract). The cortical senile cataract may start as cuneiform (more commonly) or cupuliform cataract.

It is very common to find nuclear and cortical senile cataracts coexisting in the same eye; and for this reason, it is difficult to give an accurate assessment of their relative frequency. In general, the predominant form can be given as cuneiform 70%, nuclear 25% and cupuliform 5%.

ETIOLOGY

Senile cataract is essentially an ageing process. Though its precise etiopathogenesis is not clear, the various factors implicated are described below.

A. RISK FACTORS

Risk factors affecting age of onset, type and maturation of senile cataract are:

1. ***Age.*** Age is the most important risk factor that is why, it is also termed 'age-related cataract'. As mentioned above, it usually occurs after the age of 50 years. When it occurs before 45 years of age, the term *presenile cataract* is used. By the age of 70 years, over 90% of the individuals develop senile cataract.

2. ***Sex.*** It is unequivocal doubt that, the senile cataract affects males as well as females. However, in many studies, it is reported that prevalence of cataract is greater in females than in males at all ages. In a population-based prevalence survey in Beaver Dam, Wisconsin, women had more cortical opacities compared to men within similar age groups. The possible explanation put forward are as below:

- *Longer life span of women* vis-a-vis men and, therefore, their over-representation in the age group where cataract is common.
- *Hormonal imbalance* due to menopause may be the factor, since a protective effect of hormone replacement therapy (HRT) on occurrence of cortical cataract is also reported.
- *Other factors,* more commonly associated with age in women than men, which may have some biologically independent impact on the rise of cataracts include diabetes, current overweight, history of clinically relevant obesity, hypertension and hyperlipidaemia.

3. ***Heredity.*** It plays a considerable role in the incidence, age of onset and maturation of senile cataract in different families. Studies of identical and fraternal twins and of familial association suggest that a large proportion of the risk of age-related cataract is inherited. Inheritance has been reported to be responsible for more than 50% of the risk of cortical cataract and 35–50% of the risk of nuclear cataract. Though the genes responsible have not yet been identified, most of this risk is associated with variation at a single locus, both for cortical and nuclear cataract. Identification of these genes will be important, because understanding the biochemical pathway in which they function may suggest way to slow the progression or prevent the development of age-related cataract in a large number of cases.

4. ***Ultraviolet irradiations.*** More exposure to UV irradiation from sunlight has been implicated for early onset and maturation of cortical senile cataract in many epidemiological studies. Sunlight exposure accounts for only 10% of the total risk of cortical cataract in general population. Further, there is sufficient experimental evidence that exposure to artificial source of UVB can cause lens opacities in the laboratory animals. Studies also report that nuclear cataracts are not casually associated with exposure to solar UVB, while posterior subcapsular cataracts may be.

It is being considered one of the important causes of the high prevalence of cataract in Third World (tropical) countries. This hypothesis led to many experimental studies to ensure the role of UV irradiation in causation of cataract. Recently, from animal experiments, it has been confirmed that UV radiation between 290 and 320 nm could induce lens opacification.

It has been proposed that prolonged exposure to ultraviolet rays may initiate photo-oxidative damage in the lens. Current views are that oxidative events are the most likely mechanism of cataract formation. Near UV light is absorbed by tryptophan, which in sunlight is converted to N-formyl-kynurenine, a fluorescent chromophore similar to 3-OH-kynurenine, a second UV absorbent molecule in the lens. Both these compounds can act as photosensitizers and lead to production of the free radical single oxygen. This free radical single oxygen down regulates the function of critical lens enzymes such as Na^+/K^+ ATPase and lead to lens swelling and opacification, at least in the rat model. Other free radicals generated by near UV light such as hydrogen peroxide have been implicated in the dysfunction of hexokinase, an enzyme central to glucose utilization in the lens. Lipid peroxidation may also play a role in cataractogenesis. Fatty acid radicals can ultimately produce the compound malondialdehyde, a well-known cross-linking agent, which can attach enzymes and membrane components.

Oxygen increases the rate of photo-oxidation and vitamin E, ascorbic acid and glutathione reduce the effects of light damage.

The role of UV light in human cataract is still unclear, although some interesting epidemiological evidence has emerged from a study of Chesapeake Bay, Watermen, which showed the importance of exposure to UV-B in cortical but not in nuclear cataract formation. A similar study found an association between UV-B and posterior subcapsular cataract. Interestingly, aged human lenses appear to absorb more UV-A and even visible light than young lenses.

5. ***Dietary factors.*** Diet deficient in certain proteins, amino acids, vitamins (riboflavin, vitamin E, vitamin C), and essential elements have also been blamed for early onset and maturation of senile cataract.

6. ***Dehydrational crisis.*** An association with prior episode of severe dehydrational crisis (due to diarrhoea, cholera, etc.) and age of onset and maturation of cataract is also suggested.

7. ***Smoking*** has also been reported to have some effect on the age of onset of senile cataract. In numerous studies worldwide, smoking has consistently been associated with an increase in the frequency of nuclear opacities. Smoking causes accumulation of pigmented molecules—3 hydroxykynurinine and chromophores, which lead to yellowing. Cyanates in smoke cause carbamylation and protein denaturation. Thus, smoking or the use of smokeless tobacco products is the most significant avoidable risk factor for cataract.

B. CAUSES OF PRESENILE CATARACT

The term presenile cataract is used when the cataractous changes similar to senile cataract occur before 50 years of age. Its common causes are:

1. *Heredity.* As mentioned above because of influence of heredity, the cataractous changes may occur at an earlier age in successive generations.

2. *Diabetes mellitus.* Age-related cataract occurs earlier in diabetics. Nuclear cataract is more common and tends to progress rapidly.

3. *Myotonic dystrophy* is associated with posterior subcapsular type of presenile cataract.

4. *Atopic dermatitis* may be associated with presenile cataract (atopic cataract) in 10% of the cases.

C. CONCEPT OF SYN- AND CO-CATARACTOGENIC FACTORS

It has been conceptualized that cataract is the result of multiple subthreshold cataractogenic stresses acting in a concert. Age has been implicated as one of these cataractogenic stresses and that superimposition of other toxic stresses on the ageing lens may accelerate the rate of cataract formation. Conversely, the elimination of one or more subcataractogenic stresses may delay the cataract formation.

D. MECHANISM OF LOSS OF LENS TRANSPARENCY

Mechanism of loss of lens transparency is basically different in nuclear and cortical senile cataracts.

Cortical cataract

The cortical senile opacification is accompanied by progressive decrease in lens proteins and free amino acids levels in lens and important alterations in electrolytes and water content of the lens with the maturity of cataract from immature to hypermature stage.

Water content of the lens (normal 65%) is increased with the maturation of cortical cataract from immature (about 68–70%) to hypermature morgagnian stage (about 78–80%). The increase in the water content of the lens is parallel with the increase in wet weight of the lens. Most of the water responsible for lens hydration is extralenticular. However, there also occurs a release of bound water from the conformationally altered lens proteins (syneresis).

Protein content of the lens in total (normal 34%) is decreased with the maturation of cortical senile cataract while there occurs an increase in the water-insoluble fraction of the proteins. The major protein change in cataractous lens is the loss of α-crystallin and the selective loss of γ-crystalline. In addition, there are numerous degradation peptides detectable in the water-soluble component. Following possible mechanisms have been suggested for the decrease in soluble proteins.

- Leakage of low molecular weight proteins from the lens into surrounding tissue.
- Conversion of soluble proteins into insoluble proteins.
- Decreased synthesis of lens proteins.
- An increased protein catabolism.

However, there is no conclusive evidence for any of the proposals.

Free amino acids. A progressive decrease in the level of total free amino acids has been reported with the maturation of cortical cataract. Proteogenic amino acids diminish much more than the non-proteogenic amino acids. Decrease in amino acid level has also been attributed to leakage from the disrupted lens membrane.

Sodium and potassium. The sodium content of the lens is progressively increased while the potassium levels are decreased with maturation of cortical cataract.

Calcium. The calcium content increases with the maturation of cataract. In normal lens, the ash contains 1.0% calcium, in immature cataract 5.5%. Salit classified cataracts on the basis of calcium content as incipient (those with calcium content below 10 mg% of net weight), immature (with calcium content between 10 and 35 mg%) and mature (those with a calcium content above 35 mg%). Increase in the calcium concentration of the lens is not a primary change in the cataractous process. The probable course of events leading to senile opacification of cortex is shown in Fig. 5.1.

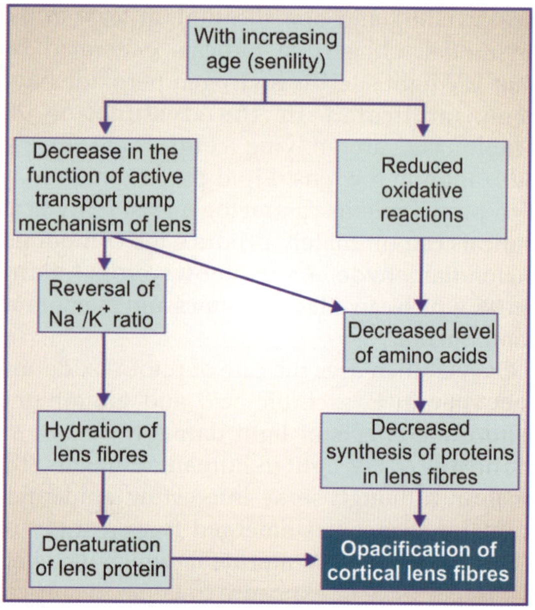

Fig. 5.1. *Flow chart depicting probable course of events involved in the occurrence of cortical cataract.*

Nuclear Cataract

In nuclear cataract, the usual degenerative change is intensification of the age-related nuclear sclerosis associated with dehydration and compaction of the nucleus resulting in a hard cataract. It is accompanied by a significant increase in water-insoluble proteins. However, the total protein content and distribution of cations (Na^+ and K^+) remain normal. There may or may not be associated deposition of pigment urochrome and/or melanin derived from the amino acid in the lens. It may, therefore, be possible that in nuclear cataract the lens transparency depends upon both—the light scattering by macromolecular complexes of the insoluble proteins and the light absorption by brown-coloured proteins of the lens.

E. ROLE OF GLUTATHIONE AND ASCORBIC ACID IN CATARACTOGENESIS

The lens has protective mechanisms against oxidative damage caused by various oxidants generated in vivo such as superoxide anions (O_2^-), hydrogen peroxide (H_2O_2), lipid peroxides and lipid hydroperoxides. Superoxide radicals may be most toxic to lens proteins. It has been suggested that there is a possible role of lens ascorbate as physiological scavenger of superoxide (O_2^-) radicals. Ascorbic acid converts highly reactive superoxide to less reactive hydrogen peroxide. High glutathione levels might have a similar protective function. Oxidants such as hydrogen peroxide, superoxide anions and hydroxyl radicals, if not disposed because of decreased concentration of ascorbic acid and glutathione, can cause oxidation of protein hydrals such as enzymes, crystallins and membrane proteins (Fig. 5.2). Thus, it can be concluded that oxidative damage to the lens because of decreased concentrations of glutathione and ascorbic acid may lead to the cataract formation. The prevention of experimental cortical cataract by vitamin E and glutathione supports this contention.

The following factors (Fig. 5.3) have been reported to contribute to a fall in the level of glutathione in a cataractous lens:

- Decrease in the synthesis of this tripeptide, since reduced glutathione is not permeable and aqueous contains a very little amount of glutathione.
- Increased permeability of lens membranes to reduced glutathione.
- Relative deficiency of enzyme glutathione reductase (since level of glutathione is upon this enzyme) as well as an increase in dependent disulphide formation with protein sulphhydryls.

F. COMMON PATHWAYS IN HUMAN CATARACT

The epidemiological studies have revealed that in addition to ageing, most of the patients with so-called age-related (senile) cataract have been exposed to more than one risk factor. An average of four risk factors have been reported by Clayton *et al.*

These considerations lead to the notion that there may be a common pathology in human cataract. A speculative scheme for some of these pathways (as described by Harding) is shown in Fig. 5.4. Harding stated that the postulated common pathways not only help towards an understanding of cataractogenesis but also have implications for anti-cataract therapy. A drug which acts on the common pathways is likely to be much more useful than one acting against a single insult to the lens.

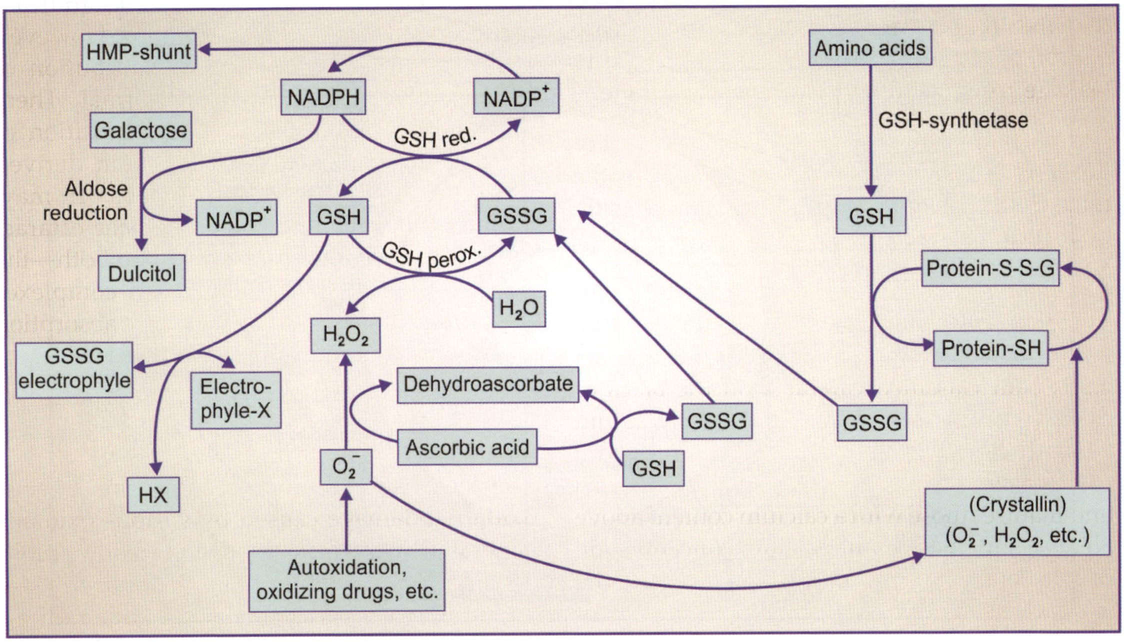

Fig. 5.2. *Glutathione scavenging pathway in the crystalline lens.*

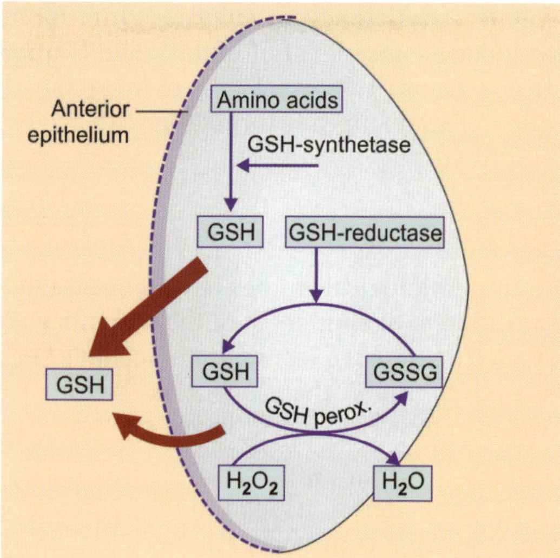

Fig. 5.3. *Depletion of glutathione (GSH) during cataract formation.*

STAGES OF MATURATION

A. MATURATION OF THE CORTICAL TYPE OF SENILE CATARACT

1. Stage of lamellar separation

The earliest senile change is demarcation of cortical fibres owing to their separation by fluid. This phenomenon of lamellar separation can be demonstrated by slit-lamp examination only. These changes are reversible.

2. Stage of incipient cataract

In this stage, early detectable opacities with clear areas between them are seen. Two distinct types of senile cortical cataracts can be recognised at this stage. They are:

a. ***Cuneiform senile cortical cataract.*** It is characterized by wedge-shaped opacities with

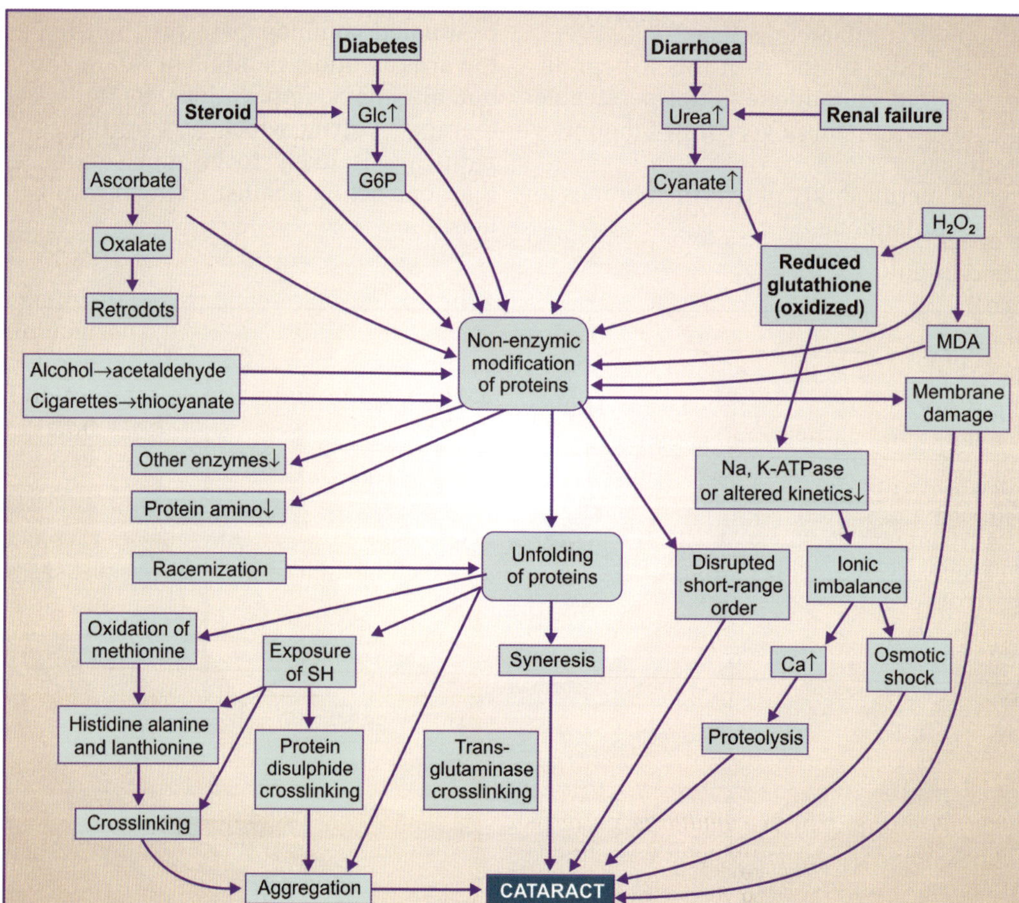

Fig. 5.4. *Possible common pathways in human cataract. G6P–glucose-6-phosphate, MDA–malondialdehyde. (Adapted from Harding).*

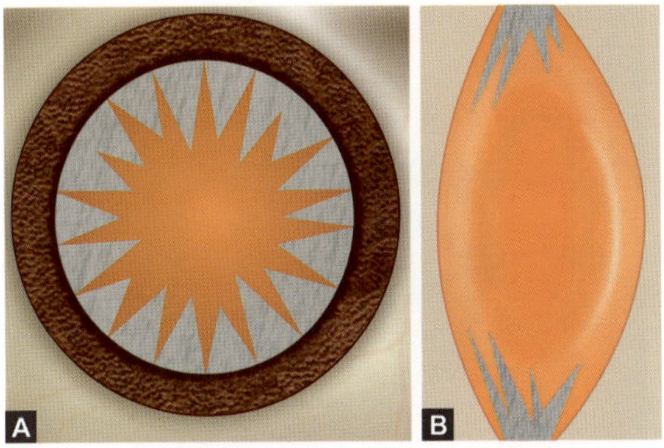

Fig. 5.5. *Diagrammatic depiction of immature senile cortical cataract (cuneiform type): **(A)** As seen on oblique illumination; **(B)** In optical section with beam of the slit-lamp.*

clear areas in between. These extend from equator towards centre and in early stages can only be demonstrated after dilatation of the pupil. They are first seen in the lower nasal quadrant. These opacities are present both in anterior and posterior cortices and their apices slowly progress towards the pupil. On oblique illumination, these present a typical radial spoke-like pattern of greyish white opacities (Fig. 5.5). On distant direct ophthalmoscopy, these opacities appear as dark lines against the red fundal glow.

Since the cuneiform cataract starts at periphery and extends centrally, the visual disturbances are noted at a comparatively late stage.

b. *Cupuliform senile cortical cataract.* Here a saucer-shaped opacity develops just below the capsule usually in the central part of posterior cortex (*posterior subcapsular cataract*), which gradually extends outwards. There is usually a definite demarcation between the cataract and the surrounding clear cortex. Cupuliform cataract lies right in the pathway of the axial rays and thus causes an early loss of visual acuity.

3. Immature senile cataract (ISC)

In this stage, opacification progresses further. The *cuneiform* (Fig. 5.5) or *cupuliform* patterns can be recognised till the advanced stage of ISC when opacification becomes more diffuse and irregular. The lens appears greyish white (Fig. 5.6) but clear cortex is still present and so iris shadow is visible.

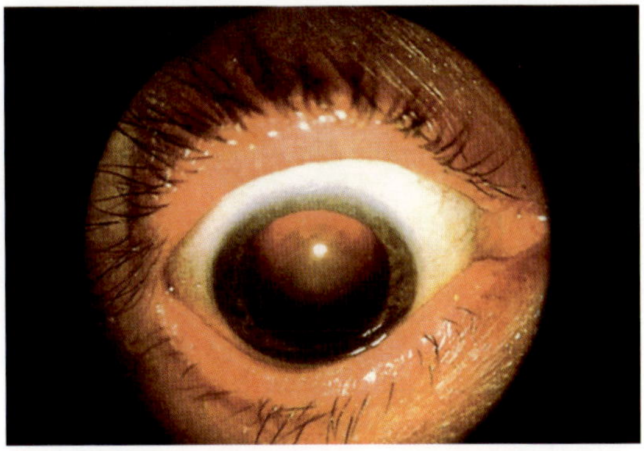

Fig. 5.6. *Immature senile cortical cataract.*

In some patients, at this stage, lens may become swollen due to continued hydration. This condition is called *'intumescent cataract'*. Intumescence may persist even in the next stage of maturation. Due to swollen lens, anterior chamber becomes shallow.

4. Mature senile cataract (MSC)

In this stage, opacification becomes complete, i.e. whole of the cortex is involved. Lens becomes pearly white in colour. Such a cataract is also labelled 'ripe cataract' (Fig. 5.7).

5. Hypermature senile cataract (HMSC)

When the mature cataract is left in situ, the stage of hypermaturity sets in. The hypermature cataract may occur in any of the two forms:

a. *Morgagnian hypermature cataract.* In some patients, after maturity, the whole cortex liquefies and the lens is converted into a bag of

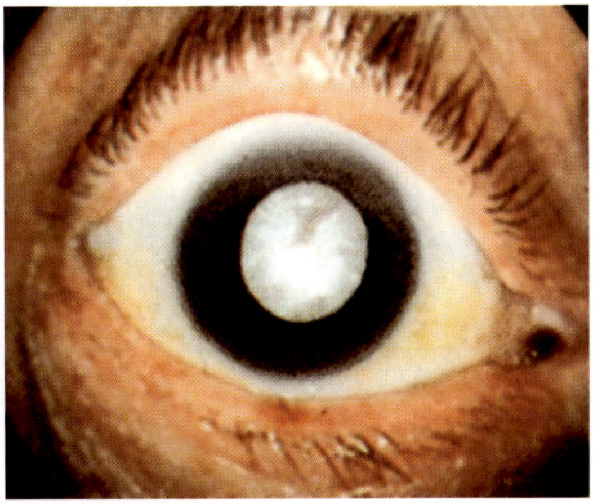

Fig. 5.7. *Mature senile cortical cataract.*

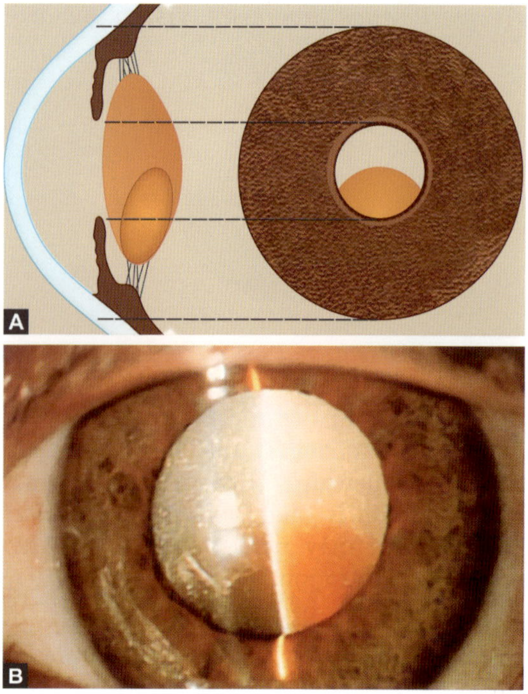

Fig. 5.8. *Morgagnian hypermature senile cortical cataract: **(A)** Diagrammatic depiction; **(B)** Clinical photograph.*

milky fluid. The small brownish nucleus settles at the bottom, altering its position with change in the position of the head. Such a cataract is called *Morgagnian cataract* (Fig. 5.8). Sometimes in this stage, calcium deposits may also be seen on the lens capsule.

b. ***Sclerotic type hypermature cataract.*** Sometimes after the stage of maturity, the cortex becomes disintegrated and the lens becomes shrunken due to leakage of water. The anterior capsule is wrinkled and thickened due to proliferation of anterior cells and a dense white capsular cataract may be formed in the pupillary area. Due to shrinkage of lens, anterior chamber becomes deep and iris becomes tremulous (iridodonesis).

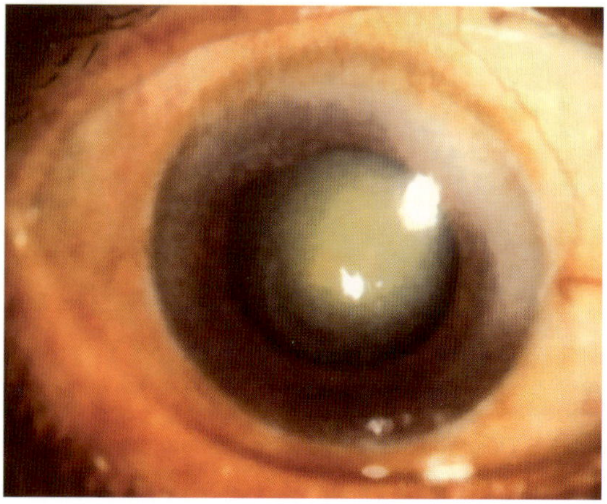

Fig. 5.9. *Early senile nuclear cataract.*

B. MATURATION OF NUCLEAR SENILE CATARACT

Progressive nuclear sclerotic process renders the lens inelastic and hard, decreases its ability to accommodate and obstructs the light rays. These changes begin centrally (Fig. 5.9) and slowly spread peripherally almost up to the capsule when it becomes mature; however, a very thin layer of clear cortex may remain unaffected.

The nucleus may become diffusely cloudy (greyish) or tinted (yellow to black) due to deposition of pigments. In practice, the commonly observed pigmented nuclear cataracts are either amber, brown (*cataracta brunescens*) or black (*cataracta nigra*) and rarely reddish (*cataracta rubra*) in colour (Fig. 5.10).

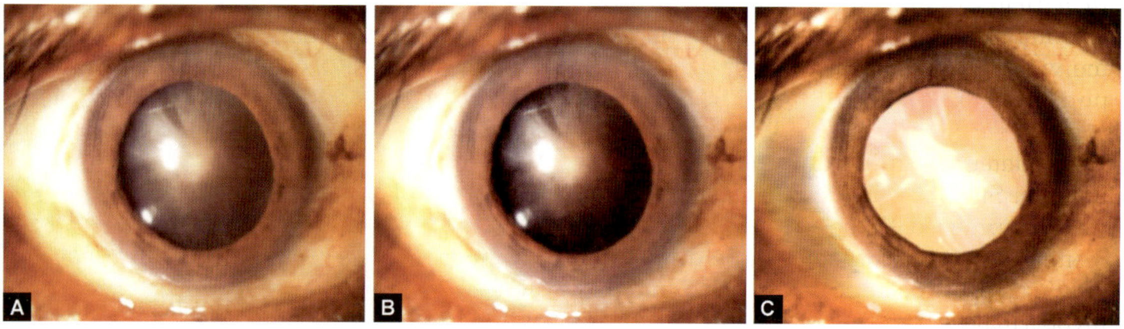

Fig. 5.10. *Nuclear cataract: **(A)** Cataracta brunescens; **(B)** Cataracta nigra; **(C)** Cataracta rubra.*

CLINICAL FEATURES

SYMPTOMS

An opacity of the lens may be present without causing any symptoms; and may be discovered on routine ocular examination. Common symptoms of cataract are as follows:

1. ***Glare.*** One of the earliest visual disturbances with the cataract is glare or intolerance of bright light; such as direct sunlight or the headlights of an oncoming motor vehicle. The amount of glare or dazzle will vary with the location and size of the opacity being particularly prominent with posterior subcapsular opacities (PSCs) and occasionally anterior cortical lens changes.

2. ***Uniocular diplopia or polyopia*** (i.e. doubling or trebling of objects): It is also one of the early symptoms. It occurs due to irregular refraction by the lens owing to variable refractive index as a result of cataractous process.

3. ***Coloured halos.*** These may be perceived by some patients owing to breaking of white light into coloured spectrum due to presence of water droplets in the lens.

4. ***Black spots in front of eyes.*** Stationary black spots may be perceived by some patients.

5. ***Image blur, distortion of images and misty vision*** may occur in early stages of cataract.

6. ***Loss of vision.*** Visual deterioration due to senile cataract has some typical features. It is painless and gradually progressive in nature.
   - *Patients with central opacities* (e.g. cupuliform cataract, i.e. posterior subcapsular cataract) have early loss of vision. These patients see better when pupil is dilated due to dim light in the evening *(day blindness).*
   - *In patients with peripheral opacities* (e.g. cuneiform cataract), visual loss is delayed and the vision is improved in bright light when pupil is contracted.
   - *In patients with nuclear sclerotic cataracts*, distant vision deteriorates due to progressive index myopia. Such patients may be able to read without presbyopic glasses. This improvement in near vision is referred to as *'second sight'*. Asymmetric development of induced myopia may produce intolerable anisometropia prompting consideration of cataract extraction.
   - *As opacification progresses*, vision steadily diminishes, until only perception of light and accurate *projection of rays* remain in the stage of mature cataract.

SIGNS

Following examination should be carried out to look for different signs of cataract:

1. ***Visual acuity testing.*** Depending upon the location and maturation of cataract, the visual acuity may range from 6/9 to just PL+ (Table 5.1).

2. ***Contrast sensitivity testing.*** Contrast sensitivity, i.e. the ability of the eye to perceive subtle changes in the shading, may be markedly decreased in patients with cataract even before the decrease in the Snellen's visual acuity is detected. However, the abnormal contrast sensitivity is a non-specific sign and can occur in many other ocular conditions. It can be tested with the use of specially designed charts with letters or stripes represented in various shades of grey, which includes:
   - Arden grating,
   - Cambridge low-contrast grating,
   - Pelli-Robison charts,
   - Functional acuity contrast test (FACT), and
   - Visittrak chart.

3. ***Oblique illumination examination.*** It reveals colour of the lens in pupillary area which varies in different types of cataracts (Table 5.1).

4. ***Test for iris shadow.*** When an oblique beam of light is thrown on the pupil, a crescentric shadow of pupillary margin of the iris will be formed on the greyish opacity of the lens, as long as clear cortex is present between the opacity and the pupillary margin (Fig. 5.11). When lens is completely transparent or completely opaque, no iris shadow is formed. Hence, presence of iris shadow is a sign of immature cataract.

5. ***Distant direct ophthalmoscopic examination.*** A reddish yellow fundal glow is observed in the absence of any opacity in the media. Partial cataractous lens shows black shadow against the red glow in the area of cataract. Complete cataractous lens does not even reveal red glow and the papillary area shows white reflex due to total reflection of light (Table 5.1).

Table 5.1 *Signs of senile cataract*

Examination	*Nuclear cataract*	*ISC*	*MSC*	*HMSC(M)*	*HMSC(S)*
1. Visual acuity	6/9 to PL+	6/9 to FC+	HM+ to PL+	PL+	PL+
2. Colour of lens	Grey, amber, brown, black or red	Greyish white	Pearly white with sinking brownish nucleus	Milky white	Dirty white with hyper-white spots
3. Iris shadow	Seen	Seen	Not seen	Not seen	Not seen
4. Distant direct ophthalmoscopy with dilated pupil	Central dark area against red fundal glow	Multiple dark areas against red fundal glow	No red glow but white pupil due to complete cataract	No red glow milky white pupil	No red glow
5. Slit-lamp examination	Nuclear opacity clear cortex	Areas of normal with cataractous cortex	Complete cortex is cataractous	Milky white sunken brownish nucleus	Shrunken cataractous lens with thickened anterior capsule

ISC: Immature senile cataract, MSC: Mature senile cataract, HMSC(M) Hypermature senile cataract (Morgagnian) HMSC(S): Hypermature senile cataract (Sclerotic), PL: Perception of light, HM: Hand movements, FC: Finger counting

6. ***Slit-lamp examination*** should be performed with a fully-dilated pupil. The examination reveals complete morphology of opacity (site, size, shape, colour pattern and hardness of the nucleus).

Grading of nucleus hardness in a cataractous lens is important for setting the parameters of machine in phacoemulsification technique of cataract extraction. The hardness of the nucleus, depending upon its colour on slit-lamp examination, can be graded as shown in Table 5.2 and Fig. 5.12.

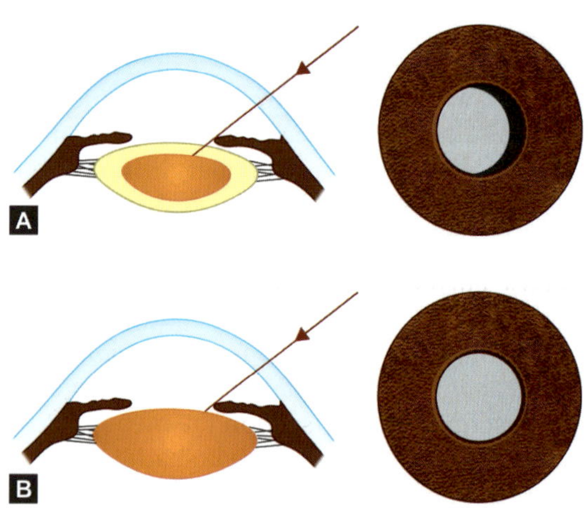

Fig. 5.11. *Diagrammatic depiction of iris shadow in immature cortical cataract **(A)** and no iris shadow in mature cortical cataract **(B)**.*

Table 5.2 *Grading of nucleus hardness on slit-lamp biomicroscopy*

Grade of hardness	*Description of hardness*	*Colour of nucleus*
Grade I	Soft	Greyish white
Grade II	Soft-medium	Yellowish
Grade III	Medium-hard	Amber
Grade IV	Hard	Brownish
Grade V	Ultrahard (rock-hard)	Blackish

The signs observed on above examinations in different stages of senile cataract are shown in Table 5.1.

DIFFERENTIAL DIAGNOSIS

I. ***Immature senile cataract (ISC)*** can be differentiated from the nuclear sclerosis without any cataract as shown in Table 5.3.

II. ***Mature senile cataract*** can be differentiated from other causes of white pupillary reflex (leukocoria) as shown in Table 5.4.

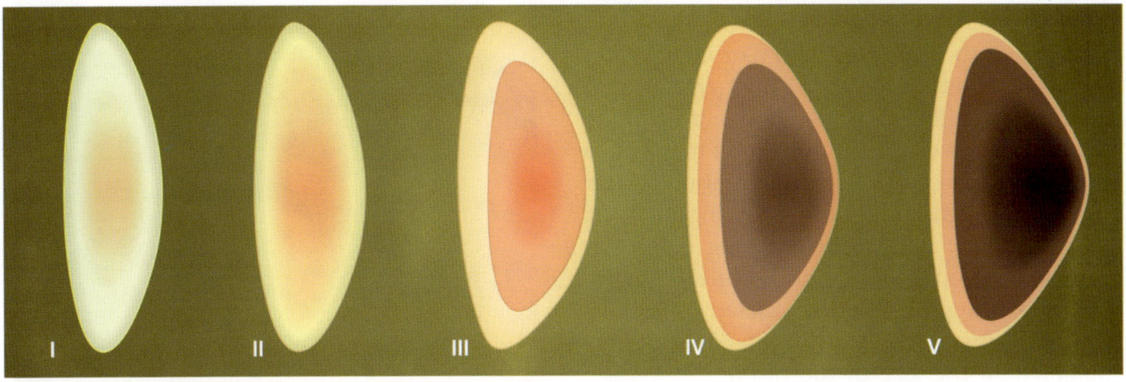

Fig. 5.12. *Slit-lamp biomicroscopic grading of the nucleus hardness in cataractous lens.*

Table 5.3 *Immature senile cataract versus nuclear sclerosis*

ISC	*Nuclear sclerosis*
1. Painless progressive loss of vision	1. Painless progressive loss of vision
2. Greyish colour of lens on oblique illumination examination	2. Greyish colour of lens
3. Iris shadow is present	3. Iris shadow is absent
4. Black spots against red glow are observed on distant direct ophthalmoscopy	4. No black spots are seen against red glow
5. Slit-lamp examination reveals area of cataractous cortex	5. Slit-lamp examination reveals clear lens
6. Visual acuity does not improve on pin-hole testing	6. Visual acuity usually improves on pin-hole testing

COMPLICATIONS

1. ***Phacoanaphylactic uveitis.*** A hypermature cataract may leak lens proteins into anterior chamber. These proteins may act as antigens and induce antigen–antibody reaction leading to phacoanaphylactic uveitis.

2. ***Lens-induced glaucoma.*** It may occur by different mechanisms, e.g. due to intumescent lens *(phacomorphic glaucoma)* and leakage of proteins into the anterior chamber from a hypermature cataract (*phacolytic glaucoma*).

3. ***Subluxation or dislocation of lens.*** It may occur due to degeneration of zonules in hypermature stage.

Table 5.4 *Differences between mature senile cataract and leukocoria*

MSC	*Leukocoria*
1. White reflex in pupillary area	1. White reflex in pupillary area
2. Size of pupil usually normal	2. Pupil usually semidilated
3. Fourth Purkinje image is absent	3. Fourth Purkinje image is present
4. Slit-lamp examination shows cataractous lens	4. Slit-lamp examination shows transparent lens with white reflex behind the lens
5. Ultrasonography normal	5. Ultrasonography reveals opacity in the vitreous cavity

TRAUMATIC CATARACT

Literally speaking, traumatic cataract refers lens opacification occurring as a result of traumatic lens damage caused by either mechanical injury or physical forces such as radiation (radiation cataract), chemicals and electric current (electric cataract). However, in clinical practice, the term traumatic cataract is used for the cataract occurring due to mechanical injuries; and so only such cataracts are described in this section.

TYPES AND PATHOGENESIS OF TRAUMATIC CATARACT

Traumatic cataracts caused by different modes of mechanical trauma are given as follows.

1. Cataract caused by closed globe injury

A blunt non-penetrating injury or concussion trauma (concussion cataract) may cause lense opacification either as an acute event or a late sequel. In some cases, blunt trauma may cause both dislocation and cataract formation. After blunt trauma, lens may show following changes:

i. ***Vossius ring.*** It is a circular ring of brown pigment seen on the anterior capsule. It occurs due to striking of the contracted pupillary margin against the crystalline lens. It is always smaller than the size of the pupil.

ii. ***Concussion cataract.*** It occurs mainly due to imbibition of aqueous and partly due to direct mechanical effects of the injury on lens fibres. It may assume any of the following shapes:

- *Discrete subepithelial opacities* are of most common occurrence.
- *Early rosette cataract* (*punctate*). It is the most typical form of concussion cataract. It appears as feathery lines of opacities along the star-shaped suture lines; usually in the posterior cortex (Fig. 5.13).
- *Late rosette cataract.* It develops in the posterior cortex 1–2 years after the injury. Its sutural extensions are shorter and more compact than the early rosette cataract.
- *Traumatic zonular cataract.* It may also occur in some cases, though rarely.
- *Diffuse (total) concussion cataract.* It is of frequent occurrence.
- *Membranous cataract* may occur after trauma, especially in children due to absorption of lens matter.

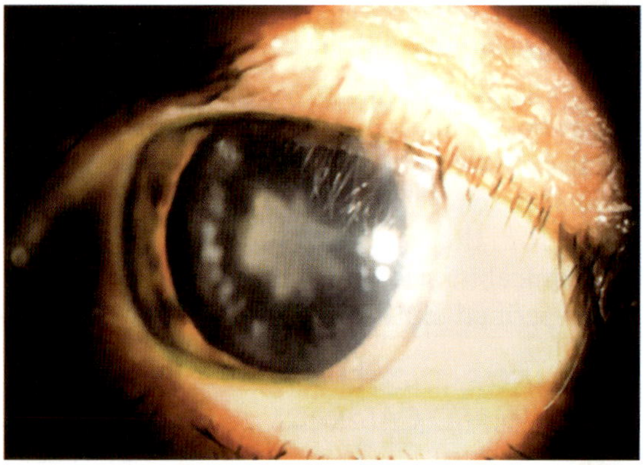

Fig. 5.13. *Rosette-shaped cataract following blunt trauma.*

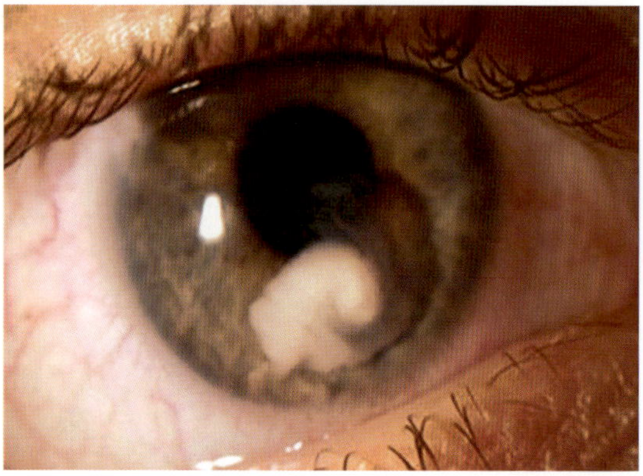

Fig. 5.14. *Free floating lens particles in the anterior chamber of a patient with open globe injury.*

iii. ***Early maturation of senile cataract*** may follow blunt truma.

2. Cataract caused by open globe injury

Open globe injuries include perforating and penetrating injuries. Such direct injuries to the lens may cause:

- Massive perforation of the lens capsule leading to release of free floating lens particles in the anterior chamber which becomes cataractous (Fig. 5.14).
- Perforating injuries of the lens often result in opacification of cortex at the site of rupture, usually progressing rapidly to complete opacification.
- A small perforation of lens capsule may occasionally heal resulting in a stationary focal cortical cataract (Fig. 5.15).

3. Cataract caused by intraocular foreign bodies

The retained intraocular foreign bodies may produce cataract by following mechanisms:

i. *Direct injuries to the lens* produce effects of perforating/penetrating injury as described above.

ii. *Retained intraocular bodies* may either produce an opaque track in the lens or the lens may become completely cataractous.

iii. *Specific reactions of the foreign body* include siderosis bulbi or chalcosis.

- *Siderosis bulbi* refers to the degenerative changes produced by retained iron foreign body. *Lenticular changes* include rusting

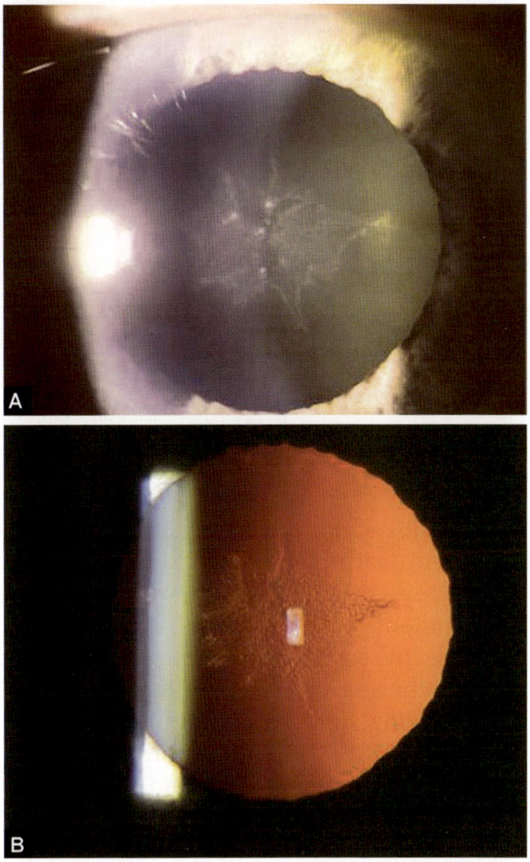

Fig. 5.15. *Stationary focal cortical cataract secondary to small perforation in the anterior capsule: **(A)** As seen on diffuse illumination; **(B)** As seen on retroillumination.*

deposits arranged radially in the anterior epithelium and lens capsule (Fig. 5.16). Eventually there occurs complete cortical cataract.

- *Chalcosis* refers to the specific changes produced by a retained copper–alloy foreign body. *Sunflower cataract* is produced by deposition of copper ions under the posterior capsule. It is brilliant golden green in colour and arranged like the petals of sunflower (Fig 5.17).

METABOLIC CATARACTS

These cataracts occur due to endocrine disorders and biochemical abnormalities. A few common varieties of metabolic cataracts are described here.

SUGAR CATARACTS

DIABETIC CATARACT

Diabetes is associated with two types of cataracts:

1. ***True diabetic cataract.*** The classical diabetic cataract is also called *'snow-flake cataract'* or *'snow-storm cataract'*. It is a rare condition, usually occurring in young adults due to osmotic over-hydration of the lens. Osmotic over-hydration of the lens occurs due to accumulation of sorbitol, when glucose is metabolised by aldose reductase. Initially, a large number of fluid vacuoles appear underneath the anterior and posterior capsules, which is soon followed by appearance of bilateral snowflake-like white opacities initially in the superficial and posterior lens cortex (Fig. 5.18). Such opacities usually mature rapidly and there occurs swelling of the lens (intumescence).

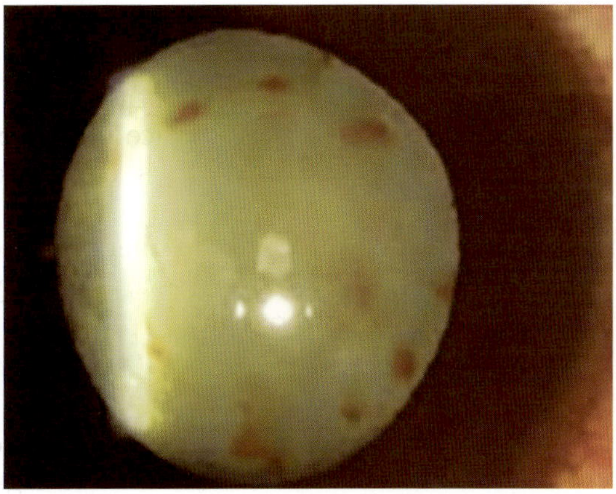

Fig. 5.16. *Siderotic cataract.*

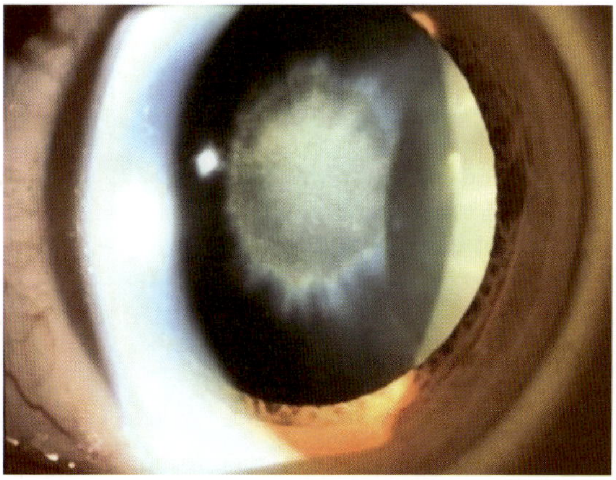

Fig. 5.17. *Sunflower cataract.*

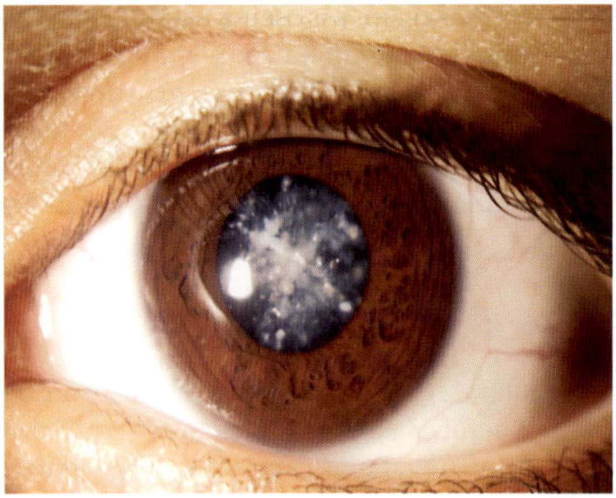

Fig. 5.18. *Snow-flake cataract.*

2. ***Senile cataract in diabetics*** appears at an early age and progresses rapidly. The increased risk or earlier onset of age-related cataracts in diabetic patients may be a result of the accumulation of sorbitol within the lens and accompanying changes in hydration, increased non-enzyme glycosylation (glycation) of lens proteins or greater oxidative stress from alteration in the lens metabolism.

GALACTOSAEMIC CATARACT

It is associated with inborn error of galactose metabolism. Galactosaemia occurs in two forms:

1. *Classical galactosaemia* occurs due to deficiency of galactose-1 phosphate uridyl-transferase (GPUT); and
2. A related disorder occurs due to *deficiency of galactokinase (GK).*

Characteristic features. Galactosaemia is frequently associated with the development of bilateral cataract (*oil droplet central lens opacities*). The lens changes may be reversible and occurrence of cataract may be prevented, if milk and milk products are eliminated from the diet when diagnosed at an early stage.

PATHOGENESIS OF SUGAR CATARACT

Three major mechanisms proposed to explain the formation of sugar-induced cataract are as follows.

1. Sorbitol, aldose reductase and the osmotic hypothesis

The course of chemical events in sugar cataract as studied by Kinoshita is depicted in Fig. 5.19. The salient features are as follows:

The key biochemical feature in the development of sugar cataract is aldose reductase, the sorbitol pathway enzyme which converts the excess sugar in the lens to the corresponding sugar alcohol (glucose sorbitol, galactose dulcitol). This only occurs at unusually high levels of sugar in blood and aqueous (*see* Fig. 5.20 and focus on sorbitol pathway of glucose metabolism). The resultant alcohol is then unable to escape from the lens nor is it readily metabolized, and thus it accumulates within the cells making the cytoplasm markedly hypertonic. This induces a large movement of water into the lens, alteration of Na^+/K^+ ratio and concomitant lens swelling. The normal lenticular architecture is thus disrupted, leading

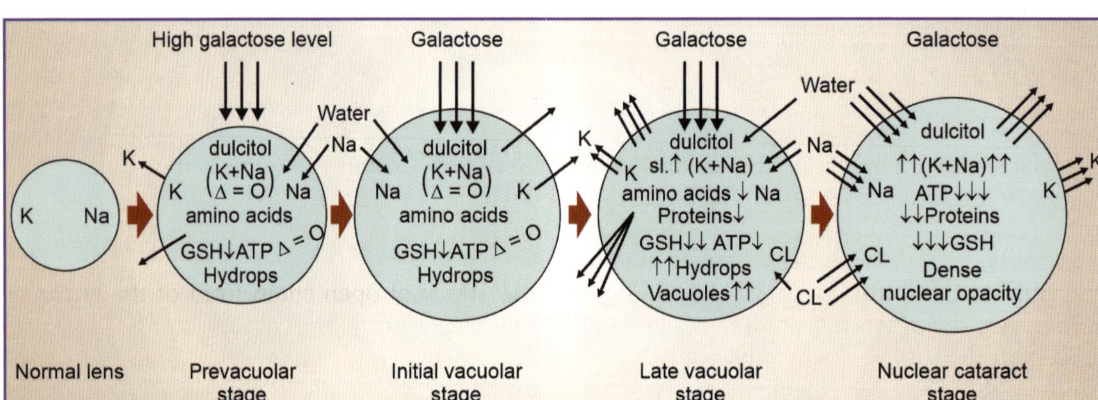

Fig. 5.19. *The course of events in sugar cataract (Kinoshita, 1965).*

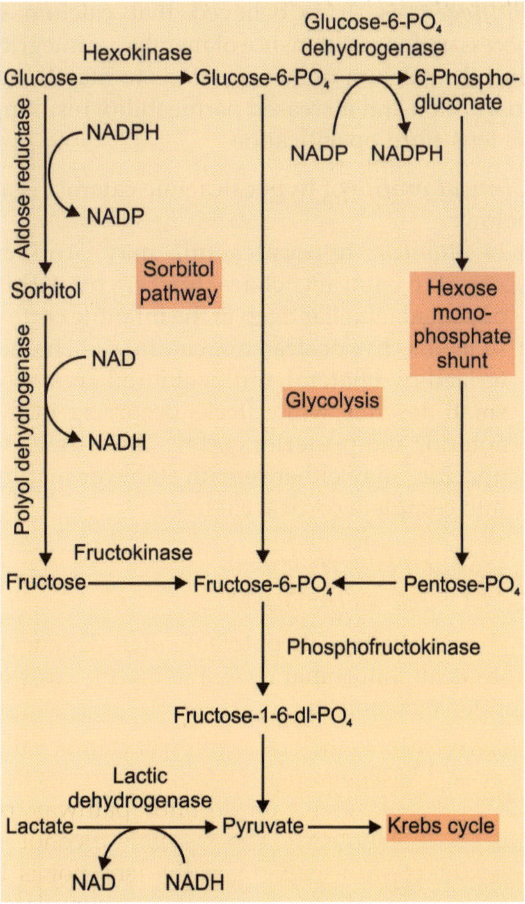

Fig. 5.20. *Pathways of glucose metabolism in the crystalline lens.*

to the formation of foci of interfibrillar and intracytoplasmic light scattering (i.e. water clefts and vacuoles) with resultant opacification.

In animal studies, inhibitors of the enzyme aldose-reductase have been shown to delay and prevent cataract formation. Thus, in near future, it might be possible to prevent occurrence of sugar cataracts (diabetic as well as galactosaemic). The active agents which have inhibitory effect on aldose-reductase include fatty acids, tetramethylene glutamic acid, flavonoids, and the synthetic compounds alrestatin and sorbinil.

However, there are several difficulties with this osmotic hypothesis especially when applied to human cataract. It is possible that the osmotic effect of accumulated polyol plays a role in cataract in the glactose-fed rat. Points put forward against any role of the osmotic damage in human diabetes are as follows:

- Osmotically significant levels of sorbitol have never been found in human lens.
- Human lens contains only tiny amounts of aldose reductase activity—unmeasurable with glucose as substrate and with no increase in diabetes.
- Human lens has a relatively high activity of polyol dehydrogenase so that any sorbitol formed would be rapidly converted into fructose to be further metabolized.
- Human lenses (normal, diabetic and cataractous) incubated in glucose at concentration between 5 and 35.5 mM accumulate negligible amounts of sorbitol.

2. Hypothesis of auto-oxidation of sugars

The possible role of auto-oxidation of sugars in the etiopathogenesis of sugar-induced cataract has been suggested by many workers. However, the balance of the evidence indicates that although the auto-oxidation of glyceraldehyde can explain some peculiarities of the usual assay for aldose reductase, the role of auto-oxidation in cataract formation is uncertain. Some of the important points disfavouring the hypothesis of auto-oxidation are as follows:

- Significant auto-oxidation of glucose has not been established.
- An alternative physiological monosaccharide has not been identified and nor has any specific damage by either free radicals or the α-oxoaldehydes been demonstrated.

3. Theory of non-enzymic glycosylation (glycation)

Till date, this theory seems more important in the aetiology of diabetic cataract than either auto-oxidation or the osmotic effect of sorbitol. According to this hypothesis, the non-enzymic glycosylation (glycation) plays an important role in the causation of sugar-induced cataracts. It has been reported that the initial reaction is the attack of open chain form of the sugar on the amino groups of lens proteins. The initial attack leads on to a variety of chemical entities and induces structural changes to enzymes, membrane proteins and crystallins in the lens. These changes start from conformational alterations progressing to thiol oxidation, aggregation, formation of disulphide and other covalent crosslinks and inactivation of enzymes. Harding reported that the non-enzymic glycosylation of the proteins is not only responsible for development of diabetic cataract but also for that of retinopathy, nephropathy, cardiovascular disease and neuropathy (Fig. 5.21).

Speculative scheme for sugar cataracts

A speculative scheme linking together changes found in the experimental diabetic cataract studies, as described by Harding, is shown in Fig. 5.22.

HYPOCALCAEMIC (TETANIC) CATARACT

Etiology. Hypocalcaemic cataract may be associated with any condition that results in hypocalcaemia. Hypocalcaemia may be due to:
- Idiopathic,
- Infantile tetany,
- Hypoparathyroidism due to atrophy or inadventential removal of parathyroid glands during thyroidectomy.

Pathogenesis. It is believed that calcium is necessary for maintenance of membrane integrity and the calcium deficiency leads to membrane disruption and increased permeability resulting in lens fibre opacification.

Clinical profile of hypocalcaemic cataract is as below:
- *In infantile,* hypocalcaemia may produce zonular cataract, characterized by a thin opacified lamellar deep in the infantile cortex.
- *In adults,* hypocalcaemia cataract is characterized by bilateral, multicoloured crystal or small descrete white flecks occurring in the anterior and posterior cortex. These descrete opacities may either remain stable or mature into complete cortical cataract.

CATARACT DUE TO ERROR OF COPPER METABOLISM

Wilson's disease (hepatolenticular degeneration) is an autosomal recessive inborn error of copper metabolism.

Ocular features include sunflower cataract and 'Kayser-Fleischer' ring.

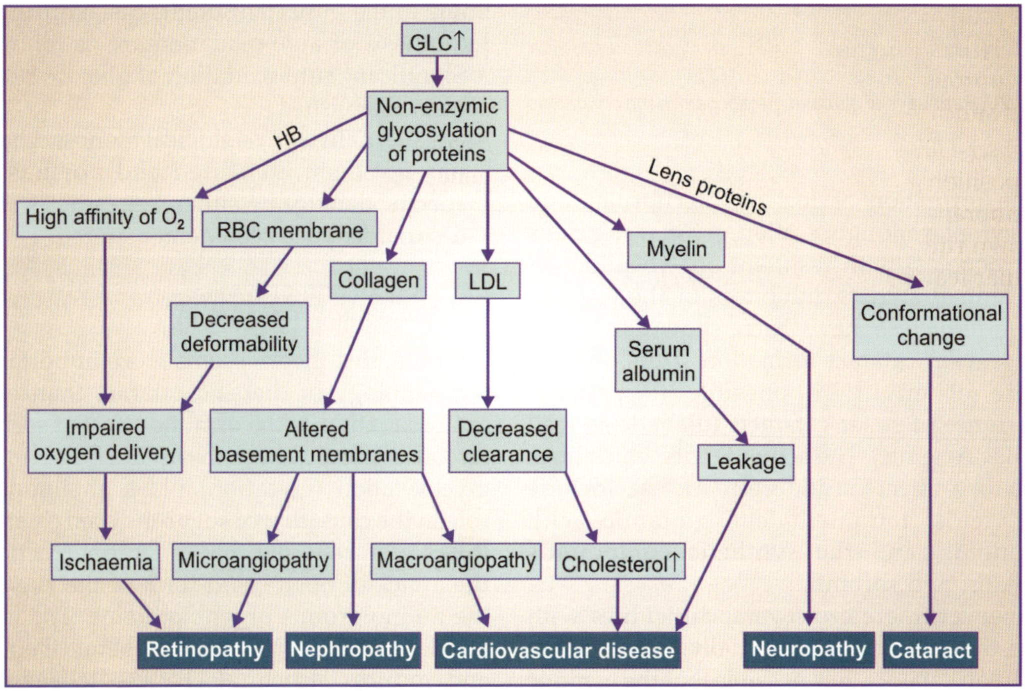

Fig. 5.21. *Possible relationships between non-enzymic glycosylation of proteins and the sequelae of diabetes. Factors other than glycosylation have been implicated in these sequelae (Adapted from Harding, 1967).*

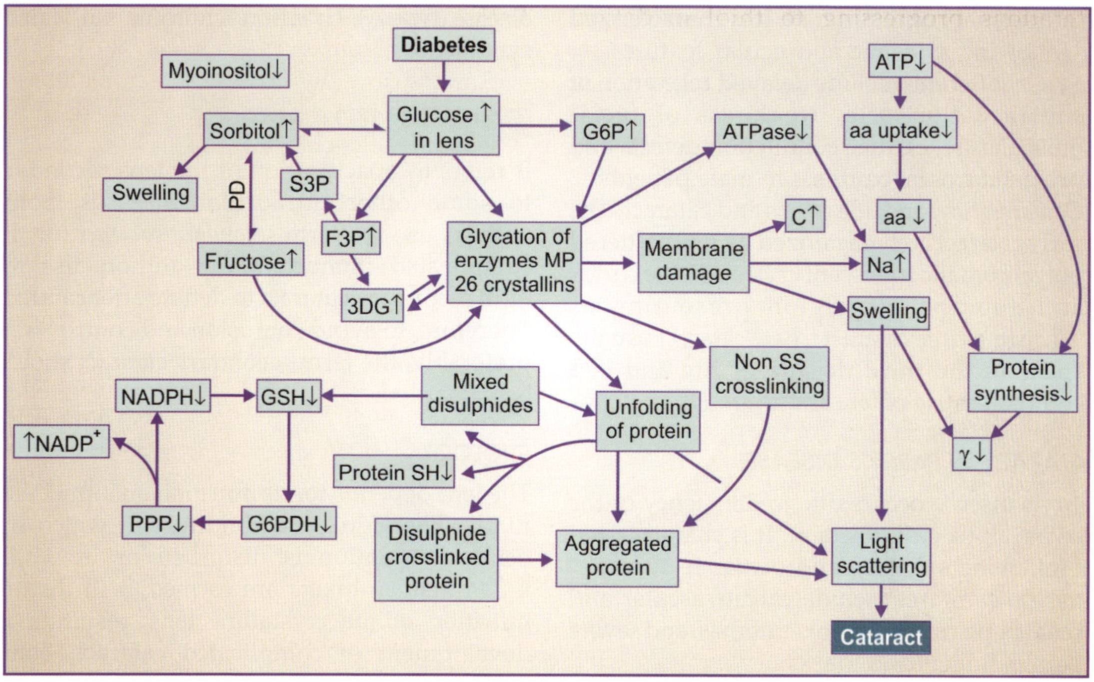

Fig. 5.22. *Speculative scheme linking together changes found in experimental diabetic cataract. F3P: fructose-3-phosphate; G6P: glucose-6-phosphate; S3P: sorbitol-3-phosphate; aa: amino acid; 3DG: deoxyglucosone; γ: γ-crystalline; PD: polyol dehydrogenase; PPP: pentose phosphate pathway (Adapted from Harding).*

- *'Sunflower cataract'* (Fig. 5.17) is characterized by yellowish brown dots may be observed rarely in such patients due to the deposition of cuprous oxide in the anterior lens capsule and subcapsular cortex in a stellate pattern.
- *'Kayser-Fleischer ring'(KF ring)* occurs due to deposition in the peripheral part of Descemet's membrane in the cornea. It is seen as a golden-brown ring and is more commonly observed ocular feature of Wilson's disease (Fig. 5.23).

CATARACT IN LOWE'S SYNDROME

Lowe's (oculo-cerebral-renal) syndrome is a rare X-linked recessive inborn error of amino acid metabolism which predominantly affects boys. It is characterized by the following ocular and systemic features:

- *Ocular features* include congenital cataract, congenital glaucoma and blue sclera. The lens is usually small (microphakia) and thin disc-like cataract seen is usually bilateral and may be capsular, lamellar, nuclear (more common) or total. Mothers of the affected children may also show multiple punctuate lens opacities.
- *Systemic features* of this syndrome are mental retardation, dwarfism, osteomalacia, muscular hypotonia and frontal prominence.

CATARACT IN MYOTONIC DYSTROPHY

Myotonic dystrophy occurs due to defect in the gene encoding myosin protein. It is inherited as

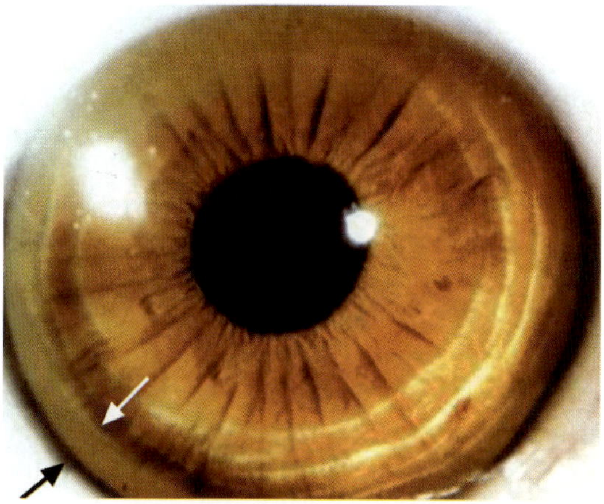

Fig. 5.23. *Kayser-Fleischer ring*

an autosomal dominant trait. It is characterized by following systemic and ocular features:

- *Systemic features* include delayed relaxation of contracted muscle, weakness of facial musculature, cardiac conduction defects and proximal frontal baldness in male patients.
- *Ocular features* include ptosis and cataract. The early cataract is characterized by fine scattered polychromatic iridescent crystals in the cortex and subcapsular region presenting as 'Christmas tree cataract'. Late cataract usually starts in the third decade of life and is a common cause of *'pre-senile catarct'*.

CATARACT IN FABRY'S DISEASE

Fabry's disease occurs due to deficiency of the enzyme alpha galactosidase. It is characterized by following systemic and ocular features:

- *Systemic features* include cardiovascular and renal impairment, angiokeratomas, and severe pain in fingers and toe.
- *Ocular features* of Fabry's disease include spoke-like lens opacities and cornea verticillata.

CATARACT IN MONGOLIAN IDIOCY AND HYPOTHYROIDISM

Punctate subcapsular cataract may be seen in patients with cretinism (due to hypothyroidism) and Mongolian idiocy.

CATARACT IN MANNOSIDOSIS

Mannosidosis occurs due to deficiency of the enzyme alpha mannosidase resulting in accumulation of mannose rich oligosaccharides in the body tissue. It is characterized by following systemic and ocular features:

- *Systemic features* include short stature, skeletal changes, hepatosplenomegaly and mental retardation.
- *Ocular features* include spike-like or wheel-like posterior subcapsular opacities

CATARACT IN SOME OTHER METABOLIC CONDITIONS

Cataract may be associated with number of other metabolic conditions. A few conditions include Hurler's disease, Fanconi's syndrome, phenylketonuria, neurofibromatosis type II, mucolipidosis, Refsum's disease, Niemann-Pick disease (type A), Thomson syndrome and Millar's syndrome.

COMPLICATED CATARACT

It refers to opacification of the lens secondary to some other intraocular diseases. Some authors use the term *secondary cataract* for the complicated cataract. Many authors use the term secondary cataract to denote after cataract. Therefore, to avoid confusion and controversy, preferably, the term secondary cataract should be discarded.

ETIOLOGY

The lens depends for its nutrition on intraocular fluids. Therefore, any condition in which the ocular circulation is disturbed or in which inflammatory toxins are formed, will disturb nutrition of the crystalline lens, resulting in development of complicated cataract. Some important ocular conditions giving rise to complicated cataract are listed here.

1. ***Inflammatory conditions.*** These include uveal inflammations (e.g. iridocyclitis, parsplanitis, choroiditis), hypopyon corneal ulcer and endophthalmitis. Complicated cataract often occurs as a result of chronic uveitis and/or associated corticosteroid therapy. About 70% cases of Fuch's heterochromic uveitis are associated with complicated cataract. Specially a posterior subcapsular cataract (PSC) begins in uveitis. Anterior subcapsular cataract associated with thickening of the anterior lens capsule may occur due to formation of posterior synechiae in uveitis.

2. ***Degenerative conditions*** such as retinitis pigmentosa, other pigmentary retinal dystrophies, myopic chorioretinal degeneration, essential iris atrophy and chronic hypotony. The complicated cataract usually begins as PSC and may progress to total lens opacification. The mechanisms responsible for cataractogenesis in degenerative ocular disorders are not well understood.

3. ***Retinal detachment.*** Complicated cataract may occur in long-standing cases.

4. ***Glaucoma (primary or secondary)*** may sometimes result in complicated cataract. The

underlying cause here is probably the embarrassment to the intraocular circulation, consequent to the raised pressure. *Glaucoma fleckns* are grey white epithelial and anterior cortical lens opacities that occur following an episode of markedly elevated IOP, as in acute angle closure glaucoma. Histopathologically, glaucoma fleckns are composed of necrotic lens epithelial cells and degenerated subepithelial cortex.

5. ***Intraocular tumours*** such as retinoblastoma or melanoma or metastatic tumours involving the choroid or anterior segment may give rise to complicated cataract in late stages.

6. ***Ischaemic ocular conditions.*** Such as pulse less disease (Takayasu arteritis), thromboangitis obliterans (Buerger disease), and anterior segment necrosis, may cause posterior subcapsular cataract (PSC). The cataract may progress rapidly to total opacification of lens.

CLINICAL FEATURES

Posterior cortical complicated cataract

Typically the complicated cataract (Fig. 5.24) starts as *posterior subcapsular cortical cataract.* The opacity is irregular in outline and variable in density. In the beam of slit-lamp, the opacities have an appearance like *'bread-crumb'*. A very characteristic sign is the appearance of iridescent-coloured particles the so-called *'polychromatic lustre'* of reds, greens and blues. A diffuse yellow-haze is seen in the adjoining cortex. Slowly the opacity spreads in the rest of the cortex, and finally the entire lens becomes opaque, giving chalky white appearance. Deposition of calcium is common in the later stages.

Anterior cortical complicated cataract

Anterior cortical complicated cataract may also occur in anterior segment lesion such as glaucoma, hypopyon corneal ulcer and acute iritis. Earliest change is appearance of vacuole below the anterior capsule followed by opacities in the neighbouring cortical fibres and thickening of anterior capsule.

DRUG-INDUCED CATARACTS

CORTICOSTEROID-INDUCED CATARACT

Posterior subcapsular cataracts (PSCs) are associated with the use of topical as well as systemic steroids. The exact relationship between dose and duration of corticosteroid therapy with the development of cataract is still unclear. However, in general, prolonged use of steroids in high doses may result in cataract formation. Children are more susceptible than adults. The increasing use of high dose intraocular steroids to treat retinal neovascularization, and inflammation has resulted in substantial rise in the incidence of PSC.

Pathogenesis

Harding and Crabbe reported that the corticosteroids could induce cataract by any of the following mechanisms:

- Elevation of glucose
- Inhibition of Na, K-ATPase
- Increased cation permeability
- Inhibition of glucose 6-phosphate dehydrogenase
- Inhibition of RNA synthesis
- Loss of ATP
- Covalent binding of steroids to lens proteins

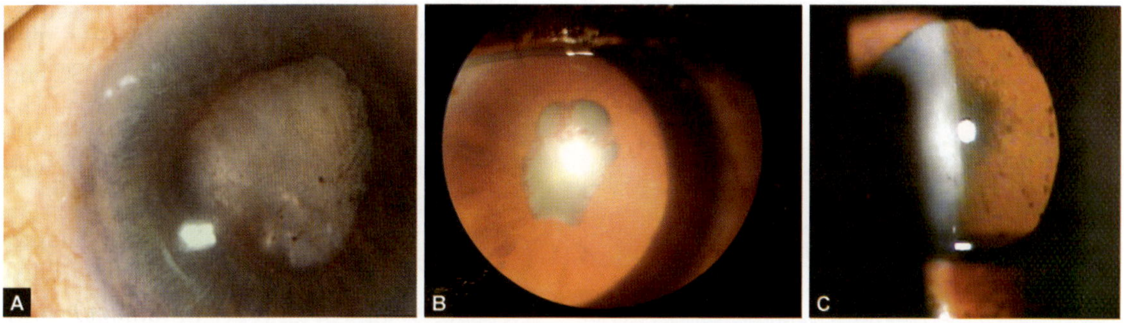

Fig. 5.24: *Complicated cataracts*

The speculative scheme of changes occurring during steroid cataract, as described by Harding, is depicted in Fig. 5.25.

Clinical and histopathological features of the corticosteroid PSCs are similar with the age-related PSCs. The first indication of PSC formation is a subtle iridescent seen in the posterior cortical layers visible with slit-lamp. In later stages, granular opacities and plaque-like axial opacity of the posterior subcapsular cortex appears.

Histopathologically, PSC is associated with posterior migration of the lens epithelial cells from the lens equator to the axis on the inner surface of posterior capsule. These cells undergo aberrant enlargement. These swollen cells are called wedl or bladder cells.

Prevention. It is recommended that all patients with diseases requiring prolonged corticosteroids therapy should be regularly examined on slit-lamp by an ophthalmologist. Further, intermittent regimes should be preferred over regular therapy and whenever possible steroids should be substituted by non-steroidal anti-inflammatory drugs (NSAIDs). Some steroid-induced PSCs in children may resolve with cessation of the drug.

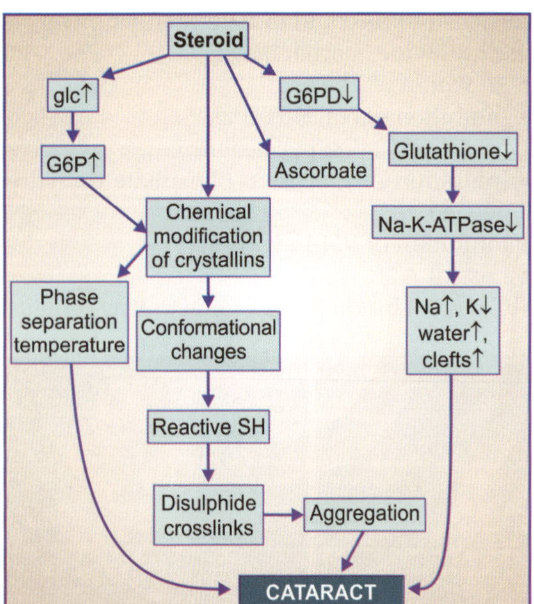

Fig. 5.25. *Speculative scheme of changes occurring during steroid cataract (G6PD: glucose-6-phosphate dehydrogenase). (Adapted from Harding).*

MIOTICS-INDUCED CATARACT

Anterior subcapsular granular type of cataract may be associated with long-term use of miotics, particularly long acting cholinesterase inhibitors such as echothiophate, demecarium bromide, disopropyl fluorophosphate (DFP). The initial changes include appearance of anterior subcapsular vacuoles which are best appreciated on retroillumination with the slit-lamp. Removal of the drug may stop progression and occasionally may cause reversal of cataract.

PHENOTHIAZINES-INDUCED CATARACT

Prolonged use of phenothiazines specially chlorpromazine and thioridazone may cause deposition of fine pigmented (yellowish-brown) granular under the anterior capsule in an axial configuration. The depositions are directly related to the dose and duration of administration of the drugs but are rarely dense enough to interfere with vision.

AMIODARONE-INDUCED CATARACT

- *Anterior subcapsular stellate shape axial pigmented opacities* have been reported to occur following the use of amiodarone drug. Usually, such opacities are visually insignificant.
- *Amiodarone is also deposited* in the corneal epithelium and is the cause of a rare optic neuropathy.

OTHER DRUG-INDUCED CATARACTS

Other drugs associated with fine toxic cataract are:

- *Busulphan,* used for treatment of chronic myeloid leukaemia.
- *Gold,* used for the treatment of rheumatoid arthritis.
- *Allopurinol,* used for treatment of gout.
- *Nitrocompounds,* such as dinitrophenol, trinitrophenol, naphthalene, thalium, carbromal, triparanol, and tetracaine.

RADIATIONAL CATARACT

Exposure to almost all types of radiant energy is known to produce cataract by causing damage to the lens epithelium. Following types are known.

1. INFRARED RADIATION (HEAT) CATARACT

Prolonged exposure (over several years) to infrared radiations may cause discoid posterior subcapsular opacities and true exfoliation of the anterior capsule. In true exfoliation, the exfoliated outer lamella of the lens capsule flake off and tends to scroll up on itself. Such a condition is rarely seen nowadays. The infrared radiation cataract is typically seen in persons working in glass industries, so also called as *'glass-blower's* or *glass-worker's cataract'*.

2. IONISING RADIATION CATARACT

Exposure to X-rays, gamma-rays or neutrons may be associated with irradiation cataract. There is usually a latent period ranging from 6 months to as much as 20 years between exposure and development of the cataract. This period of latency is related to the dose of radiation and to patient's age: Younger patients are more susceptible because they have more actively growing lens cells.

Degree of cataract formation is also related to the dose of radiation. A little single dose of 300–400 rad may lead to cataract formation. Neutrons and alpha beam produce greater ionization and pose the greater risk of cataract formation. As gamma and X-rays are most frequently used forms of radiation, so these are more linked to cataract formation.

People prone to get such cataracts are inadequately protected technicians, patients treated for malignant tumours and workers of atomic energy plants.

Pathogenesis

Radiations appear to cause an increase in the lens membrane permeability, affect metabolism and synthesis of protein and cell division. Alterations in glutathione and RNA metabolism have also been reported. The severity of lens changes is dependent upon the age of the animal and whether the whole lens or part of the lens is irradiated. A speculative scheme of pathways to cataract following X-irradiation, as suggested by Lipman *et al.*, is shown in Fig. 5.26.

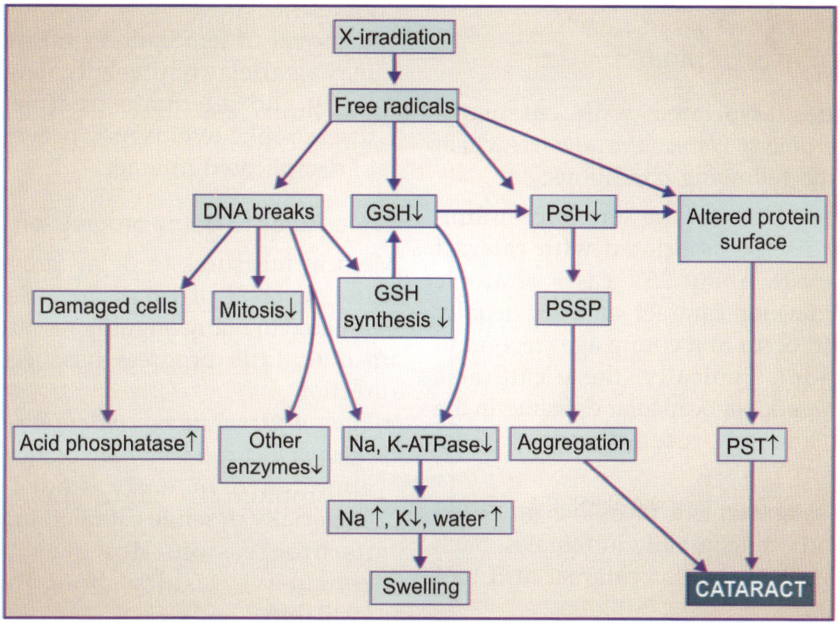

Fig. 5.26. *Flow chart showing possible pathways to cataract following X-irradiation. (Based on a flow chart by Lipman et al., 1988). PSH: protein thiol; PSSP: protein disulphide; PST: phase separation temperature. (Adapted from Harding).*

Clinical characteristics

Radiation-induced cataract specially presents as punctuate opacities within the posterior capsule and feathery anterior subcapsular opacities that radiate towards the equator of the lens. These opacities may progress to complete opacification of the lens.

3. ULTRAVIOLET RADIATION CATARACT

Long-term exposure to ultraviolet radiation has been linked with senile cataract in many studies (*see* page 60).

ELECTRIC CATARACT

Electric cataract is known to occur after passage of powerful electric current through the body. Cataract formation is more likely when the transmission of current involves patient's head. Usually more extensive cataract is formed on the side with greater electrical burns. The cataract usually starts as punctate subcapsular opacities followed by linear opacities in anterior subcapsular cortex. The electric cataract may regress, remain stationary or mature to complete cataract over months or years. The source of current can be a live electricity wire or a flash of lightning.

SYNDERMATOTIC CATARACT

Lens opacities associated with cutaneous disease are termed *syndermatotic cataracts* which are seen in the following conditions:

- *Atopic dermatitis* is the most common cutaneous disease associated with cataract *(atopic cataract)*. About 25% cases of atopic dermatitis develop cataract such are usually bilateral and occur at a young age (second to third decade). Typically, these cataracts present as anterior subcapsular opacities in the pupillary and are resemble shield-like plaques.
- *Rothmund syndrome* is a recessive inherited disorder and occurs mainly in females. Such patients develop zonular cataract at 3 to 4 years of age.
- *Werner's syndrome* is associated with formation of posterior subcapsular cataract.
- *Other skin disorders* associated with cataract include poikiloderma, vasculare atrophicans, scleroderma and keratotis follicularis.

MANAGEMENT OF CATARACT IN ADULTS

Treatment of cataract essentially consists of its surgical removal. However, certain non-surgical measures may be of help, in peculiar circumstances, till surgery is taken up.

A. NON-SURGICAL MEASURES

1. Treatment of associated disease

In acquired cataracts (other than age-related), a thorough search should be made to find out the associated causative disease. Treatment of the causative disease, many a time, may stop progression and sometimes in early stages may even cause some regression of cataractous changes and thus defer the surgical treatment. Some common examples include:

- Adequate control of diabetes mellitus, when discovered.
- Removal of cataractogenic drugs such as corticosteroids, phenothiazines and strong miotics, may delay or prevent cataractogenesis.
- Removal of irradiation (infrared or X-rays) may also delay or prevent cataract formation.
- Early and adequate treatment of ocular diseases like uveitis may prevent occurrence of complicated cataract.

2. Measures to delay progression

Medical measures to delay progression or to cause reversal of cataractogenesis, are being evaluated in many ongoing research. However, till date, little progress has occurred in this direction.

- *Topical preparations containing iodide salts of calcium and potassium* are being prescribed in abundance in early stages of cataract (especially in senile cataract) in a bid to delay its progression. However, till date, no conclusive results about their role are available.
- *Aldose reductase inhibitors,* which block the conversion of glucose to sorbitol, have been

shown to prevent cataract in animals with experimentally induced diabetes.

- *Sorbitol lowering agents, aspirin and glutathione raising agents* are still under investigation.
- *Antioxidant, vitamins E, C, beta-carotene and zinc* do not slow cataract progression.

3. Measures to improve vision in the presence of incipient and immature cataract

Measures to improve vision in the presence of incipient and immature cataract may be of great solace to the patient. These include:

- *Refraction,* which often changes with considerable rapidity, should be corrected at frequent intervals.
- *Arrangement of illumination.* Patients with peripheral opacities (pupillary area still free), may be instructed to use brilliant illumination. Conversely, in the presence of central opacities, a dull light placed beside and slightly behind the patient's head will give the best result.
- *Use of dark goggles* in patients with central opacities is of great value and comfort when worn outdoors.
- *Mydriatics.* The patients with a small axial cataract, frequently may benefit from pupillary dilatation. This allows the clear paraxial lens to participate in light transmission, image formation and focussing. Mydriatics such as 5% phenylephrine or 1% tropicamide; 1 drop b.i.d. in the affected eye may clarify vision.

4. Low vision aids for cataract patients

Low vision aids for cataract patients may be required when surgical management is not feasible. These include:

- *Handheld monoculars* of 2.5x, 2.8x, and 4x facilitate spotting objects at a distance.
- *High add spectacles, magnifiers, closed circuit television and telescope loops* may be used for reading and close work.

B. SURGICAL MANAGEMENT

Surgical management can be discussed under following headings:

- Preoperative work-up and prepration for cataract surgery (*see* Chapter 12 page 176).
- Anaesthesia for cataract surgery (*see* Chapter 8, pages 98–106).
- Types and choice of surgical techniques (*see* page 184)
- Steps of common surgical techniques (*see* Chapters 13 to 15).
- Complications of cataract surgery and their management (*see* Chapter 20).

BIBLIOGRAPHY

1. Barber, GW. Free amino acids in senile cataractous lenses Invest Ophthalmol 7, 564–583;1968.
2. Charlton, JM, and van Heyningen R. An investigation into the loss of proteins of low molecular size from the lens in senile cataract Exp Eye Res 7,47–55;1968.
3. Clayton, RM, Cuthbert, J, Seth, J, et al. Epidemological and other studies in the assessment of factors contributing to cataractogenesis Ciba Fdn Symp, 106,25–47;1989.
4. Creighton, MO and Trevithick. Cortical cataract formation prevented by vitamin E and glutathione Exp Eye Res, 29:689;1979.
5. Grant, WM. Toxicology of the Eye, 2nd ed Springfield Ill, CC Thomas, 103;1974.
6. Harding, J. Cataract: Biochemistry, epidemiology and pharmacology, Chapman and Hall, London.
7. Harding, JJ, Dilley KJ. Structural proteins of the mammalian lens. A review with emphasis on changes in development aging and cataract Exp Eye Res 22,1–73;1976.
8. Harding, JJ. Nonenzymic covalent post-translational modification of proteins in viva Adv Protein Chem 37:247–334;1985.
9. Jeduniak, JA, Chylack, LT, Cheng, HM, et al. The sorbitol pathway in the human lens: aldose reductase and polyol dehydrogenase Invest Ophthalmol Vis Sci, 20,314–326;1981.
10. Khurana AK, Lal H, Chauhan BS, Parmar IPS, Saini AS. Protein and Electrolyte Alterations in Human Senile Cataract, Academic Press Inc London Limited 35,131–135;1982.
11. Kinoshita, J. Cataracts in galactosemia. Invest Ophthalmol 4:786–799;1965.
12. Kinoshita, JH. Annual review Selected topics in Ophthalmic biochemistry Arch Ophthal, 72: 554;1964.
13. Kinoshita, JH, Dvornik, D, Kraml, M, Gabbay, KH. The effect of an aldose reductase inhibitor on the galactose-exposed rabbit lens, Biochem Biophys Acta 158:472–475;1968.

14. Lerman, S, Moran, M, Matthews, N Photographic and spectroscopic correlation of human cataracts Ophthalmic Res, 21:18–26;1989.
15. Maraini, G, Mangili, R. Cited by Ciba Foundation Symposium, Human lens in relation to cataract, 19:79–97;1973.
16. Maraini, G, Carta, F, Pescatori, A, Prosperi, L. Protein metabolism in human senile cataract Exp Eye Res 11,83–8;1971.
17. Segal, S. Disorders of galactose metabolism In Stanbury JB et al (eds): The Metabolic Basis of Inherited Disease, 3rd ed New York McGraw-Hill, 174–1965;1972.
18. Srivastava SK, Lal AK, Ansari NH. Defence system of the lens against oxidative damage: Effect of oxidative challenge on cataract formation in glutathione peroxidase deficient-Acatalasemic mice Exp Eye Res, 31:425;1980.
19. Stevens VJ, Rouzer CA, Monnier VM, Cerami A. Diabetic cataract formation: potential role of glycosylation of lens crystallins Proc Natl Acad Sci USA, 75:2918–2922;1978.
20. van Heyningen, R. The lens: metabolism and cataract In Davson, H (ed): The Eye, Vol 1, 2nd ed New York, Academic Press 381–488;1969.
21. Varma SD, TK and Richards, RD. Protection against supreside radicals in rat lens Ophthalmic Res, 9:421;1977.
22. White JH, Cinotti AA. Streptozotocin-produced cataracts in rats. Invest Ophthalmol 11:56–57, 1972.

DISPLACEMENTS OF LENS

CHAPTER 6

INTRODUCTION

Displacement of the lens from its normal position (in patellar fossa) results from partial or complete rupture or looseness of the lens zonules. Displacements of the lens can be classified as below:

- Clinico-etiological types
- Topographical types.

CLINICO-ETIOLOGICAL TYPES OF LENS DISPLACEMENTS

Clinico-etiological types of lens displacements include:

- Congenital displacements
- Traumatic displacements
- Consecutive or spontaneous displacements.

I. CONGENITAL DISPLACEMENTS

These may occur in the following forms:

- Simple ectopia lentis
- Ectopia lentis et pupillae
- Ectopia lentis with systemic anomalies.

A. *SIMPLE ECTOPIA LENTIS*

In this condition, displacement is bilaterally symmetrical and usually upwards. It is transmitted by autosomal dominant inheritance.

B. *ECTOPIA LENTIS ET PUPILLAE*

It is an autosomal recessive disorder characterized by displacement of the lens associated with slit-shaped pupil which is displaced in the opposite direction and dilates poorly (Fig. 6.1).

The displaced lens may either bisect the pupil or may be completely luxated from the papillary area. The condition is bilateral but usually not symmetric.

Other ocular associations are common and include persistent pupillary membrane (87%), abnormal iris transillumination (66%), cataract, glaucoma, retinal detachment, axial myopia and macrocornea.

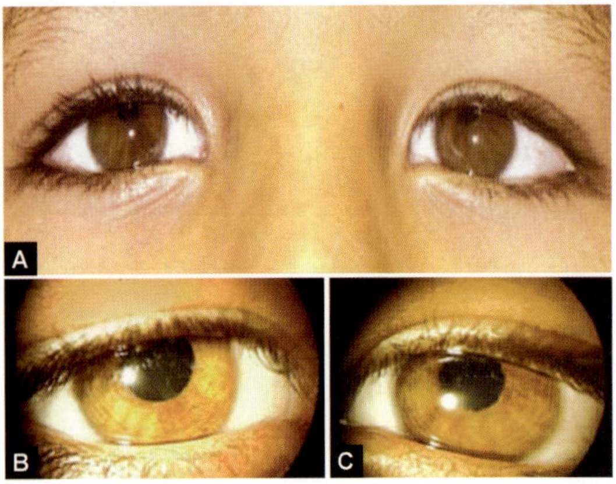

Fig. 6.1. *Ectopia lentis et pupillae showing:* ***(A)*** *Ectopic pupil;* ***(B and C)*** *Inferiorly subluxated lens.*

C. ECTOPIA LENTIS WITH SYSTEMIC ANOMALIES

Some of the common conditions are described below.

1. MARFAN'S SYNDROME

Described by Antonne Marfan in 1896, Marfan's syndrome is the commonest systemic condition associated with ectopia lentis. The syndrome comprises ocular, skeletal, and cardiovascular anomalies.

Prevalence

- It occurs in 4–6 per 1,00,000 live births.
- *Ocular involvement* is seen in 50–60% cases.
- *Cardiovascular involvement* occurs in 80% cases.
- *Skeletal anomalies* are seen in 100% cases.

Genetics

- *Autosomal dominant inherited* disorder with near complete penetrance but variable expressivities.
- *New mutations,* seen in 5–35% cases, are associated with increased paternal age.
- *Mesodermal dysplasia* occurring due to abnormal biosynthesis of fibrillin, a 350 kd cysteine rich glycoprotein. Fibrillin is a major constituent of microfibrils which are present in the connective tissue of suspensory ligaments of crystalline lens.
- *Fibrillin locus (FBN)* lies within the long arm of chromosome15 (15q21).

Clinical features

Many manifestations of the Marfan's syndrome are maturation related. Cognitive performance is usually normal. Clinical features can be described into ocular features and systemic manifestations.

I. *Ocular features*

Ocular features includes the following.

A. Anterior segment anomalies

1. ***Ectopia lentis.*** Ectopia lentis, seen in 50–80% cases of Marfan's syndrome, is by far the major ocular manifestation. Features of ectopia lentis are:

- *Laterality.* Usually bilateral and symmetric.
- *Time of onset.* Usually congenital occurring in utero; however, progression of lens subluxation is observed in some patients over time, whereas in many patients the lens position remains stable.
- *Direction.* Almost always there is bilateral-superotemporal subluxation (Fig. 6.2) but rarely can occur in any direction.
- *Zonules.* The zonular attachments commonly remain intact, but become stretched and elongated.
- *Accommodation* is possible, since zonules are mostly attached.
- *Visual acuity.* It is usually not markedly reduced, usually better than 6/18 in 60% cases. Reduced visual acuity may be due to *lenticular astigmatism* and associated myopia. Cataract formation has also been reported in some cases.

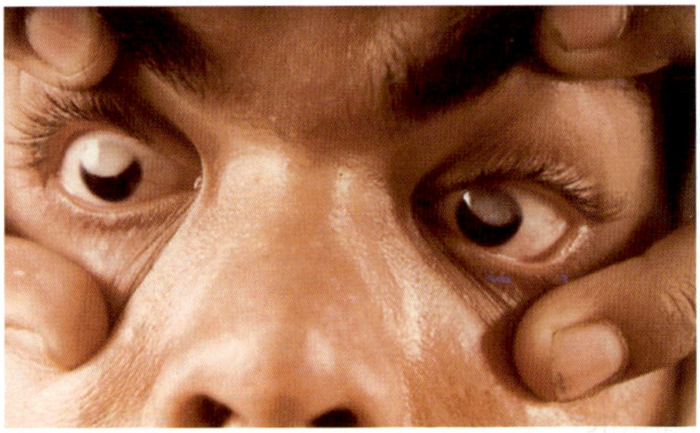

Fig. 6.2. *Subluxated cataractous lens in Marfan's syndrome.*

2. ***Other anterior segment anomalies*** include:

i. *Cornea* may be flat and its diameter may be increased. Keratoconus has been reported occasionally.

ii. *Pupils and iris* pupil dilate poorly as dilator muscle is hypoplastic. Occasionally, pupils are miotic and eccentric. Iris transillumination is seen in 10% cases. Iridodoneses may be noted. Heterochromia iridis has also been seen.

iii. *Reiger anomaly* characterized by prominent anterior Schwalbe's line, anterior stromal hypoplasia has been reported.

iv. *Secondary glaucoma* may occur due to lens dislocation or congenital angle anomaly.

B. Posterior segment anomalies

1. *Retinal detachment* is reported in 9% cases.
2. *Choroid* may be thin, but staphyloma is rare.
3. *Peripheral retinal degenerations,* associated in a few cases, include lattice degeneration, retinoschisis, retinal holes, and areas of white without pressure.
4. *Retinal arterial occlusion* has also been reported.

C. Other ocular and related anomalies

1. *Myopia* of moderate to severe degree may be there. Myopia is lenticular as usually the axial length is normal.
2. *Anisometropia with amblyopia* is also reported.
3. *Strabismus* is reported in 20% cases.
4. *Acquired Brown syndrome* occurring due to inflammation of microfibrillar fibres of superior oblique tendon accompanied by diplopia and pain in upgaze is reported.
5. *Nystagmus* may be associated, occasionally.
6. *Down slanting palpebral fissure* is also reported.
7. *Enophthalmos* may be seen.

II. *Systemic manifestations*

1. Musculoskeletal anomalies

Typical presentation is that of a tall individual with a long face (Fig. 6.3) associated following musculoskeletal anomalies (common):

- *Dolichosternomalia,* i.e. long and thin limbs.
- *Arm span to height ratio* is >1.05.
- *Upper segment of body* (head to pubic bone) is shorter than lower segment (ratio is <0.86 in adults).
- *Arachanodactly,* i.e. long spider-like fingers.

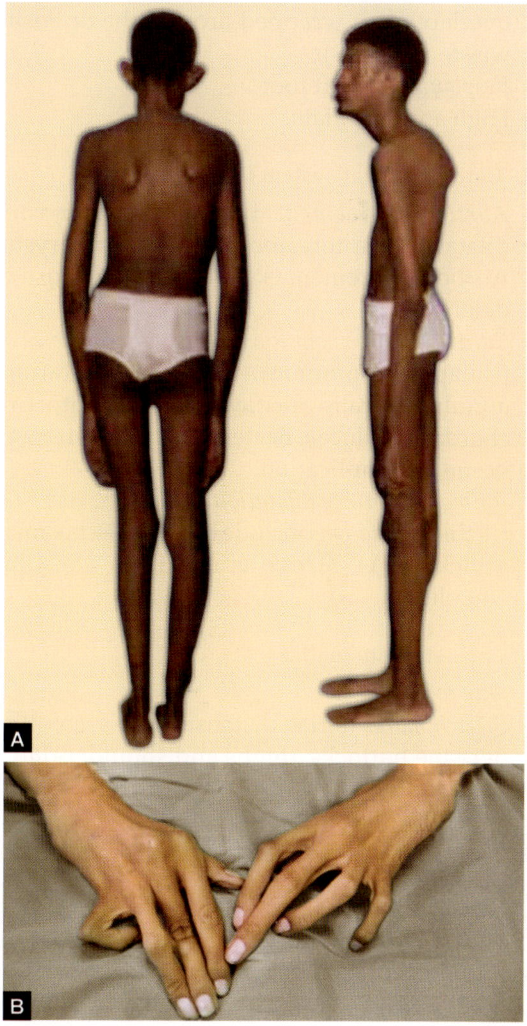

Fig. 6.3. *A patient with Marfan's syndrome **(A)**; Note arachnodactyly **(B)**.*

- *Chest wall deformities* include pectus excavatum (funnel chest) and pectus carinatum (pigeon chest).
- *Hyperextensibility* of joints is seen as hypermobility.
- *Scoliosis,* usually more than 20°, is most frequent and most debilitating of all skeletal anomalies.
- *Thumb sign and wrist sign* are positive. The thumb sign is considered positive when the thumb projects beyond the ulnar border when making a fist (thumb wrapped under fingers). The wrist sign is considered positive when the distal phalanges of the first and fifth digit

overlap when wrapped around the opposite wrist.
- *Pesplanus*, i.e. flat foot
- High arched palate.

2. Cardiovascular system (CVS) anomalies

- *Aortic involvement* includes aortic root dilatation, rupture and dissecting aneurysm. Aortic involvement is most common cause of death.
- *Cardiac involvement* may occur as mitral valve prolapsed (common), mitral regurgitation, annulus mitralis calcification, and rupture of chordae tendineae. Bacterial endocarditis may occur as complication.
- *Pulmonary artery dilatation*
- *CVS manifestations* include transient ischaemiac attack (TIA), stroke and retinal vascular emboli.

3. Cutaneous anomalies

- *Skin folds*
- *Stretch marks* (striae distensae) are seen often over the buttocks, thighs and shoulders.

4. Central nerve system (CNS) anomalies

- *Dural ectasia* seen as lumbosacral meningocele, usually diagnosed on CT/MRI.
- *Dilated cisterna magna*
- *Learning disability*
- *Attention deficit hyperactivity disorder*
- *Schizophrenia* may be associated.

5. Pulmonary system anomalies (rare)

- *Pneumothorax*, occurring spontaneously
- *Bullous emphysema*, usually apical blebs, diagnosed by X-ray chest
- *Sleep apnoea*

Management

Systemic involvement, need to be treated by periodic referral to interdisciplinary centre.

Management of ectopia lentis: *see* page 268.

2. HOMOCYSTINURIA

Homocystinuria is an autosomal recessive, inborn error of methionine metabolism due to deficiency of enzyme cystathionine synthetase. The prevalence of this disorder is 1:2000,000 births. It is characterized by systemic and ocular features.

Systemic features

Affected individual are healthy at birth but over the period develop following systemic features:
- *Skeletomuscular features.* Patients are usually tall with typical facies characterized by fair complexion, malar flush and light-coloured hair. Muscular weakness and spastic gait are common features. Scoliosis, pectus excavatum and joint laxity may be seen.
- *CNS features* include seizures, mental retardation and poor motor control.
- *Cardiovascular (CVS) complications* are secondary to thrombosis and occlusion mainly of medium sized arteries and veins. Thromboembolic episodes are reported myocardial infarction, pulmonary embolism and cerebrovascular occlusive disorder. Surgery and general anaesthesia are thought to involve the risk of thromboembolism with fatal complications.

Ocular features

- *Bilateral subluxation of the lens*, usually downwards and nasally, appears in infancy in 30% of affected individuals, and by the age of 15 years in 80% of the individuals. Subluxation occurs due to abnormal zonular development owing to deficiency of the cysteine in these conditions.
- *Accommodative power of the lens is decreased* markedly due to disintegration of the zonules.
- *Glaucoma* may be associated in about 25% cases.
- *Myopia and retinal detachment* may also be associated.

Diagnosis

Diagnosis is established by:
- *Homocysteine in the urine* detected by sodium nitroprusside test.
- *Homocysteine and methionine* raised levels in the serum, detected by amino acid analyser.

Management

Management of homocystinuria includes:
- *Medical management* in the form of low-methionine high cysteine diet and vitamin supplementation with the co-enzyme pyridoxine (vitamin B_6) in infants with

homocystinuria is reported to reduce the incidence of ectopia lentis.

- *Management of ectopia lentis. See* page 290.

3. WEILL-MARCHESANI SYNDROME

Weill-Marchesani syndrome (spherophakia–brachymorphia) is a condition of autosomal recessive (however, autosomal cases have been reported) mesodermal dysplasia, characterized by following systemic and ocular features.

Systemic features

Systemic features include:

- *Skeletal features* are brachycephaly, short stature with short and stubby fingers (brachydactyly), broad thorax and hyperextensible joints.
- *Mental retardation.*

Ocular features

- *Microspherophakia,* i.e. small and round lens (Fig. 6.4A).

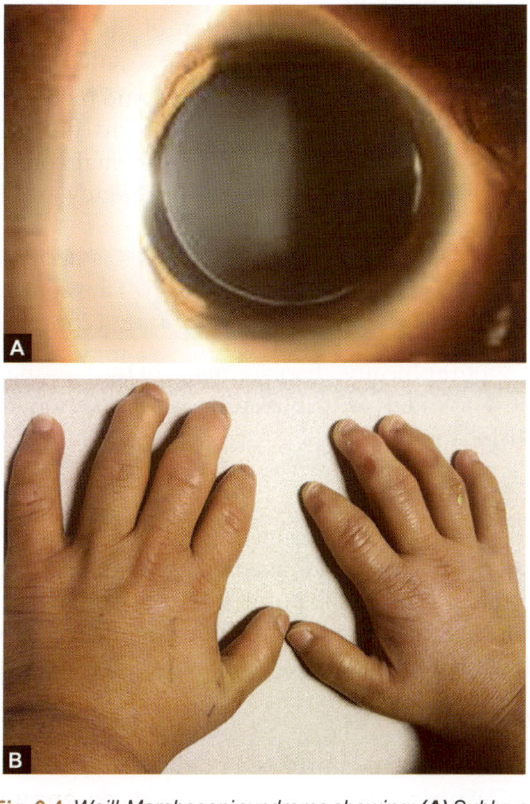

Fig. 6.4. *Weill-Marchesani syndrome showing: **(A)** Subluxation with microspherophakia; **(B)** Short webbed finger.*

- *Lenticular myopia* occurs due to steep lens.
- *Forward subluxation of lens,* which may cause pupil block glaucoma.
- *Pupil block glaucoma* is treated by mydriasis and so also called paradoxical glaucoma or glaucoma inversus. So always suspect Weill-Marchesani syndrome in children who present with unilateral or bilateral pupil block and secondary angle closure glaucoma.

Management

- *Laser peripheral iridectomy* is recommended in all cases to prevent pupillary block glaucoma.
- *Miotics* are recommended to prevent anterior dislocation of the lens.

4. EHLERS-DANLOS SYNDROME

Ehlres-Danlos syndrome, also known as fibrodysplasia hyperelastica, is an autosomal dominant hereditary disorder, characterized by following systemic and ocular features.

Systemic features

Systemic features are:

- Hyperextensibility of joints, and
- Loose skin with folds.

Ocular features

Ocular features include: Subluxation of lens, blue sclera, angioid streak, keratoconus, epicanthus, ptosis, and strabismus. Laxity of palpebral tissue shows unusual ease of everting of the upper lid (Meterier's sign).

5. HYPERLYSINAEMIA

It is an autsomal recessive inborn error of metabolism occurring due to deficiency of the enzyme lysine alpha-ketoglutarate reductase. It is an extremely rare condition.

- *Ectopia lentis* is an occasionally associated finding.
- *Systemic features* include lax ligaments, hypotonic muscles, seizures and mental handicap.

6. STICKLER SYNDROME

Ectopia lentis is occasionally associated in this condition.

7. SULPHITE OXIDASE DEFICIENCY

It is a very rare autosomal recessive disorder of sulphur metabolism.

- *Ectopia lentis* is a universal *ocular feature*.
- *Systemic features* include progressive muscular rigidity, decerebrate posture, and mental handicap. It is a fatal disease, death usually occurs before 5 years of age.

II. TRAUMATIC DISPLACEMENT OF THE LENS

Traumatic displacement of lens is most common of lens displacement constituting more than half of the cases. Traumatic displacement of lens can occur in following circumstances.

A. Concussion injury to the eyeball

Concussion injury to the eyeball is not infrequently associated with minimal subluxation to posterior dislocation of the lens.

Forces involved in causing traumatic displacement of the lens include:
- Backward thurst and rebounding of the lens,
- Pressure wave of the aqueous that forces root of the iris backward,
- Forcible recoil of the vitreous body, and
- Complimentary sudden enlargement of the corneoscleral ring.

Types of traumatic displacement of the lens

Depending upon the degree of zonular tear and the impact of the force, lens may be:
- *Retained in the patellar fossa,* even in the presence of zonular tear, due to its attachment to anterior vitreous phase.
- *Subluxation,* either lateral (superior, inferior, inward or outward) or axial (anterio-posterior) may occur when some zonules are intact.
- *Dislocation* or complete traumatic luxation of the lens may occur at any of the following sites:
  - Anterior chamber
  - Vitreous cavity
  - Subretinal space
  - Subconjunctival

Association of traumatic displacement of the lens

Associations of traumatic displacement of the lens include often traumatic lesion of concussion injury to the eyeball, namely commotio retinae, choroidal tear and retinal detachment.

Frenkel syndrome

Ocular contusion syndrome, characterized by subluxation of the lens associated with mydriasis and a tear of iris regulating from blunt trauma to eyeball was first described by a French ophthalmologist Henri Frenkel in 1931, and, therefore, also known as Frenkel syndrome.

B. Intrasurgical posterior dislocation of the lens

Nucleus drop in cataract surgery, specially in phacoemulsification has become very common.

C. Couching

Seldom practiced now, couching refers to an iatrogenic posterior dislocation of the lens which was performed as a treatment of cataract in older days.

III. CONSECUTIVE OR SPONTANEOUS DISPLACEMENT

It results from intraocular diseases giving rise to mechanical stretching, inflammatory disintegration or degeneration of the zonules. A few common conditions associated with consecutive displacements are: hypermature cataract, buphthalmos, high myopia, staphyloma, intraocular tumours, uveitis, retinitis pigmentosa and retinal detachment.

TOPOGRAPHICAL TYPES OF LENS DISPLACEMENTS

Topographically, displacements of the lens may be classified as subluxation and luxation or dislocation.

I. SUBLUXATION

It is partial displacement in which lens is moved sideways (up, down, medially or laterally), but remains behind the pupil. It results from partial rupture or unequal stretching of the zonules (Figs 6.2 and 6.5).

Clinical features

Clinical features are:
- *Defective vision* occurs due to marked astigmatism or lenticular myopia.

- *Uniocular diplopia* may result from partial aphakia.
- *Anterior chamber* becomes deep and irregular.
- *Iridodonesis* (tremulous iris) is usually present.
- Dark edge of the subluxated lens is seen on distant direct ophthalmoscopy.

Complications

Complications of subluxated lens include:

- Cataractous changes
- Uveitis
- Complete dislocation into anterior chamber or pupil which may cause papillary block and angle closure secondary glaucoma, and
- Complete dislocation into the vitreous.

Management

A. *Non-surgical management*

1. *Spectacle or contact lens correction* for phakic or aphakic area (whichever gives better visual results) is helpful in many cases. *Reading aid* is often necessary because the subluxated lens lacks sufficient accommodation.
2. *Miotics/mydriatics* may be tried to give better visual results as per individual case.
3. *Laser pupiloplasty* has been tried with controversial results.

B. *Surgical management*

Indications are:

- *Decreased visual acuity*, uncorrectable by spectacles or contact lens due to either irregular astigmatism, large lenticular astigmatism, or peripheral aberration or cataractous changes.
- *Progressive posterior subluxation*, and
- *Dislocation of lens into the anterior chamber*

Surgical options for subluxated lens, each having its own indication, include:

- Lensectomy with anterior vitrectomy
- Phacoemulsification with CTR, with PCIOL
- Intracapsular lens extraction with scleral fixation PCIOL
- Intracapsular lens extraction with ACIOL.

For details *see* page 186–188.

II. DISLOCATION OR LUXATION OF THE LENS

In it, all the zonules are severed from the lens. A dislocated lens may be:

- Incarcerated into the pupil, or
- Present in the anterior chamber (Fig. 6.5B), or
- Present in the vitreous (Fig. 6.5C) (where it may be floating – *lens nutans;* or fixed to retina – *lens fixata),*
- Present in the subretinal space, present in subscleral space or
- Extrude out of the globe, partially or completely.

Clinical features

Clinical features of posterior dislocation include:

- Deep anterior chamber

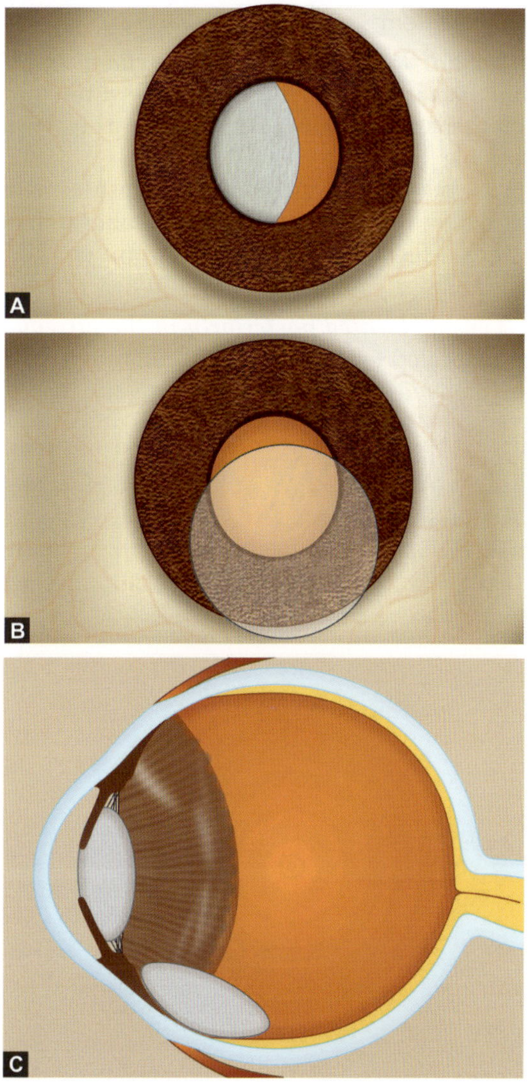

Fig. 6.5. *Diagrammatic depiction of displacements of lens: **(A)** Subluxation; **(B)** Anterior dislocation; **(C)** Posterior dislocation.*

- Aphakia in pupillary area
- Iridodonesis
- Ophthalmoscopic examination reveals lens in the vitreous cavity.

Clinical features of anterior dislocation are:
- Deep anterior chamber, and
- Presence of lens in the anterior chamber. Clear lens looks like an oil drop in the aqueous.

Complications

Complications associated with dislocated lens are *uveitis* and *secondary glaucoma.*

Management

A. ***Lens dislocated in the anterior chamber and that incarcerated in the pupil,*** constitutes an emergency and should be removed as early as possible.

Surgical options include intracapsular lens extraction with either anterior chamber IOL or scleral fixated posterior chamber IOL implantation.

B. ***Lens dislocated posteriorly in the vitreous.*** A dislocated lens from the vitreous cavity can be removed after total vitrectomy and use of perfluorocarbon liquids (PFCL) followed by any of the following methods:
- With the help of an insulated vitreous cryoprobe, or
- By aspiration facility of vitrectomy probe (only soft cataract), or
- With phacofragmentation.

Visual rehabilitation can be achieved by any of the following methods:
- Sclera fixated posterior chamber IOL, or
- Use of anterior chamber IOL, or
- Use of contact lens.

BIBLIOGRAPHY

1. Bilateral dislocation of the lens. SN Mitter. Br J Ophthalmol 40(4):253;1956 April.
2. Duker, Jay S; Myron Yanoff MD; Yanoff, Myron; Jay S. Duker MD. Ophthalmology; 2009. St. Louis, Mo: Mosby/Elsevier. ISBN 0-323-04332-1.
3. Eifrig CW, Eifrig DE. "Ectopia Lentis". eMedicine. com. November 24, 2004.
4. Peter Nicholas Robinson; Maurice Godfrey (2004). Marfan syndrome: a primer for clinicians and scientists. Springer. p.5. ISBN 978-0-306-48238-0. Retrieved 12 April 2010.

CATARACT SURGERY

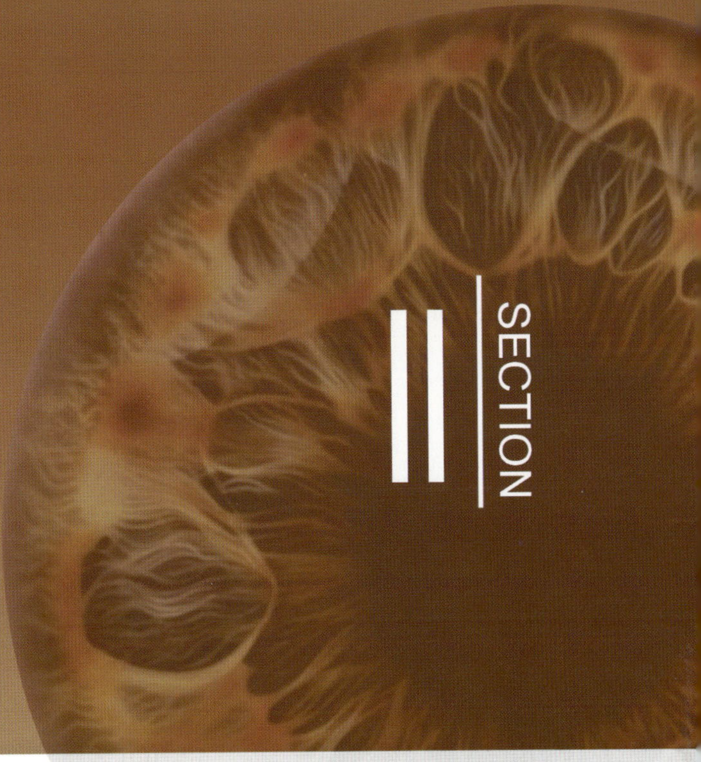

SECTION II

EVOLUTION OF CATARACT SURGERY

7 CHAPTER

EVOLUTION OF SURGICAL TECHNIQUES

Over the period, cataract surgery has evolved from couching to the latest femtosecond laser-assisted microincision cataract surgery (MICS). Before embarking on the intricacies of the present day cataract surgery, it will be worthwhile to briefly review the history of cataract surgery which can be considered under following phases:

- Era of Couching (600 BC to 18th century)
- Era of early extracapsular cataract extraction (1745–1877)
- Era of intracapsular cataract extraction (1877–1980)
- Evolution of modern extracapsular cataract extraction:
  - Planned ECCE
  - Phacoemulsification
  - Manual small incision cataract surgery (M-SICS)

ERA OF COUCHING

Era of couching started in 600 BC when ***Sushruta*** from India popularized its practice. This is the first documented surgery of cataract in the literature. Soon it became popular in the Egypt, Greek, Roman, medieval Europe sub-Saharan Africa and remained popular worldwide till 18th century. It was practised in some remote areas of the world even in the 19th century.

Definition of couching

The term couching, derived from the French word *'couche'* which means 'to put to bed' refers to displacement of the abnormal material obstructing vision. In the ancient literature, the terms 'Reclination' and 'Depression' have been used as synonyms for couching describing the surgical procedure consisting of pushing the lens into the vitreous cavity.

Procedure of couching

The couching was practiced in fully mature and hypermature cataracts. The surgeon used to sit in front of the patient with an assistant

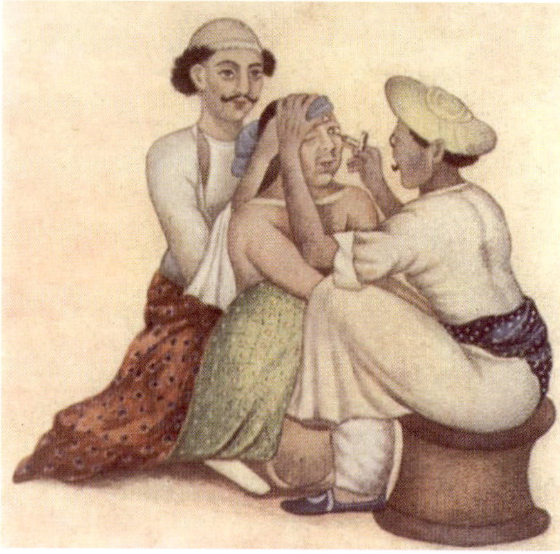

Fig. 7.1. *Painting depicting position of surgeon, patient and assistant during couching.*

holding the patient's head from behind while opening the eyelids (Fig. 7.1). The technique involved making a hole (sclerotomy) somewhere posterior to the corneoscleral junction followed by pushing the cataractous lens inferiorly with the help of the so-called couching needle (Fig. 7.2). Later many surgeons started using two instruments—a sharp one to make sclerotomy and another blunt instrument to produce disinsertion of the zonular fibres without breaking the capsule. The surgery was performed without anaesthesia and asepsis. The surgeons used to travel from town to town to perform the surgery.

Outcome and complications

Immediately following surgery, the bilaterally blind patient used to get some useful vision.

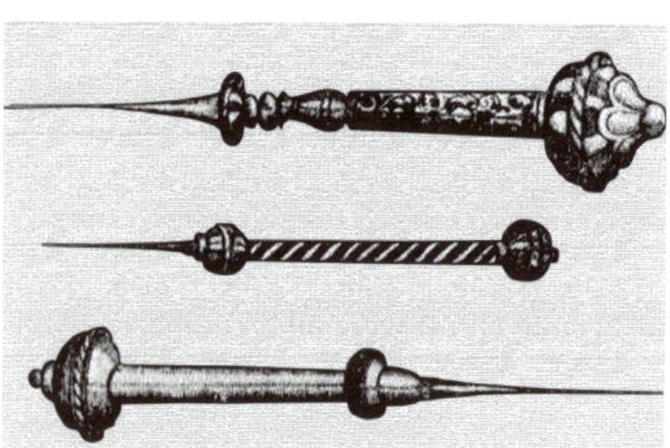

Fig. 7.2. *A set of couching needles.*

These miraculous results made the procedure popular. However, over the period, many patients used to develop complications such as lens matter induced inflammation, infection and raised intraocular pressure. In spite of frequent complications, the technique remained prevalent throughout the millennia until the arrival of knowledge derived from dissection and the study of the anatomy of the eyeball.

ERA OF EARLY EXTRACAPSULAR CATARACT EXTRACTION (1745–1877)

Daviel in 1745 made the first attempt to remove the cataract rather than displacing it inside the eye. He performed a limbal section in the lower half of the eye with a triangular knife and enlarged this incision either with scissors or a blunt-ended knife. The corneal flap was lifted, the capsule incised and the cataract was extracted by applying pressure to the eyeball (Fig. 7.3). The complications like infection, wound healing, prolapse of uveal tissue and vitreous, and lens matter induced inflammation were deterrent to the widespread practice of Daviel's extracapsular cataract extraction (ECCE). This technique was performed by many surgeons between 1750 and 20th century with many improvizations.

von Graefe in 1865 made a number of technical improvements which increased the surgical outcome (Fig. 7.4). He made following contributions:

- Designed the so-called Graefe' cataract knife (which remained very popular for a long time over making ab-interno incision in extracapsular as well as later in intracapsular technique),
- Made the section in the superior limbus, and
- Advocated the iridectomy to prevent pupillary block glaucoma.

Williams (1867) was the first to use a corneal suture, and since then many variations in the application of sutures have been described with the advantages of finer sutures and materials giving more accurate and secure wound healing.

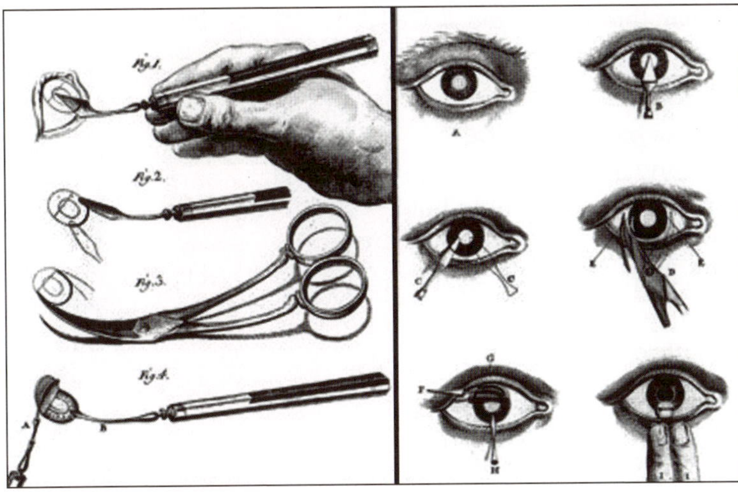

Fig. 7.3. *Daviel's method of extracapsular cataract extraction.*

ERA OF INTRACAPSULAR CATARACT EXTRACTION (1877–1980)

Because of the increased incidence of lens matter induced inflammation, pupillary membrane (after cataract) formation and rise of IOP (secondary glaucoma), following extracapsular cataract extraction, efforts started to remove the lens in its entirety.

Samuel Sharp (1773), an Englishman was the first surgeon to advocate intracapsular cataract extraction (ICCE), through a limbal incision using pressure from his thumb. However, this technique did not become popular for the coming next 100 years.

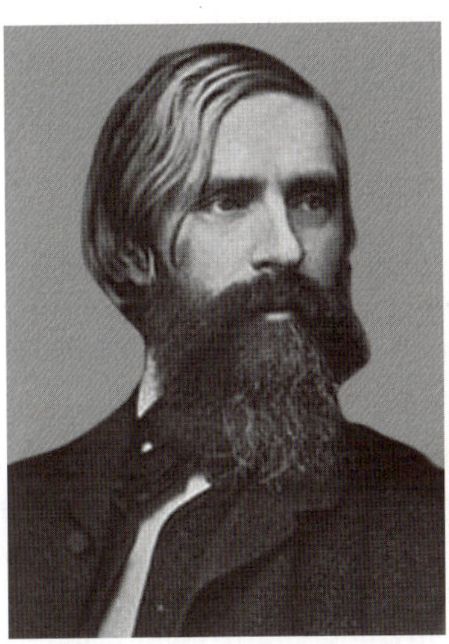

Fig. 7.4. *Prof. Albrechi von Graefe (1828–1870).*

Pagenstecher (1877) popularized the technique of ICCE. He advocated the delivery of lens complete in its capsule by indenting the cornea in front of the limbus below with fixation forceps and depressing the scleral edge of the section above so as to introduce a spatula behind the lens.

Established techniques of intracapsular cataract extraction

The intracapsular cataract extraction reached the height of its popularity in the beginning of 19th century and remained popular until around 1980. Over the years, various techniques of ICCE were evolved and established.

1. *Smith-Indian expression technique (1910)*

Col. Henry Smith, an English ophthalmologist, while serving in Punjab, India described his expression technique of ICCE in 1910 known as 'Smith-Indian operation'. This technique remained very popular throughout the era of ICCE. Surgical technique of this method is described at pages 186–187.

2. *Capsule forceps method*

Stanculeam (1911), Knopp (1914), Torok (1916) and Elshnig (1924) were all great masters who developed the technique of ICCE using various patterns of capsule forceps. In later years, Arruga, Verhoff, and Kirby added much to the capsule forceps technique of ICCE. This technique also remained very popular throughout the ICCE era. The surgical technique of this method is described in Chapter 13 page 187.

3. *Barraquer's erysiphake method of ICCE*

Barraquer (Fig. 7.5) in 1917 devised suction cap-like device called erysiphake (Fig. 7.6) to hold the lens by pneumatic suction and extract with traction or tumbling. This technique gained limited popularity.

4. *Cryoextaraction method of ICCE*

Introduced in 1961 by the Polish ophthalmologist Tadeusz Krawawics and later refined by many workers led to the discovery of a cryo-machine (Fig. 7.7) for cataract extraction. This technique became very popular all over the world soon after its description and became the preferred choice till the end of era of ICCE. The technique of cryoextraction is described in Chapter 13, page 187.

Use of L-chymotrypsin to dissolve the zonules (advocated by Barraquer in 1959) became popular especially in patients with strong zonules and markedly reduced the incidence of vitreous prolapse and accidental rupture of the lens capsule in ICCE. Cryoextraction of the lens with the use of L-chymotrypsin became very safe and very popular method of ICCE.

5. *Wire vectis method*

This method was developed to extract the subluxated and dislocated cataractous lenses (page 188).

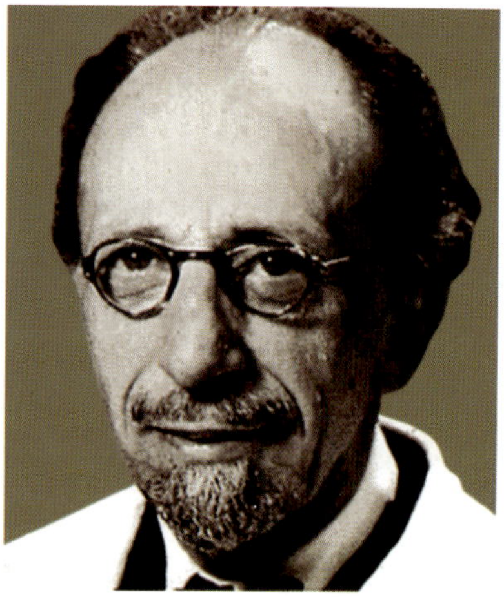

Fig. 7.5. *Prof. Ignacio Baraquer (1884–1965).*

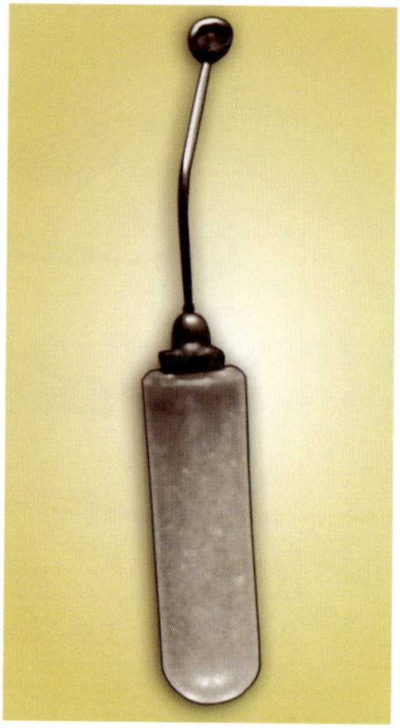

Fig. 7.6. *Erysiphake.*

Place of ICCE in the present scenario

Intracapsular cataract extraction (ICCE) still has a place in today's surgical environment, but that place is restricted mainly to eyes with dislocated or subluxated crystalline lens in the first world environment. Unfortunately, there are places in the world where ICCE is still performed.

EVOLUTION OF MODERN EXTRACAPSULAR CATARACT EXTRACTION

The ICCE has stood the test of time and had been widely employed for about 100 years (1877–1980) all over the world. From 1945 onwards, at many places, the planned ECCE was being practised and both ICCE and planned ECCE were equally popular till early 1980s. However, since 1980 over the years, the ICCE has been almost entirely replaced by planned extracapsular cataract extraction (ECCE) because of the evolution of modern techniques with obvious advantages.

Established techniques of ECCE

The ECCE techniques have improved greatly with the availability of newer instruments, use of microscopes, better techniques of anterior capsulotomy, and improved infusion/aspiration modalities.

In true sense, the term 'extracapsular cataract extraction' includes all the techniques of cataract extraction mentioned below in which posterior capsule is left intact. Therefore, the different techniques of ECCE, which have evolved and established over the years, include the following:

- Planned modern ECCE procedure
- Phacoemulsification
- Manual small incision cataract surgery (SICS).

Planned modern extracapsular cataract extraction

As mentioned above, extracapsular cataract extraction, strictly speaking, includes all the techniques in which posterior lens capsule is left intact. However, by convention, the term 'extracapsular or planned extracapsular cataract extraction' refers to an operation in which lens nucleus is delivered intact through a limbal incision of about 8 mm. With the introduction of microsurgical techniques, this improved modern ECCE technique was being adopted increasingly. In 1949, Sir Harold Ridley placed, with relative success, a posterior chamber intraocular lens using refined ECCE procedure. Though the IOLs did not soon become popular, but the planned ECCE had replaced the ICCE as the surgical choice for cataract over the years. The surgical steps for this technique are described in Chapter 13, pages 188–190.

Technique of lens aspiration for congenital and traumatic soft cataracts was standardized and popularized by Harold Scheie in 1960.

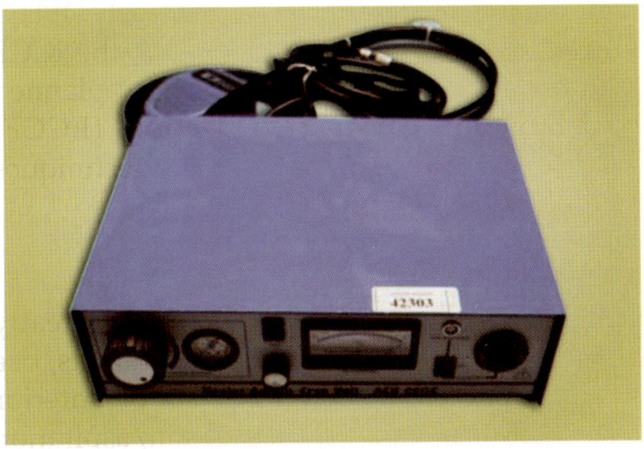

Fig. 7.7. *Cryomachine.*

Present status of planned ECCE. The planned ECCE with posterior chamber IOL implantation is still practiced by some surgeons from the developing countries with good visual results. Further, in certain circumstances, e.g. very hard black cataract, it is still considered an option all over the world.

Phacoemulsification

Charles D. Kelman introduced the concept of phacoemulsification as early as 1948, but it was accepted after 1967 and became well established and popular after 1980. The original equipment known as Cavitron-Kelman Phacoemulsifier Mark I was an equipment almost of the size of a household refrigerator (Fig. 7.8). In the last few years, tremendous advances have occurred in the phaco-machines.

The surgical technique of phacoemulsification have also evolved over the years, which are reviewed at page 256. Presently, phacoemulsification is the surgery of choice for cataract removal. In this technique, the surgery is performed through a 3 mm or smaller incision and the lens is aspirated after phacoemulsification. Phacoemulsification basically acts

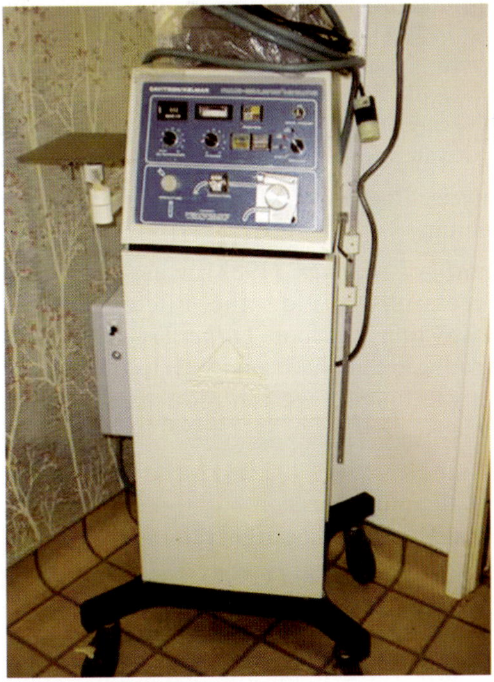

Fig. 7.8. *Cavitron-Kelman phacoemulsifier mark I.*

through a hollow 1 mm titanium needle which vibrates by piezoelectric crystal in its longitudinal axis at an ultrasonic speed of 40000 times a second thus emulsifying the nucleus.

Microincision cataract surgery. Recent advances have led to microincision cataract surgery (MICS), in which phacoemulsification can be performed through an incision below 1 mm in size.

Femtosecond cataract surgery. The US FDA cleared femtosecond laser for cataract surgery in 2010. Use of femto laser causes 43% reduction in phacoemulsification energy and 51% reduction in time which improves the safety profile.

Manual small incision cataract surgery (M-SICS)

Even after the establishment of phacoemulsification, many surgeons in early 1980s were performing planned extracapsular cataract surgery with posterior chamber IOL implantation with 5–7 sutures. It was because of the fact that the phacoemulsification machine was expensive, even unreliable, the learning curve was tedious and instrumentation-related complications were unacceptable to many surgeons. Hence, efforts were made to divide the nucleus by alternative methods intracamerally. The credit for developing manual small incision cataract surgery (M-SICS) over the years (1983–2003) goes to Keener, Fry, Kansas, Bluementhal, Mc Intyre, Carmona and Hennig.

Gerald T Keener (1983) was the first to successfully divide the nucleus using a constricting wire loop. ***Luther Fry*** subsequently introduced the phacosandwich technique. Later many techniques were introduced to divide the nucleus.

Richard Kratz (1990) introduced the concept of scleral tunnel incision for the small incision sutureless cataract surgery.

Michael Mc Farland (1990) demonstrated that the subsequent closure of scleral tunnel incision was due to posterior corneal lip which acted as one way valve imparting self-sealing characteristics.

Over the years, many modifications have been made in the incision and method of nucleus management, which are discussed in Chapter 14, pages 192–220. The credit for the presently prevalent techniques of SICS goes to the following:

- Irrigating vectis method: Steinert (1982)
- Phacofracture with wire loop: Gerald Keener (1983)
- Phacosandwich technique: Luther Fry (1985)
- Manual phacofragmentation: Kansas (1988)
- Bluementhal mini-nucleus technique: Bluementhal (1993)
- Fish-hook technique: Albrecht Hennig (1998).

EVOLUTION OF ANAESTHETIC TECHNIQUES FOR CATARACT SURGERY AND INTRAOCULAR LENSES (IOLs)

EVOLUTION OF ANAESTHETIC TECHNIQUES

Along with the advances in the techniques of cataract extraction, there occurred simultaneous advances in the techniques of anaesthesia for cataract surgery which are reviewed in the chapter on anaesthesia for cataract surgery (Pages 98–106).

EVOLUTION OF INTRAOCULAR LENSES

The marvellous success of cataract surgery occurred due to discovery of intraocular lens implantation by Sir Harold Ridley in 1949. Since then IOL designs have changed progressively. The history of IOLs is briefly reviewed in Chapter 11, Pages 151–175.

SUMMARY

The evolution of cataract surgery starting from couching till date is summarized in Table 7.1.

BIBLIOGRAPHY

1. Agapitos PJ. Cataract surgical techniques. Curr Opin Ophthalmol 2:16–27;1991.
2. Apple D. Sir Harold Ridley and His Fight for Sight: He Changed the World So That We May Better See It. Thorofare, NJ: Slack Incorporated; 2006.

Table 7.1 *Evolution of cataract surgery at a glance*

S.no.	*Technique*	*Year*	*Inventor*
1.	Couching	600 BC	Sushruta (India)
2.	Early ECCE (inferior incision)	1745	Daviel (France)
3.	Early ECCE (superior incision)	1865	Von Graefe
4.	ICCE	1877	Pogenstecher
5.	ICCE (tumbling)	1910	Col. Smith (English based in India)
6.	Planned ECCE with PCIOL	1949	Sir Harold Ridley (Britain)
7.	Phacoemulsification	1967	Charles D. Kelman (USA)
8.	Foldable IOLs	1984	Mazzooco
9.	Phacofracture with wire loop	1983	Gerald Keener
10.	Phacosandwich technique (SICS)	1985	Luthar Fry
11.	Manual phacofragmentation	1988	Kansas
12.	Capsular surgery	1992	David Apple (USA)
13.	Mini-nucleus technique (SICS)	1993	Bluementhal (Israel)
14.	Fish-hook technique (SICS)	1998	Hennig
15.	Accommodating IOLs	1997	Cummings/? Kamman
16.	Phaconit	1998	Amar Agarwal (India)
17.	MICS	1998	Alio
18.	Micro-phaco	1998	Olson
19.	Dye-enhanced cataract surgery	2000	Pandey/Werner/Apple
20.	Nd:YAG laser phacolysis (experimental)	1991	Dodick JM
21.	Erbium:YAG laser photoablation	1996	Berger
22.	Femtosecond laser phacolysis	2010	Zoltan Z. Nagy in 2008

3. Cataract Surgery in Antiquity. American Academy of Ophthalmology. 2008. http://www.aaofoundation.org/what/heritage/exhibits/online/cataract/antiquity.cfm. Accessed May 25, 2008.
4. Cataract Surgery in the Modern Era. American Academy of Ophthalmology. 2008. http://www.aaofoundation.org/what/heritage/exhibits/online/cataract/modern.cfm. Accessed May 25, 2008.
5. Linebarger EJ, Hardten DR, Shah GK, et al. Phacoemulsification and modern cataract surgery. Surv Ophthalmol 44:123–147;1999.
6. Priya Vrat Sharma, *Susruta-Samhita with English translation of text and Dalhana's commentary along with critical notes. Vol II (Kalpasthâna and Uttaratantra)* (Varanasi, India: Chaukhambha Visvabharati Oriental Publishers & Distributors, 2001), pp. 202–204.
7. Sanders DR, Sanders ML. Visual performance results after Tetraflex accommodating intraocular lens implantation. Ophthalmology 114:1679–1684;2007.
8. The History of Modern Cataract Surgery. Marvin L. Kwitko, Charles D. Kelman, Kugler Publications; 1998.
9. Vijaya Deshpande, "Ophthalmic surgery: a chapter in the history of Sino-Indian medical contacts," *Bulletin of the School of Oriental and African Studies* 63.3:370–388;2000. See also, Vijaya Deshpande, "Indian influences on early Chinese ophthalmology: glaucoma as a case study," *Bulletin of the School of Oriental and African Studies* 62.2:306–322;1999.

CHAPTER 8

ANAESTHESIA FOR CATARACT SURGERY

REGIONAL (LOCAL) ANAESTHESIA

Ocular surgery may be performed under topical anaesthesia, local block anaesthesia or general anaesthesia. Local anaesthesia is more frequently employed as it entails little risk and is less dependent upon patient's general health. It is easy to perform, has got rapid onset of action and provides a low intraocular pressure with dilated pupil. Above all, in developing countries like India, with a large number of cataract cases, it is much more economical.

Indications. Almost all ocular operations, namely, cataract extraction, glaucoma surgery, keratoplasty and other corneal surgeries, iridectomy, squint and retinal detachment surgery in adults can be performed under local anaesthesia.

Goals. The main goals of regional anaesthesia for successful ocular surgery are: globe and conjunctival anaesthesia, orbicularis akinesia, ocular akinesia and low intraocular and intraorbital pressure.

These goals can be achieved by a local anaesthesia comprising either surface anaesthesia, facial block and retrobulbar block or a combination of surface anaesthesia and peribulbar block.

HISTORICAL BACKGROUND

Historically, cataract surgery started with no anaesthesia and after completing a full cycle once again has reached to no anaesthesia cataract surgery. The events which occurred during completion of the cycle are as below:

- *No anaesthesia cataract surgery technique,* the couching, was popularized by the Indian surgeon *Sushruta* in the year 800 AD.
- *First local anaesthetic agent,* the cocaine, was discovered in the year 1884, and lidocain the most commonly used local anaesthetic agent in 1948.
- *Topical anaesthesia for eye surgery with cocaine,* for the first time, was used by *Karl Koller* in 1884 in Austria.

- *Retrobulbar block anaesthesia* was introduced by *Herman Knapp* in 1884, for the first time using 4% cocaine, for enucleation of the eye-ball.
- *Block for the peripheral branches of facial nerve* to produce orbicularis akinesia to supplement topical and subconjunctival anaesthesia was for the first time introduced by *Van Lint* in *1914*.
- *Technique of facial nerve trunk block* was introduced by *O' Brien* in 1934. He also introduced the use of procaine for retrobulbar anaesthesia.
- *Modern technique of retrobulbar anaesthesia* was introduced by *Atkinson* in 1948. He reported that larger volume of local anaesthesia can be injected without much increasing the orbital pressure by addition of *hyaluronidase*. Following this, the retrobulbar anaesthesia became very popular and remained so till the introduction of peribulbar anaesthesia in 1986. Atkinson also introduced his technique (Atkinson's block) for blocking the superior branches of the facial nerve.
- *Peribulbar block* was, for the first time, introduced by Davis and Mandel in 1986. Many workers including Wein and Deichman (1989) and Bloomberg (1999) reported further modifications in the technique. It is still the most popular technique for eye surgery.
- *Subconjunctival anaesthesia* for cataract surgery was reintroduced by Furate et al. (1990). The term *pin point anaesthesia* was introduced by Fukaswa (1992) for the subconjunctival anaesthesia for small incision cataract surgery.
- *Topical anaesthesia* using tetracain for cataract surgery by phacoemulsification was reintroduced by Fichman in 1993, and by now it has become the preferred choice by many phaco surgeons worldwide.
- *Topical plus intracameral anaesthesia* for phaco cataract surgery was introduced by Gills in 1997.
- *No anaesthesia cataract surgery* by phaco-chop technique was introduced by Amar Aggarwal in 1998.

REGIONAL ANAESTHETIC AGENTS

Regional anaesthetic agents available for use in ophthalmology can be grouped as given:

- *Esters*, e.g. procaine, oxybuprocaine (Benoxinate HCl), chlorprocaine, tetracaine, proparacaine, butacaine, and piprocaine.
- *Amides* which include: lidocain, prilocaine, mepivacaine, bupivacaine, etidocaine, and centbueridine.

Essential features of regional anaesthetic agents are summarized in Table 8.1

TECHNIQUES OF LOCAL ANAESTHESIA

Techniques of local anaesthesis used for ocular surgery include:

- Facial block,
- Retrobulber block,
- Peribulbar block,
- Sub-Tenon's anaesthesia, and
- Topical (surface) anaesthesia.

FACIAL BLOCK

For ocular surgery, it is necessary to block the facial nerve which supplies the orbicularis oculi muscle, so that patient should not squeeze the eyelids.

Orbicularis akinesia can be achieved by blocking the facial nerve at its terminal branches (van Lint block), superior branches (Atkinson block) or proximal trunk (O' Brien or Nadbath block).

1. Blocking the peripheral branches of facial nerve (van Lint's block)

This technique blocks the terminal branches of the facial nerve, producing localized akinesia of the orbicularis oculi muscle without associated facial paralysis.

In this technique, 2.5 ml of anaesthetic solution is injected in deeper tissues just above the eyebrow and just below the inferior orbital margin, through a point about 2 cm behind the lateral orbital margin, level with outer canthus (Fig. 8.1).

2. Facial nerve trunk block at the neck of mandible (O' Brien's block)

In this technique, facial nerve is blocked near the condyloid process. The condyle is located 1 cm anterior to the tragus. It is easily palpated, if the patient is asked to open and close the mouth with the operator's index finger located

Table 8.1 *Essential features of regional anaesthetic agents*

Agent	*Commercial preparation*	*Conc (%)*	*Relative potency*	*Onset of action*	*Duration of action*	*Max dose mg/kg*	*Used for type of anaesthesia*
Esters							
Procaine	Novacaine	0.5–2	1	2–5 min	1hr	14	Infiltration
2-Chloroprocaine		0.5–2		2–5 min	1–1/2 hr	14	Infiltration
Tetracaine and topical	Amethocaine	0.25–2		20 sec	12 min	1.5	Infiltration
Oxybuprocaine	Benoxinate HCl	0.4		10 sec	15 min		Topical
Proparacaine		0.5–0.75		15–20 sec	15 min	10	Topical
Butacaine		2		10–15 sec	15 min	10	Topical
Piprocaine		2		10–15 sec	15 min	10	Topical
Proxy methacaine	-	-	rapid				
Amides							
Lidocaine	Xylocaine	1–2	2	4–5	1 hr	7	Infiltration
		2–4		30 sec	10 min		
Mepiracaine	Carbocaine	1–2	2	3–5	2–1/2 hr		Topical
Bupivacaine	Sensoricaine Maracaine	0.75	8	5–10	3–5 hr	2	Infiltration
Centibucridine		0.5	15	2–5	1–1½ hr		
Levobupivacaine	-	-	-	5–10 min	3–5 hr	-	Infiltration
Prilocaine		0.5–3	8	5–15	1–3 hr	10	Infiltration
Etiducaine	Duranest	1–1.5	8	3–5	3–5 hr		Infiltration
Articaine	-	-	-				

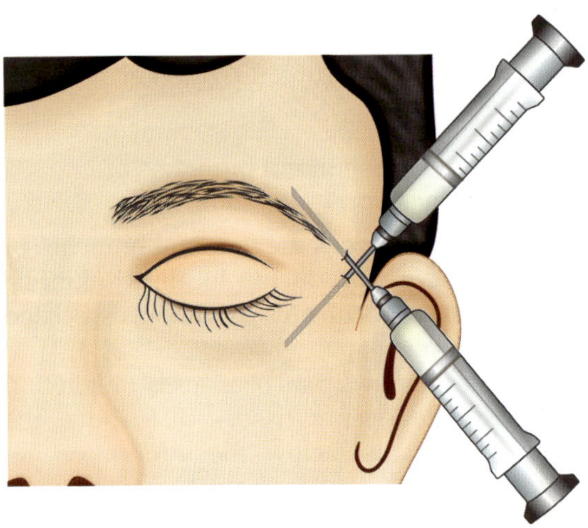

Fig. 8.1. *Technique of van Lint's block.*

across the neck of the mandible. At this point, the needle is inserted until contact is made with the periosteum and then 4–6 ml of local anaesthetic is injected while the needle is withdrawn (Fig. 8.2). This technique is associated with pain at the injection site and unwanted facial paralysis.

3. Nadbath block

In this technique, the facial nerve is blocked as it leaves the skull through the stylomastoid foramen. This block is also painful.

4. Atkinson's block

In this technique, superior branches of the facial nerve are blocked by injecting anaesthetic solution at the inferior margin of the zygomatic bone.

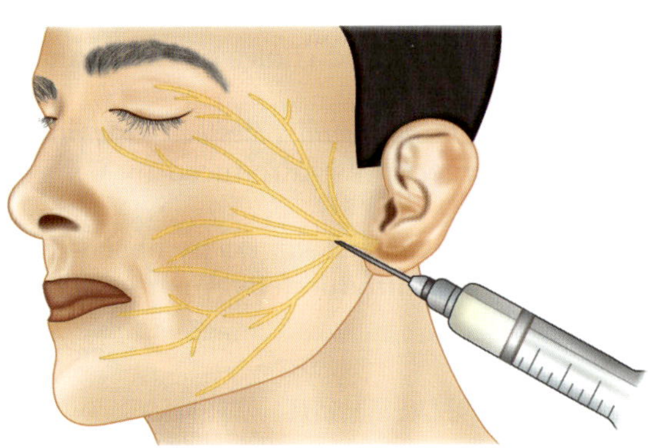

Fig. 8.2. *Diagrammatic distribution of the facial nerve and technique of O' Brien's block.*

Note. Facial nerve block may be required along with topical anaesthesia or retrobulbar block anaesthesia. However, it is sparingly used nowadays, since peribulbar block anaesthesia provides orbicularis akinesia also along with globe anaesthesia and akinesia.

RETROBULBAR BLOCK

Retrobulbar block was introduced by Herman Knapp in 1884.

Anaesthetic solution

Anaesthetic solution injected for retrobulbar block includes 2–4 ml of 2% xylocaine with added hyaluronidase 5 IU/ml and with or without adrenaline one in one lac.

Hyaluronidase *is* added for better diffusion of the anaesthetic solution to the tissues. It is an enzyme capable of depolimarizing hyaluronic acid found in the interstitial spaces. Depolimarization of hyaluronic acid allows more easily diffusion of the fluid between the tissues. It also improves the onset and quality of the block in the sub-Tenon procedure by promoting diffusion to the periorbital and retro-orbital tissues and alleviating the need for a facial nerve block, which can be painful. Hyaluronidase helps to prevent a decrease in retinal circulation, an increase in intraocular pressure (IOP) and also reduce the risk for muscle toxicity from local anaesthetic agents.

Adrenaline, 1 in 100000 concentration is added to prolong the anaesthetic effect as the adrenaline causes sufficient vasospasm to reduce significantly rate of removal of local anaesthetic agent.

Technique

It is usual to give the injection for retrobulbar block in the muscle cone (Fig. 8.3 postion A) through the inferior fornix or the skin of outer part of lower lid with the eye in primary gaze (Fig. 8.4 position A). The needle is first directed straight backwards then slightly upwards and inwards towards the apex of the orbit, up to a depth of 2.5–3 cm.

Retrobulbar block anaesthetizes the ciliary nerves, ciliary ganglion and third and sixth cranial nerves thus producing globe akinesia, anaesthesia and analgesia. The superior oblique muscle is not usually paralyzed as the fourth cranial nerve is outside the muscle cone.

Complications

Complications encountered with it include retrobulbar haemorrhage, globe perforation, optic nerve injury, and extraocular muscle palsies.

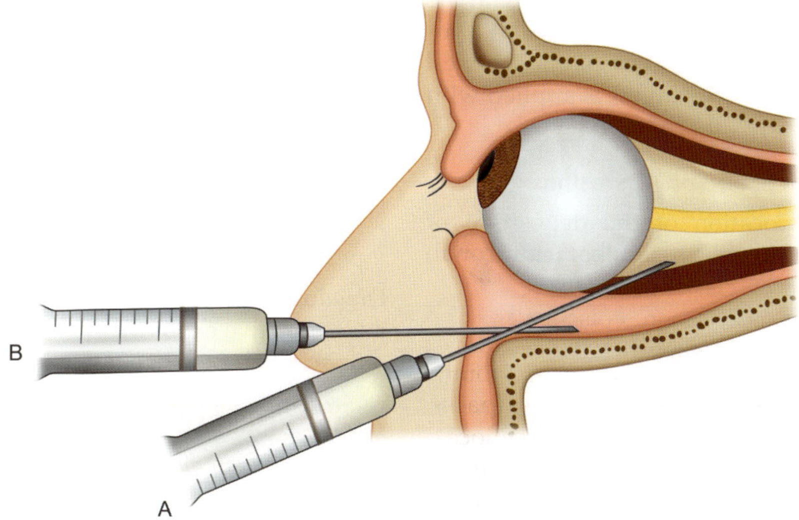

Fig. 8.3. *Position of needle:* ***(A)*** *For retrobulbar block in the muscle cone;* ***(B)*** *For peribulbar block in the peripheral orbital space.*

Note. Because of the above mentioned complications, the retrobulbar block anaesthesia is not preferred nowadays.

PERIBULBAR BLOCK

Peribulbar (extraconal) anaesthesia, described in 1986 by Davis and Mandel, has almost replaced the time-tested combination of retro-bulbar and facial blocks, because of its fewer complications and by obviating the need for a separate facial block.

Anaesthetic solution

Anaesthetic solution used for peribulbar anaesthesia consists of a mixture of 2% lignocaine, and 0.5–0.75% bupivacaine (in a ratio of 2:1) with hyaluronidase 5 IU/ml and adrenaline one in one lac. Bupivacaine increases the duration of anaesthesia and postoperative analgesia.

Technique

Primarily the technique involves the injection of 6–7 ml of local anaesthetic solution in the peripheral space of the orbit (Fig. 8.3 position B), from where it diffuses into the muscle cone and lids; leading to globe and orbicularis akinesia and anaesthesia. Classically, the peribulbar block is administered by two injections; first through the upper lid (at the junction of medial one-third and lateral two-thirds) and second through the lower lid (at the junction of lateral one-third and medial two-thirds (Fig. 8.4 position B). After injection, orbital compression for 10–15 minutes is applied with superpinky or any other method.

Classification of peribulbar anaesthesia

Based on the location of the deposition of anaesthetic solution, the peribulbar (extraconal) anaesthesia can be classified as:

- Circumocular (sub-Tenon, episcleral)
- Periocular (anterior, superficial)
- Periconal (posterior, deep)
- Apical (ultra-deep).

Efficacy and advantages

Efficacy of peribulbar anaesthesia depends on the proximity of the deposition of anaesthetic solution to the globe or the orbital apex.

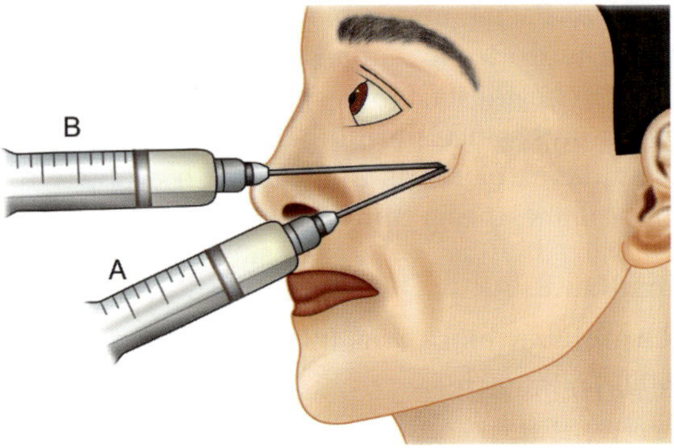

Fig. 8.4. *Position of the needle on the skin:* ***(A)*** *For retrobulbar block;* ***(B)*** *For peribulbar block.*

Advantages of peribulbar anaesthesia include:

- Provides superior globe anaesthesia and akinesia.
- Provides adequate orbicularis akinesia.
- Leads to significant reduction in pulsatile ocular blood flow and IOP, which may be of benefit in certain operations.
- Extremely low risk for globe penetration, damage to optic nerve and orbital haemorr-hage as compared to retrobulbar anaesthesia.

SUB-TENON ANAESTHESIA

In this technique, 2% lidocaine is injected into the sub-Tenon space under the effect of topical anaesthesia with 26 gauge needle. Alternatively, sub-Tenon's anaesthesia can be given using curved or flexible blunt tipped cannula after incising the conjunctiva and Tenon's capsule under topical anaesthesia.

Advantages of sub-Tenon anaesthesia include:

- Provides anaesthesia as well as globe akinesia.
- Lack of elevation of blood pressure and transitory cardiac arrhythmia
- No postoperative rise of IOP (as seen with peribulbar block)

Disadvantages include:

- Conjunctive chemosis
- Subconjunctival haemorrhage.

TOPICAL (SURFACE) ANAESTHESIA

Anaesthetic solutions

Topical anaesthesia can be achieved by topical instillation of any of the following anaesthetic solutions:

Lidocaine (xylocaine) 2–4% solution is instilled 2–3 times every 5 minutes before suegery. Due to stinging sensation produced, it is now less commonly preferred.

Proparacaine 0.5–0.75% solution, used 2–5 minutes before surgery, is one of the most commonly used agent for topical anaesthesia, because it does not cause stinging sensation.

Benoxinate HCl (oxybuprocaine) 0.4% solution, used 2–3 time 5–10 minutes before surgery, is the most suitable agent for short-term topical anaesthesia because of high degree of safety.

Tetracaine. 0.5% solution used 2–5 minutes before surgery, is also one of the most popular topical anaesthetic agents currently used in ophthalmology. However, like lidocaine, it also produces stinging sensation for 30 seconds.

Bupivacaine. 0.75% solution in used 2–3 times 5–10 minutes before surgery. It provides comparatively deep topical anaesthesia.

Alternative to eyedrops for topical anaesthesia

An alternative to eyedrops for topical application is the use of *viscous lidocaine gel*. The gel is often mixed with dilating medications, antibiotics and non-steroidal anti-inflammatory agents. It is reported that 5 ml of 2% lidocaine gel mixed with 4 drops tropicamide, 4 drops cyclopentolate 1%, 4 drops phenylephrine 10%, 10 drops moxifloxacin, and 4 drops ketorolac, applied to the operative eye twice before the surgery typically achieves excellent dilation and anaesthesia. However, drug absorption and corneal epithelial safety of this mixture have not been fully investigated.

Mechanism of action

Topically instilled anaesthetic agents block conduction of afferent nerve impulses in the cornea and conjunctiva, thereby abolishing sensation and producing local anaesthesia. Basically, the anaesthetic agents prevent the sodium flux by closing pores through which the ions migrate in the lipid layer of nerve cell membrane.

Indications and contraindications

Indications

Topical anaesthesia is used for any short duration diagnostic or surgical procedure on the eye.

Cataract surgery by phacoemulsification is being performed under topical anaesthesia by increasing number of eye surgeons. Prerequisites include informed and cooperative patient and skilled surgeon. Topical anaesthetic agents block the nerve endings in the cornea and conjunctiva only, leaving the intraocular structures in the anterior segment unanaesthetized. Thus, manipulation of the iris and stretching of the ciliary and zonular tissues during surgery can irritate the ciliary nerves resulting in discomfort. For this reason, recently, use of preservative free intracameral lidocaine as an adjunct is getting popularity.

Masket technique of topical anaesthesia for clear corneal phacoemulsification includes the use of 4% lidocaine topical drops, 0.5% tetracaine swab to the limbus and 0.5 ml of 1% preservative free lidocaine into the anterior chamber after paracentesis.

Other ocular indications of topical anaesthesia include LASIK surgery, excimer laser PRK, gonioscopy, tonometry, fundus contact lens biomicroscopy, forced duction test, electroretinography, lacrimal dilatation and irrigation, superficial foreign body removal, minor surgery of conjunctiva, suture removal, corneal epithelial debridment, etc.

Contraindications

Since topical anaesthesia does not provide akinesia and may even give inadequate sensory blockade for the iris and ciliary body, so it is contraindicated in:

- Unmotivated, uncooperative, anxious and deaf patients,
- Very hard cataract,
- Less experienced surgeon, and
- Known hypersensitivity to anaesthetic agents are other contraindications.

Advantages and disadvantages

Advantages of topical anaesthesia in cataract surgery include:

- Less cost
- Immediate visual recovery
- Avoidance of postoperative ptosis
- Avoidance of sight-threatening complications such as globe perforation, and optic nerve damage.

Disadvantages of topical anaesthesia include:

- *Toxicity to corneal epithelium* occurs by high or prolonged doses of local anaesthetic agents, and this prolongs wound healing and causes corneal erosion.
- *Clouding of cornea* occurs due to repeated administration of topical anaesthetic drops, rendering surgery more difficult.

INTRACAMERAL ANAESTHESIA

Intracameral anaesthesia is a common adjunct to topical anaesthesia in phacoemulsification. Normally preservative free lidocaine 1% is injected into the anterior chamber through the corneal incision at the beginning of the operation. It probably provides sensory blockage of the iris and ciliary body and thereby relieves discomfort experienced during IOL placement. Intracameral lidocaine alone dilates the pupil well, and this is believed to be due to the direct action of lidocaine on the iris, which in turn causes muscle relaxation. Preservative-free lidocaine 1% with 1:100 000 epinephrine enhances pupillary dilation more than lidocaine 1% alone and thus obviates the need for preoperative dilating drops.

CRYO-ANAESTHESIA

As a step towards 'drug free' anaesthesias, cold/chilled BSS has been used in patients allergic to paracaine or tetracaine. Preoperative administration of 2 drops of topical, cold BSS at 4°C gave similar results as topical anaesthesia. Along with this, came the added advantage of reduced inflammation due to decreased uveal flow and stabilization of the blood-aqueous barrier.

COMPLICATIONS OF LOCAL ANAESTHESIA

I. Local complications

The use of retrobulbar and peribulbar anaesthesias is decreasing primarily because of the increased risk and severity of complications such as globe perforation and retrobulbar haemorrhage, especially as other modalities have been found to be as effective.

1. *Orbital haemorrhage.* Orbital haemorrhage is not an uncommon complication encountered with local anaesthesia blocks. Orbital haemorrhage can be reduced by avoiding injection into the apex (vascular area), using fine and short needles (25-gauge and 25 mm needles). The use of needles longer than 31 mm is not recommended.

2. *Globe perforation.* Globe perforation is a rare complication, more likely to occur in myopic eyes (which are thinner and longer), especially when carrying out retrobulbar and peribulbar blocks. A significant proportion of globe penetrations are not detected during administration of the anaesthetic agent but are noticed following the development of hypotony, poor red reflex, and vitreous haemorrhage during surgery.

During delivery of the anaesthetic agent, patients are often asked to move their eyes from side to side to ensure that no contact with the globe has occurred. The risk with this is that a patient will move his or her head instead and in doing so run the risk of deepening the depth of penetration.

3. *Toxicity to the corneal epithelium* can occur due to high or prolonged doses of local anaesthesia and this prolongs wound healing and causes corneal erosion.

4. *Corneal cloudiness.* Repeated administration of topical local anaesthetic agents frequently sting and occasionally cause temporary clouding of the cornea, rendering surgery difficult.

5. *Persistent diplopia* lasting over a month and due to direct damage to the inferior rectus muscle, can occur as a result of the retrobulbar technique. Muscle palsy (diplopia and ptosis) can be prevented by not using high concentrations of local anaesthesia, which can become both neurotoxic and myotoxic.

II. Systemic complications

Systemic risks include:

1. *Brainstem anaesthesia* can occur with local anaesthesia. For this reason, the patient must be monitored carefully after administration of the anaesthesia and also during surgery. Symptoms such as drowsiness and loss of or confused verbal contact often suggest brainstem anaesthesia, which can lead to respiratory and cardiac arrest. The onset usually occurs within 8–10 minutes of local anaesthesia delivery. Resuscitation equipment and personnel trained to use it must be available.

2. *Oculocardiac reflex,* i.e. episodes of bradycardia provoked by eye surgery or eye manipulation are blocked when the ciliary ganglion is anaesthetized. The oculocardiac reflex is rare with local anaesthesia because blockade of the ciliary ganglion ablates the afferent oculocardiac reflex, but rapid distension of the tissues by volume or haemorrhage can occasionally provoke it.

3. *Allergic reactions.* Toxicity (arising because of overdose or intravascular injection) and allergic or vasovagal reactions are the most common complications associated with local anaesthesia and can lead to systemic complications. There have been several case reports of allergy from use of local anaesthesia or proparacaine eyedrops. Although cross-sensitization between proparacaine and other related topical ophthalmologic anaesthetic agents such as tetracaine is a rare occurrence, some studies suggest that allergic sensitization and possible cross-reaction to topical anaesthetic agents in ophthalmologists is an occupational hazard. The development of amide local anaesthetic agents has effectively reduced allergic reactions, and amides are now considered rare allergens; only about 1% alleged reactions are believed to be caused by a truly immune-mediated process. Hyaluronidase, an additive used to promote the onset and quality of the block, may rarely cause allergic reactions.

4. *Dysphagia or respiratory obstruction* can occur due to facial nerve blocks from spread of the anaesthesia to the glossopharyngeal nerve and should be used only in the presence of severe blepharospasm. Adjuvant IV anaesthetic agents for the reduction of pain are normally associated with an increase in medical events.

5. *Perioperative myocardial ischaemia* in elderly patients having cataract surgery is significantly less under local anaesthesia than general anaesthesia.

6. *Death* last but not the least, death can result from local anaesthesia as a consequence of spread of the anesthetic agent along the optic nerve sheath or intra-arterial injection of the anaesthetic solution with retrograde flow, giving rise to systemic toxicity that causes brainstem anaesthesia. This is more likely to occur with retrobulbar anaesthesia; it rarely occurs with peribulbar and short needles, as they avoid the cone of the extraocular muscles. This risk is also reduced, if short needles are used in primary gaze to avoid rotation of the needle towards the nerve, which reduces the incidence of direct trauma to the optic nerve.

GENERAL ANAESTHESIA FOR OCULAR SURGERY

INDICATIONS

- Infants and children
- Anxious and uncooperative and mentally retarded adults
- Perforating ocular injuries
- Major operations like exenteration and the patients willing for operation under general anaesthesia.

IMPORTANT CONSIDERATIONS

Important points to be considered during various steps of general anaesthesia for ocular surgery are as below:

Induction of anaesthesia should preferably be done with thiopental or propofol, since onset is smooth and safe and these agents do not cause rise in IOP. Ketamine should not be used, as it causes sustained rise of IOP, blepharospasm and eyeball movements.

Intubation. Suxamethonium (1–1.5 mg/kg body weight) should be given intravenously to ensure the adequate condition for intubation. Endotracheal intubation and controlled ventilation should be preferred.

Maintenance of anaesthesia should be achieved with oxygen and nitrous oxide (33–66%) with intermittent pancuronium and halothane (0.5–1.5%)

Halothane should be preferred since it:

- Offers rapid induction to sufficient depth, which causes small fall in IOP and is not irritating to trachea.
- Provides good operating condition, and is associated with a low incidence of post-operative nausea and vomiting.
- Allows early return of consciousness when the anaesthesia is withdrawn.
- *Intermittent positive pressure ventilation* should also be given while under anaesthesia to ensure good hypotony. Otherwise, carbon dioxide retention may lead to swelling of choroid (to many times its normal value) and prolapse of ocular contents as the eye is opened, especially in conventional surgery with IOL implantation.
- *At the conclusion of surgery reversal with intravenous neostigmine* (50 µg/kg) preceded by atropine (20 µg/kg) is done and spontaneous ventilation is established.

Extubation and recovery from general anaesthesia

- *To prevent coughing during extubation,* an adequate halothane concentration should be maintained until the closure of surgery.
- *Pharynx should be suctioned* and a few breaths of oxygen should be given followed by the removal of tube.
- *Administration of oxygen via a disposable face mask* should be ensured to all elderly patients until they are fully awaken.

Note. In perforating injuries and other ocular emergency cases, use of suxamethonium should always be preferred over non-depolarizing relaxants as the risk of vomiting and regurgitation of stomach contents is less with it.

BIBLIOGRAPHY

1. Alhassan MB, Kyari F, Ejere HO. Peribulbar versus retrobulbar anaesthetsia for cataract surgery. Cochrane Database of Systematic Reviews, 16, No.3; 2008. CD004083. ISSN 1469–1493X.
2. Almubrad TM, Ogbuehi KC. Clinical investigation of the effects of topical anesthesia on intraocular pressure. Clinical Ophthalmology, V.1, pp. 305–309;2007. ISSN 1177–5467.
3. Atkinson WS. Retrobulbar injection of anesthetic within the muscular cone. The Archieves of Ophthalmology, V.16, pp.494–503;1936. ISSN 0003–9950.
4. Bacon DR. Seeing an anesthetic revolution: ocular anesthesia in history. In Ocular Anesthesia, Moster MR, Azuara-Blanco A, (eds). Ophthalmology Clinics of North America, V.19, No.2, pp.151–154; 2006. ISSN 0896–1549.
5. Cass GD. Choices of local anesthetics for ocular surgery in Ocular Anesthesia, Moster MR, Azuara-Blanco A, (eds). Ophthalmology Clinics of North America, V.19, No.2, pp. 203–207; 2006. ISSN 0896–1549.
6. Chandradeva K, Nangalia V, Hugkulstone CE. Role of the anaesthetist during cataract surgery under local anaesthesia in the UK: a national survey. British Journal of Anaesthesia, V.104, No.5, pp.577–581;2010. ISSN 0007-0912.
7. Fanning GL. Orbital regional anesthesia. In Ocular Anesthesia, Moster MR, Azuara-Blanco A, (eds). Ophthalmology Clinics of North America, V.19, No.2, pp.221–232;2006. ISSN 0896–1549.
8. Feldman MA, Patel A. Anesthesia for eye, ear, nose, and throat surgery In Miller's Anesthesia Miller RD ed Churchill-Livingstone (7th ed.) p. 2189; 2010. ISBN 978-0-44306959-8, Philadelphia.
9. Fry RA, Henderson J. Local anesthesia for eye surgery. the periocular technique. Anaesthesia, 45, No.1, pp.14–17;1990. ISSN 1365–2044.
10. McGoldrick KE, Gayer SI. Anesthesia and the eye. In Clinical anesthesia (5th ed.) Barash PG, Cullen BF, Stoelting RK (eds). Lippincott Williams and Wilkins, 995;2006. ISBN-13:970-07817-5745-4, Philadelphia.
11. Reah G, Bodenham AR, Braitwaite P, Esmond J, Menage MJ. Peribulbar anesthesia using a mixture of local anesthetic and vecuronium. Anaesthesia, V.53, No.6, pp. 551–554; 1998. ISSN 1365-2044.
12. Ripart, J, Nouvellon, E, Chaumeron, A. Regional anesthesia for eye surgery. Regional Anesthesia and Pain Medicine, V.30, No.1, pp.72–82,2005. ISSN 1098-7339.
13. Stevens JD. A new local anaesthesia technique for cataract extraction by one quadrant sub-Tenon's infiltration. British Journal of Ophthalmology, V.76, No.11, pp.670–674;1992. ISSN 1468-2079.

BIOMETRY: CALCULATION OF IOL POWER

CHAPTER 9

INTRODUCTION

Calculation of accurate IOL power is an important step in modern cataract surgery with successful IOL implantation. The refractive power of the pseudophakic is final, and the patient must live with any mistake committed or be subjected to repeat operation, i.e. the removal/replacement of the IOL with all the potential risks. Later correction, in other words, can only be achieved with lens exchange or extraocular aids like glasses or contact lenses, or corneal refractive surgery.

To ensure that patients will have the optimal correction, the power of the lens to be implanted must be determined individually in every case. The development of modern ultrasonography units has made it possible to conveniently and accurately measure the AL of the eye. In the absence of ultrasonography in the past, IOL power was determined using an intelligent guess-work approach. However, now various formulae have been developed to calculate the IOL power on the basis of various measurements (biometry).

CRUDE IOL POWER CALCULATIONS IN THE PAST

In the 1980s, IOL power was a guesswork based on the patient's previous refractive status. However, ethically as well as legally 'guess-work' approach for calculating IOL power should not be employed presently since it is a far less accurate method, and its widespread use rapidly revealed that there were occasional unexpected and unsatisfactory results, deviating very widely from the targeted final refraction.

GUESSWORK APPROACH

The use of 'guesswork' approach for determining IOL power in the past led to the development of following concepts:

- IDEM lenses
- Standard lens
- Emmetropia lens

Note. These concepts have no place in the present day practice. However, they are described here as historical events and to help us in odd situations.

IDEM LENSES

These lenses are so named since the pre- and postoperative refraction with them is the same. Therefore, IDEM lenses were recommended for the patients who were emmetropic before the onset of cataract. Gernet and Zorkendorfer (1982) have shown that the refractive power of the natural lens is 23.70 D. The cardinal plane of this lens is approximately 6 mm behind the corneal apex. The distance for the cardinal plane of the posterior chamber lens is less; that is, it is further removed from the retina. In order to focus parallel rays of light on the retina, it must be weaker than the natural lens. Therefore, a 20 D artificial lens in the posterior chamber will restore the preoperative refractive error. Similarly IDEM lenses can be calculated for other sites of implantation as shown in Table 9.1. Here, it is must to mention an important limitation. An IDEM artificial lens will restore the preoperative refractive error, only if the natural lens indeed had about 23.70 D refractive power. This, however, is not always the case. The refractive power of an eye is the result of the combination of different factors, such as the corneal curvature, the distance of lens from the cornea (the depth of anterior chamber), the dioptric power of the lens and the length of the eye. Each of these values can deviate and still an eye can be emmetropic as the different components compensate for each other. Therefore, deviations of 2 D are common and of more than 3 D are rare with the concept of IDEM lens.

STANDARD LENS

The standard lens is one that is approximately 2 D stronger than the IDEM lens, thereby rendering the pseudophakic eye about 1.5 D myopic as compared to preoperative emmetropic refraction. Since 80% of eyes are less than 1 D nearsighted or farsighted, this will be a correct, or at least not an incorrect, result for the majority of patients. Further, in emmetropic patients, these were useful in keeping a balance between the distance and near visions. Because these lenses were the most commonly used implants, they were called standard lenses.

- The standard PCIOL had a refractive power of +22.0 D.
- The standard ACIOL had a refractive power of 20 D.

One has to know, however, that the standard lens is good only for a majority of, but by no means for all, eyes.

EMMETROPIA LENS

The emmetropia lens was used with the intention of restoring emmetropic status in previous ammetropic patients. The power of an 'emmetropia lens' was calculated by multiplying primary refractive error by 1.25 and then adding (for hypermetropia) or subtracting (for myopia) this number from the IDEM lens power. Thus,

- *Power of emmetropia lens in hypermetropic patients.* Power of IDEM lens + (Preoperative refractive error × 1.25).
- *Power of emmetropia lens in myopic patients.* Power of IDEM lens – (Preoperative refractive error × 1.25).

For this, a careful history has to be taken, including the kind of glasses the patient wore

Table 9.1 *Power of different IDEM lenses*

Description of lens	*Description of lens in short*	*Power (D)*
1. Angle-supported lenses	AACl	+17.0
2. Iris clip lenses	ACL	+18.0
3. Iris plane lenses		+19.0
4. Posterior chamber lens (convexity of optic: anterior)	PCL	+20.0
5. Posterior chamber lens (nodal point closer to retina than with PCL)	PPCL	+21.0
6. Posterior chamber lens (convexity of optic: posterior)	PPPCL	+22.0

comfortably in the past. Old refractive values should be accepted only if they come from reliable records or unequivocal history, or if they match our clinical findings. However, as mentioned in 'IDEM lens' description, deviation of 2–3 D is not rare; therefore, using primary refraction as the basis to determine the power of IOL to be implanted also entails the possibility of significant errors.

IOL POWER CALCULATION WITH BIOMETRY

With the advent of mini-science of biometry, now it is possible to calculate the power of IOL fairly accurately. *Three major components of IOL power calculation* are:

- Biomerty,
- Formulae for calculating IOL power
- Clinical variables.

Other aspects for IOL power calculation in the biometry are:

- IOL power calculation in special situations.
- Biometry: Important considerations

BIOMETRY

Biometry essentially includes:

- Keratometry (K-reading), i.e. measurement of refracting power of corneal
- Measurement of axial length (AL)
- Effective IOL position.

I. MEASUREMENT OF REFRACTING POWER OF CORNEA

The central corneal power is the second most important factor in the calculation formulae, with a 1.0 D error in corneal power resulting in 1.0 D postoperative refractive error. Central corneal power can be measured by:

- *Keratometry or corneal topography*, neither of which measures the corneal power directly.
- *Pentacam* is relatively new imaging system that uses a single Scheimpflug camera to measure the radius of curvature of the anterior and posterior corneal surfaces, as well as corneal thickness, for the calculation of corneal power.
- *Galilei*, an another device, which measures corneal power in a similar fashion as pentacam.

Keratometry

It is the most frequently used method to measure the refractive power of cornea.

Important points to be considered for keratometry are summarized here:

- The keratometer should be *calibrated* for each observe.
- Should be ideally *reclibrated after 20* cases for single observer.
- Adjust eyepiece to make mires coincide.
- Always do keratometry first before tonometry or any other corneal contact procedures.
- While performing keratometry, the patient should be instructed to look into the keratometer. Majority of the patients with immature cataracts can fixate the reflection of their own eye, so they should be instructed to fixate into the centre of this reflection. Patients with mature cataract can be instructed to fixate the pin with the other eye.
- Mires should be focused in the centre of the eye to take care of the refractive error of the observer.
- Both the minus signs and the vertical component of the plus signs should be superimposed completely. If there is any angle between them, rotate the keratometer till they can be completely superimposed.
- Keratometry may be difficult or impossible in conditions with irregular or distorted corneal surface. In such cases, keratometric readings of opposite eye may be used or K-reading may be calculated from the corneal topography map.

Re-measure the corneal curvature of both eyes, if:

- Corneal curvature is *less than 40 D* or *more than 47 D*.
- The difference in corneal cylinder is *more than 1 D* between eyes.
- The corneal cylinder correlates *poorly with the refraction cylinder*.

II. MEASUREMENT OF AXIAL LENGTH AND ESSENTIALS OF BIOMETERS

Axial length is the most important factor in biometric calculations. As 1 mm error in AL measurement results in a refractive error of approximately 2.35 D in a 23.5 mm eye, the error with wrong AL assessment being less in case of longer eyes as compared to shorter eyes.

METHODS OF MEASUREMENT OF AXIAL LENGTH

1. ***Ultrasonic measurement*** of axial length can be made by applanation method or immersion technique, the latter being more accurate. A-scans measure the time required for a sound pulse to travel from the cornea to retina. In eyes more than 25 mm, staphyloma should be suspected especially when multiple disparate readings are obtained. To measure these eyes and to obtain the true measurement to the fovea, a B-scan technique must be used.

2. ***Optical measurement of axial length*** uses partial coherence laser. The IOL master measures time required for infrared light to travel to the retina. This technique does not require contact with the globe, so corneal compression artifacts are eliminated.

Essentials of a biometer

Settings of the biometer

Calibration check. The calibration of the biometer using the model eye provided with it should be checked from time to time to ensure accuracy. Instructions for the calibration check are specific and are provided with each instrument by the manufacturer.

Gain or sensitivity setting. Gain refers to the electronic amplification of the sound waves received by the transducer. The amplification factor is called a decibel (dB).

- Normal setting of gain is 70% in most of the biometers.
- Increase in gain may be required when the height of echoes achieved is inadequate as in very dense cataracts, other ocular opacities and high myopia. Increase in the gain produces taller echoes.
- Decrease in the gain is done when artefacts are seen near the retinal echoes, e.g. in silicone-filled eyes and pseudophakic eyes.

Sound velocity setting should be done appropriately according to the type of eye, i.e.

- Normal,
- Cataractous (mild, moderate or dense),
- Aphakic, and
- Pseudophakic (silicone or acrylic)

Note. Change in the sound velocity due to materials like silicone oil in the eye can produce an error of 3–4 D.

Operative instructions

Operative instructions to be kept in mind while performing the A-scan for measuring AL are as follows:

Placing of probe on the anaesthetized cornea should be such that:

- It points towards macula, this is specially important in myopes, who may have a staphyloma.
- There is no fluid bridge between the probe and cornea.
- Cornea should not be depressed, otherwise it will result in inadvertent shortening of AL.

Mode settings may be manual or automatic, depending on the operator's preference:

- Manual mode setting allows the examiner to choose the best echo pattern produced by the eye. However, there may be delay in pressing the foot pedal, and one may miss the right reading.
- Automatic mode is operated by a software algorithm inside the instrument which controls the interpretation of echo pattern. Most of the surgeons use this mode. It is particularly useful in uncooperative patients.

Note. (1) It is always better to have an observer who should decide whether the best echo pattern has been selected by the automatic mode or not. In this way, one can have advantage of manual dynamic biometry as well as that of static graph of automatic biometry. (2) AL of both eyes should be measured for comparison.

Characteristics of a good scan

A-scan produces one-dimensional images in which echo strengths are displayed as vertical deflections or spikes of varying heights, on a display screen. Characteristics of a good scan are:

- Corneal echo is seen as a tall single peak.
- Aqueous chamber does not produce any echo.
- Anterior and posterior lens capsules produce tall echoes.
- Vitreous cavity produces few to no echoes.
- Retina produces tall, sharply rising echoes with no staircase at the origin.
- Orbital fat produces medium to low echoes.

The echo heights show the quality of the scan. The person doing the scan should be aware of it and check whether the echo heights are adequate:

- Anterior lens echo is 90% or more of maximum height.
- Posterior lens echo is between 50% and 75% of maximum height.
- Retinal echo is 75% or more of maximum height.
- In addition check, whether each rise angle is clear; the take off of the retinal spike must be clean and form a 90° angle from the baseline.

To get good results, obtain at least three scans (ideally 5–10) on each eye that are within 15 mm of one another. Average the 5–10 most consistent results giving the lowest standard deviation (ideally <0.06 mm).

Selection of the scan

The scan with the maximum AL, within the range obtained, should be selected.

Measure the axial length of both eyes, if:

- Axial length measurement *is less than 22 mm or more than 25 mm* in either eye.
- The difference between the two eyes is *more than 0.3 mm.*

III. EFFECTIVE IOL POSITION

Effective IOL position is influenced by several factors:

1. ***Anatomical factors*** include axial length, the steepness of cornea, limbal white to white measurement, preoperative anterior chamber depth and lens thickness. Holladay showed in a study that the depth of anterior chamber had a positive and partial relationship to the limbal white-to-white measurement.

2. ***IOL-related factors*** include shape, length, flexibility, anterior angulation (if any) and the material of the haptic of IOL.

3. ***Surgeon-related factors.*** Surgeon's individual surgical technique can also influence the effective lens position (ELPo).

4. ***Bag to sulcus shift*** in situations like posterior capsule rent or loss of anterior capsule integrity, the IOL needs to be placed in ciliary sulcus instead of the normal "in the bag" position. This requires deduction from the calculated IOL power in order to compensate for increase in effective IOL power, depending upon the base power of IOL, empirically taken 0.50–0.75 D less by most surgeons.

OPTICAL BIOMETERS

The introduction of optical biometry has significantly improved the accuracy of AL measurement from 0.12 mm in immersion ultrasound to 0.02 mm in optical methods. The fact that the retinal pigment epithelium is the end-point of an optical measurement (refractive AL), whereas the interface between the vitreous and the neuroretina is the end-point of an ultrasonic measurement (anatomical AL), makes measurements by optical methods longer than those taken with ultrasound. In general, optical biometers are reported to give accurate measurement of IOL power as compared to conventional A-scan biometry. However, in eye with dense cataract and posterior staphyloma the AL measurement is more accurate with immersion A/B- scan (Holladay or Shamma's method) than with optical biometer. Commercially available optical biometer include the following:

IOL MASTER

IOL MASTER 500

IOL Master 500 (Zeiss Humphrey System) is a combined biometric instrument that measures quickly and precisely parameters of human eye needed for IOL power calculation by a non-contact technique. It also incorporates the software to calculate IOL power from various formulae.

Working Principle

It is a non-contact optical device that measures the various parameters based on the following principles:

1. ***AL measurement*** is based on a patented interference optical method known as 'partial coherence interferometry (PCI)'. This technique relies on a laser Doppler technique to measure the echo delay and intensity of infrared light reflected back from the tissue interfaces – cornea and retinal pigment epithelium. The instrument is calibrated against the ultrahigh resolution 40 MHz Grieshaber Biometric System. An internal algorithm approximates the distance to the vitreoretinal interphase for the equipment of an immersion A-scan ultrasonic AL.

2. ***Corneal curvature (K)*** is determined by measuring the distance between reflected light images as in conventional keratometry (principle of reflection).

3. ***Anterior chamber depth (ACD)*** is determined as the distance between the optical sections of the crystalline lens and the cornea produced by lateral slit illumination.

4. ***White-to-white*** is determined from the image of the iris.

5. ***Calculation of IOL power*** by the software incorporating internationally accepted calculation formulae.

Advantages of the IOL Master

Operative advantages

1. *Patient comfort*, as the technique involves non-contact measurements.
2. *User-friendly*, as the operator can learn the technique very quickly.
3. *Single instrument* for measuring AL, corneal curvature (K) and ACD.
4. *Cross-infection* risk is not there, as the technique is non-contact.

Technical advantages

1. *LC display* functions both for monitoring patient's eye alignment and displaying the results of calculation of IOL power.
2. *Safety features* are extensively integrated.
3. *More accurate AL measurement* as compared to A-scan (five times) of the eyes, with AL ranging between 14.0 and 40.0 mm.
4. *Specially useful in certain ocular conditions* where conventional methods are not so accurate, which include:
   - Small corneal scars
   - Anterior cortical spokes
   - Posterior subcapsular plaques
   - Other localized media capacities
   - High to extreme myopia with a type 1, peripapillary posterior staphyloma (ability to measure to the fovea in such a condition is an enormous advantage over conventional A-scan ultrasonography)
5. *Incorporates five IOL power calculating formulae* in an integrated manner. These include Haigis, Hoffer Q, Holladay, SRK-II and SRK-T formulae.
6. *Individual optimization of formulae* is possible for every user. Data of the desired lenses need to be entered in the database. On the basis of postoperative refraction results, the lens constants that are entered in the calculation formulae may be personalized (i.e. individually optimized).
7. *Biometry in patients undergone corneal refractive surgery* is possible by use of:
   - Refractive history or contact lens method

Procedure

- The procedure and operational details of the instrument are beyond the scope. The interested readers may consult the company's manual.

IOL MASTER 700

IOL Master 700 (Fig. 9.1) is a biometry device based on swept-source OCT (SS-OCT) technology that enables full-eye length tomography, providing good fixation control. It uses high frequency 1,055 nm tuneable laser source for AL, LT, ACD and central corneal thickness (CCT) measurements. Light is projected onto the cornea at three zones (1.5, 2.5 and 3.5 mm). PS and WTW are obtained using an LED light source.

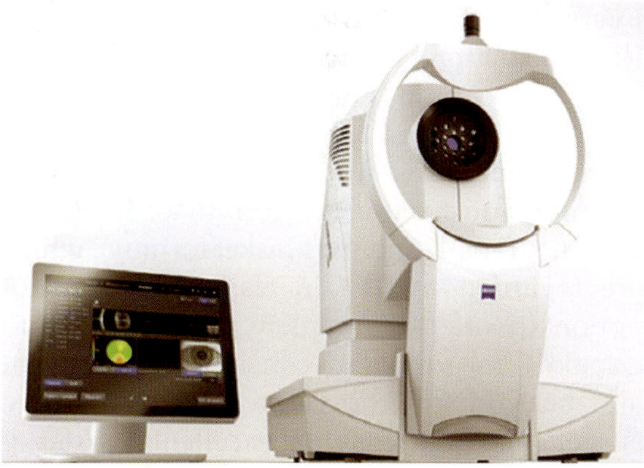

Fig. 9.1. IOLMaster 700

Advantages of IOL Master 700

- It provides 1 mm horizontal scan of the retina to ensure that the measurements are on the visual axis by using the presence of foveal pit.
- Keratometry measurements are distance dependent.
- The measurement speed of IOL Master 700 is faster than IOL Master 500.
- IOLMaster 700 high repeatability and reproducibility.
- IOLMaster 700 penetrates the opaque media better and measure the AL with fewer drop-outs compared with the LenStar and IOLMaster 500 even in dense cataracts

LENS STAR

LenStar LS900 (Haag-Streit diagnostics) provides highly accurate laser optic measurements for every section of the eye and is the first optical biometer that can measure the thickness of the crystalline lens. With its integrated Olsen formula and the optional Toric Planner featuring the Barrett toric calculator, the LenStar provides the user with latest technology in IOL prediction for any patient.

WORKING PRINCIPLE

It is a non-contact optical device which measures multiple parameters based on the following characteristics:

1. ***CCT.*** As for every other LenStar axial measurement, optical coherence biometry is used to measure CCT with stunning reproducibility of 62 mm. CCT is a key parameter in glaucoma diagnosis, and is also used for laser refractive surgery and/or to differentiate prior myopic or hyperopic LASIK procedures when there is no patient history.

2. ***Keratometry/topography.*** LenStar's unique dual zone keratometry, featuring 32 marker points, provides perfect spherical equivalent, magnitude of astigmatism and axis position, making it the biometer of choice for toric IOLs. With the optional T-Cone topography add-on, LenStar provides full topography maps of the central 6 mm optical zone that are crucial for cataract planning.

3. ***White-to-white.*** Based on high-resolution colour photography of the eye, every white-to-white measurement can be reviewed and adjusted by the user, if necessary. As such, it is fully reliable for use with anterior chamber and sulcus-fixated phakic IOLs. It can also be used to determine advanced IOL calculation formulae.

4. ***Pupillometry.*** Measurement of the pupil di-ameter in ambient light conditions can be used as an indicator for the patient's suitability for apodized premium IOLs, as well as for laser refractive procedures.

5. ***Lens thickness (LT).*** Accurate measurement of the LT is key to optimal IOL prediction accuracy when us-ing the latest IOL calculation formulae, Olsen or Holladay II. Measuring the LT with LenStar significantly improves the IOL prediction accuracy of Holladay II and leads to a different IOL power selection in 30% of cases.

6. ***ACD.*** Like all axial dimensions captured by the LenStar, ACD is measured by optical coherence biometry, providing more precision and reproducibility. This allows ACD to be measured on phakic as well as on pseudophakic eyes. Additionally, the LenStar is able to display the anatomical ACD (endothelium to anterior lens surface).

7. ***Axial length (AL).*** It uses a superluminescent diode as the laser source which enables measurement of the AL of the patient's eye, precisely on the patient's visual axis and in the presence of dense media. The user can review and move all of the measuring gate positions on the A-scan, if necessary.

8. ***Special eye conditions.*** All of the described measurements are available for use on the regular eye, as well as for aphakic, pseudo-aphakic and silicone oil-filled eyes. In case of error, users may even change the selected eye condition after completion of the measurement procedure.

Advantages

In addition to all the advantages provided by IOLMaster, LenStar also allow the user to calculate power for toric IOL implantation using Barrett toric calculator, which is incorporated in its software.

LenStar LS900

An easy-to-use manual selection of the retinal peaks in the A-scan enables the user to measure RT (distance between the ILM and the RPE) and to calculate IOL based on the individual RT. A typical value for the RT is automatically displayed and employed for IOL calculation. LenStar delivers results comparable to existing ultrasound and optical biometers.

Upgrades to LenStar LS900

Automated positioning system (APS) kit added onto the LenStar LS900 for automated dynamic eye tracking.

Easier mechanical tracking minimizes user delay and error, full measurement with single click, quicker measurement with single click, quicker measurement for improved tear stability and support T-Cone measurement through the latest through the latest EyeSuite.

T-Cone toric platform complements Len- Star's comprehensive measurement palette with true 11-ring Placido topography of the central 6 mm of the anterior cornea, and highly accurate K-readings of the 2.3 and 1.65 mm rings. This offers reassurance of axis location and determines regularity and symmetry of the astigmatism.

With the integrated Barrett toric calculator taking cornea front and back surface into account, you achieve excellent toric IOL calculation. And, the software enables you to plan the surgery on high-resolution images of the eye that can be transferred to the surgery room via EyeSuite for improved outcomes

EyeSuite IOL software offers latest generation IOL calculations such as the Hill-RBF method and Barrett and Olsen for standard IOL, enabling improved results with any patient. It further includes a comprehensive set of premium post-refractive formulae, including Barrett's True-K and the Masket formula, which are regarded as best in class. For torics, it optionally offers a complete planning suite to calculate the implant, considering the front and back of the cornea and create intuitive surgery sketches, enabling excellent transfer of the plan to surgery.

IOLMASTER VERSUS LENSTAR

The LenStar LS900 device enables to perform accurate and repetitive biometric measurements and implant power calculations. Implant calculation results obtained using the LenStar LS900 device are comparable to those achieved using the IOLMaster V.5 device, which has been commonly accepted as standard for over a decade.

- IOLMaster 500 is based on the principle of PCI with 780 nm infrared diode as the source, which emits a dual beam and a short coherence length of 160 µm. LenStar is based on the principle of low coherence reflectometry with 820 nm super luminescent diode as the light source and a 3 dB fibre coupler.
- The use of both devices is limited by significant lens opacification, posterior capsule calcification and in presence of posterior staphyloma. In such cases, additional ultrasound biometry should be performed.
- Keratometry results obtained using both devices should not be used alternatively because of the different measurement methods and different refraction indices.
- The LenStar takes two sets of keratometric readings: one at 1.65 mm and one at 2.3 mm, with 16 points each which is more accurate than IOLMaster which takes a single set at 2.5 mm with six points each.
- The LenStar LS900 device comparing to the IOLMaster additionally enables pachymetry, macular retinal thickness, lens thickens and pupil diameter measurement.

- Newer IOL power calculation formulae like the Barrett universal II formula, Olsen formula and Hill-RBF are available in LenStar LS900 but not in IOLMaster V.5.
- LenStar can also calculate power for toric IOL implantation using Barrett toric calculator, which is not possible in the case of IOLMaster.
- LenStar software runs on an external PC, which allows direct communication with electronic medical record programs; the software can automatically fill in data fields in a chosen formula.

AL-SCAN (Nidek) 2012

AL-Scan (Nidek) 2012 uses an 830 nm infrared laser diode for AL measurement with PCI. With AL-Scan in 10s, six values for cataract surgery are measured:

- AL
- Corneal curvature radius
- ACD
- CCT
- White-to-white distance
- Pupil size.

The AL-Scan incorporates a 3D autotracking and auto shot. The 3D auto tracking follows eye movements along the X–Y–Z directions to ensure accurate alignment of the eye. Once correct alignment is completed, the auto shot immediately captures the image and data.

Anterior segment observation with Scheimpflug imaging and double mire ring keratometry. The AL-Scan provides sectional lens image, pupil image and reflected image of double mire rings projected onto the cornea. It measures keratometry (K) at 36 measurement points in two circles with diameters of 2.4 and 3.3 mm, reflected from the corneal surface.

WTW and PS are obtained by analysing the image of the iris and fitting the best circle with the lowest error square to the detected edge. ACD and CCT are measured with an incorporated Scheimpflug camera with a 470 nm monochromatic light, the light source used for WTW measurements is green (wave-length 525 nm). The sectional lens image assists in the evaluation of the severity of the cataract. The pupil image assists in the assessment for multifocal IOL. The reflected image of mire rings assists in detecting an irregular corneal surface.

In cases where the optical biometer cannot measure an eye with an extremely dense cataract, the AL-Scan provides an optional built-in ultrasound biometer, allowing measurement of virtually any cataractous eye with a combined model. The AL-Scan requires no connection with an external ultrasound unit. IOL power calculation formula on AL-Scan SRK, SRK II, SRK/T, Binkhorst, Hoffer Q, Holladay 1, Formula/H, Camellin-Calossi, Shammas-PL with additional Barrett formulae available for the NAVIS-EX AL-Scan Viewer Barrett Universal II, Barrett True-K and Barrett toric calculator.

NAVIS-EX is the image filing software that enables data from the NIDEK diagnostic devices to be centralized in the NAVIS-EX database.

PENTACAM AXL WAVE (OCULUS)

The Pentacam AXL Wave (Fig. 9.2) device consists of a Scheimpflug camera which rotates around the eye and a PCI-based optical biometer. It was introduced in autumn 2015. In addition to anterior segment tomography, ACD, CCT and WTW measurements, corneal topography, anterior and posterior corneal surface and SAs, it also has integrated AL measurement. Calculation of toric IOLs is based on the total corneal refractive power and it

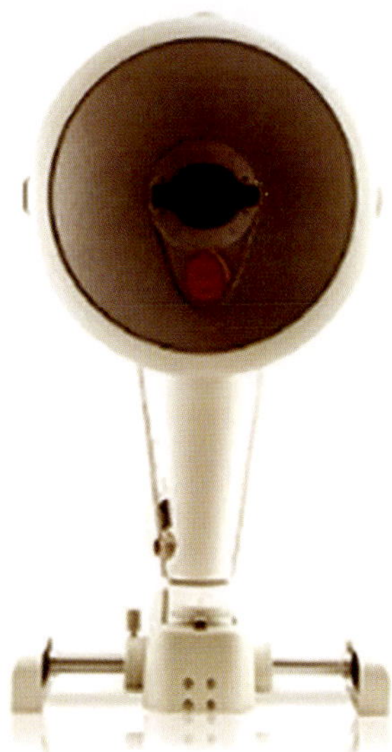

Fig. 9.2. The Pentacam AXL Wave (OCULUS)

takes into account the influence of the posterior corneal surface. The latest model, the Pentacam AXL Wave, includes a Hartmann-Shack wavefront sensor to measure total eye aberrations and objective refraction, as well as retroillumination for preoperative assessment of crystalline lens opacities in the non-dilated pupil and postoperative control of IOL position and inclination. In all, this one device performs five major functions in one measurement routine on the same measuring axis and using the same alignment navigation: objective refraction, total eye wavefront, retroillumination, optical biometry and anterior segment tomography.

ALADDIN/ALADDIN LT (TOPCON)

Aladdin/Aladdin LT (Fig. 9.3) is an optical biometer based on optical low-coherence interferometry (OLCR) with an 830 nm super luminescent diode and Placido topography system. It allows to perform eight measurements in one acquisition: AL, keratometry, corneal topography, ACD, pupillometry, WTW, CCT and LT, although the last two parameters (measured by OLCR) are available only on the Aladdin LT. Pupillometry can be measured in three modes: dynamic, photopic and mesopic. Corneal topography is based on the reflection of 24 Placido disc rings with a diameter of 8 mm. Topography-based keratometry is obtained by analysing approximately 1,024 data points of four dedicated Placido rings whose diameters range between 2.4 and 3.4 mm. Aladdin provides also Zernike analysis and keratoconus screening.

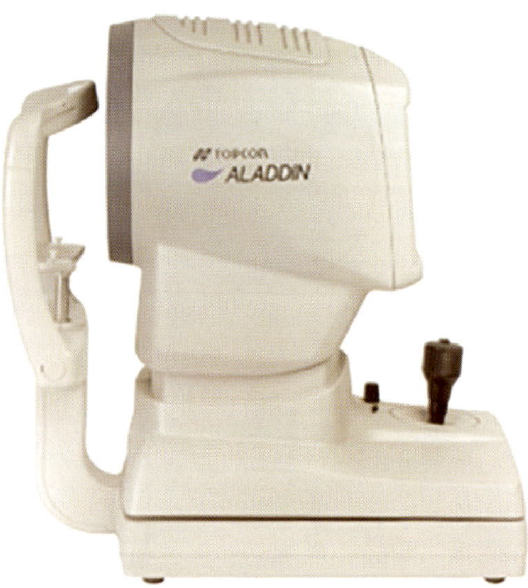

Fig. 9.3. Aladdin/Aladdin LT

OA-2000 (TOMEY)

OA-2000 (Fig. 9.4) combines Placido-disc to-pography and OLCR biometry. It measures AL, CCT, LT and ACD using the OLCR technique. Corneal curvature is measured by Placido-disc topography with nine rings each 256 points in a 5.5 mm zone projected onto the cornea. It also measures WTW and PS.

GALILEI G6 ColorZ (ZIEMER)

Galilei G6 ColorZ (Fig. 9.5) combines OLCR optical biometry, dual-Scheimpflug imaging

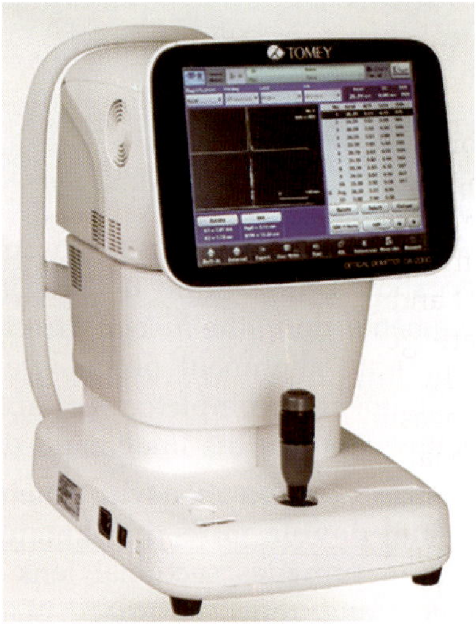

Fig. 9.4. OA-2000

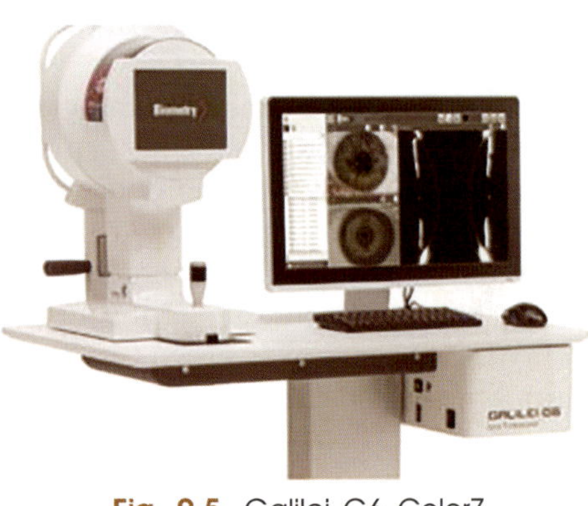

Fig. 9.5. Galilei G6 ColorZ

and Placido-disc topography measures AL, LT, ACD, CCT, corneal topography, PS and WTW. In addition to biometry, Galilei G6 provides high-definition pachymetry, total corneal wave-front, curvature and astigmatism data of the anterior and posterior cornea—complete data required to plan cataract or refractive surgery. ColorZ has high-contrast top view image in vibrant colours for more intuitive and advanced diagnostics so as to give enhanced visualization of a range of details such as blood vessels, iris pattern and pupil. Color Eye Metrics Report with improved overlays measurement in high resolution. It has new biometry software adding customized, biometry peak detection for AL measurement. Toric IOL calculator for premium IOL selection. Addition of state-of-the-art IOL calculation formulas (i.e. Barrett Universal II, Barrett Toric, Holladay II export, PANACEA export

ARGOS BIOMETER (MOVU)

Argos biometer (Fig. 9.6) uses a 1,060 nm wavelength and 20 nm bandwidth swept-source technology to collect two-dimensional OCT data of the full eye (SS-OCT). It measures AL, LT, ACD and CCT with SS-OCT. Keratometry values are generated by illumination from a ring of 16 infrared LEDs. In addition, the device measures PS by analysing the two-dimensional OCT image.

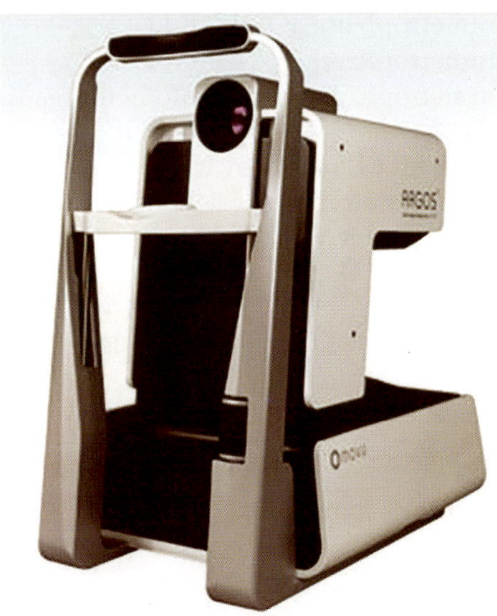

Fig. 9.6. Argos Biometer

ANTERION (HEIDELBERG ENGINEERING)

Anterion (Fig. 9.7) utilizes the power of high-resolution SS-OCT images to provide the most important anterior segment examinations and measurements in one modular, upgradeable platform. The single workflow-efficient solution brings together corneal topography and tomography, anterior segment metrics, AL measurement and IOL calculation to transform the day-to-day routine of busy practices and clinics.

SS-OCT that uses a 1300 nm wavelength with a scanning rate of 50,000 scans/s, 14 mm scan depth and 10 mm of axial resolution. Anterior and posterior corneal curvature is measured using 65 B-scans on 8 mm considering an RI of 1.3375 and 1.376, respectively. It measures the horizontal WTW distance using an 820 to 890 nm LED light source.

APPLICATIONS

1. **Cornea applications.** Generate high-resolution images and detailed maps, including camera image, OCT image, anterior and posterior axial curvature maps, tangential maps, elevation maps, total corneal power map, corneal wave-front maps and pachymetry map.
2. **Cataract applications.** The data obtained in the cornea analysis combined with the ACD and width, LT and AL determines the parameters for IOL calculations. View the camera image and OCT image to confirm your measurements.
3. **Metric applications:** Measure ACD, volume and angle, spur-to-spur, white-to-white and

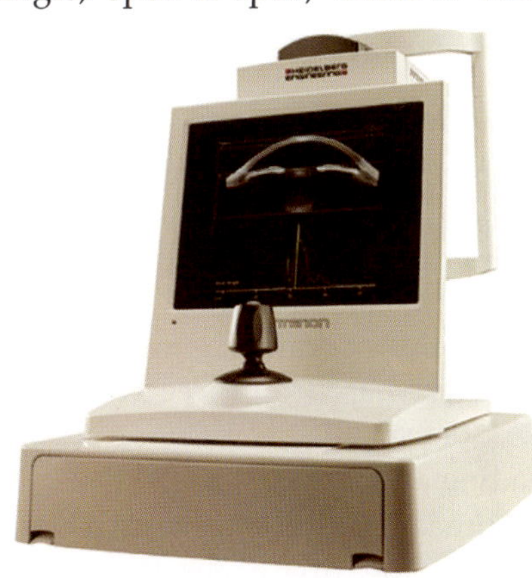

Fig. 9.7. Anterion (Heidelberg Engineering)

angle opening distances, trabecular iris space area (TISA) and LT parameters all in one application.

4. Imaging applications: Visualize anterior segment pathologies and signs of surgical interventions, e.g. keratoplasty, LASIK, implanted IOLs and phakic lenses using the versatile anterior segment imaging application.

FORMULAE FOR CALCULATING IOL POWER

Depending upon the basis of their deviation, the various formulae for calculating IOL power have been grouped into theoretical formulae and regression formulae.

- *Theoretical formulae.* These are based on mathematical principles revolving around the 'schematic eye'.
- *Regression formulae.* These were arrived at by looking at postoperative outcomes retrospectively.

Taking into consideration the time when they were evolved and the corrections incorporated into them with newer developments, the IOL power calculating formulae have been grouped into various generations, i.e.:

- First-generation formulae
- Second-generation formulae
- Third-generation formulae
- Fourth-generation formulae, and
- Fifth-generation formulae.

A. FIRST-GENERATION FORMULAE

The earliest formulae used for IOL power calculation were the first-generation theoretical and regression formulae.

I. THEORETICAL FORMULAE

Various theoretical formulae derived from the geometric optics as applied to the schematic eyes, using theoretical constants, had been developed to calculate the power of IOL required for postoperative emmetropia. These formulae were based on three variables:

- The AL of eyeball,
- K-reading and
- The estimated postoperative ACD.

A few of the first-generation theoretical formulae include the following.

1. Binkhorst formula

$$P = \frac{1336\,(4r - a)}{(a - d)\,(4r - d)}$$

where

P is the IOL power in dioptres.

r is the corneal radius in millimetres (average)

a is the AL in millimetres.

d is the assumed postoperative ACD plus corneal thickness.

2. Colenbrander–Hoffer formula

$$P = \frac{1336}{a - d - 0.05} = \frac{1336}{\frac{1336}{K} - d - 0.05}$$

where K is the average keratometry in diopters

3. Gill's formula

$$\begin{aligned} P &= 129.40 + (+108 \times K) \\ &= +(-2.79 - L\ \text{eye}) + (0.26 - \text{LCL}) + (-0.38 \times \text{Ref}) \end{aligned}$$

where

P is the desired IOL power.

K is refractive power of cornea in dioptres.

L eye is the AL in millimetres.

LCL is the distance of apex of anterior corneal surface to apex of IOL in millimetres.

Ref is the desired postoperative refraction.

4. Clayman's formula

Assume

Emmetropizing IOL = 18 D

Emmetropic AL = 24 mm

Emmetropic average keratometer reading = 42.0 D

1 mm in AL = 3 D of IOL power

1 D in keratometry = 1 D of IOL power

If IOL power >21 D, deduct 0.25 for every dioptre >18.0 D.

For example: AL = 22 mm; K = 43.0 D.

It leads to 6 D hyperopia in length; 1.0 D myopia in keratometry.

Hence, IOL power = 18 + 6 – 1 = 23.0 D – (23 – 18) × 0.25 D = 21.75 D.

5. Fyodorov's formula

$$P = \frac{1336 - LK}{(L - C) - \frac{CK}{1336}}$$

where
P is the implant power for emmetropia.
L is the AL in millimetres.
K is the corneal curvature in dioptres.
C is the estimated postoperative ACD.

Algebraic transformation of theoretical formulae

These apparently different formulae are in fact identical except for the correction factors. They can all be algebraically transformed into:

$$P = \frac{N}{L - C} = \frac{N}{N - KC}$$

where
P is the implant power for emmetropia
N is the aqueous and vitreous RI.
C is the estimated postoperative ACD in millimetres
L is the AL in millimetres.
K is the corneal curvature in diopters

Drawbacks of theoretical formulae

Although the theoretical formulae in practice generally are reliable for eyes with AL between 22 and 24.5 mm, they have following drawbacks:

1. They tend to predict too large an emme-tropic value in short eyes (<22 mm) and too small a value in long eyes (>24.5 mm).
2. They are too cumbersome to apply without the assistance of a calculator or a computer.
3. They still require a guess about the ACD, and the ultimate result depends on the accuracy of that guess.
4. Most of these formulae were developed and iris-supported lenses were commonly used. So, the estimate for the distance between the cornea and the implant (postoperative ACD) are dif-ferent for the presently used PCIOLs.
5. These formulae are based on theoretical simplistic assumption about the optics of the eye.

II. REGRESSION FORMULAE

In view of the drawbacks of theoretical formulae, there had been a tendency to use the simpler empirical formulae in clinical practice. The empirical formulae are based on regression analysis of the actual post-operative results of implant power as a function of the variables of corneal power and AL. In other words, a 'best-fit' line or curve is plotted from the known ALs and K-readings and is subsequently used to predict the implant power needed for future patients.

A number of regression formulae are available. The commonly used are the SRK formula and its modifications.

SRK-I formula

It was introduced by Sanders, Retzlaff and Kraff (SRK), based on the regression analysis, taking into account the retrospective computer analysis of a large number of postoperative refractions. The postoperative ACD was not included but was replaced with A-constant which is unique to each different type of IOL and is determined by the manufacture depending upon its material, position of the eye and optic and haptic design angulation, etc. The SRK formula is as follows:

$$P = A - 2.5\ L - 0.9\ K$$

where
P is the IOL power.
A is the constant specific for each lens.
L is the AL in millimetres.
K is the average keratometry in dioptres.

This formula has become the most widely used formula for IOL power calculation. However, like theoretical formulae, it also performs well for eyes with AL between 22 and 24.5 mm. In converse to theoretical formulae, the regression formula tends to predict too small a value in short eyes and too large a value in long eyes. To address this problem, SRK-I formula has been modified twice.

B. SECOND-GENERATION FORMULAE

I. THEORETICAL FORMULAE

Modified Binkhorst formulae

Binkhorst in 1981 improved the prediction of ef-fective lens position (ELP) by using a single variable predictor, the AL, as a scaling factor for ELP and presented a formula to better predict ACD.

II. REGRESSION FORMULAE

SRK-II formula

The basic equation of the formula is same, i.e. P = A – 2.5 L – 0.9 K, but the A-constant is modified on the basis of the AL as follows:

- If L is <20 mm: A + 3.0
- If L is 20–20.99 mm: A + 2.0
- If L is 21–21.99 mm: A + 1.0
- If L is 22–24.5 mm: A
- If L is >24.5 mm: A – 0.5

Modified SRK-II formula

In this formula, based on the AL, A-constant is modified as given:

- If L is <20 mm: A + 1.5
- If L is 20–21 mm: A + 1.0
- If L is 21–22 mm: A + 0.5
- If L is 22–24.5 mm: A
- If L is 24.5–26 mm: A – 1.0
- If L is >26 mm: A – 1.5

C. THIRD-GENERATION FORMULAE

Most of the third-generation formulae are a hybrid of both theoretical and regression (empirical) formulae.

HOLLADAY I FORMULA

In 1988, Holladay proved that the use of a two-variable predictor (AL and keratometry) could significantly improve the predictor of ELP, particularly in unusual eyes. He proposed the formulae based on geometric relationship of the anterior segment (third-generation theoretical formula). However, soon this formula was modified and now the Holladay I formula, though theoretical, also uses an empirically derived constant, which is then added to the ACD estimate.

HOFFER'S Q FORMULA

Hoffer's Q formula is a third-generation theoretical formula, optimized with regression techniques for ACD. This formula performs best for short eyes.

SRK/T FORMULA

It is a non-linear theoretical optical formula, empirically optimized for postoperative ACD, retinal thickness and corneal RI. It thus combines the advantages of both the theoretical and empirical analyses. This formula seems to be significantly more accurate for extremely long eyes (>28 mm).

D. FOURTH-GENERATION FORMULAE

Holladay II Formula

It is being considered more accurate because of its enhanced ability to predict the position of the implants. Software programs are available in the modern biometers to use the Holladay formulae. Otherwise, the Holladay formulae are very exhaustive. The various constants and equations used in this formula are as follows:

Measured Values

K = average K-reading (dioptres)
R = average corneal radius (millimetres) = 337.5/K
AL = measured ultrasonic axial length (millimetres)

Recommended Constants

C = RI of cornea = 4/3
A = RI of aqueous = 1.336
RT = retinal thickness factor = 0.200 mm

Chosen Values

V = vertex distance of pseudophakic spectacles (millimetres); default = 12 mm
Ref = desired postoperative spherical equivalent refraction (SER) (dioptres)
SF = 'surgeon factor' = distance (millimetres) from aphakic anterior iris plane to optical plane of IOL. It is analogous to A-constant of SRK formula

Definitions of Other Variables

AG = anterior chamber diameter from angle to angle (millimetres)
ACD = anatomic ACD (millimetres), distance from corneal vertex to anterior iris plane
Alm = modified AL (millimetres) 5 AL + retinal thickness factor (RT)
I = power of IOL (dioptres)
A Ref = actual postoperative spherical equivalent refraction (SER) (dioptres)

HOLLADAY CONSULTANT IOL PROGRAM

It uses Holladay II formula with seven variables.

REFRACTIVE FORMULA

It is a theoretical formula described by Holla-day to calculate IOL power for aphakic, ametropic, pseudophakic and PRLs. According to this formula, AL measurement is not required. This formula calculates IOL power from the following parameters:

- Preoperative refractive power,
- Corneal power,
- Desired postoperative refraction, and
- Vertex distance.

However, this formula was not found to be very good for aphakic eyes, as it is difficult to measure the vertex distance accurately, and this may result in high errors.

HAIGIS FORMULA

Haigis introduced his formula in 1999. The formula is built on the same theoretical base as all others, and differs only in the way the ELP is calculated. Haigis proposed using three different constants to better define the ELP. These constants are called the a0, the a1 and the a2 constants. The three constants can be used as standard, optimized or triple optimized. In the standard form, none of the constants is opti-mized. The first constant, a0, is derived from the A-constant using a standard equation (a0 = 0.62467 × A-constant – 72.434). The a1 and a2 constants are set at default values, a1 = 0.4 and a2 = 0.1. Single or triple optimization of the Haigis constants can improve prediction accuracy, but requires a large number of cases.

WANG-KOCH ADJUSTMENT

A Wang-Koch (WK) adjustment can be applied to some third- and fourth-generation IOL formulae to optimize the calculation for AL >25 mm.

- *For the Holladay II formula*, adding AL adjustment can improve the accuracy of the lens calculation.
- *When applied to other IOL formulae*, the WK adjustment has yielded differing results, improving the accuracy of some formulae while worsening the error in others. The adjustment seems to improve Holladay I, and shifts the hyperopic errors at longer ALs to more myopic errors.

Overall, the effect of the WK adjustment is to shift refractive outcomes in long eyes from hyperopic to myopic, and can be considered as an adjunct to the use of the Holladay I, Hoffer Q, SRK/T, and Haigis formulae in long eyes. However, the Barrett is still the more accurate formula.

E. FIFTH-GENERATION FORMULAE

HOFFER H-5 FORMULA

The Hoffer H-5 formula is the first fifth-generation IOL power formula introduced in 2013, which uses the structure of the Holladay II formula and takes into account the demographic specifics of the individual patient based on race and gender. Fourth-generation formulae use arbitrary average biometric values. These values are completely different in males and females and in different races. The gender/race-specific average is used for a specific patient rather than the overall human average.

NEWER IOL POWER CALCULATION FORMULAE

1. BARRETT SUITE

It is a combination of five formulae.

i. *Barrett Universal II Formula:* Barrett universal II formula determines lens position via anatomical depth, utilizes a lens factor related to the physical position of the principal planes of the IOL and calculates the change in principal planes for positive and negative IOLs. It is termed as 'universal formula' because it is designed for use with multiple lens styles and with short, medium and long ALs. The Barrett universal II for non-toric IOL calculation with keratometry (K) values. It is available in LenStar optical biometer.

ii. *Barrett toric for toric IOL calculation* with keratometry (K) values.

iii. *Barrett true K for non-toric IOL calculation* for post-Laser Vision Correction cases (LASIK, LASEK, PRK) and RK with keratometry (K) values. Better results with this formula are seen if pre-refractive surgery refraction and post-refractive surgery refraction is known.

iv. *Barrett TK toric for toric calculation* with total keratometry (TK) values.

v. *Barrett treatment for IOL exchange and piggy-back selection* after surgical surprises.

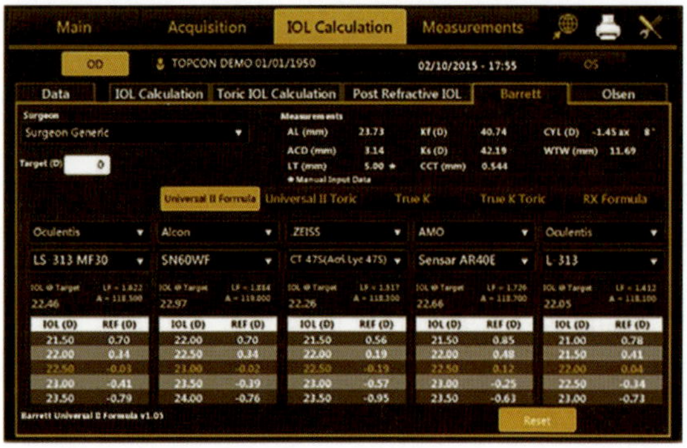

Fig. 9.8. Display of Barrett Suite

Figure 9.8 is the display of Barrett formula.

2. OLSEN FORMULA

The Olsen formula uses exact ray tracing which allows better prediction ELP as a function of LT and ACD to account for the true physical dimensions of an eye's optical system. It uses the same technology employed by physicists to design telescopes and camera lenses.

A key feature of the Olsen formula is accurate estimation of the IOL's physical position using a newly developed concept, the C-constant (Fig. 9.9). The C-constant can be thought of as a ratio by which the empty capsular bag will encapsulate and fixate an IOL following in the bag implantation. This approach predicts the IOL position as a function of preoperative ACD and LT. It is also available in LenStar optical biometer.

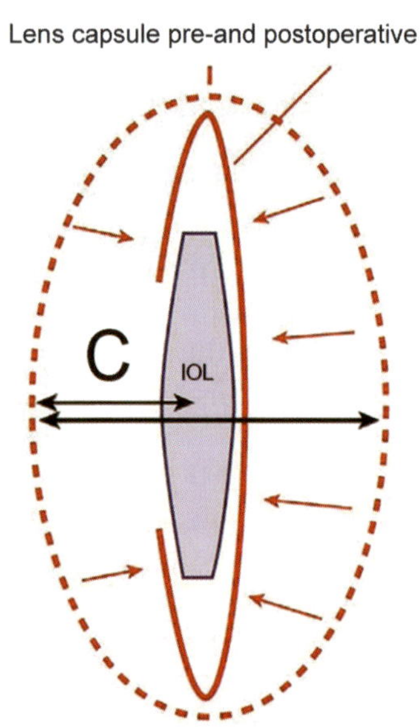

Fig. 9.9. Concept of C-constant in Olsen formula

3. HILL-RBF FORMULA

The new Hill-RBF method is a pure data-driven IOL calculation approach and, therefore, it is free of the limitation of lens-position estimation. RBF stands for *Radial Basis activation Function*. It is driven by an advanced, self-validating method using pattern recognition based on artificial intelligence and sophisticated data interpolation. Starting with a large number of cases where the biometry and the outcomes are known, RBF is capable to find distinct patterns in the apparently random cloud of data points.

The current algorithm is based on outcome data of more than 3400 eyes, with LenStar biometry data and the Alcon SN60WL IOL implanted. It works best with this combination of biometry device and IOL but works also very good with biometry data from other optical biometry devices and with other biconvex IOLs from +6 to +30 D.

Reliable calculation results are labelled with 'in bounds', results that deserve more attention of the surgeon, since the prediction algorithm was not able to determine the desired level of reliability, are labelled 'out of bounds'. An out of bounds labelled result does not need to be inaccurate, but the Hill-RBF method informs the surgeon that the respective pattern of biometric measurements is not well studied by the algorithm and it is recommended to use the Olsen and the Barrett formula to confirm the proposed IOL.

Hill-RBF 2.0 was derived from a large data set with expanded 'in bounds' biometry ranges. Version 2.0 is based on more than 12,000 eyes and, opposite of the original version, can calculate IOL power for a target different than zero. Required inputs are AL, K and ACD (LT, CCT and CD are optional).

Hill-RBF 3.0 was trained on an even more enlarged and refined data set compared to previous versions and provides more reliable predictions in extreme cases, i.e. long and short eyes, than ever before.

New patient parameters, i.e. LT, white-to-white corneal diameter, CCT and the patient's gender refine the spherical and toric IOL power calculations even further.

4. KANE FORMULA

Based on the theoretical optics and incorporates regression and artificial intelligence (AI) to further refine its predictions.

Uses AL, K, ACD and patient gender along with LT and CCT to predict refractive outcome Focus of formula is to decrease the errors in eyes with extreme dimensions. It maintains its accuracy at extreme AL, resulting in 25.1% reduction in absolute error in long eyes (≥26 mm), compared to SRK/T; and 25.5% reduction in absolute error in short eyes (≤22 mm), compared with Hoffer Q.

Figure 9.10 is the display of Kane formula.

5. EVO 2.0 FORMULA: DEVELOPED BY Dr Tun Kuan Yeo

EVO stands for emmetropia verifying optical, is a new thick lens formula that is based on the theory of emmetropization and generates an 'emmetropia factor' for each eye. It uses AL, keratometry and ACD with optional variables for LT and white-to-white distance.

The **EVO toric formula** is a toric IOL formula based on the EVO formula. It combines theoretical posterior cornea astigmatism prediction, thick lens modelling for different types of toric IOLs, and a dynamically interconnected prediction of IOL power and toricity.

Figure 9.11 is the display of EVO formula.

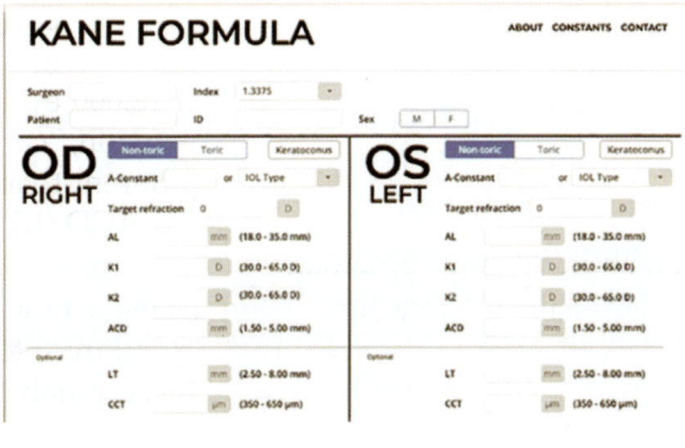

Fig. 9.10. Display of Kane formula

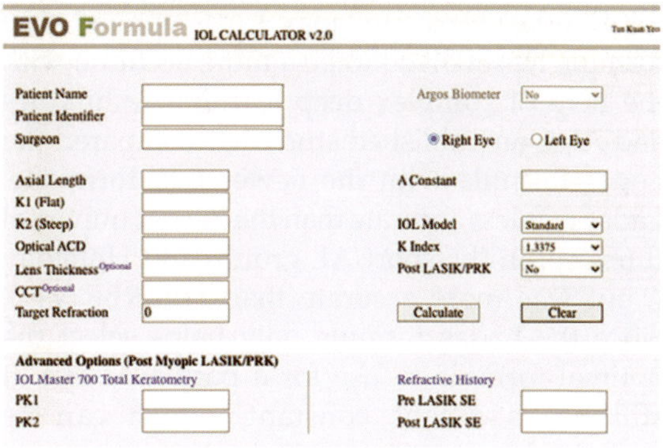

Fig. 9.11. Display of EVO formula, IOL calculator v2.0

6. PEARL-DGS FORMULA: DEVELOPED USING OPTICAL AND MACHINE LEARNING MODELLING

PEARL stands for Prediction Enhanced by Artificial Intelligence and output Linearization. *DGS* named after the formula developers: Debelle-manière, Gatinel, and Saad.

The PEARL formula is based on thick lens equations and uses machine learning models to predict the posterior corneal radius and the *theoretical internal lens position* (TILP).

The Postoperative spherical Equivalent Prediction using Artificial Intelligence and Linear algorithms (PEARL) project aims to assess the potential of AI techniques in the IOL calculation field, to determine the optimal architecture of those formulae, and to encourage open research in this field by publishing the experiments and the related code under an open-source license. *Calculator is not designed for meniscus IOL calculations. This calculator works best with PhysIOL FineVision IOLs.*

7. LADAS FORMULA

As different IOL formulae perform more accurately for certain eye dimensions. The Ladas formula works by combining the most accurate portions of the IOL formulae to make a 'super formula'.

Depending on the AL or corneal power of the patient, this super formula will choose, among the available formulae, the most ideal one to use. The formulae incorporated into the Ladas are SRK/T, Hoffer Q, Holladay I, Holladay with WK adjustment and the Haigis. For AL <21.49 mm, the Hoffer Q was used. For AL >25 mm, Holladay I with WK adjustment was used, and for all other eyes, Holladay I was applied. The formula has evolved to be a more accurate with the help of complex deep learning techniques and AI. One published study has compared the Ladas formula with the newer IOL formulae. Ladas was less accurate than the Barrett universal II (except in the short AL group) and Holladay I, but was more accurate than Hill-RBF V1.0. Since the Ladas formula only helps select the optimal formula to use for a particular eye, it still needs a lens constant, which can be optimized as per the surgeon.

8. NAESER 2 FORMULA

This is a thick-lens formula developed by Kristian Naeser, MD. The original Naeser 1 formula was based on the manufacturer's cutting-card for the IOL anterior and posterior curvatures. The Naeser 2 uses calculated data for the architecture of the IOL. AL measurements are optimized so that the refractive outcomes are equally good in short, medium and long eyes. The results reported by the author were as good as those obtained with the BUII formula.

USES OF DIFFERENT FORMULAE

Most of the IOL calculation formulae work well for eyes with ALs between 22 and 24.5 mm. However, in case of longer and shorter ALs, their inaccuracy needs to be compensated by optimization.

Optimization is the process of increasing the accuracy of a formula by altering and refining the manufacturer's lens constant. It is worked out by analysing post-operative outcomes with respect to targeted refraction for a particular surgical technique, in a specified IOL design and for a given range of ALs.

Albeit controversial, some guidelines have been developed for which formulae to use under specific circumstances. Although earlier widely used, the SRK-II and older ones now obsolete. Appropriate calibration of settings and adjustments of constants is a must before IOL power prediction. No single formula has been found to be useful in all circumstances. So depending upon the circumstances, possible recommendation is as follows:

Circumstance	*Choice of formulae*
AL–<20 mm	Holladay II/Hoffer Q
–20–22 mm	Hoffer Q
–22–24.5 mm	SRK/T; Hoffer Q; Holladay
–24.5–26 mm	Holladay I
>26 mm	SRK/T
Myopic LASIK	Haigis L
Piggyback	Holladay's refractive formula

The newer formulae Barrett universal II formula; Olsen's formula, Hill-RBF formula and Hoffer H-5 formula are still not widely available in the biometry software. Due to the absence of compelling comparative evidence of the superiority of these formulae over each other, it is justifiable to continue using an appropriate combination (according to AL) of the two variable–single constant formulae.

Note. Ultimately, the choice of formula is up to the surgeon, but whatever the method, every effort should be made to ensure the highest possible accuracy.

ERRORS IN IOL POWER CALCULATION

Even with the recent advances like IOLMaster and Orbscan, which have greatly improved the accuracy of ocular biometry, errors in the prediction of IOL power still exist in almost all the methods. These could be subjective or intrinsic in nature.

Most of the existing methods of IOL power calculation are based on the mean zero error (MZE) concept, where the empirically fit parameters (such as ELPo) are defined by regression formulae with one-constant optimization. The current MZE methods have personalized the following factors for improved accuracy:

1. *AL.* The factor with maximum contribution to error. Sources of error in AL include: Corneal indentation,

- Improper calibration,
- Anatomical thickness of retina and
- Failure to recognize appropriate echo pat terns on A-scan ultrasound.

2. ***Corneal power errors.*** These can arise due to inaccuracies in keratometric evaluation.

3. ***Estimated lens position,*** also known as effective ACD, this can result in an error of 0.5–2.5 D for every 1 mm error in calculating ELPo. This parameter takes into account both placement of the IOL during surgery and thickness of the lens to be implanted.

4. ***Errors from formula used.*** As discussed above, certain formulae have more accuracy in the setting of long and short ALs. Selecting inappropriate formula can produce an error of 0.50–2.5 D in the final IOL power.

5. ***Manufacturer labelling error.*** The higher the IOL power, the higher will be the error.

BIOMETRY IN SPECIAL CONDITIONS

1. BIOMETRY FOR TORIC IOLs

For toric IOL power calculation, commonly used calculators are (Fig. 9.12):

- ASSORT calculator,
- Holladay IOL Consultant toric planner and
- Barrett toric calculator

The ASSORT calculator has a unique feature of calculating the most effective implant available and to compare IOLs based on the target postoperative refraction. The software also

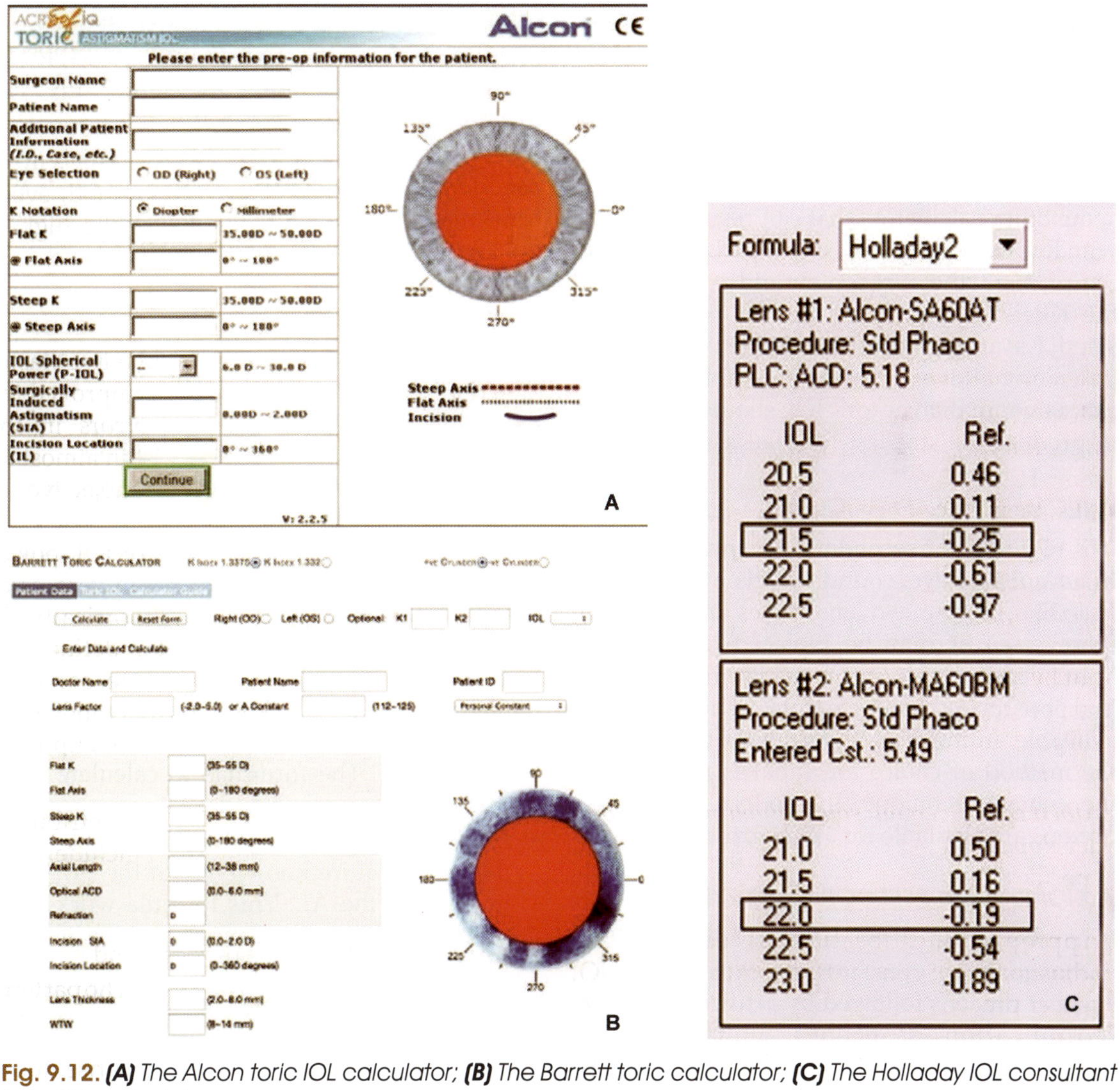

Fig. 9.12. ***(A)*** *The Alcon toric IOL calculator;* ***(B)*** *The Barrett toric calculator;* ***(C)*** *The Holladay IOL consultant toric IOL calculator*

includes optimized lens constants for commonly used formulae, such as Hoffer, Haigis, Holladay and SRK/T, to obtain the ELP. The astigmatic effect of the phaco incision can be dynamically adjusted based on the incision placement. The new parameter of corneal topographic astigmatism (CorT Total) can be employed to include an accurate measure of corneal astigmatism with inclusion of the posterior cornea. So, it displays all pre- and postoperative toric implant requirements.

The Holladay IOL consultant software features both a ToricPreOp planner for forward calculation and a ToricPostOp Back Calculator for back calculation. The ToricPreOp planner allows the user to determine the ideal toricity and axis of placement for a toric IOL using K-readings and the expected SIA from the cataract incision. It does not use a constant ratio of 1.46 to determine the ideal toricity of the IOL from the corneal astigmatism, which is used by some other calculators that can result in errors with low- and high-powered IOLs. Before using the planner, the surgeon should confirm that the K-readings and the axes for the flat and steep Ks are correct. The ToricPostOp Back Calculator allows the surgeon to determine the exact amount that the toric IOL should be rotated to produce the smallest residual astigmatism.

2. BIOMETRY IN APHAKIC EYES

It is required for secondary IOL implantation. In an aphakic eye, sound travels at the speed of 1532 m/s. The two lens spikes are absent in these cases or may be replaced by a single spike obtained by the anterior vitreous face and posterior lens capsule. Therefore, if available, immersion technique of biometry is the method of choice for aphakes rather than the contact technique. In modern biometers, options are available for aphakic mode as well.

3. BIOMETRY IN PSEUDOPHAKIC EYES

It is required in those cases, needing an IOL exchange. Such eyes have an extremely high spike at the lens followed by artificial chain of reduplication of echoes which can be misinterpreted as spikes from the retina. This can be avoided by lowering the gain, which eliminates the artificial spikes and increases the retinal spikes. In cataractous eye, the velocity of sound speed is about 1550 m/s but this is not so in pseudophakic eye. In such an eye, sound speed depends on the sound transmission characteristics and the centre thickness of the IOL in that particular eye. In modern biometers, options are available for phakic, pseudophakic or aphakic mode. This should be rechecked while measuring routine cataract cases to avoid miscalculation of IOL power.

Apparent axial length (AAL) and true axial length (TAL). When AL is measured in apseudophakic eye with an ultrasonic probe with a velocity setting of 1550 m/s, which is the standard setting for the normal cataractous eye, the result obtained is labelled as AAL. This is not TAL because unlike the cataractous eye the average sound speed in the pseudophakic eye is not 1550 m/s. Sound speed in pseudophakic eye depends both on the 'sound transmission characteristic' and the 'centre thickness' of the IOL in that particular eye.

Holladay formula for pseudophakic biometry

$$TAL = (0.988\ AAL) + T\ [1 - (1532/V)]$$

where TAL is true axial length, AAL is apparent axial length measured at 1550 m/s, T is the thickness of IOL and V is the velocity of sound in the IOL.

Secondary piggyback IOL for pseudophakia

It has been suggested that in patients who have a significant residual refractive error following the primary IOL implantation, it is often easier surgically and more predictable optically to leave the primary implant in place and calculate the secondary piggyback IOL power to achieve the desired refraction; rather than doing the IOL exchange. The formulae to calculate IOL power in such cases include:

- ***Holladay's refractive formula.*** This method does not require knowledge of the primary implant or the AL. This formula works for plus as well as minus lenses.
- ***Gill's nomogram.*** The power of piggyback secondary 10 L can also be calculated from the residence spherical refrector error (SE) based on the axial length incorporating Gill nomogram (Table 9.2).

Table 9.2 Gill's nomogram for secondary piggyback IOLs power

Axial length (mm)	*IOL power*
For residual hyperopia	
<22	P = 1.5 × SE + 1
22–25	P = 1.4 × SE + 1
>25	P = 1.3 × SE + 1
For residual myopia	
<22	P = 1.5 × SE – 1
22–25	P = 1.4 × SE – 1
>25	P = 1.3 × SE – 1

4. BIOMETRY IN VITRECTOMIZED EYES

Measuring the AL of eyes in which the vitreous has been replaced with silicone oil is difficult because sound attenuation within the liquid silicone causes the retinal spike to be small and confusing to identify. The difficulty can be overcome simply by increasing the 'system gain'. The result obtained is the AAL, which must be converted to TAL.

Formula suggested by Professor John Shammus: Velocity of sound wave in silicone oil medium is 990 m/s in an average eye.

TAL = 1133/1550 AAL

e.g. a cataractous eye containing silicone oil

AAL = 30.00 mm

TAL = 1133/1550 AAL

= 1133/1550×× 30 = 21.93 mm.

As the silicone oil alters the optics of the eye due to its index of refraction, further adjustment is required after calculation of IOL power using the TAL. Usually, these eyes require an IOL which is 2–3 D stronger than indicated by standard power calculation.

5. PAEDIATRIC BIOMETRY AND IOL POWER CALCULATION

Management of childhood cataract is a very complex and controversial topic. The optical outcome of paediatric aphakia is also not very satisfactory.

Factors that affect the optical outcome in childhood IOL implantations are as follows:

- Unilateral versus bilateral cataract,
- Time of surgery,
- Problem of preventing/treating amblyopia,
- Difficulties in IOL power calculation,
- Significant change in refractive status with growth and
- High incidence of PCO, secondary membrane formation and other IOL-related complications.

Recommendations for childhood cataract at present are as follows:

i. ***Surgery should be done at an early date*** to avoid irreversible amblyopia. In unilateral cataracts, it should be planned as early as possible, preferably within 6 weeks of birth.

ii. ***Surgery of choice*** is to perform lens aspiration with primary posterior capsulorrhexis with or without anterior vitrectomy.

iii. ***Correction of paediatric aphakia*** is still an unsolved query. Presently, common views are as follows:

- *Children above the age of 2 years* can be corrected by implantation of PCIOL during surgery.
- *Children below the age of 2 years* should preferably be treated by extended wear contact lens. Spectacles can be prescribed in bilateral cases. Later on, secondary IOL implantation may be considered. Present trend is to do primary implantation at the earliest possible especially in unilateral cataract, i.e. in all cases because most surgeons have reported negative experience in the compliance with glasses and contact lenses.

iv. ***Paediatric IOL: size, design and power.*** The main concerns regarding the use of IOL in children are the growth of the eye, IOL power considerations, increased uveal reaction and long-term safety. Present recom-mendations are as follows:

- *Size of IOL* above the age of 2 years may be standard 12–12.75 mm diameter for in the bag implantation.
- *Design of IOL*, presently, most surgeons are preferring foldable IOLs made of hydrophobic acrylic material (e.g. Acrys of IOL manufactured by Alcon Labs).
- *Power of IOL*. Most surgeons follow the following protocol:
  - In older children (>8 years), emmetropia is the target.
  - In children between 2 and 8 years of age, 10% under-correction from the calculated biometric power is recommended to counter the myopic shift.

- In children below 2 years, an under-correction by 20% is recommended from the biometric readings.

Note. *Most surgeons follow Dahan et al.'s simplified approach* based on the AL only, which is as follows:

Axial length	*IOL power*
17 mm	28 D
18 mm	27 D
19 mm	26 D
20 mm	24 D
21 mm	24 D
22 mm	23 D
23 mm	23 D
>24 mm	Axial length –1 D

Similarly, Vasavada et al. have suggested the following approach:

Age	*Undercorrection*
0–3 months	35%
3–6 months	30%
6–12 months	25%
1–2 years	20%
2–4 years	15%
4–6 years	10%
>6 years	5%

v. *Amblyopia is must to be prevented/treated.* The appropriate schedule and its importance must be stressed upon the parents.

6. BIOMETRY AND CALCULATION OF IOL POWER AFTER KERATOREFRACTIVE SURGERY

Routine IOL power calculation based on the AL and the keratometry is often inaccurate in eyes that have undergone previous keratorefractive surgery and often leads to an unacceptable hyperopic error, which inconveniences the patient for both near and distance visions. This incorrect IOL power is due to three errors: instrument error, index of refraction error and formulae error.

1. *Instrument error.* Keratometers and corneal topographers used to calculate corneal power cannot obtain accurate measurements in eyes that have undergone corneal refractive surgery. The major cause of error is that the most keratometers measure at the 3.2 mm zone of central cornea, which often misses the central flatter zone of effective corneal power; the flatter the cornea, the larger the zone of measurement.

2. *Index of refraction error.* The assumed index of refraction (IR) of normal cornea is based on the relationship between the anterior and posterior corneal curvature. This relationship is changed in PRK, LASIK and LASEK eyes but not in RK eyes. The manual keratometers measure only the front surface curvature leading to error in calculation.

3. *Formula errors.* All modern formulae except the Haigis formula use AL and K-reading to predict position of IOL postoperatively (ELP). In post-corneal refractive surgery, eyes flatter K causes error in calculation.

Hence special methods need to be adopted to measure the actual corneal power after any keratorefractive procedure.

SPECIAL METHODS TO CALCULATE IOL POWER

There are more than 20 methods proposed over the years to calculate true corneal power or adjust the calculated IOL power to account for the errors caused. A few of them are:

i. Calculation method
ii. Trial hard contact lens method
iii. Corneal topographic/keratometric method
iv. Intraoperative retinoscopy method
v. DBR method
vi. Aramberri double K method

i. *Calculation method.* This is the most accurate method, but requires that the keratometry and refraction prior to the keratorefractive procedure be known, in addition to the stabilized postoperative refraction. In this method, the change in refraction at the corneal plane is subtracted from the original K-reading prior to the procedure, to obtain a calculated postoperative K-reading. Although this is the most accurate method, the preoperative parameters may not be available since there is usually a long time interval between the refractive surgery and the cataract extraction. In addition, one must be careful to measure the postoperative refraction before any myopic shift occurs due to nuclear sclerosis.

Mean postoperative K = (Mean preoperative K) – (Change in refraction at corneal plane).

- Convert the pre- and postoperative refraction into spheral equivalents [sphere 0.5 (cylinder)].
- Now convert these SERs at the spectacle plane (SEQS) with a given vertex distance (V) (in millimetres) into SER at the corneal plane (SEQC)

  SEQC = 1000/ [(1000/SEQS) – V]

  Therefore, the change in refraction at the corneal plane = Preoperative SEQC – Postoperative SEQC.
- Now subtract this from the mean preoperative K-reading to get the mean postoperative K-value. This is to be used for IOL power calculation.

ii. *Trial hard contact lens method.* In this method, the SER is determined by normal refraction and then repeated with a hard contact lens in place. If the SER does not change with the contact lens, then the K-reading of the cornea must be equal to the base curve of the plano contact lens. If the patient has a myopic shift in refraction with the contact lens, then the base curve of the contact lens is greater than that of the cornea by a magnitude equal to the amount of the shift. If there is a hyperopic shift in refraction with the contact lens, then the base curve of the contact lens is less than that for the cornea by the amount of the shift.

For example: A patient with current SER = +0.5 sphere.

SER with plano contact lens = –2.0 D (myopic shift)

Therefore, the corneal power is lower than the base curve (e.g. 35.0 D) of the contact lens by 2.5 D, i.e. 35.0 –>2.5 = 32.50 D. Hence, mean K = 32.50 D.

Use this K for IOL power calculation.

This is also an accurate method for determining the K-value, but the main limitation is that the cataract itself may prevent an accurate refraction. The formula for corrected K value can be summarized as below:

$$K = B + P + R_{CL} - Rb_{are}$$

iii. *Corneal topography/keratometry method.* These systems are based on the assumption that the posterior radius of curvature of the cornea averages 1.2 mm less than the anterior surface and use an index of refraction of 1.33. This assumption is no longer true in corneas subjected to keratorefractive surgery and it leads to an overestimation of the keratometry by 14% of the change induced by the refractive surgery, i.e. after LASIK, if there is a 7 D change in the refraction at the corneal plane with a preoperative K = 44 D, the actual power of the cornea is 37 D, but the topography/keratometric system reads 38 D. Hence, there is a 1 D overestimation for a change of 7 D, and a 2 D overestimation for a change of 14 D. Therefore, whatever the change in postoperative K-reading, undercorrect it by 14% to get an accurate postoperative K-reading. If this correction is not made, then the end result will be a hyperopic refractive error due to an underestimation of the IOL power.

iv. *Intraoperative retinoscopy method.* In this technique, retinoscopy is performed intraoperatively in the aphakic eye after completion of the cataract extraction. The IOL power is then calculated from the aphakic refraction.

Advantage. Theoretically, it seems to be a simple method.

Disadvantages. Asepsis during surgery may be jeopardized and inaccuracy is possible in retinoscopy specially in the eyes which had refractive surgery for hyperopia.

v. *DBR method.* In this method, like calculation method, preoperative patient data is essential. For it, the refractive surgeons need to measure AL along with refraction and keratometry during refractive surgery and keep a record of the IOL power calculated for emmetropia. The record of residual refractive error after stabilization of the post-surgery refraction is also needed. The calculation is explained with an imaginary example:

Pre-refractive surgery data
- Refraction: –5.25 D
- Keratometry: 46.20 D
- Axial length: 25.00 mm
- IOL power for emmetropia (A-constant 118.0): 16.80 D

Post-refractive surgery data
Refraction: Plane

Calculation

0.7 D change at spectacle plane (known fact) = 1.0 D change at IOL plane

Therefore, 5.25 D change at spectacle plane = 5.25/0.7 = 7.5 D change at IOL plane

Thus, IOL power for emmetropia = 16.8 + 7.5 = 24.3 D

vi. *Aramberri double K method.* It is one of the most important methods. It uses pre-LASIK corneal power (or 43.5, if unknown) for calculation of ELP and post-LASIK corneal power for the calculation of the IOL power. This can be done automatically in the Hoffer programmes (for the Hoffer Q, Holladay I, SRK-T formulae) and in the Holladay IOL consultant programme (for the Holladay II).

CONCLUSION

For accurate calculation of IOL power in patients who have undergone keratorefractive surgery, an access to pre- and postoperative patient data is essential. Therefore, it becomes mandatory for the refractive surgeons to maintain detailed records. It may also be prudent to provide all the patients undergoing refractive surgery with a copy of the relevant data, in case they approach another ophthalmologist for cataract surgery. This endeavour will definitely result in more accurate refractive outcomes following cataract surgery and IOL implantation, in patients who had undergone keratorefractive surgery.

Note. Always use more than one modern third-generation and fourth-generation formula (SRK-T, Hoffer Q, Holladay-II, Haigis) to calculate IOL power in such patients and choose the highest value. Never use a regression formula (SRK-I or SRK-II).

BIOMETRY: IMPORTANT CONSIDERATIONS AND FINAL SELECTION IOL POWER

BIOMETRY: IMPORTANT CONSIDERATIONS

- The surgeon should prefer to do biometry himself or herself, or should have a reliable technician.
- Take care to select the correct mode/velocity.
- Data input should be done very carefully.
- Selection of the appropriate formula is very important.
- Always check and compare the ALs of both eyes.
- To minimize errors in IOL power calculation, recheck the preoperative measurement under following circumstances:
  - AL <22 mm or >25 mm.
  - Average corneal power <40 D or >47 D.
  - Calculated emmetropic implant power is
  - >3 D from the average for the specific style used.
  - The difference in corneal power >1 D, AL
  - > 0.5 mm and emmetropic implant power
  - >1 D is found between two eyes.
- IOL power choosen should be compatible with history.
- Always choose a power that is suitable for patient (age, profession and needs).
- Surgeon factor should always be estimated.

FINAL SELECTION OF IOL POWER

After the measurements have been obtained, and the implant power formula chosen has been applied, the surgeon armed with the calculated emmetropizing and ammetropizing values for the patient must make the final decision as to what strength implant to place in the patient's eye. The following factors should be considered:

1. *Fellow-eye refraction and cataract,* if any. If the refractive error of opposite eye lies between –2.0 and +2.0 D, then emmetropia should be aimed for. These patients can usually tolerate an anisometropia of 2.0 D. If the refractive error is more than ±2.0 D and both eyes have got cataract, then stepwise reduction can be done by choosing suitable implant powers; e.g. –4.0 D preoperative refraction can be reduced by aiming for 2.0 D undercorrection in one eye and then emmetropia in the other.

2. *Lifestyle of patient.* Active patients are best served by near emmetropia; sedentary patients may prefer myopia.

3. *Hedging.* It has been found that the actual postoperative refraction varies by more than 1 D from the calculated refraction in over 10% of the cases, and so it is preferable to hedge towards myopia.

RECOMMENDATIONS FOR SELECTION OF IOL IN THE OPERATING ROOM

1. The surgeon and a responsible assistant should personally select the primary and backup implants from stock.
2. IOL power and style to be used should be mentioned in the OT list against each patient's name and fixed on the operating room wall.
3. OT staff should be made aware of the importance of proper IOL power.
4. Avoid using varieties of IOL styles.
5. Corresponding ACIOL power should also be calculated preoperatively for use in case of need.
6. Before IOL implantation, the assistant and the operating surgeon must recheck the IOL power.

BIBLIOGRAPHY

1. Borasio E, Stevens J, Smith GT. Estimation of true corneal power after keratorefractive surgery in eyes requiring cataract surgery: BESSt formula. J Cataract Refract Surg 2006;32:2004–2014. The BESSt formula may be a useful technique to more accurately predict IOL power after kerato-refractive surgery.
2. Gelender H. Orbscan II-assisted intraocular lens power calculation for cataract surgery following myopic laser in situ keratomileusis. Trans Am Ophthalmol Soc 2006;104:402–413. The effective corneal power measured by 1.5 mm Orbscan II in the laser in-situ keratomileusis-altered cornea can be used to accurately predict the IOL power.
3. Haigis W, Lege B, Miller N, et al. Comparison of immersion ultrasound biometry and partial coherence interferometry for intraocular lens calculation according to Haigis. Graefes Arch Clin Exp Ophthalmol 2000;238:765–773.
4. Holladay JT, Prager TC, Ruiz RS, et al. Improving the predictability of intraocular lens power calculations. Arch Ophthalmol 1986;104:539–541.
5. Lavanya R, Teo L, Friedman DS, et al. Comparison of anterior chamber depth measurements using the IOLMaster, scanning peripheral anterior chamber depth analyser, and anterior segment optical coherence tomography. Br J Ophthalmol 2007;91:1023–1026. The study showed that differences in ACD measurements were small between the anterior segment OCT and IOL Master. These differences were unlikely to be clinically important.
6. Nemeth G, Vajas A, Kolozsvari B, et al. Anterior chamber depth measurements in phakic and pseudophakic eyes: Pentacam versus ultrasound device. J Cataract Refract Surg 2006;32:1331–1335. ACD measured with the Pentacam and ultrasound were comparable; however, further evaluation of ACD data is necessary in pseudo-phakic patients.
7. Nemeth G, Vajas A, Tsorbatzoglou A, et al. Assessment and reproducibility of anterior chamber depth measurement with anterior segment optical coherence tomography compared with immersion ultrasonography. J Cataract Refract Surg 2007;33:443–447. Repeatability of ACD measurements was better with anterior segment OCT than with immersion ultrasound and reproducibility was equal.
8. Olsen T. Calculation of intraocular lens power: a review. Acta Ophthalmol Scand 2007;85:472–485.
9. Olsen T. Improved accuracy of intraocular lens power calculation with the Zeiss IOL Master. Acta Ophthalmol Scand 2007;85:84–87. Study that shows the accuracy of IOL power calculation can be improved with IOL Master and current ACD prediction algorithms.
10. Prinz A, Neumayer T, Buehl W, et al. Influence of severity of nuclear cataract on optical biometry. J Cataract Refract Surg 2006;32:1161–1165. This study showed that the severity of nuclear cataract did not alter the axial length measurements obtained with the IOL Master.
11. Qazi MA, Cua IY, Roberts CJ, et al. Determining corneal power using Orbscan II videokeratography for intraocular lens calculation after excimer laser surgery for myopia. J Cataract Refract Surg 2007;33:21–30. Study that show the Orbscan II axial length and optical power can be used to more accurately predict true corneal power.

CHAPTER 10

OPHTHALMIC VISCOSURGICAL DEVICES, IRRIGATING FLUIDS, AND SURGICAL INSTRUMENTS

OPHTHALMIC VISCOSURGICAL DEVICES

Ophthalmic viscosurgical devices (OVDs), also known as viscoelastic substances, refer to the solutions having viscous, elastic and pseudoplastic properties. These substances, in real sense, have revolutionized the ocular surgery in general and anterior segment surgery in particular. *Viscosurgery* is the term coined by Prof. Endre Balasz to describe the use of OVDs during ocular surgery.

RHEOLOGICAL AND PHYSICAL PROPERTIES OF OVDs

1. ***Viscosity*** refers to the solution's resistance to flow. It is the function of concentration, molecular weight, and the size of flexible molecules in the material. Higher the viscosity of the substance, better is its ability to maintain its shape and difficult to be displaced. An ideal OVD should have enough viscosity to provide sufficient space for manipulation within the eye.

2. ***Viscoelasticity*** refers to the property of a substance to resume its original form after having been stretched, compressed or deformed. The degree of elasticity increases with increasing molecular weight and the chain length. Under low frequency impact, a viscoelastic substance behaves in a primarily viscous manner, while at the increased frequency of the applied force, it behaves as an elastic substance. This property affords the protection to the tissues against high frequency mechanical insults such as vibrations associated with phacoemulsification or other turbulence induced by rapidly delivered irrigating stream. Sodium hyaluronate is more elastic than chondroitin sulphate or HPMC.

3. ***Pseudoplasticity*** refers to the ability of viscoelastic substance to transform from the gel into liquid-like substance when under pressure. Sodium hyaluronate has more pseudoplasticity than chondroitin sulphate and HPMC. Because of this reason, it is easy to inject the sodium hyaluronate even through a

30G needle while HPMC needs a larger bore needle usually 23–25G.

4. ***Surface tension*** describes the ability of an OVD to coat a surface. Lower surface tension provides better coating and a low contact angle. HPMC has lower surface tension than sodium hyaluronate and thus better coats the cornea and IOL.

5. ***Cohesiveness and dispersiveness.*** Cohesiveness describes the tendency of a material's constituent molecules to adhere to one another and form a mass. In general, the substance with higher molecular weight, higher surface tension and higher pseudoplasticity are more cohesive. Dispersive agents, conversely are substance with little tendency for self-adherence. In general, substances with low molecular weight, low surface tension (better coating ability) and low pseudoplasticity are dispersive. Sodium hyaluronate is more cohesive than HPMC, and therefore, while aspirating out from the eye it comes out as a single blab while HPMC breaks into small pieces and thus takes much longer to get aspirated.

6. ***Viscoadaptability*** refers to the ability of a substance to change from a supraviscous cohesive profile at low shear rate to fracturable (pseudo-dispersive) substance at higher shear rates. This property of recently introduced Healon 5 (a commercially available OVD) has revolutionized the qualities of an OVD.

7. ***Rigidity,*** also known as a complex viscosity, refers to the sensation of resistance felt by the surgeon to the movement of an object through a viscoelastic substance. Mathematically, rigidity "R" is equal to the square root of the sum of the squares of the dynamic viscosity(v) and the elasticity (E), i.e.

$$R = \sqrt{v^2 + E^2}$$

An ideal OVD

Though near ideal OVDs are available, the ideal OVD is yet awaited. The ideal OVD should have following characteristics:

- *Optical clarity* should be par excellence to provide enhanced visibility.
- *Chemically inert,* i.e. non-toxic, non-inflammatory and non-antigenic.
- *Ability of retention under pressure,* i.e. should be highly cohesive with high viscosity.
- *Ability to protect endothelium* should be high.
- *Interference with instruments* and IOL should be minimum.
- *Removal of OVD* from the anterior chamber should be easy.
- *Obstruction to aqueous outflow* should not be caused, i.e. should not cause postoperative rise in IOP.
- *Cost* should be low, i.e. last but not the least, the OVD should be inexpensive.

PHARMACOLOGICAL CONSTITUENTS OF OVDs

Commonly used ophthalmic viscosurgical devices contain one or more of the following substances in varying concentrations: sodium hyluronate, chondroitin sulphate or hydroxypropyl methylcellulose.

1. Sodium hyaluronate (NaHa)

It is a salt of hyaluronic acid that is found in all connective tissues of living organism from bacteria to humans. In humans, it is extensively found in soft connective tissues throughout the body especially in the skin and also in the synovial fluid and vitreous humour. The pioneer of OVDs Mayer and Palmer isolated this substance from vitreous of cows and named it hyaluronic acid because they extracted it from the hyaloids and it contains uronic acid. Commercially available sodium hyaluronate as OVDs is extacted from rooster combs or streptococcal bacterial cultures.

Chemical characteristics of the sodium hyaluronate.

- *Molecular weight* is higher (2.5–4 million Daltons).
- *Protein content* is low and carries a single negative charge for the disaccharide unit.
- *Viscosity* is 100,000–300,000 centipoise.
- *Half-life* is approximately 1 day in aqueous and 3 days in vitreous.

2. Chondroitin sulphate

It is viscoelastic substance like sodium hyaluronate. Physical and chemical properties and molecular structure of chondroitin sulphate are similar to sodium hyaluronate with the difference of presence of a sulphated group and double negative charges per molecular subunit. Commercially available chondroitin sulphate as OVD is obtained from the shark cartilage.

Preparations

a. *Chondroitin sulphate (20%)* alone is available. But alone it has a low viscosity because of which it cannot maintain space. So it is more a surface than a space tectile tool. Its viscosity is increased as 50% solution but causes damage to the corneal endothelium.

b. *Chondroitin sulphate in combination with sodium hyaluronate (viscoat)* forms a more viscous substance which increases its coating ability.

c. *Chondroitin sulphate in combination with HPMC (Ocugel)* has a good coating property and does not require refrigeration.

3. Hydroxypropyl methylcellulose (HPMC)

It does not occur naturally in animal tissues. It is prepared from the cellulose which is widely distributed in plant fibres such as cotton and wood. Commercially available HPMC is a cellulose polymer modified by the addition of hydroxyl-propyl and methyl groups to increase the hydrophilicity of the compound.

Characteristic features of HPMC are as below:

a. *Viscosity* is 3000–4000 centipoise. It is somewhat viscous but not a true viscoelastic.

b. *Molecular weight* is about 86000.

c. *Osmolarity* is 285 mOsm and pH is 7.2.

d. *Sterilization* with autoclaving is well tolerated by HPMC and its shelf-life at room temperature is about 2 years.

CLASSIFICATION AND COMMERCIALLY AVAILABLE PREPARATIONS OF OVDs

Classification and essential characteristics of some common commercially available OVDs are depicted in Table 10.1.

Table 10.1 *Classification and essential features of commercially available ophthalmic viscosurgical devices (DVDs)*

Viscosurgical agent	*Manufacture*	*Molecular Wt(D)*	*Source*	*Chemical compound*	*Osmolality*	*Viscosity*	*Vo(mPa-s)*
1. **Viscoadaptive OVDs**							
Healon-5®	Pharmacia Inc.	5.0 M	Rooster combs	Hyaluronic acid	322	2.4 NaHa (23 mg/ml)	7.0 M
2. **Viscocohesive OVD**							
a. Super Viscous							
Healon–GV®	Pharmacia Inc.	5.0 M	Rooster combs	Hyaluronic Acid	310	1.4 NaHa (14 mg/ml)	4.8 M
b. Viscous							
Hyal 2000®	L9	4.0 M	Microbial fermentation	Hyaluronic acid	307	1.0 NaHa (10 mg/ml)	280 k
Healon®	Pharmacia Inc.	4.0 M	Rooster combs	Hyaluronic acid	302	1.0 NaHa (10 mg/ml)	230 k
Provisc®	Alcon	2.0 M	Microbial fermentation	Hyaluronic acid	307	1.0 NaHa (10 mg/ml)	280 k
c. Medium viscosity							
Viscoat®	Alcon	500 k	Bacterial fermentation Shark fin	Hyaluronic acid Chondroitin sulphate	325	3.0 NaHa (40 mg/ml) 4.0 CDS	41 K
3. **Viscous-dispersive OVDs**							
Visilon®	Shah&Shah	86 k	_	_	_	2.0 HPMC (20 mg/ml)	4 k

Vo (mPa-s) = Zero shear viscosity (millipascal seconds); (D) = Daltons; M = Millions; k = Thousand; NaHa = Sodium hyaluronate; HPMC = Hydroxypropyl methylcellulose; CDS = Chondroitin sulphate

ADVANTAGES AND DISADVANTAGES OF DIFFERENT OVDs

As described in Table 10.1, the OVDs are broadly of three types:
- Viscoadaptive OVDs,
- Viscocohesive OVDs, and
- Viscodispersive OVDs.

Their advantages and disadvantages are summarized below.

1. Viscoadaptive OVDs

Viscoadaptive OVDs are those super-viscous cohesive substances at low shear rate which can change their profile to pseudo-dispersives at higher shear rate. Healon-5, a commonly available viscoadaptive OVD, consists of sodium hyaluronate 2.3%.

Advantage of viscoadaptive OVD (Healon-5) over others is that it allows superior space maintenance as it can be injected by 30G needle and can be trapped in the concavity of cornea while phacoemulsification is performed in the capsular bag, enhancing endothelial protection.

Disadvantages. Since at higher flow settings, the Healon-5 breaks up and resembles a dispersive OVD, so its removal requires more time and more attention to avoid postoperative rise of IOP.

2. Viscocohesive OVDs

Viscocohesive OVDs include super-viscous, viscous and medium viscosity cohesive OVDs.

i. *Super-viscous cohesive OVDs*

Super-viscous cohesive OVDs refer to a subclass of higher viscosity cohesive OVDs that show extremely high zero shear viscosity greater than 1 million mPa-s (millipascal seconds). Healon-GV is a commercially available super-viscous cohesive OVD, that consists of 1.4% sodium hyaluronate.

Advantages
- Create and maintain adequate operative space. Therefore, it is quite useful for capsulorhexis in a shallow chambered hyperope, especially when operating under topical anaesthesia.
- Displaces and mobilizes tissues, i.e. so useful in achieving intraocular stability.
- Pressurizes the anterior chamber properly.
- Provides clear view of the posterior capsule during phacoemulsification.

Disadvantages
- Provides suboptimal endothelial protection during phacoemulsification and during irrigation and aspiration it leaves the anterior chamber quickly.
- Unable to partition spaces
- More difficult to remove at the end of the procedure.

ii. *Viscous cohesive OVDs*

Viscous cohesive OVDs have zero-shear viscosity between 100,000 and 1000,000 mPa-S. Healon, Hyal 2000 and Provisc are the examples of commercially available viscous cohesive OVDs. These consist of 1% sodium hyaluronate. Uses and drawbacks of viscous cohesive are similar to super-viscous cohesive OVDs, but generally are not quite as effective.

iii. *Medium viscosity cohesive OVDs*

Viscoat is a medium viscosity cohesive OVDs available commercially. It consists of 3% sodium hyaluronate and 4% chondroitin sulphate.

3. Viscodispersive OVDs

These are less viscous and more dispersives when injected as a bolus into the eye. These are more likely to disperse into fragments in the anterior chamber as compared to the cohesive OVDs. HPMC 2% preparations commercially available by various names, e.g. Visilon, Moisol PFS, etc. are examples of lower viscosity dispersive OVDs.

Advantages of 2% HPMC are:
- Remains adjacent to the corneal endothelium throughout the phaco procedure.
- Selectively moves and isolates.
- Partition the spaces.

Disadvantages
- Does not maintain the spaces.
- Fractures easily and the irregular fractured boundaries obscure view of the posterior capsule.

USES, REMOVAL AND COMPLICATIONS OF OVDs

Uses of OVDs

1. Uses of OVDs in cataract surgery

OVDs are essential for each and every step of the modern cataract surgery using phacoemulsification with IOL implantation as below.

a. *Capsulorhexis* can be performed under OVDs as compared to air and BSS. For performing good capsulorhexis, the OVDs should have following features:

- High viscosity and high molecular weight at zero shear rate to maintain the anterior chamber.
- High transparency to provide excellent visibility.
- High elasticity and pseudoplasticity, to make surgical manoeuvres easy.
- Should have a good capsular flap control to provide soft and permanent spatula effect.

Note. Capsulorhexis becomes difficult in paediatric cases due to high capsular elasticity, low sclera rigidity and greater intravitreal pressure. Therefore, use of high density viscoelastic such as Healon–GV® is recommended.

b. *Hydraulic separation of nucleus and cortex* is best preformed with the use of OVDs. The ideal viscoelastic material keeps the anterior chamber shape unchanged during BSS injection and also avoids increase in pressure, which can be produced with excessive amount of BSS, known as capsular blockage.

c. *During nuclear emulsification,* the OVDs help in:

- Preserving the space, and
- Protecting the corneal endothelium.

d. *During irrigation and aspiration,* the OVDs helps in protecting the corneal endothelium. This is possible due to high adhesiveness. In case of posterior capsular break, the OVD plugs it and allows dry aspiration of the cortex.

e. *During IOL implantation,* the OVD keeps the capsular bag expanded and formed thus allowing the easy implantation of IOL. The OVD also helps in correct positioning and centring by allowing the possible IOL rotation manoeuvres. Besides posterior chamber IOL, the OVD is also helpful in implanting various phakic and aphakic IOL designs in the anterior chamber and ciliary sulcus.

Summary. The OVD requirements during cataract surgery (phacoemulsification) are summarized in Table 10.2.

2. Use of the OVDs in glaucoma surgery

a. *In trabeculectomy surgery,* intracameral use of Healon-5® protects corneal endothelial cells, maintains anterior chamber depth and if left into the anterior chamber, avoids immediate postoperative hypotony and choroidal detachment. A subconjunctival OVD injection helps in getting a diffuse bleb.

b. *Viscocanalostomy* is a new glaucoma surgery in which canal of Schlemm is opened up with

Table 10.2 *Summary of requirement of OVDs during phacoemulsification*

S.no.	*Surgical procedure*	*Primary function OVD required*	*Essential properties of OVDs for required function*	*Category of OVDs*	*Compound of OVDs*
1.	Capsulorhexis	Maintenance of deep anterior chamber	High viscosity at low sheer rates; elasticity	Cohesive OVD	Sodium hyaluronate (1%)
2.	Nucleotomy	Endothelial coating, stay in eye to adhesion and coat tissues	High viscosity at high shear rates with low molecular weight and low surface tension	Dispersive OVD	HPMC (2%)
3.	Cortical removal	Endothelial coating	Low surface tension	Dispersive OVD	HPMC (2%)
4.	IOL implantation	Maintenance of deep anterior chamber and inflated capsular bag	High viscosity at low shear rate; elasticity	Cohesive OVD	Sodium hyaluronate (1%)

the help of a viscoelastic substance. The OVD used for this procedure should have high pseudoplasticity to allow injection into Schlemm's canal through a small needle and should have high viscosity at shear rate of zero to maintain the space for a longer period. Healon-GV® and Healon-5® are the OVDs of choice for this procedure.

3. Uses of OVDs in corneal surgery

a. ***In penetrating keratoplasty,*** the OVD injected into the anterior chamber prior to trephination provide proper pressure for trephination and protects the intraocular structures. It also helps in releasing the anterior and posterior synechia. It coats and protects the new endothelial cells of donor corneal button.

b. ***In deep anterior lamellar keratoplasty,*** the use of air and an OVD has been reported to expose Descemet's membrane.

c. ***In femtosecond laser dissection of corneas,*** an OVD acts as a cushion to protect endothelium cells from the lasers.

4. Use of OVDs for intracameral anaesthesia

Use of OVDs for intracameral anaesthesia, i.e. viscoanaesthesia refers to intracameral use of an OVD mixed with lidocaine. It is intended to prolong the anaesthetic effect of intracameral lidocaine as a complement to topical anaesthesia.

5. Uses of OVDs in vitreoretinal surgery

Sodium hyaluronate can be used to separate membranes away from the retina for safe excision and release of traction.

6. Uses of OVDs in strabismus surgery

It has been sugested that sodium hyaluronate is useful in adjustable strabismus surgery for smooth adjustment with less force. Further, it lubricates the muscle and may decrease scarring in the epimuscular tissue postoperatively.

7. Uses of OVDs in oculoplasty surgery

a. ***In probing for congenital NLD block,*** the OVD injected into the sac helps in smooth passage of the probe and also keeps the opened NLD patent.

b. ***In DCR surgery,*** the OVD helps in identifying the sac.

c. ***In repair of severed lacrimal canaliculus,*** the OVD helps in identifying the cut ends.

d. ***In frontalis sling surgery for ptosis,*** the OVD can be used to lubricate fascia lata strips.

Removal of OVDs

A careful and thorough removal of an OVD from the capsular bag and the anterior chamber of the eye is must after the end of surgery. This is important to avoid complications such as rise in IOP, crystallization of the IOL surface and iritis.

Techniques of OVD removal

i. ***Rock-n-roll technique*** relies on the OVD being supple enough to deform and cohesive enough to follow well, allowing it to be scrolled out of the corners into the I/A tip. This technique, therefore, works best with viscous cohesive OVDs.

ii. ***Two-compartment and bimanual I/A techniques*** go directly after the OVD pieces, wherever they are, and do not rely on scrolling or cohesion.

Note. Studies have shown that complete removal of the OVD from the capsular bag can be more difficult when some hydrophobic acrylic lenses are used because of the tacky surface of the IOL.

Complications of OVDs

1. ***Rise in IOP.*** OVD, if not thoroughly removed from the anterior chamber at the end of surgery, may lead to rise in IOP, usually within 6–24 hours. The IOP rises due to mechanical resistance of the trabecular meshwork to the large molecule of OVD material. Usually, it resolves spontaneously within 72 hours. The significant rise in IOP should be treated appropriately

2. ***Capsular block syndrome*** *(CBS) or capsular bag distension syndrome.* The CBS refers to collection of fluid in the capsular bag behind the lens nucleus or IOL, which are pushed forward blocking the capsulorhexis opening of the capsular bag. Depending upon the time of onset, CBS is classified as below:

- *Intraoperative CBS* occurs following hydrodissection.

- *Early postoperative CBS* occurs due to the OVD left behind the IOL at the end of surgery.
- *Late onset CBS* is usually associated with the use of high density OVDs such as Healon-GV®. Main ingredient in the transparent liquid in the capsular bag is sodium hyaluronate. Usually, the distension is caused by aqueous humour being drawn into the capsular bag by an osmotic gradient across the capsule.

3. ***Postoperative inflammation*** *(iritis and hypopyon)* induced by OVD has also been reported sometimes.

4. ***Corneal oedema and corneal decompensation*** have also been reported.

5. ***Hypersensitivity reactions.*** As the sodium hyaluronate is extracted from the rooster combs or streptococcal bacterial cultures, and contains minute amounts of protein, so potential risk of hypersensitivity may exist.

INTRAOCULAR IRRIGATING SOLUTIONS

FUNCTIONS

Intraocular irrigating solutions are the most essential tools for the modern cataract surgery and other intraocular surgeries. These are aqueous solutions which sub-serve the following functions:

- Clear and maintain moisture of the ocular tissues.
- Maintain physiological and anatomical integrity of the intraocular tissues and chamber.
- Provide cellular nutrients required for intercellular and intracellular functions during prolonged intraocular surgery.
- Maintain corneal transparency during intraocular surgery by maintaining endothelial cell metabolism and then avoiding corneal clouding.
- Maintain intraocular pressure during the surgery.

AN IDEAL IRRIGATING SOLUTION

Though near ideal irrigating solutions are available, the ideal irrigating solution is yet awaited. The ideal irrigating solution should have following characteristics:

- Optical clarity should be par excellence to provide enhanced visibility.
- Chemically inert, i.e. non-toxic, non-inflammatory and non-antigenic.
- Composition should be similar to aqueous humour, i.e. concentration of the inorganic and organic constituents should be appropriate. The endeavour will prevent corneal oedema, endothelial cell loss, crystalline lens opacification, damage to trabecular meshwork and regional oedema during intraocular surgery.
- Isotonic, i.e. should have pH of 7.4. A pH of less than 7 and more than 8 can cause cellular stress and clefts on prolonged exposure.
- Should be able to maintain the shape of the eyeball by keeping it inflated.
- Intraocular pressure–volume relationship should be maintained normal during intraocular surgery.

INDICATIONS

- ***Cataract surgery.*** Irrigating solutions are essential for each and every step of modern cataract surgery with IOL implantation.
- ***Glaucoma surgery.*** In trabeculectomy and other invasive filtration surgery, irrigation solution helps to maintain the chamber, washes delirious substances and maintains tissues moist.
- ***Corneal surgery and anterior segment reconstruction.***
- ***Vitrectomy and posterior segment surgery.***

COMMERCIALY AVAILABLE INTRAOCULAR IRRIGATING SOLUTIONS

Commercially available irrigating solutions suitable for intraocular use include:

- Lactated Ringer's solution
- Balanced salt solution (BSS)
- Balanced salt solution plus (BSS-plus)

Chemical composition

Chemical composition of commercially available intraocular irrigating solution is shown in Table 10.3.

Functions of chemical ingredients

- Sodium chloride and potassium chloride are required to maintain corneal transparency.
- Magnesium and calcium ions act as cellular nutrients for normal intracellular and

Table 10.3 *Chemical composition of intraocular irrigating solution (mmol/Litre of the solution)*

S.no	*Chemical composition pH and osmoles*	*Lactated ringers solution*	*BSS*	*BSS plus*
1	NaCl	102	110	122.2
2	KCl	4	10	5.08
3	Sodium lactate	28	–	–
4	$MgCl_2$	5	1.5	0.98
5	Sodium acetate	–	29	–
6	Sodium citrate	–	–	–
7	Sodium bicarbonate	–	0.6	25
8	Disodium phosphate	–	–	0.3
9	Dextrose	–	–	0.5–11
10	Glutathione (oxidized)	–	–	0.3
11	pH	7.2	7.4	7.4
12	Osmolality (mOsm)	277	305	305

intracellular vital barrier functioning during ocular surgery.

- Bicarbonate, added in the balanced salt solution plus, helps to maintain a normal endothelium pump function and thus a deturgesced or thin cornea by avoiding corneal clouding.
- Dextrose added in BSS plus solution, being an energy source, is essential for aerobic metabolism of endothelial cells and thus also helps to maintain its transparency.
- Glutathione (oxidised), added in the BSS plus, protects the cells against oxidative stress and helps to maintain the integrity of blood aqueous barrier and thus minimizes inflammation.

Salient features of commercially available irrigating solutions

Lactated Ringer's solution

Composition in mmol/litre is: NaCl (102), KCl(4), $CaCl_2$(3), and sodium lactate (28).

pH of lactate Ringer's solution is 7.2

Osmolality is 279.

Advantages: Maintains the integrity of intraocular tissues.

Disadvantages: Since it contains sodium lactate in much higher concentration than aqueous humour, so prolonged perfusion causes endothelial cell breakdown and corneal swelling.

Balanced salt solution (BSS)

Composition in mmol/litre is: NaCl (110), KCl (10), $CaCl_3$(3), $MgCl_2$(1.5), sodium citrate (8) and sodium acetate (29)

pH of BSS is 7.4.

Osmolality is 305.

Advantages: It is better tolerated irrigant which helps to maintain the integrity of intraocular tissues.

Disadvantages: BSS is less protective to corneal endothelial cells as compared to BSS plus as it lacks the bicarbonate, glucose and glutathione. After prolonged exposure, it may result in:

- *Polymegathism*, i.e. a significant increase in the coefficient of variation of cell area;
- *Pleomorphism*, i.e. a significant decrease in the percentage of hexagonal cells; and
- *Stressed endothelial monolayer*, which may be more susceptible to additional surgical trauma.

Balanced salt solution (BSS) plus

Composition. The concentration of constituents of BSS plus, also known as GBR (glutathione, bicarbonate, Ringer's) in mmol/l is NaCl (122.2.2), KCl (5.08)/$MgCl_2$ (0.98), disodium phosphate (2.5), dextrose (5.11), oxidized glutathione (0.30), and sodium bicarbonate (25).

pH of BSS plus is 7.4.

Osmolality (mOsm) is 305.

Advantages of BSS plus are as below:

- Iso-osmotic with intraocular tissues.
- Corneal endothelium functioning is maintained even on prolonged irrigation and thus minimal changes occur in endothelial morphologic characteristics.
- Lens clarity is maintained in posterior segment surgery.

- Blood aqueous barrier is maintained by glutathione which protects the cells against oxidative stress and thus inflammation is minimized.

SURGICAL INSTRUMENTS

As we know, over the years, the cataract surgery has evolved from couching to the femtosecond assisted microincision cataract surgery (MICS). So, is the evolution of cataract surgical instruments from a set of couching needles (*see* Fig. 7.2) to a number of sophisticated instruments.

Sugical instruments which are used in different cataract surgical techniques include:

A. Common surgical instruments
- Lid speculums
- Forceps
- Needle holders
- Knives and knife-needles
- Scissors
- Lens hook, spatula, vectis and loop
- Cannulas

B. Instruments for capsulorhexis

C. Pre-choppers, choppers, capsule polishers and iris repositor

D. Instruments used in microincision cataract surgery (MICS)

E. Instruments for intraocular lens implantation

A. COMMON SURGICAL INSTRUMENTS

I. Lid speculums

Three types of speculums in use are:

1. ***Universal metallic eye speculum*** (Fig. 10.1). It is called universal eye speculum as it can be used for both right and left eyes. It has two limbs and a spring mechanism with a screw to adjust the limbs. Its blades are open. It is a heavy instrument and cannot keep eyelashes out of the operating field.

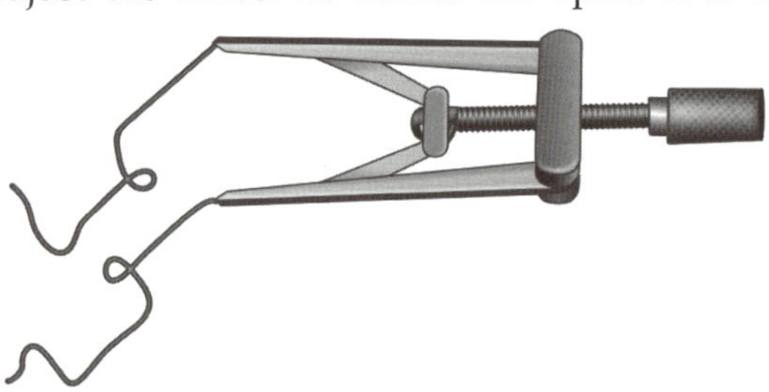

Fig. 10.1. *Universal metallic eye speculum.*

2. ***Eye speculum with guard or with solid blades*** (Fig. 10.2). It retracts the lids and its solid blades keep the lashes away from the field of operation.

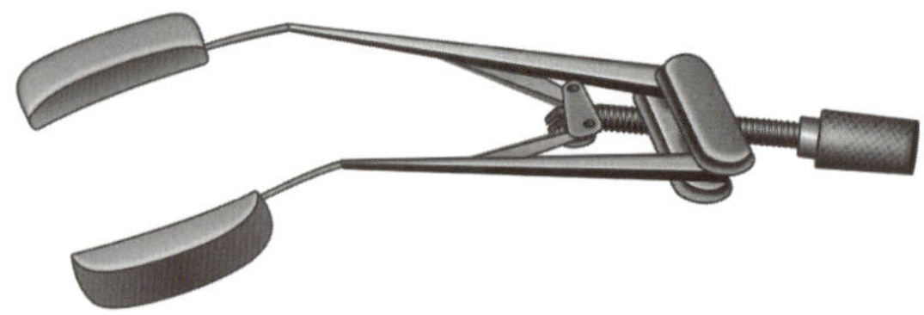

Fig. 10.2. *Eye speculum with guard.*

3. ***Barraquer's wire speculum*** (Fig. 10.3). It is very light and puts minimal pressure on the eyeball. It is also universal and is used to keep the lids apart during surgery.

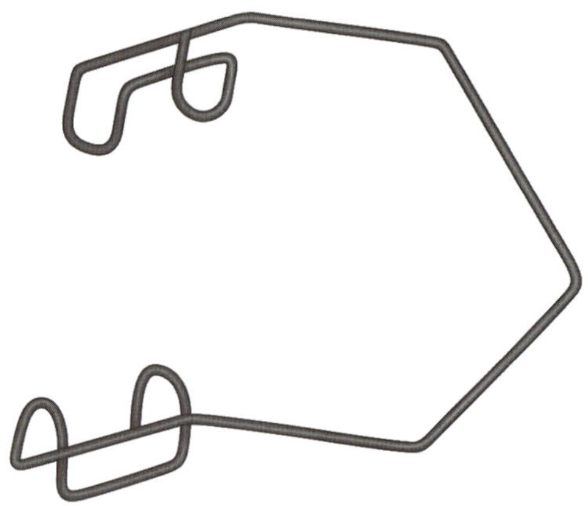

Fig. 10.3. *Barraquer's wire speculum.*

II. Forceps

Many kinds of forceps are available for different purposes. A few common ones are mentioned here.

1. *Plain forceps* (Fig. 10.4). It is simple forcep without any teeth. Serrations (either horizontal or vertical) are present near the tip.

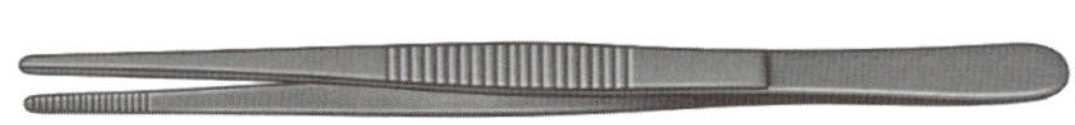

Fig. 10.4. *Plain forceps.*

Uses. To hold the conjunctiva during any surgical procedure.

2. *Globe fixation forceps* (Fig. 10.5). It has 2 × 3 or 3 × 4 teeth at the tip. It is applied near the limbus to hold the conjunctiva and episclera tissues together. It is used to fix the eyeball during operations on the eyeball.

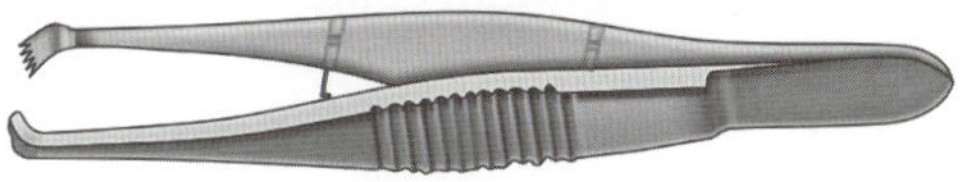

Fig. 10.5. *Globe fixation forceps.*

3. ***Superior rectus holding forceps*** (Fig. 10.6). It is a toothed forceps (1 × 2 teeth) with S-shaped double curve near the tip.

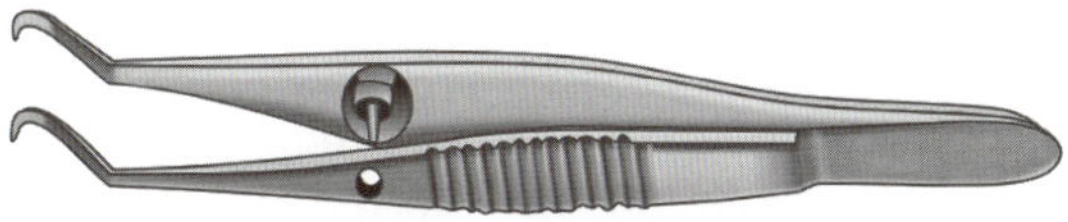

Fig. 10.6. *Superior rectus holding forceps.*

Uses. It is used to hold the superior rectus muscle while passing a bridle suture under it; to stabilize the eyeball during cataract surgery (ICCE, ECCE and SICS).

4. ***Corneoscleral forceps.*** These are available in many shapes and designs. Commonly used are. *Colibri Barraquer's forceps* (Fig. 10.7A), *Lim's forceps* (Fig. 10.7B), *Hoskin's forceps* (Fig. 10.7C) and *Pierse forceps* (Fig. 10.7D). These are forceps with very fine teeth (1 × 2) at the tip.

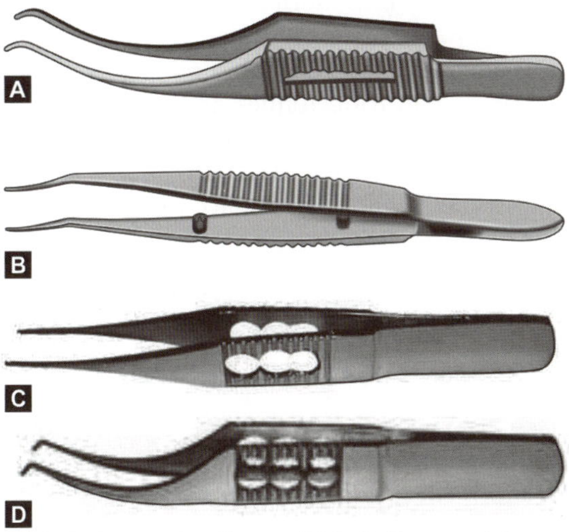

Fig. 10.7. *Corneoscleral forceps.* ***(A)*** *Colibri Barraquer's forceps;* ***(B)*** *Lim's forceps;* ***(C)*** *Hoskin's forceps;* ***(D)*** *Pierse forceps.*

Uses. These are used to hold the cornea or scleral edge (of incision) for suturing during cataract, glaucoma, repair of corneal and/or scleral tears and keratoplasty operations.

5. ***Iris forceps*** (Fig. 10.8). These are small and delicate forceps having fine 1 × 2 teeth on the inner side of the limbs. These are also available in various shapes and designs.

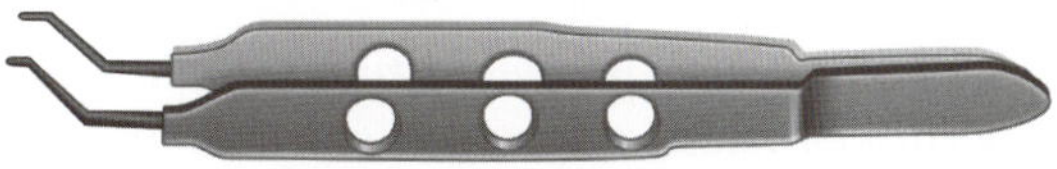

Fig. 10.8. *Iris forceps.*

Uses. These are used to catch the iris for the purpose of iridectomy when required during operations for cataract.

6. ***Arruga's intracapsular (capsule holding) forceps*** (Fig. 10.9). Intracapsular forceps have a cup on the inner side of the tip of each limb. The margins of the cup are very smooth which do not damage the lens capsule when applied.

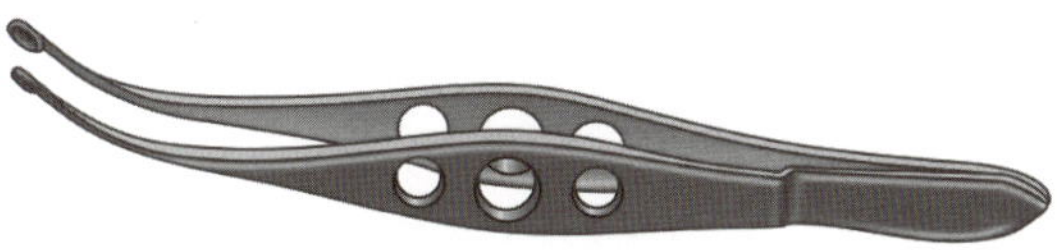

Fig. 10.9. *Arruga's intracapsular (capsule holding) forceps.*

Uses. Not used nowadays. In the era of intracapsular cataract extraction (ICCE), it was used to hold the lens capsule (usually to 6 o'clock position) during capsule forceps method of lens delivery in intracapsular cataract extraction and to grasp and remove the capsular remnants after accidental extracapsular lens extraction.

7. ***Mosquito artery (haemostatic) forceps*** (Fig. 10.10). It is a blunt-tipped stout forceps having a scissors-like configuration. It has multiple straight grooves (at right angle to the limbs) near the tip and a locking mechanism near the ringed end. These are available in large, medium and small size. The small-sized artery forceps, also called *mosquito artery forceps* are more

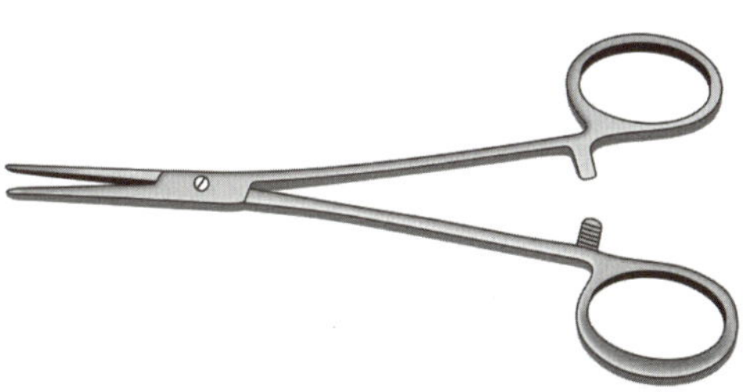

Fig. 10.10. *Mosquito artery (haemostatic) forceps.*

commonly used in ophthalmology. These can be straight or with curved ends. It is used to hold the bridle sutures.

III Needle holders

1. ***Spring action (Barraquer's type) needle holder*** (Fig. 10.11). These are available in various sizes with straight or curved tips, in different shapes and may be with or without locking system. Jaws of the needle holders are finely serrated to hold the fine needles firmly.

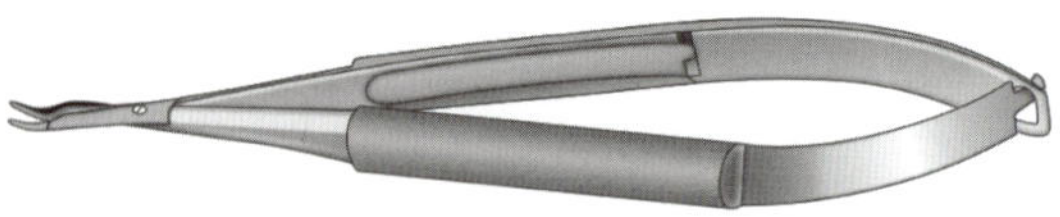

Fig. 10.11. *Spring action (Barraquer's type) needle holder.*

Uses: Spring type needle holders are used for passing sutures in the conjunctiva and cornea when required in cataract surgery.

2. ***Castroviejo's needle holder*** (Fig. 10.12). It is a medium-sized spring action needle holder with an S-shaped locking system.

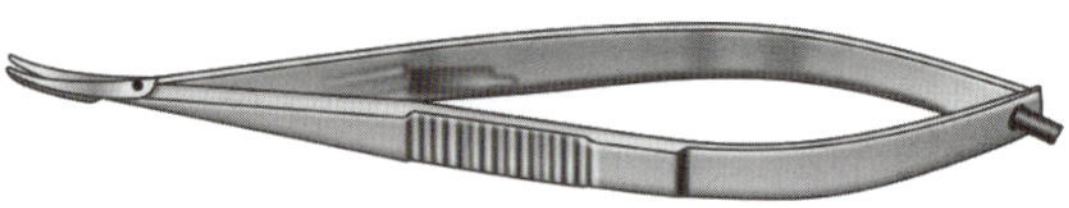

Fig. 10.12. *Castroviejo's needle holder.*

Uses. It is generally used in extraocular surgery but can also be used for intraocular surgery.

3. ***Arruga's, Steven's, Silcock's and Kelt needle holder*** (Fig. 10.13). These are large needle holders and all are of similar type with slight model differences. The upper shank of these needle holders has a flat and broad plate to accommodate the surgeon's thumb. These are available with and without locking device.

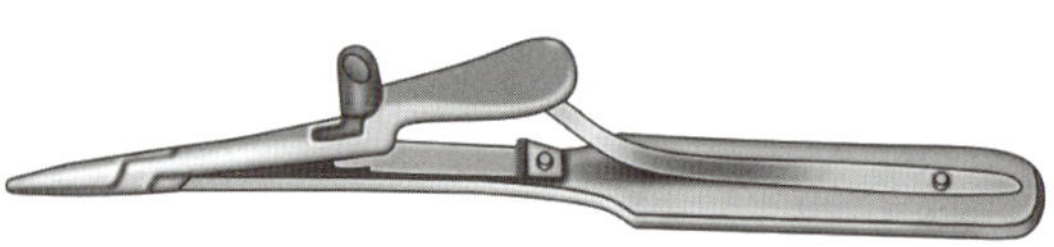

Fig. 10.13. *Arruga's, Steven's, Silcock's and Kelt needle holder.*

Uses. These are used for passing superior rectus bridle suture.

IV. Knives and knife-needles

1. ***von Graefe's knife*** (Fig. 10.14). It is a long, narrow, thin and straight blade with a sharp tip and cutting edge on one side. It is not used presently.

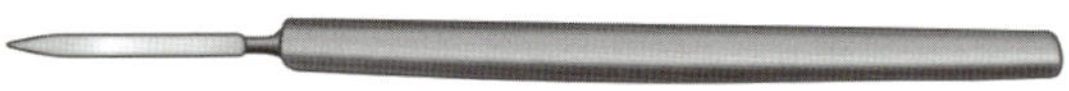

Fig. 10.14. *von Graefe's knife.*

Uses. Previously, it was used for making an ab interno corneo-scleral incision during cataract surgery and for iridectomy operation.

2. ***Keratomes*** (Fig. 10.15). A keratome has a thin diamond-shaped blade with a sharp apex and two cutting edges. Straight as well as curved keratomes are available in various sizes (2.8 mm, 3 mm, 3.5 mm, 5.5 mm). Presently disposable curved keratomes are more commonly used.

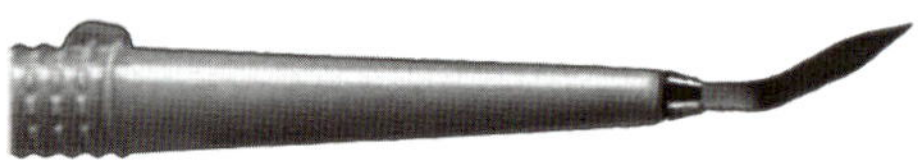

Fig. 10.15. *Keratomes.*

Uses. Keratomes are used to make valvular corneal incisions for entry into the anterior chamber for all modern techniques of cataract extraction, viz. phacoemulsification, SICS or even conventional ECCE and other intraocular surgeries, e.g. iridectomies and paracentesis.

3. ***15° side port entry blade*** (Fig. 10.16). It is a fine straight knife with a sharp pointed tip and cutting edge on one side.

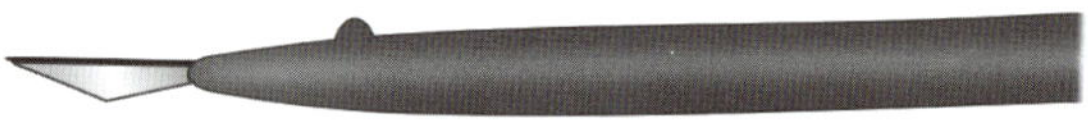

Fig. 10.16. *15° side port entry blade.*

Uses. It is used to make a small valvular clear corneal incision (commonly called as side port incision) in phacoemulsification and other intraocular surgeries including pars plana vitrectomy.

4. ***MVR*** (Fig. 10.17A) ***and Lance tip blade*** (Fig. 10.17B). These are fine straight but triangular knife similar to 15° side port entry blade but with cutting edges on both sides.

Fig. 10.17. *(A)* MVR; *(B)* Lance tip blade.

Uses: Their uses are similar to 15° side port entry blade.

5. ***Razor blade fragment with blade holder.*** Razor blade fragment holder (Fig. 10.18) is designed to hold the razor blade fragment frimly in its jaws and has a locking device. The razor blade fragments broken to a uniform size and shape have the sharpest possible metal edge with an absolute point. Presently presterilized razor blade fragments mounted on a disposable plastic handle (Fig. 10.19) are being preferred.

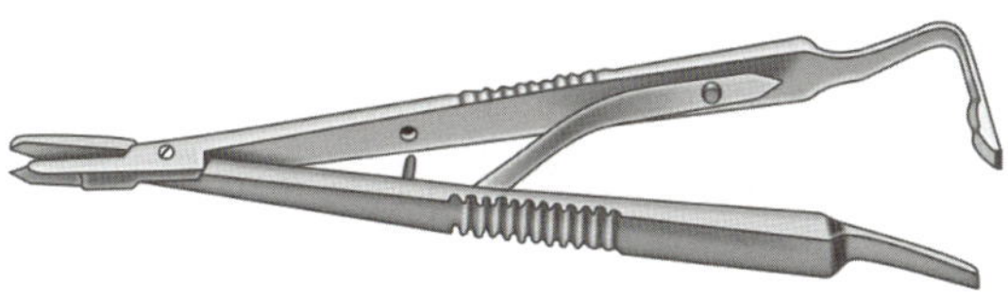

Fig. 10.18. *Razor blade fragment holder.*

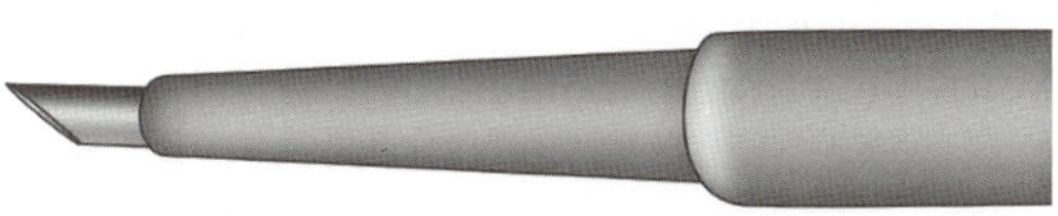

Fig. 10.19. *Presterilized razor blade.*

Uses. It is a commonly used cutting device for making incision in cataract, glaucoma, keratoplasty, sclerotomy, pterygium and many other operations.

6. ***Crescent knife*** (Fig. 10.20). It is blunt-tipped, bevel up knife having cut-splitting action at the tip and at both sides. Its blade is curved and either mounted on a plastic handle (disposable) or can be fixed with metallic handle.

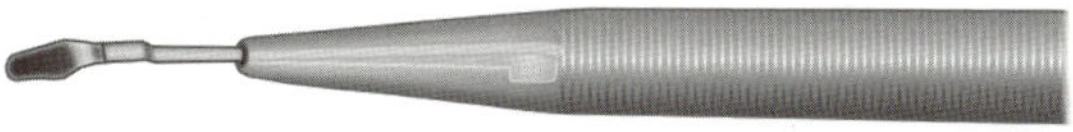

Fig. 10.20. *Crescent knife.*

Uses. It is used to make tunnel incision in the sclera and cornea for phacoemulsification, manual small incision cataract surgery (SICS) and sutureless trabeculectomy.

7. ***Diamond knives*** (Fig. 10.21). These have advantages of better and precise wound construction. Its extreme sharpness creates a more uniform internal incision that seals more consistently with minimal hydration, potentially reducing the risk of wound leak and endophthalmitis. However, they are very expensive and need special care.

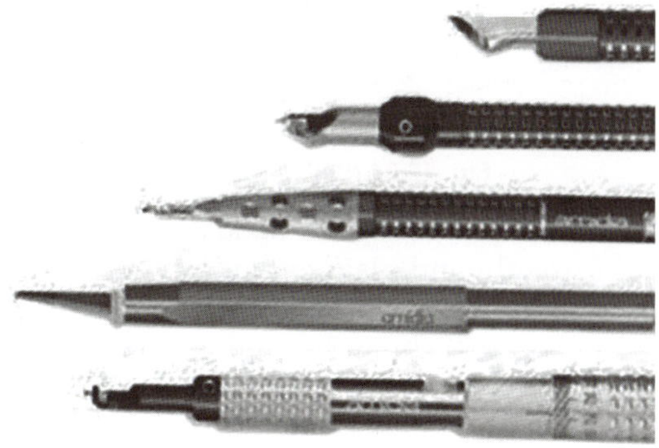

Fig. 10.21. *Diamond knives.*

V. Scissors

1. ***Plain straight scissors (ringed)*** (Fig. 10.22). It is a fine pointed scissors with straight sharp cutting blades.

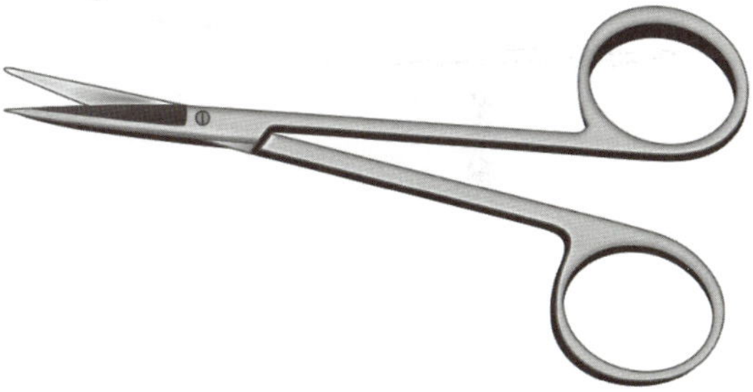

Fig. 10.22. *Plain straight scissors (ringed).*

Uses. It is used to cut conjunctival sutures, and eyelashes.

2. ***Plain curved scissors (ringed)*** (Fig. 10.23). It is a fine pointed scissors with curved, sharp cutting blades.

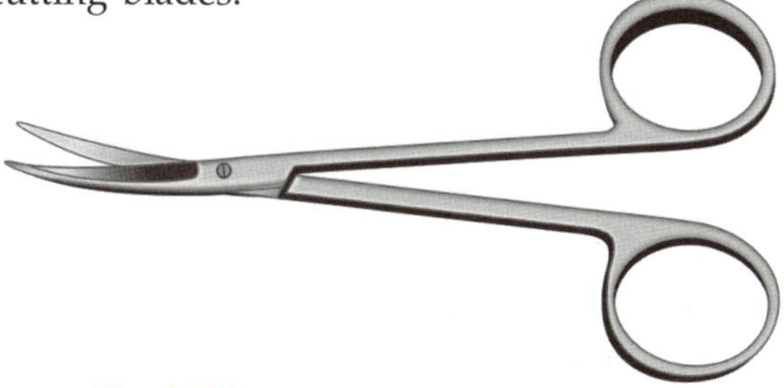

Fig. 10.23. *Plain curved scissors (ringed).*

Uses. It is used to cut and undermine conjunctiva in various operations.

3. ***Spring scissors (Westcott)*** (Fig. 10.24). They are stout scissors available with straight and curved blades with sharp or blunt tips. The blades are kept apart by spring action.

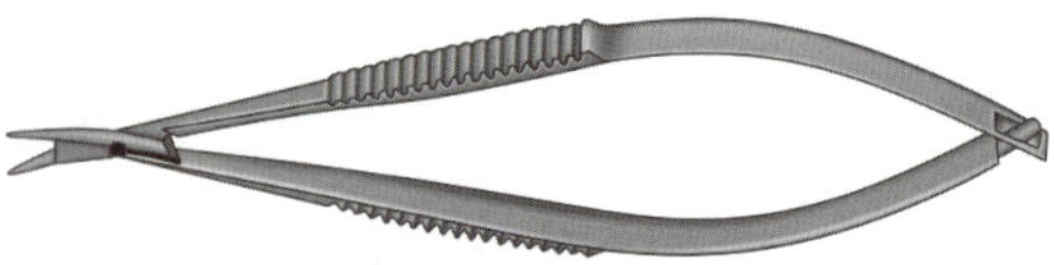

Fig. 10.24. *Spring scissors.*

Uses. They are used as a handy alternative to plain straight and plain curved ringed scissors for cutting and undermining conjunctiva in various operations and to cut the sutures.

4. ***Corneal scissors or section enlarging scissors*** (Fig. 10.25A and B). They are fine curved scissors. Their cutting blades are kept apart by spring action. They are available in various shapes and sizes. The universal corneal scissors can be used for both sides while right and left curved corneal scissors are separate for the two sides.

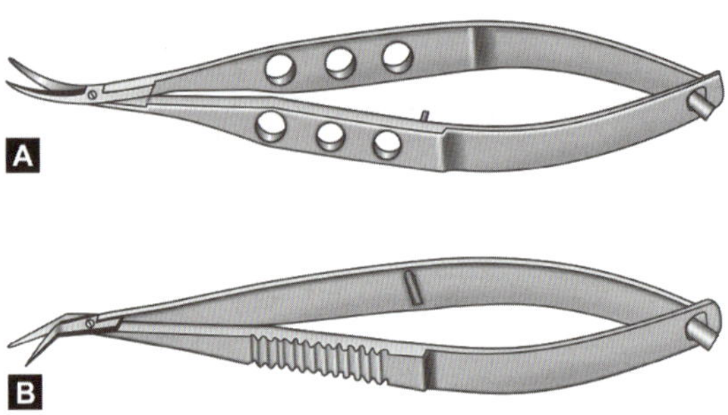

Fig. 10.25. *Corneal scissors.*

Uses. (i) These are used to enlarge corneal or corneoscleral incision for conventional intracapsular and extracapsular cataract extraction techniques (sparingly performed procedures nowadays) for cataract surgery. (ii) It can also be used for cutting and undermining conjunctiva in various operations.

5. ***de Wecker's scissors*** (Fig. 10.26). They are fine scissors with small blades directed at right angles to the arms. The blades are kept apart, making V-shape, by spring action.

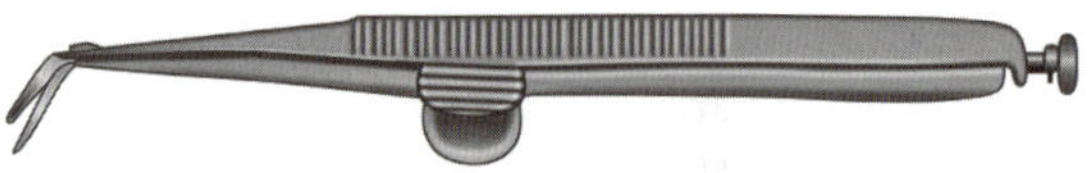

Fig. 10.26. *de Wecker's scissors.*

Uses. It is used to perform iridectomy, iridotomy and to cut the prolapsed vitreous and pupillary membranes.

6. ***Vannas scissors*** (Fig. 10.27). These are very fine delicate scissors with small cutting blades kept apart by spring action. The blades may be straight or curved or angled.

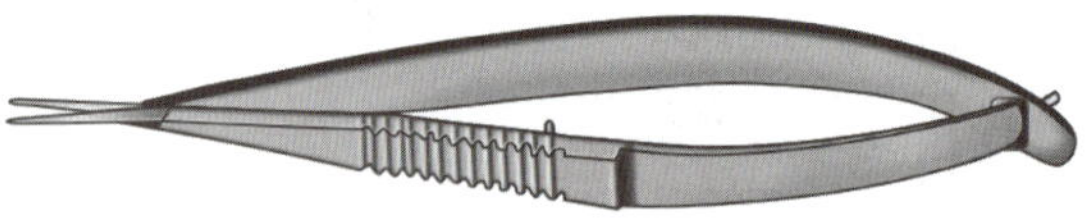

Fig. 10.27. *Vannas scissors.*

Uses. (i) These are used for cutting anterior capsule of the lens in extracapsular surgery and for cutting 10–0 nylon sutures. (ii) For doing pupillary sphincterotomy. (iii) For performing iridectomy. (iv) For cutting pupillary membranes.

VI. Lens hook, spatula, vectis and loop

1. ***Lens expressor (hook)*** (Fig. 10.28). It is a flat metal handle with a rounded curve at one end. Tip of the curve is knobbed. The plane of the handle is at right angle to the curvature of the hook.

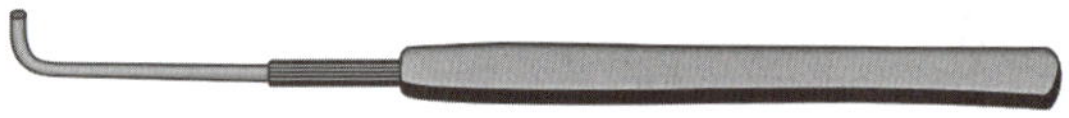

Fig. 10.28. *Lens expressor.*

Uses. (i) To express the nucleus in extracapsular cataract extraction. (ii) In the era of ICCE, it was used to apply pressure on the limbus at the 6 O'clock position during the delivery of lens in intracapsular cataract extraction with Smith's (tumbling) and capsule forceps techniques.

2. ***Lens spatula*** (Fig. 10.29). It is a flat metallic handle with tiny spoon-shaped ends. It is used

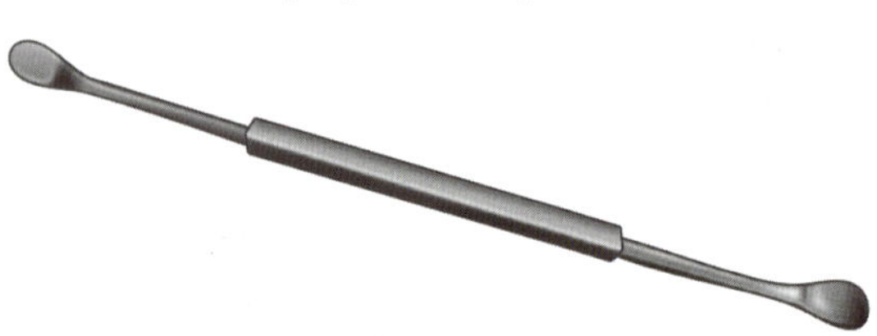

Fig. 10.29. *Lens spatula.*

to apply counter-pressure at 12 o'clock position during expression of nucleus during extra-capsular cataract extraction. In the era of ICCE, it was used in similar way to extract the cataractous lens in Smith's techniques.

3. ***Wire vectis*** (Fig. 10.30). It is a wire loop attached to a metallic handle.

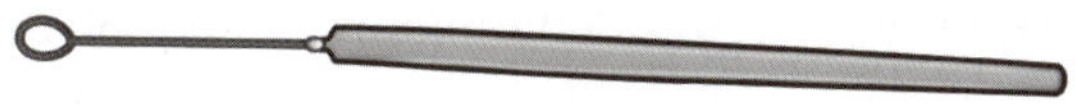

Fig. 10.30. *Wire vectis.*

Uses: It is used to remove subluxated lens and anteriorly dislocated lens in ICCE techniques and the nucleus in ECCE techinques. It is used to apply pressure on the sclera superiorly, depressing the posterior lip of the wound to facilitate lens delivery by sliding technique.

4. ***Irrigating wire vectis*** (Fig. 10.31). It is a modified vectis in which the loop is made of a thick hollow wire. The anterior end of the loop has three 0.3 mm openings. The posterior end of the loop is continuous with a hollow handle. The posterior end of the hollow handles has a hub similar to that of a hypodermic needle to which is attached a syringe or infusion set to a infusion line to assist hydraulic separation of nucleus. The size of the loop of the vectis is variable. In commonly used wire vectis, the loop is 4 mm in width and about 8–9 mm in length. The superior surface of the loop has a slight concavity to accommodate the lens nucleus.

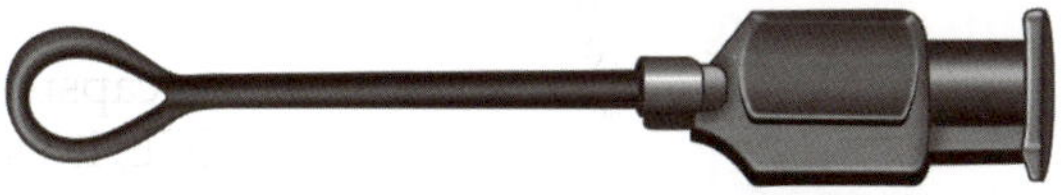

Fig. 10.31. *Irrigating wire vectis.*

Uses: Irrigation wire vectis is most commonly used to deliver nucleus in the manual small incision cataract surgery (SICS) and in conventional ECCE by hydroexpression or viscoexpression technique.

5. ***Kansas lens loop.*** It is 3 mm wide and is serrated at the loop side (Fig. 1.32) and used for nucleus fragment removal in SICS.

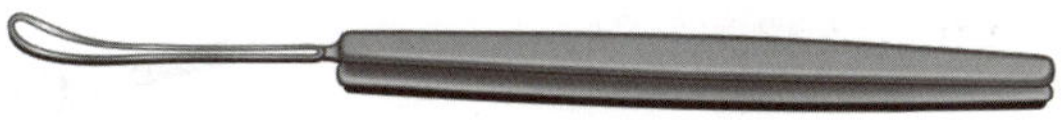

Fig. 10.32. *Kansas lens loop.*

VII. Cannulas

Cannulas are hollow, needle-like instruments with a blunt or rounded tip, that are fitted to an irrigation line or an aspiration mechanism such as syringe or vacuum bulb to either irrigate or aspirate fluid or soft material such as lens cortex.

1. ***Two-way irrigation and aspiration cannula*** (Fig. 10.33). It is available in various designs, commonly used are Simcoe's classical or reverse cannula.

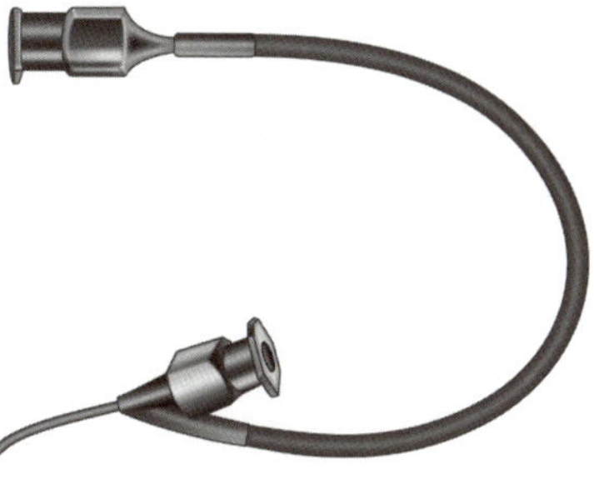

Fig. 10.33. *Two-way irrigation and aspiration cannula.*

Uses. (i) For irrigation and aspiration of the lens matter and viscoelastic mterial in extracapsular cataract extraction. (ii) Aspiration of hyphaema.

2. ***Hydrodissection cannula*** (Fig. 10.34). It is a single bore 25G, 27G or 30G cannula with a 45° angulation at about 10 to 12 mm from the free end. The tip at the free end can be flattened or bevelled.

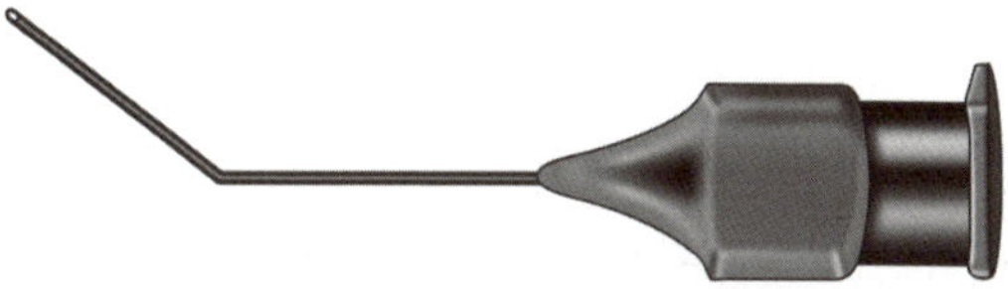

Fig. 10.34. *Hydrodissection cannula.*

Uses. It is used to perform hydrodissection (separation of cortex from the posterior capsule) and hydrodelineation (separation of cortex from the nucleus) in phacoemulsification and manual SICS. This cannula is attached to the syringe carrying irrigating fluid. For hydrodissection its tip is introduced beneath the anterior capsular margin after capsulorhexis and fluid is injected to obtain subcapsular dissection.

3. ***Akahoshi hydrosection cannula*** (Fig. 10.35). 27 gauge cannula facilitates hydrodissection.

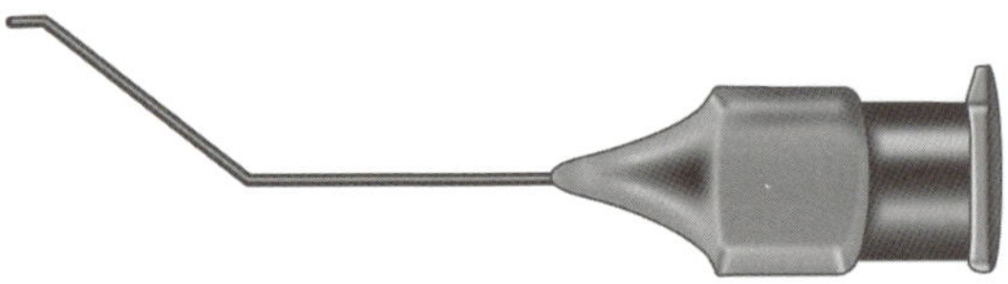

Fig. 10.35. *Akahoshi hydrosection cannula.*

Beveled tip can be easily inserted beneath the capsulorhexis edge. Tapered design easily increases the intraocular pressure for sealing the wound.

4. ***Kellan hydrodelineation cannula*** (Fig. 10.36). It is used to separate cortical matter from the nucleus.

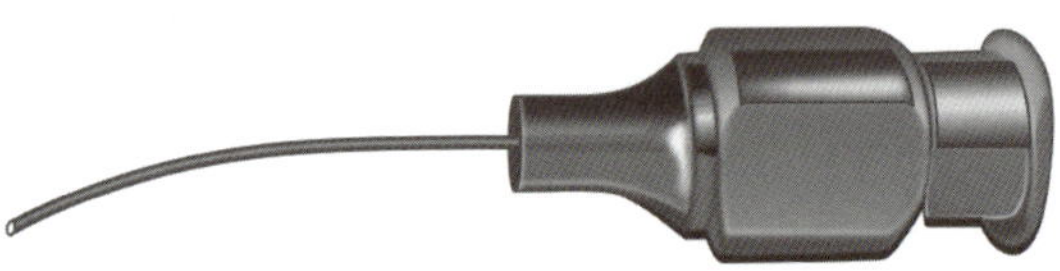

Fig. 10.36. *Kellan hydrodelineation cannula.*

5. ***Binkhorst irrigating cannula*** (Fig. 10.37). Available in 22 g, 25 g and 26 g. It is safe for the capsule, fast, simple, and the J-shaped cannula is particularly useful as loosening subincisional cortical adhesions when hydrodissection is insufficient.

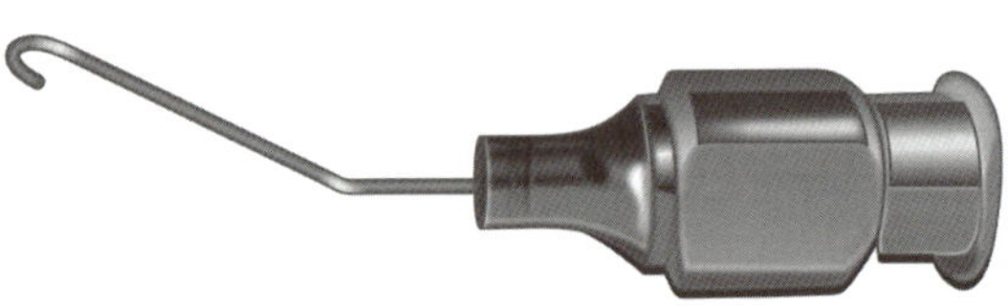

Fig. 10.37. *Binkhorst irrigating cannula.*

B. INSTRUMENTS FOR CAPSULORHEXIS

1. ***O'Gawa-Utrata capsulorhexis forceps*** are available with curved (Fig. 10.38) and straight (Fig. 10.39). These have very delicate grasping tips and extremely thin long straight shanks. They are useful for holding the lens capsule after a flap has been raised with a cystitome or bent 26-gauge needle to perform a continuous curvilinear capsulorhexis.

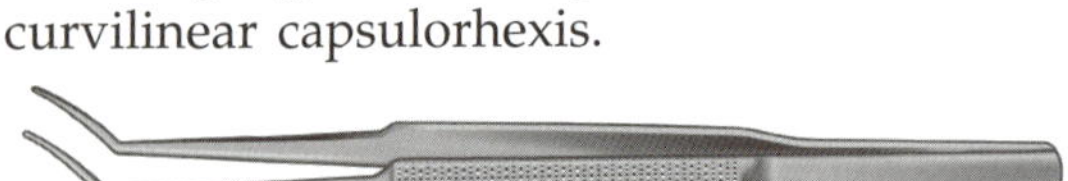

Fig. 10.38. *O'Gawa-Utrata capsulorhexis forceps—curved.*

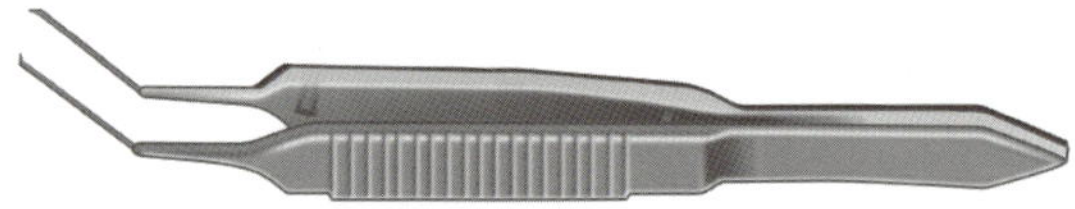

Fig. 10.39. *O'Gawa-Utrata capsulorhexis forceps—straight.*

2. ***Cystitome or capsulotome.*** It is a small needle knife with a bent tip which is sharp on both the edges (Fig. 10.40A). Presently disposable cystitome is prepared by bending the disposable 26 gauge or 30 gauge hypodermic needle (Fig. 10.40B).

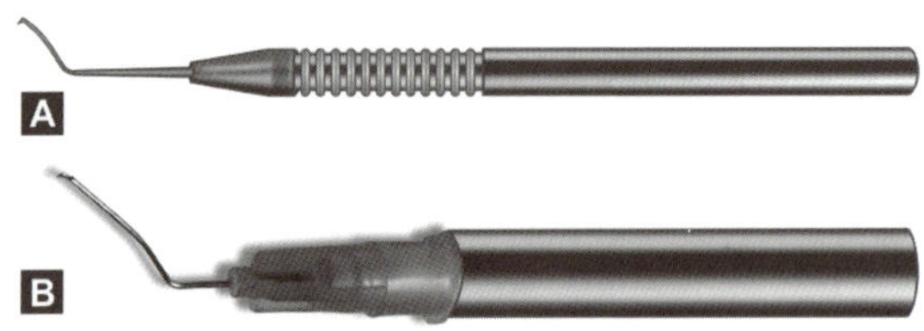

Fig. 10.40. *Cystitome or capsulotome.*

Uses. It is used for doing anterior capsulotomy or capsulorhexis during extracapsular cataract extraction.

C. PRECHOPPERS, CHOPPERS, CAPSULE POLISHERS AND IRIS REPOSITOR

1. ***Akahoshi prechopper-combo:*** It has a paddle shaped tip which has broad blunt edges on one side and thin, blunt edges on other side which merge at the tip to create a penetrating point (Fig. 10.41). The broad edges are used to completely divide a soft nucleus without harming the posterior capsule while the pointed tip and sharp edges are used to penetrate and split a hard nucleus.

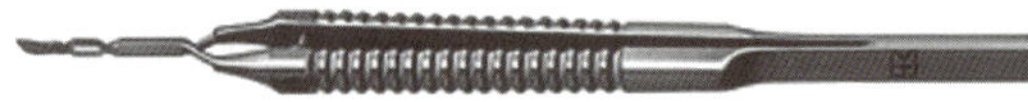

Fig. 10.41. *Akahoshi prechopper-combo.*

2. ***Choppers.*** The chopper is a fine instrument resembling Sinskey hook in shape. The inner edge of the bent tip is cutting and may have different angles.

Uses. It is used to split or chop the nucleus into smaller pieces and also for nuclear manipulation in phacoemulsification surgery.

Types of choppers

Nagahara was the first one to device the chopper, called Nagahara Karate chopper

(Fig. 10.42). Presently available choppers can be divided as:
- Blunt versus shape choppers, and
- Non-irrigating versus irrigating choppers.

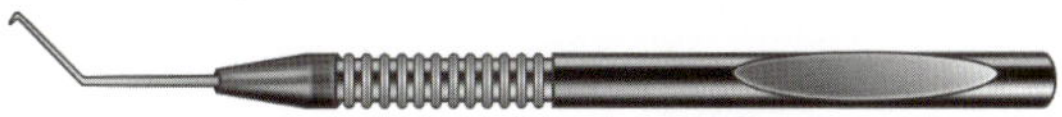

Fig. 10.42. *Nagahara Karate chopper.*

Blunt choppers (Fig. 10.43A) have a ball at their end which protects posterior capsule during manipulation, but that reduce its cutting power. ***Sharp choppers*** (Fig. 10.43B) have a sharp tip and used for cutting the nucleus.

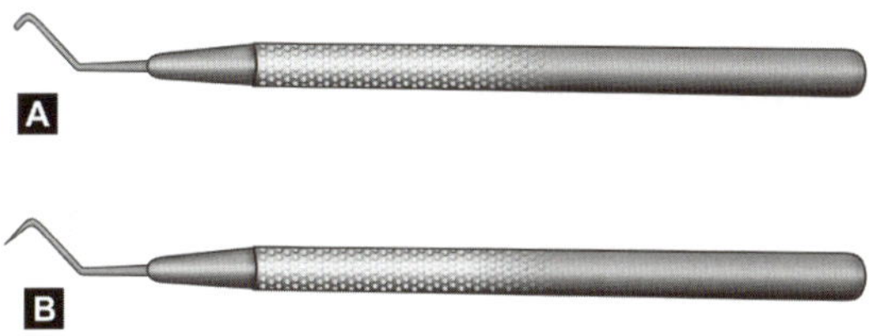

Fig. 10.43. ***(A)*** *Blunt choppers;* ***(B)*** *Sharp choppers.*

Irrigating choppers are now available, which are hollow like a needle and have a hole near the tip (Fig. 10.44). There are specially designed for use in bimanual microincision phacoemulsification.

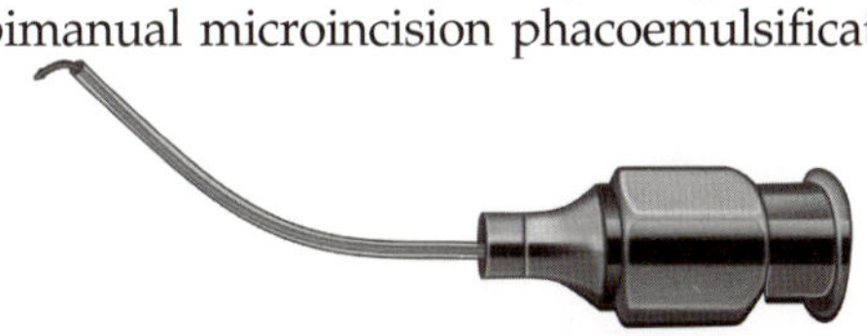

Fig. 10.44. *Irrigating choppers.*

Various modifications have been made in the design of choppers by various surgeons. A few examples are mentioned below:
- *Nagahara Karate chopper* (Fig. 10.42)
- *Agarwal's phaco chopper* (Fig. 10.45)

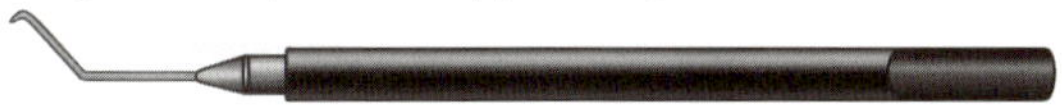

Fig. 10.45. *Agarwal's phaco chopper.*

- *Dodick nucleus chopper* (Fig. 10.46): It has a wedge- shaped inferior edge and a rounded posterior tip to avoid damage to posterior capsule.

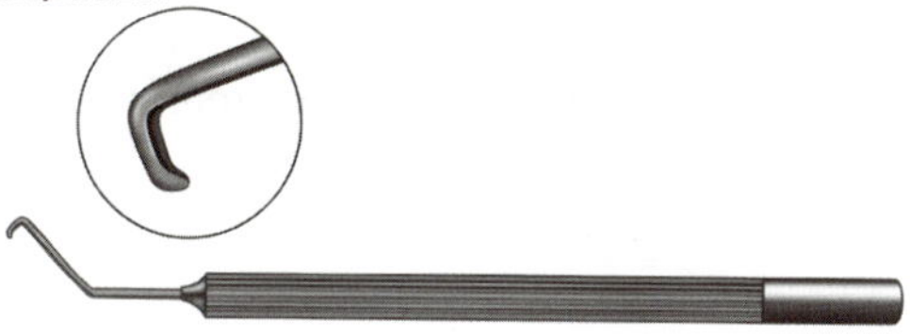

Fig. 10.46. *Dodick nucleus chopper.*

- *Kopaev phacochopper* (Fig. 10.47)

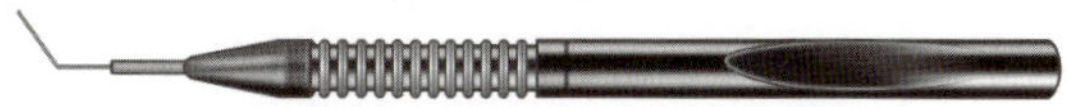

Fig. 10.47. *Kopaev phacochopper.*

- *Nucleus claw chopper* (Fig. 10.48)

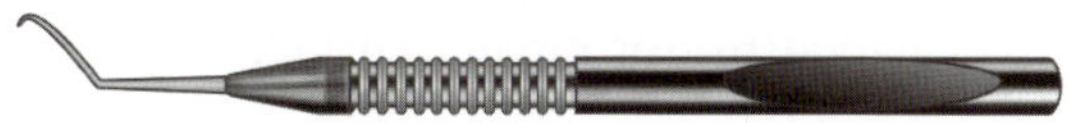

Fig. 10.48. *Nucleus claw chopper.*

- *Pyramidion universal phacochopper* (Fig. 10.49)

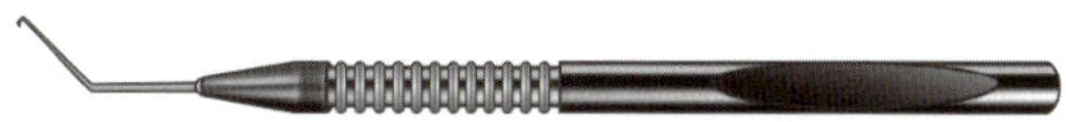

Fig. 10.49. *Pyramidion universal phacochopper.*

- *Reverse phacochopper* (Fig. 10.50)

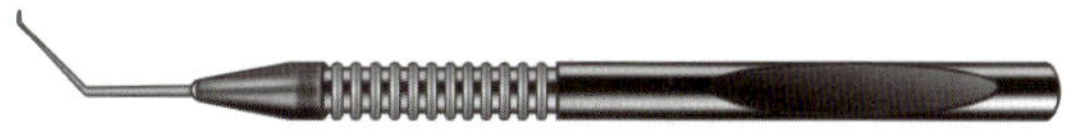

Fig. 10.50. *Reverse phacochopper.*

- *Rosen phacochopper* (Fig. 10.51)

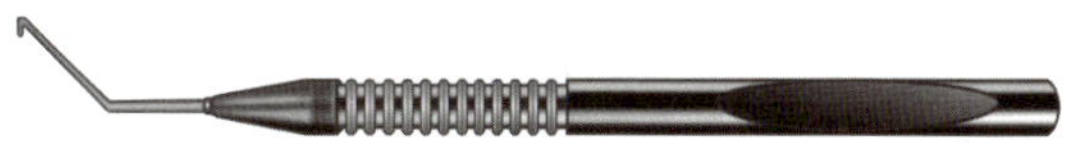

Fig. 10.51. *Rosen phacochopper.*

- *Takhtaev phacochopper* (Fig 10.52)

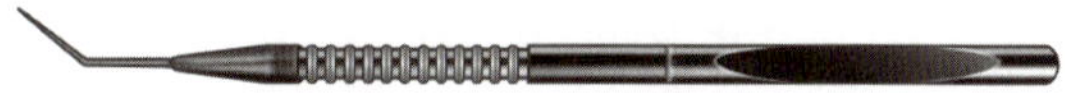

Fig. 10.52. *Takhtaev phacochopper.*

- *Tomohawk phacochopper* (Fig. 10.53)

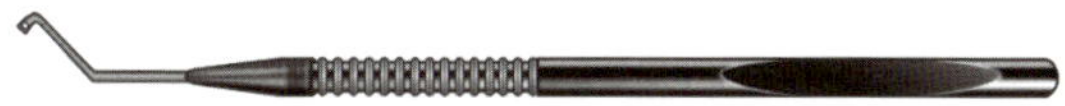

Fig. 10.53. *Tomohawk phacochopper.*

3. *Phaco spatula* (Fig. 10.54) is used to manipulate the nucleus during phacoemulsification.

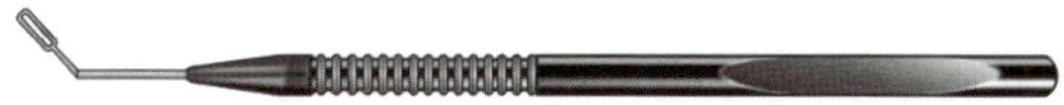

Fig. 10.54. *Phaco spatula.*

4. *Capsule polishers,* available are:

i. *Ring capsule polisher or posterior capsule polishing curette* (Fig. 10.55). It consists of a long handle and a bent slender neck. The tip of the instrument has a tiny circular ring.

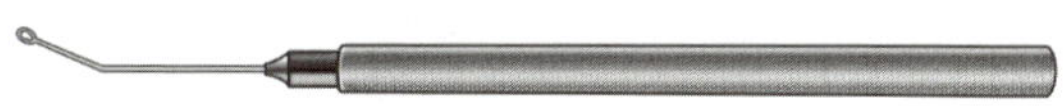

Fig. 10.55. *Ring capsule polisher.*

Uses. It is used to clear and polish the posterior lens capsule to make it more clear in the extracapsular cataract surgery. It is specially used when a plaque or sticky cortex is adhered to the posterior capsule.

ii. *Lu capsule polisher* (Fig. 10.56): It has a large olive-shaped tip for greater surface contact.

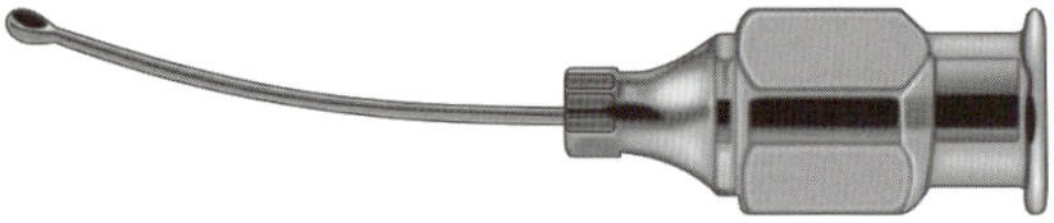

Fig. 10.56. *Lu capsule polisher.*

iii. *Round repositer* (Fig. 10.57), can also be used as posterior capsule polisher.

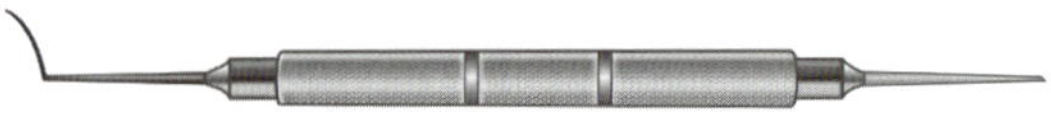

Fig. 10.57. *Round repositor.*

iv. *Sand-blasted capsule polisher* (Fig. 10.58) is very effectiver in removing the cortical matter sticking to the posterior capsule.

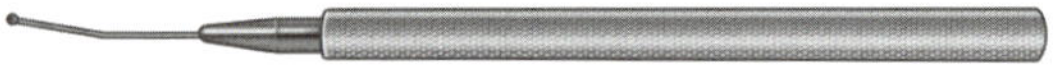

Fig. 10.58. *Sand-blasted capsule polisher.*

5. ***Iris repositor*** (Fig. 10.59). It consists of a delicate flat, malleable, straight or bent blade with blunt edges and tip attached to a handle.

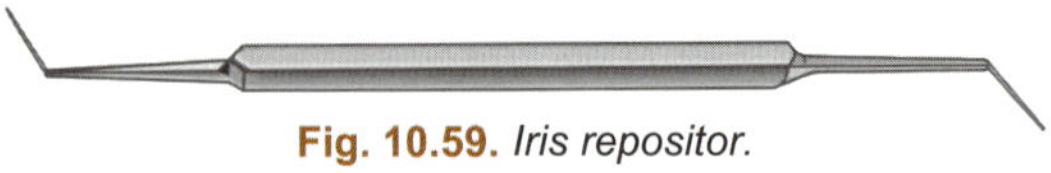

Fig. 10.59. *Iris repositor.*

Uses. (i) To reposit the iris in the anterior chamber in any intraocular surgery. (ii) To break synechiae at the pupillary margin.

D. INSTRUMENTS USED IN MICROINCISION CATARACT SURGERY (MICS)

1. ***Alio's MICS knife.*** Trapezoid-shaped. 1.25 mm/1.4 mm/2.0 mm angled, double bevel (Fig. 10.60).

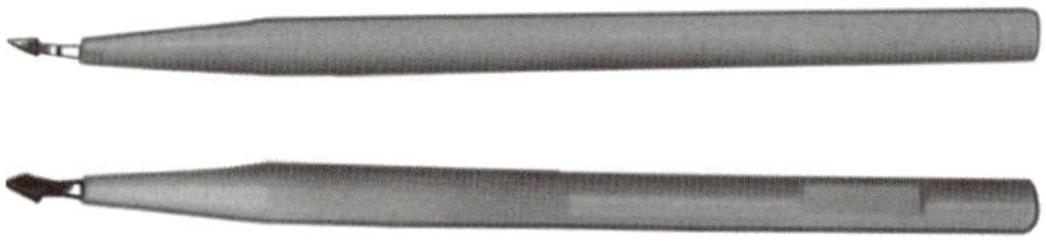

Fig. 10.60. Alio's MICS knife

2. ***MICS diamond knife.*** Trapezoid-shaped. 1.25 mm/1.4 mm/2.0 mm angled. Laser etched line indicating 1.25 mm width (Fig 10.61).

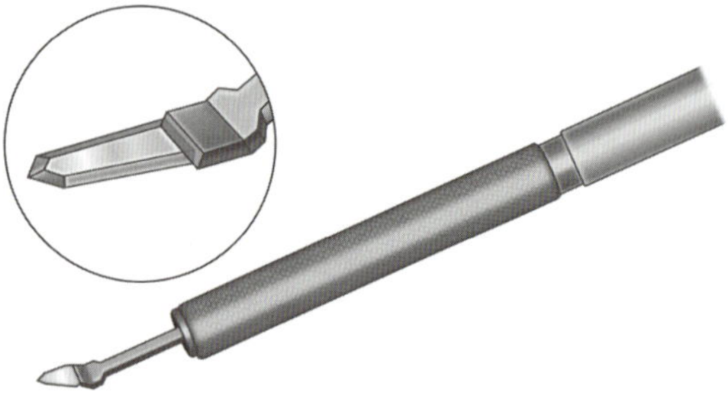

Fig. 10.61. *MICS diamond knife.*

3. ***Alio's MICS capsulorhexis forceps.*** There is a pointed hook at the end of forceps which enables controlled puncturing of anterior capsule of the lens (Fig 10.62).

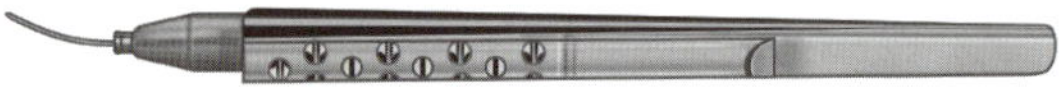

Fig. 10.62. *Alio's MICS capsulorhexis forceps.*

4. ***Gianetti MICS capsulorhexis forceps*** (Fig. 10.63)

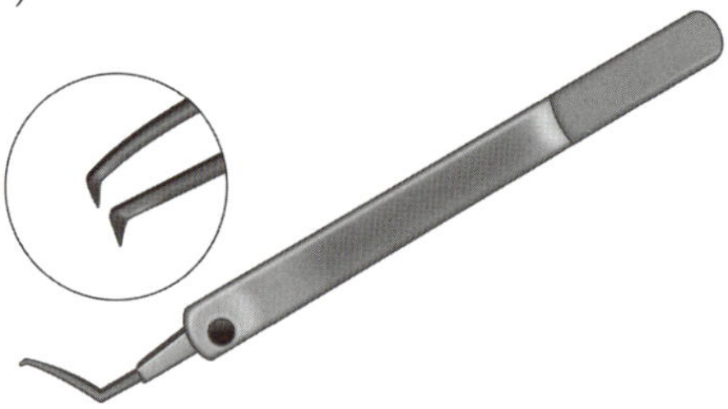

Fig. 10.63. *Gianetti MICS capsulorhexis forceps.*

5. ***Kelman MICS capsulorhexis forceps*** (Fig. 10.64)

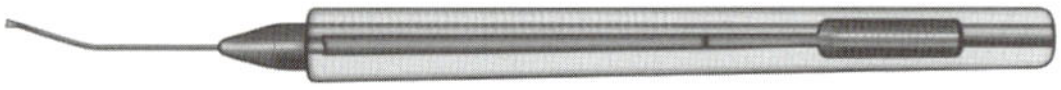

Fig. 10.64. *Kelman MICS capsulorhexis forceps.*

6. ***Hoffman MICS capsulorhexis forceps*** (Fig. 10.65)

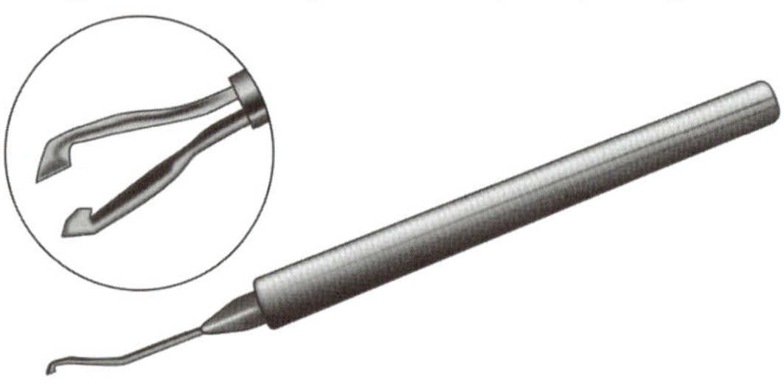

Fig. 10.65. *Hoffman MICS capsulorhexis forceps.*

7. *Alio's Rosen MICS phacochopper* (Fig. 10.66)

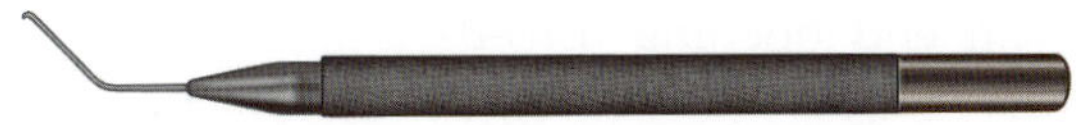

Fig. 10.66. *Alio Rosen MICS phacochopper.*

8. *Alio's MICS hydromanipulator irrigating finger nail* (Fig. 10.67). Its end is finger nail shaped. It helps to remove soft cataracts. There is 1 mm irrigation hole on the bottom lower side. It has very thin walls to increase internal diameter of instrument

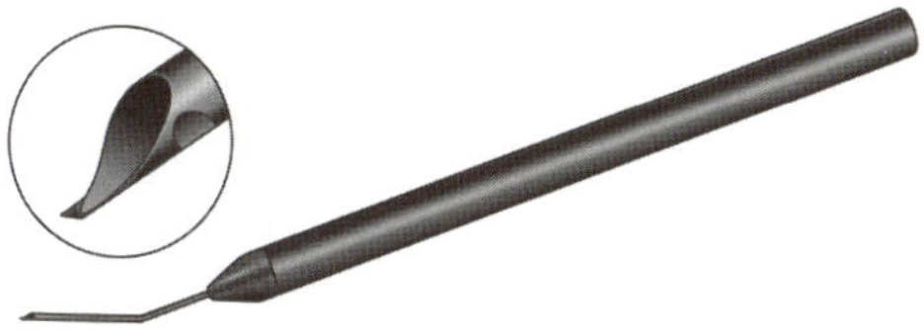

Fig. 10.67. *Alio's MICS hydromanipulator irrigating finger nail.*

9. *Alio's MICS irrigating stinger.* It is used to remove hard cataracts. It has a tip at the end which is angled downwards (Fig. 10.68). It is useful to chop off segments or dividing masses of the nucleus in the phacoemulsification tip.

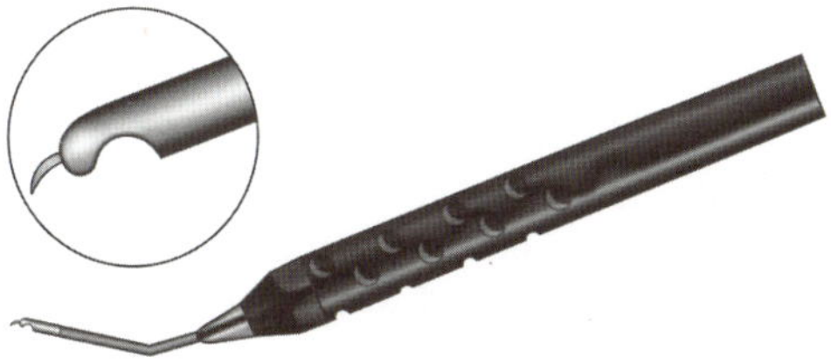

Fig. 10.68. *Alio's MICS irrigating stinger.*

10. *Alio's MICS aspiration handpiece.* Used for remaining cortical remains. It has a port diameter of 0.3 mm which assures stability of hydrodynamic of liquid within the anterior chamber (Fig. 10.69).

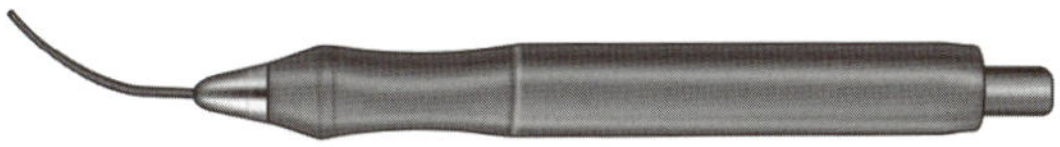

Fig. 10.69. *Alio's MICS aspiration handpiece.*

11. *Alio's MICS scissors* (Fig. 10.70). Used for complicated cataract which may require cutting within the anterior chamber.

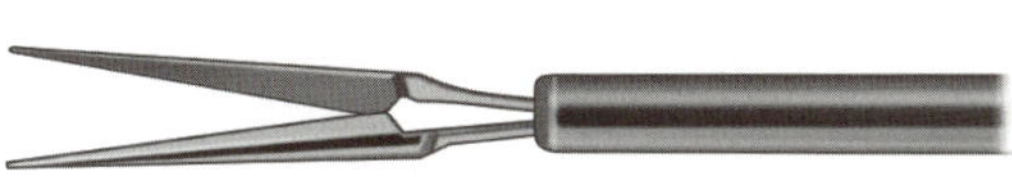

Fig. 10.70. *Alio's MICS scissors.*

Uses: It can cut delicate membranes, adhesions, to make iridotomy, and also cut the fibrosis of capsules.

E. INSTRUMENTS FOR INTRAOCULAR LENS IMPLANTATION

For IOL implantation, the cataract surgery set should contain the following basic additional instruments:

1. *IOL holding forceps.* These are spring action forceps with short, blunt and curved blades having smooth edges and tips with platform (no teeth or serrations). These are available in various designs:

- *Clayman lens forceps* (Fig. 10.71). It has curved blades with smooth edges and tips with platform but no teeth, used for holding non-foldable PMMA lenses.

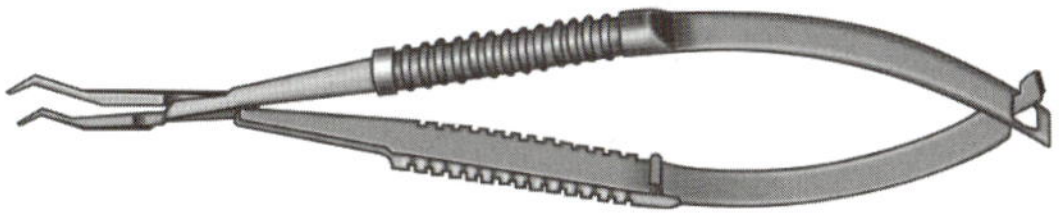

Fig. 10.71. *Clayman lens forceps.*

- *Seibel lens folding forceps* (Fig. 10.72). It is used for the implantation of foldable intraocular lenses. It allows even folding of acrylic and silicone lenses.

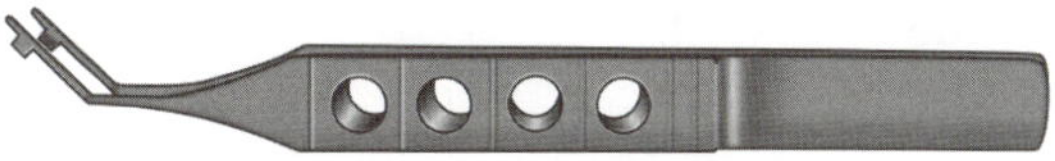

Fig. 10.72. *Seibel lens folding forceps.*

- *Anis lens holding forceps* (Fig. 10.73): They have extra delicate long smooth jaws and and 450 angulation. These are used for holding rigid lenses.

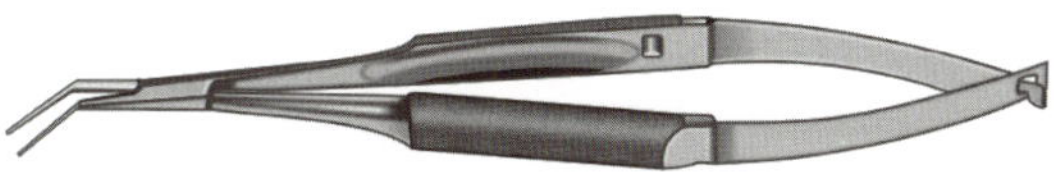

Fig. 10.73. *Anis lens holding forceps.*

2. *Kelman-McPherson forceps* (Fig. 10.74). These are fine forceps with bent limbs. They are non-toothed forceps with smooth jaws.

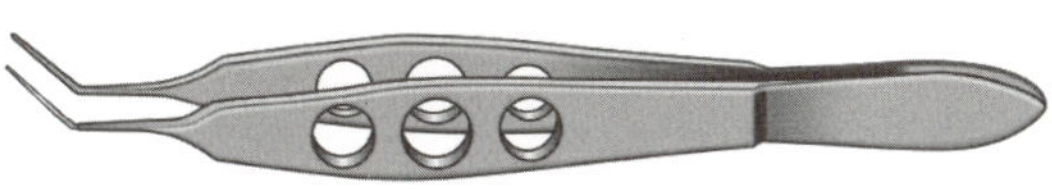

Fig. 10.74. *Kelman-McPherson forceps.*

Uses. (i) To hold the superior haptic of IOL during its placement. (ii) To tear off the anterior capsular flap in ECCE, (iii) Can be used for suture tying.

3. ***Sinskey hook*** (Fig. 10.75). It is a fine but stout instrument with a bent tip. The tip engages the dialing holes of the IOL.

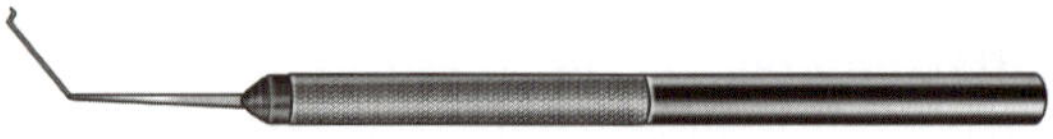

Fig. 10.75. *Sinskey hook.*

Uses. (i) It is used to dial the PMMA non-foldable IOL for proper positioning in the capsular bag or ciliary sulcus. (ii) It can also be used to manipulate the nucleus in phacoemulsification surgery. Nucleus manipulation may be in the form of nucleus rotation in the capsular bag, cracking of the nucleus and feeding of the nuclear fragments into the phaco tip.

4. ***IOL dialer*** is similar to Sinskey hook except that its tip in dumble shaped (Fig. 10.76). Its uses are similar to Sinskey hook.

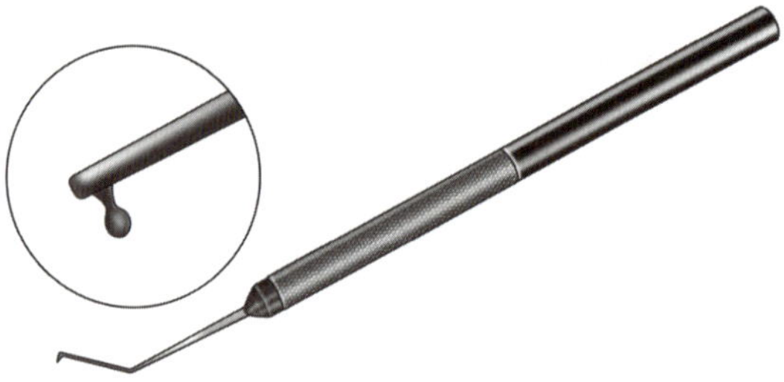

Fig. 10.76. *IOL dialer.*

5. ***Nevyas IOL manipulator*** (Fig. 10.77). The tip provides sufficient traction on the surface of the IOL to rotate it without damaging the optic.

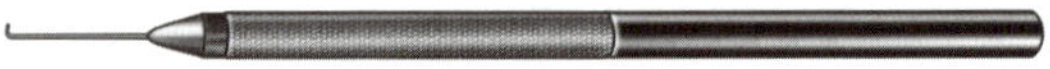

Fig. 10.77. *Nevyas IOL manipulator.*

6. ***Glued IOL forceps—Ahmed micrograsper.*** It is an end opening forceps (Fig. 10.78) from MicroSurgical Technology (MST) used for glued IOL surgery.

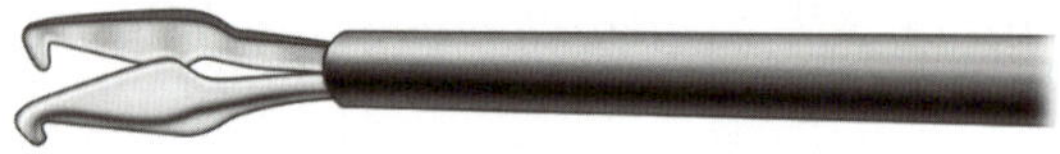

Fig. 10.78. *Ahmed micrograsper.*

BIBLIOGRAPHY

1. Arshinoff S. Dispersive and cohesive viscoelastic materials in phacoemulsification. In: Solomon L, ed. Ophthalmic Advisory Panel at the ASCRS. Montreal: Medicopea International; 28–40;1995.
2. Arshinoff SA, Jafari M. A new classification of ophthalmic viscosurgical devices (OVDs)-2005. J Cataract Refract Surg. 31(11):2167–2171;2005.
3. Arshinoff SA. Comparative physical properties of ophthalmic viscoelastic materials. Ophthalmic Pract. 7(1):16–19,36–37;1989.
4. Arshinoff SA. Dispersive and cohesive viscoelastic materials in phacoemulsification. Ophthalmic Pract. 13:98–104;1995.
5. Arshinoff SA. Dispersive-cohesive viscoelastic soft shell technique. J Cataract Refract Surg. 25(2):167–173;1999.
6. Arshinoff SA. Modified SST–USST for tamsulosin-associated intraocular floppy-iris syndrome. J Cataract Refract Surg. 32:559–561; 2006.
7. Arshinoff SA. Phaco slice and separate. J Cataract Refract Surg. 25(4):474–478;1999.
8. Arshinoff SA. Using BSS with viscoadaptives in the ultimate soft-shell technique. J Cataract Refract Surg. 28(9):1509–1514;2002.
9. Arshinoff Steve A. Healon5 entering selected countries in Europe. Ocular Surgery News, International Ed. September; 9:9:11–12;1998.
10. Balazs EA, inventor; Biotrics, Inc. assignee. Ultrapure hyaloronic acid and the use thereof. US patent 4 141 973 1973. October 17, 1979.

INTRAOCULAR LENSES: AN OVERVIEW

11 CHAPTER

HISTORICAL OVERVIEW

What has happened in the past 100 years in terms of eye care makes the previous 3,000 years look like a period of dormancy. Cataract surgery has seen an exponential growth in the past decade. Intraocular lenses have evolved along with the improvement in surgical techniques for cataract. The history of the IOL is interesting and colourful. It is a classic example of the improvement of medicine with the active cooperation of science and industry.

Credit for the invention and first implantation of the IOL is given to Sir Harold Ridley of London (Fig. 11.1). It was serendipity that led him to the discovery of IOL. He noticed innocuous nature of injuries sustained by the pilots during Second World War when bullets would strike the plastic canopy of the aircraft, causing small shreds of plastic to go in their eye. He realized that this polymethylmethacrylate (PMMA) acrylic of the canopies was an inert material compatible with the eyes. Ridley's first IOL implantation was a two-step procedure

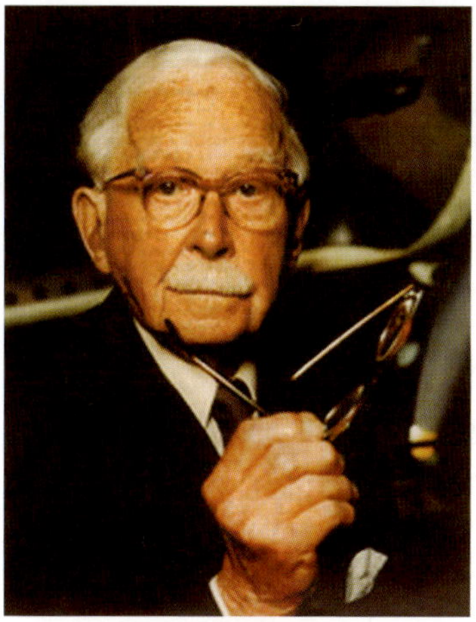

Fig. 11.1. *Sir Harold Ridley.*

carried out on a 45-year-old lady. The extracapsular removal of cataract was done on Nov 29, 1949 and IOL implantation was done as a secondary procedure on Feb 8, 1950.

The journey from Ridley's lens to the modern state of the art IOLs of today is best read divided into generations, almost coincident with the generational evolution of cataract surgery.

GENERATION I IOLs (ORIGINAL RIDLEY POSTERIOR CHAMBER LENS; 1949–54)

Ridley's lens (Fig. 11.2) was a biconvex PMMA disc designed to be implanted after extracapsular cataract extraction (ECCE). During the next 12 years after its discovery, about 1000 Ridley lenses were implanted. Modern analysis has demonstrated that Ridley's IOL passes modern optical bench examinations. These IOL implantations were described as successes in 70% cases. Dislocation (20%) and secondary glaucoma (10%) were the main causes of failure of the surgery.

GENERATION II IOLs (EARLY ANTERIOR CHAMBER LENSES; 1952–62)

As a consequence of the relatively high incidence of dislocations with the Ridley lens, a new implantation site was considered—the anterior chamber with fixation of lens in the angle recess after ICCE or ECCE. Early anterior chamber IOLs were rigid (Fig. 11.3A to D). Complications like late endothelial atrophy, corneal decompensation, pseudophakic bullous keratopathy and UGH (uveitis, glaucoma and hyphema) syndrome were observed with the initial anterior chamber IOLs.

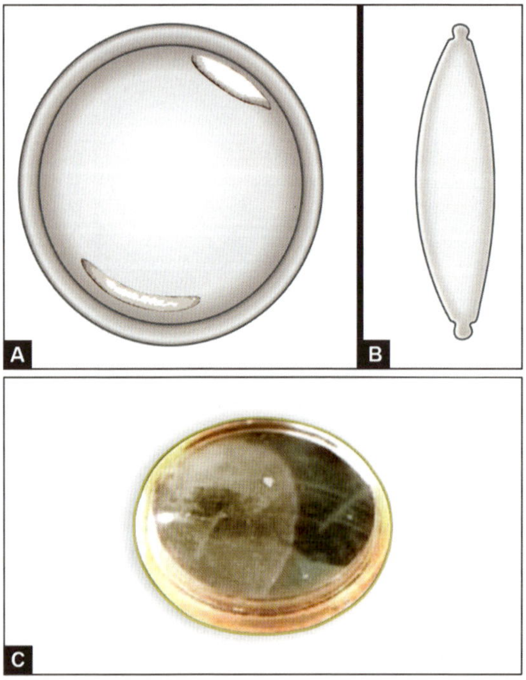

Fig. 11.2. *Ridley's original posterior chamber intraocular lens: **(A and B)** Diagrammatic depiction; **(C)** Photograph.*

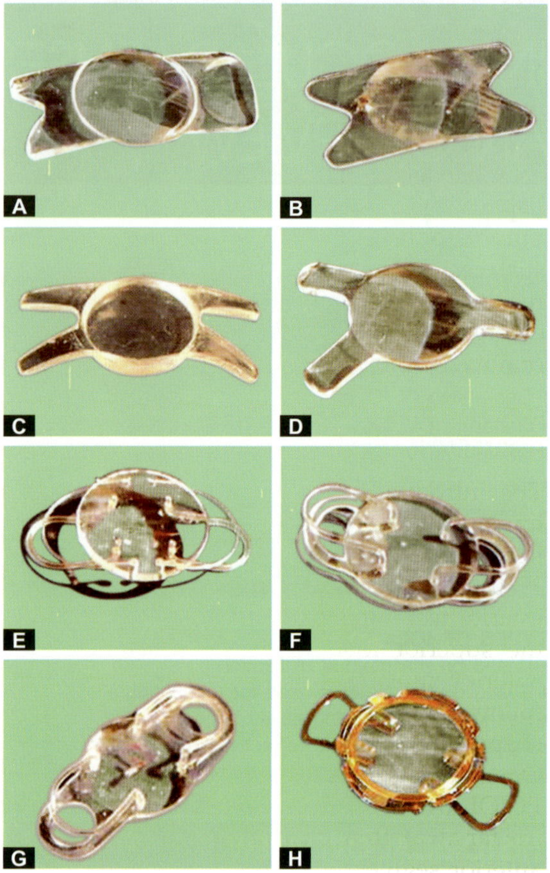

Fig. 11.3. *Earlier intraocular lenses: **(A)** AC lens with broad foot plate; **(B and C)** Four-foot AC lenses; **(D)** Three-foot AC lens; **(E and F)** Binkhorst four-loop lens; **(G)** Boberg-Ans four-loop lens (Rayner); **(H)** Two-loop Lynell glass lens.*

GENERATION III IOLs (IRIS SUPPORTED LENSES; 1953–75)

Iris supported lenses overcame the problems with Ridley's PCIOL and early ACIOLs. Initial iris supported IOLs were four-loop lenses (Fig. 11.3E to G). Iris chafing, pupillary abnormalities, and dislocation and improper sizing were reported with these lenses. This prompted a change from ICCE to ECCE and the introduction of two-loop iridocapsular IOL (Fig. 11.3H) which led to a marked reduction in incidence of above mentioned complications. These changes were a landmark in the evolution of IOLs and laid foundation for modern capsular (in-the-bag) fixation of posterior chamber IOLs.

GENERATION IV IOLs (INTERMEDIATE ANTERIOR CHAMBER LENSES; 1963–1990)

The problems of iris tissue chafing and difficulties in correct sizing with rigid IOLs were addressed by the development of anterior chamber lenses with more flexible loops and haptics made of PMMA or polypropylene. Tumble polishing of IOLs produced excellent surfaces and edges. This search of flexibility resulted in many of the disastrous lenses that emerged in 1970s and early 1980 and had to be removed from the market.

GENERATION V IOLs (RIGID PMMA POSTERIOR CHAMBER LENSES; 1975–1992)

The introduction of PCIOLs designed to be implanted following ECCE under an operating microscope gained momentum in the early 1970s. The lens was a tripod design with two inferior feet implanted in the capsular bag and the superior foot implanted in front of the anterior capsule and sutured to iris. It was followed by lens with an optic and 2 flexible J-shaped loops succeeded by C-shaped loops. One obvious major theoretical advantage of PCIOL over ACIOL is its position behind the iris far away from the delicate structures of the anterior segment.

GENERATION VI IOLs (IMPROVED, SOFT FOLDABLE AND MODERN ANTERIOR CHAMBER IOLS, 1992–PRESENT DAY)

Generation VI IOLs represent the improved rigid PMMA and soft foldable conventional (unifocal) IOLs used presently. Many changes in surgical techniques that occurred after 1980s and into the 1990s include the introduction of ocular viscoelastic devices, increased awareness of the advantages of in-the-bag fixation, the introduction of continuous curvilinear capsulorhexis (CCC), hydrodissection and the increased use of phacoemulsification. Silicone lenses were introduced followed by hydrogel and acrylic lenses subsequently. Apart from the above mentioned standard lenses, special lenses were developed to meet special requirements.

GENERATION VII IOLs

Generation VII IOLs represent the various types of multifocal IOLs being used presently.

GENERATION VIII IOLs

Generation VIII IOLs represent the various accommodative IOLs, toric IOLs and phakic refractive lenses (PRLs) being used presently.

IOL CHEMISTRY

A variety of materials have been used for IOLs including glass, but most have been made from plastics, also known as polymers. Biomaterials currently used for manufacture of IOL optics can be divided into two major groups according to the rigidity of the materials—rigid and foldable.

RIGID IOL

The rigid material for IOL optic usage is PMMA. PMMA is 'glassy' material at room and body temperature, i.e. it is both rigid and brittle. It is inert, hydrophobic and non-autoclavable. Its main disadvantages are hydrophobicity (causes adherence of cell and bacteria) and shattering caused by laser irradiation by secondary laser procedures. It is available in positive and negative optic powers and is suitable for ciliary sulcus-fixated secondary IOL implantation.

FOLDABLE IOLs

Foldable IOLs use flexible polymers which are of two types:

1. Silicones

Known chemically as polysiloxanes, derive their flexibility from both their chain as well as intermolecular structure. They have good memory and incite little inflammation. But surface deposits are common and silicone lenses are prone to decentration.

2. Acrylics

'Acrylic' is derived as any compound from acrylic acid. They are available in two varieties, hydrophobic and hydrophilic. It has all the advantages of foldable optic with none of the problems associated with silicone.

i. Flexible hydrophobic acrylic polymers

They are nearly identical to the glassy PMMA. Hydrophobic lenses have very low water content, usually less than 2%.

ii. Flexible hydrophilic acrylic polymers

They are insoluble in water but have the ability to swell like a sponge in water and retain a significant amount of water to form soft, swollen, rubbery mass. They are hydrophilic, hence repel cells and microbes and incite less reaction. Hydrophilic IOLs had occupied a backseat to silicone and hydrophobic acrylics due to technical complexities, varying degrees of biocompatibility and several case reports of whitish discolouration on the optic surface. But with technological improvement and introduction of MICS, there is a resurgence of hydrophilic IOLs.

Haptic material

Four materials are used at present for the manufacture of the haptic component (loops) of three-piece lenses: PMMA, polypropylene (prolene), polyamide (elastamide), and polyvinylidene fluoride (PVDF).

Light filters

Two classes of UV-absorbing chromophores are used in general for the manufacture of pseudophakic IOLs, namely, benzotriazole and benzophenone.

More recently, IOLs that filter both UV and short wavelength visible violet and blue light have been introduced. A yellow chromophore is incorporated into the IOL optic, which represents an attempt to more accurately mimic the light transmission characteristics of the normal crystalline lens.

TYPES OF IOLs

During the last 70 years, a large number of different types and styles of lenses have been developed. Undoubtedly, reviewing the evolution of IOLs in the last half century will be fascinating but, unfortunately, it is beyond the scope of this chapter which is devoted to the basic aspects of IOLs. However, as mentioned above from Ridley's first lens implantation to the present day, the evolution of IOLs can be arbitrarily divided into eight generations. The rigid posterior chamber IOLs belong to the fifth generation, the improved rigid PMMA IOLs and the foldable IOLs to the sixth generation, multifocal IOLs to the seventh generation and phakic refractive lenses (PRLs), toric IOLs, and accommodative IOLs to the eighth generation.

Presently available IOLs can be grouped as follows.

I. BASED ON THE METHOD OF FIXATION

The major classes of IOLs based on the method of fixation in the eye are as follows:

1. Anterior chamber IOLs (ACIOLs)

These lenses lie entirely in front of the iris and are supported in the angle of anterior chamber. ACIOLs can be inserted after intracapsular cataract extraction or extracapsular cataract extraction. These are not very popular due to comparatively higher incidence of bullous keratopathy. When indicated, 'Kelman multiflex' (Fig. 11.4A) type of ACIOL is used commonly.

2. Iris-supported lenses

These lenses are fixed on the iris with the help of sutures, loops or claws. These lenses are also not very popular due to a high incidence of postoperative complications. Example of iris-supported lens is Singh and Worst's iris claw lens (Fig. 11.4B).

3. Posterior chamber IOLs (PCIOLs)

These lenses rest entirely behind the iris. They may be supported by the ciliary sulcus or the capsular bag. Ideal is 'in-the-bag-fixation.' Commonly used models of PCIOLs are modified C-loop (Fig. 11.4C), and quadriloop (Fig. 11.4D).

4. Scleral-fixated IOLs

These IOLs are used in the absence of capsular support. There are two main techniques of scleral fixation of IOLs:

i. Sutured scleral-fixated IOLs. Commonly used IOLs are:

- *Standard one- or three-piece PCIOL.* Some suture fixation techniques involve tying knots directly to the haptic of a one- or three-piece IOL.
- *Special scleral-fixated IOLs with eyelets* in the haptic include:

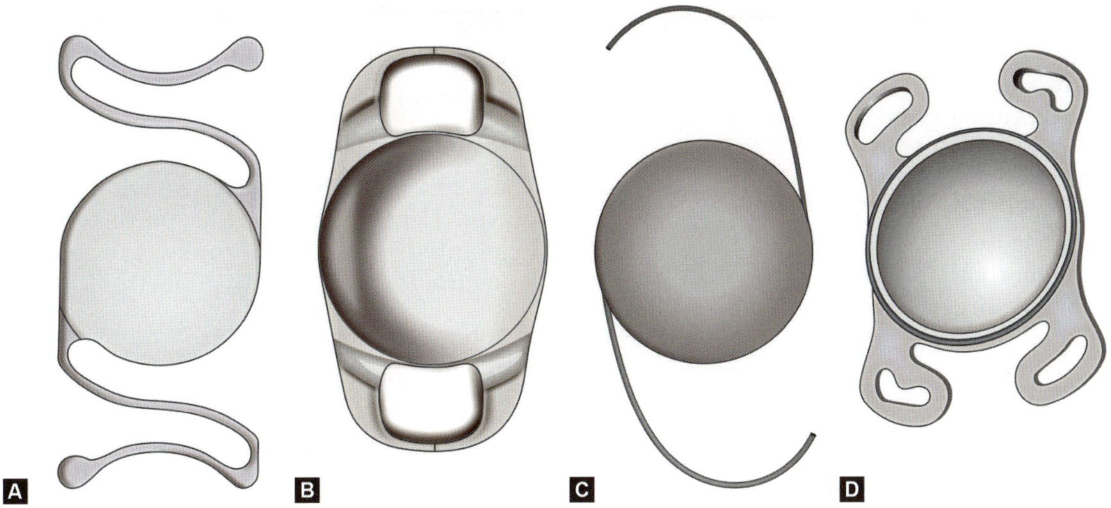

Fig. 11.4. Types of IOLs, based on the method of fixation: (A) Anterior chamber IOL (Kelman multiflex); (B) Iris-supported IOL; (C) Posterior chamber IOL (modified C-loop); (D) Posterior chamber IOL (quadriloop).

- Alcon CZ70BD PMMA lens contains eyelets along the haptics that facilitate suture fixation and requires a 7 mm incision, as it is not foldable.
- Bausch and Lomb Akreos AO60 hydrophilic acrylic lens contains four eyelets through which suture can be passed, providing 4-point fixation.
- Bausch and Lomb enVista MX60 IOL is a hydrophobic acrylic IOL that contains eyelets at the two hapticoptic junctions.
- Zeiss CT Lucia 602 is a three-piece hydrophobic acrylic IOL with poly-vinylidene fluoride (PVDF) monofilament haptics.

II. BASED ON THE MATERIAL USED FOR MANUFACTURE

1. RIGID PMMA IOLs

The commonly used material for manufacture of rigid IOLs is PMMA. It is chemically stable compound. Its excellent optical properties have been demonstrated through years of experience with PMMA contact lenses. PMMA has a relatively high index of refraction.

As with other lens materials, it may vary some what with temperature and water absorption. The specific gravity of PMMA is about 1.2 and thus is much closer to neutral buoyancy than the much heavier glass. The use of glass as an implant material has been abandoned because of its weight and its tendency to shatter when subjected to laser irradiation in the course of secondary laser procedures.

2. FOLDABLE IOLs

These lenses have become popular after the success of phacoemulsification technique of lens extraction through a small incision. The foldable lenses are available in many different designs and are made up of silicone, acrylic or hydrogel.

i. ***Silicone IOLs.*** These are made from a number of formulations of polyorgano-siloxane. Silicone polymers have a lower index of refraction (μ = 1.43) than PMMA (μ = 1.49) and thus must be thicker for the same refractive correction.

ii. ***Acrylic IOLs.*** Acrylic or hydrogel lenses are generally manufactured from polyhydroxy-ethyl methacrylate.

iii. ***Hydrogel IOLs.*** Like silicone lenses, the hydrogel lenses are also sufficiently flexible to be inserted through a small incision.

The index of refraction of hydrogels is also 1.43. These are available as hydrophilic and hydrophobic IOLs.

- Hydrophobic IOLs are comparatively tougher and have low water content (<2%).

- Hydrophilic lenses have a water content of approximately 3.8%. They are smaller in their dry state and swell upon hydration. For instance, a 4.3 mm dry optic can expand to 6 mm when implanted.

3. Rollable IOLs or ultrathin IOLs

These lenses are required to be implanted through a <2 mm incision after microincision cataract surgery or the so-called phaconit technique. Some examples of commercially available ultrathin IOLs for microincision cataract surgery are (Fig. 11.5):

- AcriSmart™ lens is a hydrophilic acrylic lens with 25% water content and a hydrophobic coating. The overall design is that of a plate haptic lens with square edges.
- ThinOptx ultrachoice™ lens. It is manufactured from off-the-shelf hydrophilic acrylic materials. The ultrathin properties of this lens are attributable to its Fresnel optic design.
- Medennium smart lens. It is made of thermoplastic hydrophobic acrylic gel polymer.
- Slimflex lens. It is made of 26% hydrophilic acrylic material. It is not of plate haptic design but has a 360° square edge optic, four haptics and 5° angulation between optic and haptics.

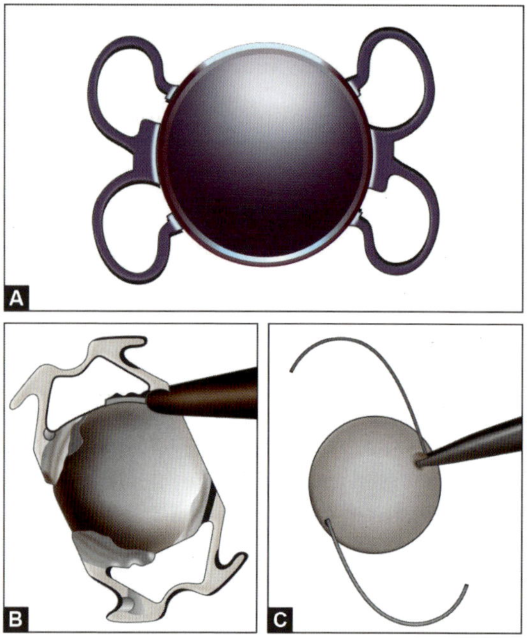

Fig. 11.5. *Ultrathin or rollable IOLs: (A) Slimflex; (B) Alcon Acrysof MA 60AC; (C) Human optics MC 611.*

III. BASED ON THE FOCUSING ABILITY

Based on the focusing ability, the IOLs are of following types:

1. Monofocal IOLs

These are the conventional IOLs having unifocal power. Depending upon the power of IOLs implanted, these can make the patient emmetropic, myopic or hypermetropic.

2. Enhanced monofocal IOLs

Recently, a new generation of monofocal IOLs called enhanced monofocal IOLs has been introduced, with the aim of providing excellent visual acuity for distant (the same as conventional monofocal lenses) while improving intermediate distant performance, without the side effects traditionally caused by multifocality.

3. Multifocal IOLs

As the name indicates, they have optics to focus for distant as well as near vision. These are based on either refractive optics or diffractive optics. These are also called simultaneous vision lenses.

4. Pseudoaccommodative IOLs

For example, the AcrySof ReSTOR (MA60D3 or SA60D3) with its apodized diffractive optic provides to the patients an excellent near visual acuity without compromising distance vision. This IOL has an anterior conventional refractive surface that provides the distance-vision power and a posterior concentric diffractive plate that provides additional near-viewing power ranging from +2.5 to +4.5 D.

5. Accommodative IOLs

These IOLs exhibit anterior movement of the optic to improve near vision. Examples of accommodative IOLs are:

- Eyeonics Crystalens AT-45, and
- AG Accommodative IOL.

6. Extended depth-of-focus

Extended depth-of-focus (EDOF) IOL, e.g. TECNIS Symfony IOL, which allows extended range of vision due to an elongated focus area (instead of several focus areas of multifocal IOLs).

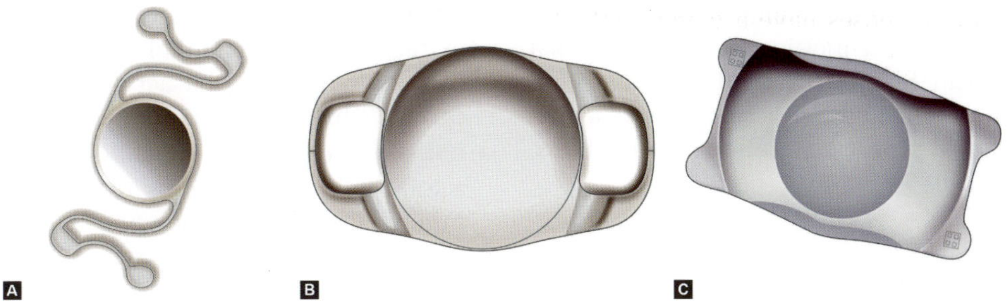

Fig. 11.6. *Phakic IOLs: (A) Angle supported PC IOL; (B) Retro iris fixed PC IOL; (C) Plate haptic IOL.*

7. Trifocal IOLs

These are newer lenses which allow distant vision, intermediate vision and near vision. Examples include Alcon PanOptix trifocal IOLs and Zeiss AT LISA Tri.

IV. APHAKIC VERSUS PHAKIC REFRACTIVE LENSES

In addition to the aphakic IOLs which are implanted after lens extraction, special phakic IOLs have been developed which are placed between the cornea and crystalline lens. Three types of PRLs are available.

1. Angle-supported PRLs

These IOLs are designed to have long legs (haptics). The best known lens is NUVITA a third-generation Baikoff lens design, by Bausch and Lomb Surgical, France (Fig. 11.6A).

2. Iris-supported PRLs

The best known as of today is Artisan lens (Fig. 11.6B).

Posterior chamber sulcus fixated PRLs

These IOLs are designed to vault the crystalline lens (Fig. 11.6C).

Examples of posterior chamber PRL are:
- ICL™ by Staar Surgical
- PRL™ by IVI-Medennium.

V. BASED ON SPHERICITY AND TORICITY

These include spheric IOLs, aspheric IOLs and toric IOLs.

1. Toric IOLs now provide the opportunity to correct corneal astigmatism, offering patients with pre-existing astigmatism optimal distance vision without the use of spectacles or contact lenses with a cylindrical correction. Shimizu *et al.* presented the first toric IOL in 1994. This was a non-foldable three-piece toric IOL made from PMMA.

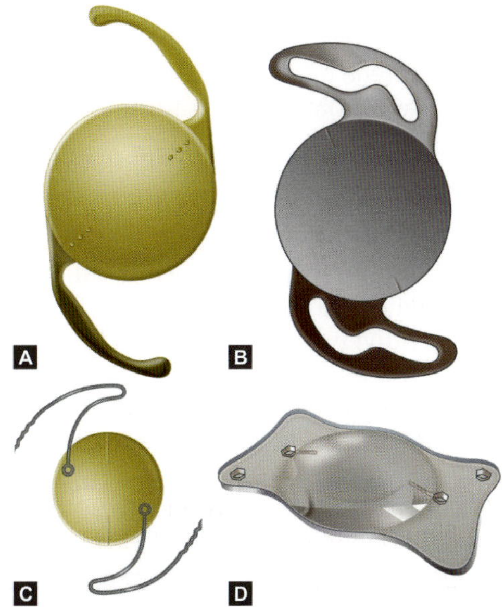

Fig. 11.7. *Toric intraocular lenses: (A) Acrysof®; (B) Rayner; (C) Zeiss; and (D) Toric multifocal.*

Currently available toric IOLs are foldable, some of the examples are as follows (Fig. 11.7):
- AcrySof (Alcon)–Hydrophobic acrylic
- T-flex (Rayner)–Hydrophilic acrylic
- STAAR (STAAR Surgical company)–Silicone
- Acri. Comfort (Carl Zeiss)–Hydrophilic acrylic

Indications for toric IOL implantation. Patients with regular astigmatism (otherwise having good vision potential and without any coexistent ocular pathology) which might need correction for astigmatism, should be considered for toric IOLs.

Toric IOL power calculation. It requires accurate keratometry and consideration for surgically induced astigmatism (SIA), which depends upon the size of the incision. AcrySof toric IOLs require a 2.2 mm incision for IOL implantation. These incisions have been shown to induce an SIA of 0.2–0.3 D for temporal incisions and 0.4 D for superior incisions. (For details of IOL power calculation for toric IOLs, see page xx.)

Technique of toric IOL implantation. IOL implantation requires a proper pre- and intra-operative marking of axis:

The first step consists of preoperative marking of the horizontal axis with the patient in upright position to correct for cyclotorsion. This may be done with the patient seated at the slit lamp and with a coaxial thin slit turned to 0–180 degrees.

- Another technique to mark the horizontal axis is by using a bubble marker, such as a Nuijts/Lane Toric Reference Marker (ASICO) or by using a gravity marker with a calibrated horizontal position.
- Intraoperatively, the preoperative horizontal marks are used to position an angular graduation instrument. The actual alignment axis is marked using a toric axis marker.

Newer techniques to ensure accurate intraoperative toric IOL alignment described are as follows:

- *Iris-fingerprinting technique,* described by Osher, in which preoperative detailed images of the eye are obtained. The desired alignment axis is drawn in this image.
- *Intraoperative wavefront aberrometry* is a device connected to the operating microscope and enables intraoperative measurement of residual refraction.
- *Verion image-guided system* uses real-time eye tracking, based on iris and blood vessel characteristics. Preoperatively, a detailed image of the eye is captured, in which blood vessel and iris characteristics are visible.

Rotational stability is a crucial factor in the safety and efficacy of toric IOLs, since as little as 10 degrees of axis misalignment reduces the efficacy of the astigmatic correction by 33%. *Factors responsible for rotational stability* include:

- *IOL material.* Hydrophobic acrylic lenses have the highest bioadhesion property between the IOL and the capsular bag followed by hydrophilic acrylic, PMMA IOLs and finally silicone IOLs. Fibronectin is the primary extracellular protein involved in adhesion to the bag in hydrophobic acrylic lenses, which provides high rotational stability.
- *IOL design.* Currently available toric IOLs have a total IOL diameter ranging from 11 to 13 mm, which has been shown to be effective in avoiding IOL rotation. Prinz et al. recently compared plate-haptic and loop-haptic acrylic IOLs and did not find a significant difference in early and late rotation. ***Postoperative assessment of the axis.*** If there is a misalignment of more than 10 degrees, then repositioning may be required. Realignment of a rotated toric IOL should ideally be performed preferably before 2 weeks because of the formation of adhesions between the capsular bag and the IOL optic.

2. Aspheric (negative spherical) IOLs have been designed to reduce SAs. SA occurs when parallel rays of light do not focus on one point. The refractive power in the periphery of the lens may either be too weak or (usually) too strong. When the peripheral rays of light focus in front of the central rays, it is called positive SA, and if behind the central rays, it is called negative SA. The cornea has positive SA which in young patient gets compensated by negative SA of the lens. The lens grows over in lifetime. In the process, it gets thicker. Its refractive error also increases. Hence, the lens develops a positive SA with age. So overall, the eye has positive SA in old age due to additive effects of the SA of cornea and lens leading to reduced contrast sensitivity. Conventional spherical IOLs have a positive SA, resulting in reduced contrast sensitivity under mesopic and scotopic conditions. Aspheric IOLs like the TECNIS (AMO), AcrySof IQ (Alcon) and Akreos AO (Bausch & Lomb) minimize the SA resulting in improved vision. Initial clinical results with these lenses have shown improvement in contrast sensitivity under low luminance and high spatial frequencies when compared with fellow eyes implanted with conventional IOLs and has improved patients' night driving simulator performance. However, decentration greater than 0.5 mm will decrease the functional vision when compared to spherical IOLs.

VI. BASED ON EDGE FINISH

Based on edge finish the IOLs are of the following types:

- Ridge IOLs,
- Square edge IOLs and
- Sharp edge IOLs.

VII. SPECIAL FUNCTION IOLs

The IOLs have been developed to provide some special function in addition to correcting aphakic special function IOLs. Examples are as follows:

1. ***Aniridia IOLs.*** These lenses were devised to cosmetically cover the defects of aniridia or partial iris loss in cases like trauma. The following two lens models are available:

- For partial iris damage, a ring with one black segment added to it can be implanted in the damaged area.
- For extensive iris damage, a multisegmented ring is available (Fig. 11.8). These lenses are best used, if these are secured within the capsular bag or when suturing of the lens is done.

2. ***Implantable miniature telescope.*** The implantable miniature telescope, manufactured by VisionCare Ophthalmic Technologies (Saratoga, California), is a unique visual prosthetic device designed specifically to improve vision of patients suffering from late-stage age-related macular degeneration (ARMD). The second-generation telescope is a wide-angle version of the device that allows for a larger view of the central visual field than previous models. This device is an optical apparatus comprises two main components: a pure glass optical cylinder and a carrying device constructed from standard biocompatible materials suitable for implantation in the eye (Fig. 11.9). The optical portion contains ultraprecise, wide-angle microlenses that provide retinal image enlargement of the central visual field. Two models are available, allowing for a magnification of ×´2.2 or ´3, with an enlarged retinal image produced over approximately 52–60 degrees of the central retina. The carry-ing device is comprised of a clear carrier and a blue light restrictor. The carrier has two modified C-loops that hold the prosthetic device in the capsular bag. Once secured inside the bag, the anterior window of the optic extends marginally through the pupil. It is designed to allow a clearance of approximately 2–3 mm from the corneal endothelium.

3. ***Piggyback IOL.*** An eye with a shorter axial length (AL) requires a stronger IOL. As IOL powers become too high however, the lens becomes too spheric and image quality decreases. Using two lenses to obtain a needed high-power correction results in an optically superior image compared with that obtainable by a single lens of required power. Thus, for short or nanophthalmic eyes so-called piggyback IOLs represent a viable solution. Piggy-back minus lenses have been used in eyes of long ALs alone or combined with high corneal curvature to achieve minus powers commercially unavailable in a single lens. Piggyback IOL can also be inserted in two

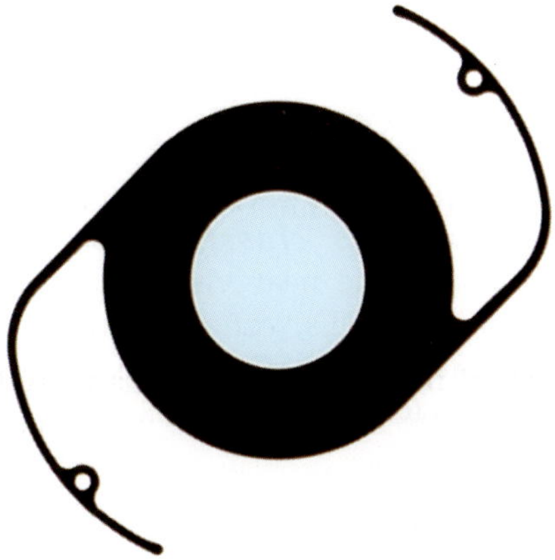

Fig. 11.8. *Aniridia lens.*

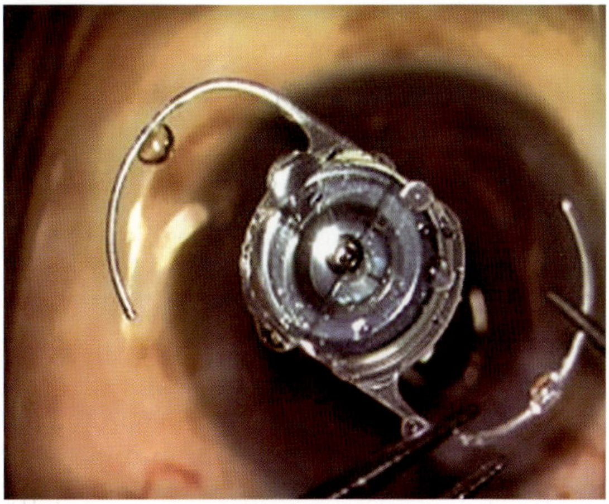

Fig. 11.9. *Telescopic IOL.*

stages, with the second IOL inserted (in the ciliary sulcus) to correct an undesirable refractive result following the initial IOL implantation. Refractive results in adding a piggybacked IOL as a second procedure should be superior to that of an IOL exchange for several reasons. First, the power of the second IOL is based only on the postoperative refraction. Second, the surgeon cannot be certain that an exchanged IOL would be in exactly the same plane as the IOL it replaced. Third, the accuracy of the power labelling of the first IOL is irrelevant, because of the first reason. Fourth, these added IOLs tend to be of lower power, and vergence distance changes are less important with lower power lenses. One occasional curious finding in piggyback lenses is an apparent increase in the depth of focus.

These advancements in IOL have transformed cataract extraction to a refractive surgery nowadays. Now the patient demands beyond 6/6 distant visual acuity from IOL implantation. Each IOL has its own pros and cons and judicious reasoning is required while deciding which IOL to implant to a particular patient. Still there is no substitute that provides all the functions of the natural lens and further research and development is required for the creation of an ideal IOL.

4. ***Smart yellow IOLs.*** These are the photochromic lenses, which have an ultraviolet (UV) near blue absorption curve similar to blue blocking lenses but only in photopic condition. Thus, they behave like a clear lens in mesopic and scotopic conditions. These are made up of hydrophobic acrylic material.

5. ***Blue blocking IOLs.*** These IOLs are based on the concept that normal human lens turns yellow with age due to oxidation of tryptophan and glycosylation of lens proteins which leads to progressive absorption of blue range wave-length. This protects the lipofuscin containing retinal pigment epithelial (RPE) cells from blue light damage, which may result in reducing the risk of ARMD.

Examples include AcrySof SN60AT IOL, which has hydroxybenzophenone, and hydroxyphenylbenzotriazole as chromophores absorbs visible blue light (200–550 nm). This may cause decrease in night vision since blue light is important for scotopic vision.

IOLs AND NEAR VISION

The conventional IOL is a single-focus device, restricting the practitioner to only a single power to select for a particular patient. A number of solutions that have been put forward which will allow the patient who has an intraocular implant to see clearly the distance as well as near, are as follows:

1. ***Implantation of an emmetropic IOL*** with use of reading glasses or bifocals/progressive as per situation.

2. ***A small amount of myopic astigmatism*** (i.e. refractive error of about –0.75 to –1.25 DC 180 degrees) would allow uncorrected visual acuity of about 20/40 for distance and near.

3. ***Monovision approach,*** i.e. one eye to be emmetropic (for distance vision) and second eye purposely made myopic by 2.5–3.0 D (for near vision). Such an approach has a patient satisfaction rating of greater than 50%.

4. ***Implantation of multifocal IOLs*** is being considered in an attempt to provide both near and distance visions without the need for spectacle correction.

5. ***Accommodative IOLs,*** used to provide best uncorrected distance and near visions, are losing popularity.

6. ***Extended range of vision IOLs,*** e.g. TECNIS Sym*f*ony IOL, which provide uncorrected distance and near visions due to its elongated focus, are gaining popularity nowadays.

7. ***Trifocal IOLs.*** These are newer lenses which allow distant vision, intermediate vison and near vision. Examples include Alcon PanOptix trifocal IOLs, Zeiss AT LISA Tri.

Classification of near vision IOLs

Coventional lens classification system. Conventionally the near vision IOLs divided into multifocal IOLs, *extended depth of focus IOLs*, and Accommodative IOLs:

I. Multifocal IOLs
   1. Refractive
      a. Zonal refractive IOL, e.g., ReZoom (AMO) and Array (AMO)
      b. Aspheric IOLs

2. Diffractive
   a. Bifocal diffractive, e.g. ReSTOR (Alcon)
   b. Trifocal diffractive IOLs, e.g. Alcon PanOptix, RayOne trifocal IOL (Rayner, Sussex, UK), AT LISA tri 839 MP (Carl Zeiss)
3. Combined, e.g. Acrysof ReSTOR IOL (Alcon)

II. Extended depth of focus (EDOF), e.g. Symfony IOL (Johnson & Johnson Vision/ AMO, ZXR00), Vivity IOL (Alcon)

III. Combined Trifocal and EDOF IOLs, e.g. Synergy IOL (Johnson & Johnson Vision)

IV. Accommodative IOLs, e.g. Crystalens.

Functional lens classification system, based in the AUC (Area under defocus curve), has recently been recommended by J. Fernández (2021). With this classification system, AUCs can be compared between multifocal IOLs in four possible regions:

- Total AUC (+1.00 to –4.00 D in 0.50 D steps);
- Distance AUC (+0.50 to –0.50 D);
- Intermediate AUC (–0.50 to –2.00 D); and
- Near AUC (–2.00 to -4.00 D). Use of the Multifocal Lens Analyzer to classify multifocal IOLs based on their performance at total distance, intermediate, and near.

Summary of commercially available near vision IOLs is summarized in Table 11.1

MULTIFOCAL IOLs

At present, two general styles of multifocal IOLs are in vogue. Both rely on the eye's ability to select one clear image from two or many unfocused images. This inherent limitation will exist until there is a novel method for actually altering the power of an implanted lens according to the user's immediate need. The currently available multifocal IOLs using either refractive or diffractive principles are as follows.

1. Refractive optics multifocal IOLs

These IOLs, also termed as bull's-eye design lenses, have concentric rings of different powers. These lenses, using concentric zone philosophy, are available in two styles:

i. ***Two-zone lenses.*** These have a central near-vision segment surrounded by a distance-vision segment (Fig. 11.10) and so also may be called a bifocal IOL. Since the pupil constricts during near focus, the central section is about 2 mm in diameter. Optimally when the pupil dilates during distance viewing, the peripheral distance segment is exposed. This design has a disadvantage in bright sunlight, since the constricted pupil blocks the distant segment of the lens. It is thus poorly tolerated by patients who enjoy outdoor sports in which clear vision is required.

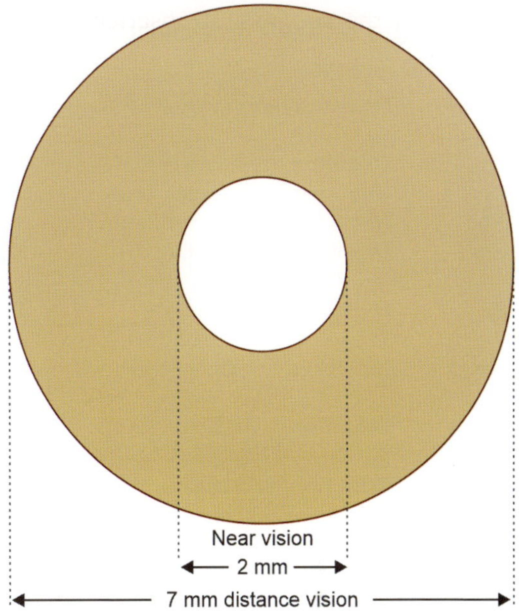

Fig. 11.10. *Two-zone type of bifocal intraocular lens.*

ii. ***Annulus type or bull's eye lens.*** The pupils constrict not only during near task but also for distance visual tasks in bright light. Therefore, it becomes imperative that the central zone must function for both distance and near. Thus, in annulus design multifocal IOLs, the central portion of the optics contains the distance-vision refraction and there is a near-vision ring outside it, which is in turn surrounded by another distance-vision ring (Fig. 11.11). With this lens style, even marked pupillary constriction allows distance vision and mild constriction allows distance and near visions, and all the three lens segments are exposed when the pupil is dilated. However, excessive constriction during reading in bright light blocks the add portion of the lens, thus preventing clear near vision.

Table 11.1 Summary of commercially available near-vision IOLs

Industry	*Technology*	*Model*	*Addition (D)/ DOF*	*Material*	*Spherical Aberration (mm)*
Bifocal					
J&J	Diffractive	Tecnis	2.75, 3.25, 4.00	Hydrophobic acrylic	–0.27
Alcon	Diffractive	AcrySof Restor	2.50	Hydrophobic acrylic	–0.20
Alcon	Diffractive	AcrySof Restor	3.00, 4.00	Hydrophobic acrylic	–0.10
Zeiss	Diffractive	AT LISA 809	3.75	Hydrophilic acrylic with hydrophobic surface	–0.18
VSY	Diffractive	Reviol MF 613/625/611	3.75	Hydrophilic acrylic with hydrophobic surface	N/A
Alsanza	Diffractive	Alsiol 30 VF	3.75	Hydrophobic-hydrophilic acrylic	–0.09
Teleon surgical	Refractive	MPlus	2.00, 3.00	Hydrophilic acrylic	0.0
Rayner	Refractive	M-flex	3.00, 4.00	Hydrophilic acrylic	0.0
Ophtec	Refractive-CTF	Precizon	2.75	Hydrophilic/hydrophobic acrylic	–0.11
Cristalens	Diffractive-mix and match	Artis symbiose mid/plus	1.75/175	Hydrophobic	–0.23
Trifocal					
Medicontur	Diffractive-EPS	Liberty	3.50 (N)–175 (I)	Hydrophilic acrylic	0.0
8iotech	Diffractive	Optiflex Trio	3.50 (NI)–185 (I)	Hydrophobic acrylic	Negative N/A
Alcon	Diffractive	AcryS of PanOptix	3.25 (N)–2.17 (I)	Hydrophobic acrylic	–0.10
Zeiss	Diffractive	AT LiISA tri 839 MP	3.33 [NJ–1.66 (I)	Hydrophilic acrylic with hydrophobic surface	–018
Alsanza	Diffractive-sinusoidal	Alsafit Fourier	3.55 (N)–1.77 (I)	Hydrophobidhydrophilic acrylic	–0.09
PhyslOL	Diffractive	FineVision	3.50[NJ–1.75(1)	Two materials (hydrophobic and hydrophilic)	–0.11
Rayner	Diffractive	RayOne Trifocal	3.50 (N)–1.75 (I)	Hydrophilic acrylic	–0.0
8+L	Diffractive-EOOF	Versario 3F	3.00 (NJ–1.50 (I)	Hydrophilic acrylic with hydrophobic surface	–0.16
EDOF					
Zeiss	Diffractive	AT LISA	2.00, 2.25*	Hydrophilic acrylic with hydrophobic surface	0.0
PhyslOL	Diffractive	FineVision Triumf	1.50, 2.50*	Hydrophobic acrylic	N/A
J&J	Diffractive	Tecnis Symfony	IOL 1.75, 2.00*	Hydrophobic acrylic	N/A
J&J	Diffractive	Tecnis Synergy	3.50, 3.75*	Hydrophobic acrylic	N/A
Sav-IOL	Diffractive	Harmonis	1.00–2.00	Hydrophilic acrylic	N/A
Sav-IOL	Diffractive	Eden	3.00	Hydrophilic acrylic	N/A
AcuFocus	Small-aperture	IC-8	2.00*	Hydrophobic acrylic	N/A
Sav-IOL	Refractive	Lucidis EDOF	3.00	Hydrophilic acrylic	NIA
Medtech	Refractive	Mini Well Ready	2.25, 2.50*	Hydrophilic acrylic with hydrophobic surface	N/A
Teleon surgical	Refractive	Comfort	2.00*	Hydrophilic acrylic	N/A

(*Contd.*)

Table 11.1 Summary of commercially available near-vision IOLs (*Contd.*)

Industry	*Technology*	*Model*	*Addition (D)/ DOF*	*Material*	*Spherical Aberration (mm)*
Teleon surgical	Refractive	Acunex Vario AN6V	2.00*	Hydrophobic acrylic	0.0
Medicem	Refractive	WIOL-CF	2.00*	Hydrogel	N/A
8+L	Refractive	Crystalens	2.00*	Silicone elastomer (Biosill)	0.0
Alcon	Refractive	AcrySof IQ Vivity DFT015	2.00*	Hydrophobic acrylic	–0.20
B+L	Refractive	LuxSmart	1.75*	Hydrophobic acrylic	N/A
Appasamy	Refractive	Supraphob Infocus	2.00*	Hydrophobic acrylic	N/A
Monofocal-EDOF					
Santen	Diffractive	Xact ME4	1.50*	Hydrophobic acrylic	N/A
PhysIOL	Refractive	IsoPure	1.50*	Hydrophobic acrylic	N/A
J&J	Refractive	Tecnis Eyhance	1.50*	Hydrophobic acrylic	N/A
Rayner	Refractive-monovision	RayOne EMV	—	Hydrophilic acrylic	N/A

*Position of the defocus curve where the patient achieves an arreptable roonocular visual aruity of 0.3 logMAR For binocular reported defocus curves, a correction of –0.1 logMAR was applied.
Classification is based on QVision interpretation. whidl considers measuremencs on the optical bench and clinical results shared at rongresses and in peer-reviewed j)urnals and magazines.
Abbreviations: DOF. depth of field; EDOF, extended depth of focus; J&J, Johnson & Johnson Vision; Sav-IOL, Swiss Advanced Vision; Zeiss, Carl Zeiss Meditec; NIA, not available; B+L, Bausch + Lomb; CTF, continuous transitional focus; EPS, elevated phase shih; N, near; I, intermediate.

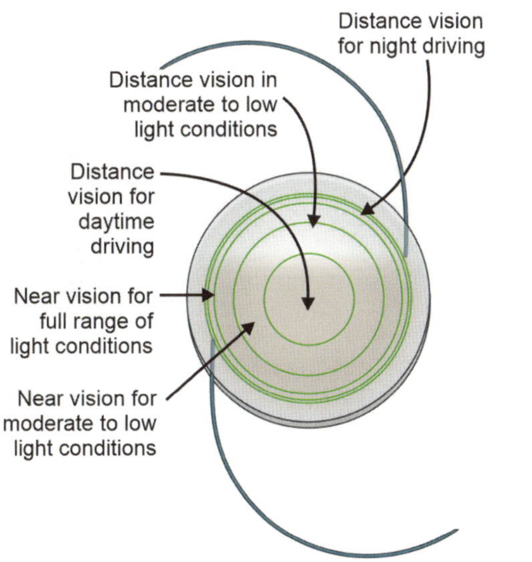

Fig. 11.11. *Annulus type of refractive optics—Multifocal IOL or Bull's-eye lens.*

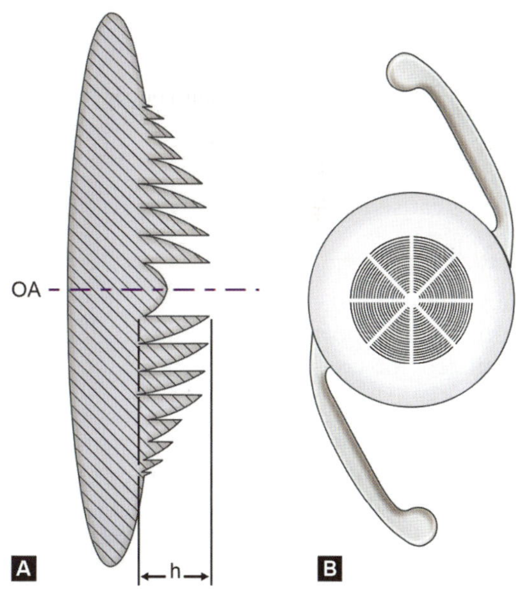

Fig. 11.12. *Diagrammatic depiction of optics of diffractive type multifocal IOLs.*

2. Diffractive optics multifocal IOLs

In these lenses, the near and distance correction is put in each of the concentric rings, using diffraction optics. The diffractive optics utilizes the principle of wavefront optics of light. The diffraction optics lens combines a standard convex curvature placed on the front surface with approximately 25 concentric annular zones cut on the posterior surface with microscopic steps between coterminous annuli (Fig. 11.12). The step height is in the range of the wavelength of light. Such a lens design produces two diffractive orders in which the incoming waves

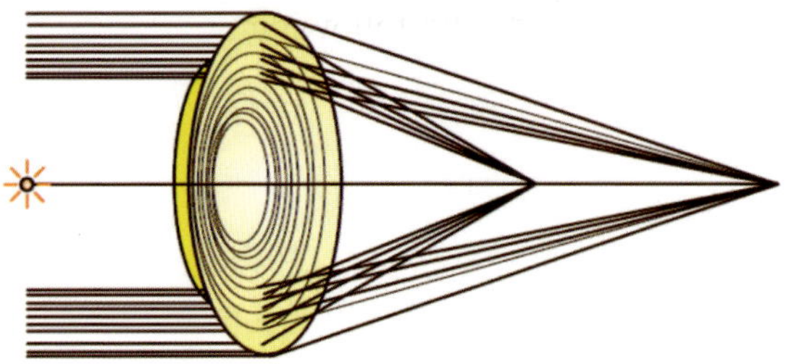

Fig. 11.13. *Optics of diffractive type of multifocal intraocular lens.*

of light will be in phase, resulting in discrete optical foci of equal intensity. Actually, 82% of the light is found in two major foci (approximately 41% of the light is in phase and focused for near vision and about another 41% is in phase and focused for distance vision) and the remaining 18% is lost (Fig. 11.13). This diffractive optical effect is present at all points (or more precisely, at all sufficiently large areas) of the lens. Thus, even if the lens is decentred or pupil is eccentric or deformed, the portion of the lens within the pupil will supply power for distance and near visions.

Drawbacks of diffractive IOLs include the following:

- The intermediate vision in these lenses has been typically compromised.
- Another problem is the problem of glare and halos caused by the randomly diffracted rays of light.
- Furthermore, the contrast and scotopic vision are compromised because at any given focal point only a portion of total light intensity is utilized for creating an image. Most of the lenses split light in the ration of 60:40 (distance: near–light distribution).

Innovative changes attempted to correct these problems include the following:

- *Height and spacing of the diffractive rings are reduced* from the centre to the periphery. This reduces the scatter from the periphery hence reducing glare.
- *Rings are also made with smooth rounded edges* in lens to reduce glare, e.g. Acri. LISA (Zeiss Germany).
- Partial optic diffractive lenses are also available, where the diffractive rings only occupy central 3 mm of the lens the peripheral lens is clear giving a better night time driving vision, e.g. ReSTOR (Alcon Labs Inc., Fort Worth, Texas).
- *Full optic diffractive lenses* are also available which provide near and far visions, e.g. TECNIS from AMO.

Apodization. Along with the above-mentioned changes in the diffractive rings from the centre to the periphery IOLs are available in which the diffractive rings are also progressively sloped greater from the centre to the periphery. This changes the angle of diffraction of light affording good intermediate vision. This is called concept of apodization, e.g. the iDIFF Plus and AcriDIFF (trifocal). The iDIFF Plus lens is a hydrophilic lens, while the AcriDIFF (trifocal) lens is hydrophobic lens.

Disadvantages of multifocal IOLs

1. *Reduced light intensity.* The light intensity entering the eye is halved. Thus, the greatest optical disadvantage of multifocal IOLs, in general, is that even in the ideal situation not all the light entering the eye reaches the retina in focus for either near or distance vision, as:

i. *In bull's eye lenses*, the amount of light transmitted for each of the focal lengths varies with pupil size (i.e. the area of the IOL exposed). Therefore, distant and near objects may be of different intensities.

ii. *In diffractive optics IOLs*, image intensity is equal for near and distance visions, but even in the ideal situation, only one-half of the light entering the eye is in focus.

2. *Reduced contrast sensitivity.* Contrast sensitivity is decreased in multifocal IOLs as compared to conventional IOLs, obviously because of decreased intensity of the light focused. Moreover, even more light may be lost due to scattering, further decreasing retinal image contrast. The patients fitted with a multifocal IOL may, therefore, need somewhat brighter light to read well, and generally function less well in dim light.

Off-axis aberrations in decentred IOLs create more problems in multifocal IOLs as compared to conventional IOLs. Although both bull's eye and diffractive IOLs require excellent centration, it is more critical with diffractive lenses since they suffer stronger off–axis aberration.

3. *Perception of rings* around point sources of light is another problem faced with use of multifocal IOLs.

Present status of multifocal IOLs

The advantage of the multifocal IOL is that it provides near and distance visions without additional refractive correction. However, this return must be weighed against the superior optical performance of conventional IOLs with the bifocal spectacles.

Nevertheless, an advance generation of multifocal IOLs (e.g. Alcon ReSTOR lens and AMO ReZoom lens) have been designed in a fashion that reduces the halo, the colour distortion and contrast sensitivity loss that occur with multifocal IOLs.

TRIFOCAL IOLs

These are newer lenses which allow distant vision, intermediate vison and near vision. Examples include Alcon PanOptix trifocal IOLs, Zeiss AT LISA Tri. Recently many other companies have come up with trifocal IOLs.

AcrySof IQ PanOptix IOL

AcrySof IQ PanOptix IOL (Alcon) FDA approved in 2019, uses ENLIGHTEN Optical Technology, a proprietary design that optimizes intermediate vision without compromising near and distance visions available in spherical (Fig. 11.14) and toric designs.

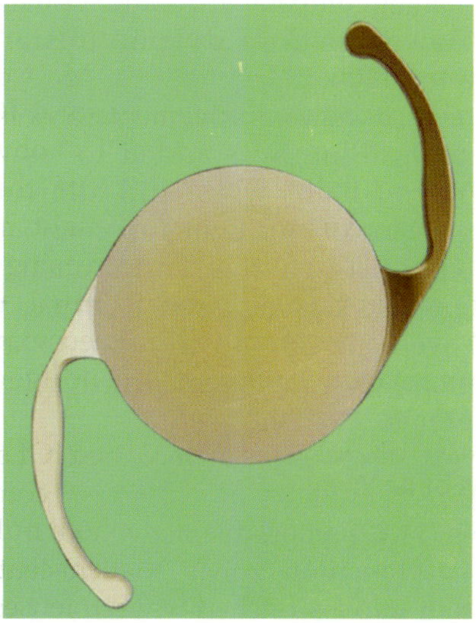

Fig. 11.14. *AcrySof IQ PanOptix Trifocal Spherical IOL.*

Features include the following:

- Hydrophobic acrylate/methacrylate copolymer
- Optic 6 mm, overall diameter 13 mm
- Non-apodized new trifocal design
- Redirects light from the third step height to distance
- Intermediate +2.17 D add
- Near +3.25 D add
- *Spherical range:* 6 to +34.0 D
- Light distribution less dependent on pupil size.

Potential side effects. These are due to the design of multifocal IOL (AcrySof IQ PanOptix Trifocal IOL) models. These may be worse than with a monofocal IOL, including visual disturbances such as glare, rings around lights, star-bursts (rays around light sources) and reduced contrast sensitivity (especially in dim lighting). These side effects may make it more difficult to see while driving at night or completing tasks in low lighting conditions such as at night or in fog, or in a dimly lit room after surgery as compared to before surgery.

AT LISA Tri and at LISA Tri Toric from ZEISS

Features. Introduced in 2012, features of these IOLs (Fig. 11.15) are as follows:

- Hydrophilic acrylate with hydrophobic surface properties
- Optic 6 mm, overall diameter 11 mm
- Trifocal over 4.34 mm, bifocal from 4.34–6 mm
- Diffractive profile using 'smooth steps'
- Intermediate +1.66 D add
- Near +3.33 D add
- Spherical range: 0.0 to +32.0 D
- Maximized pupil-independent design
- Performs well at distance and near visions.

Potential side effects. Trifocal IOLs come with certain photopic phenomena like glare and

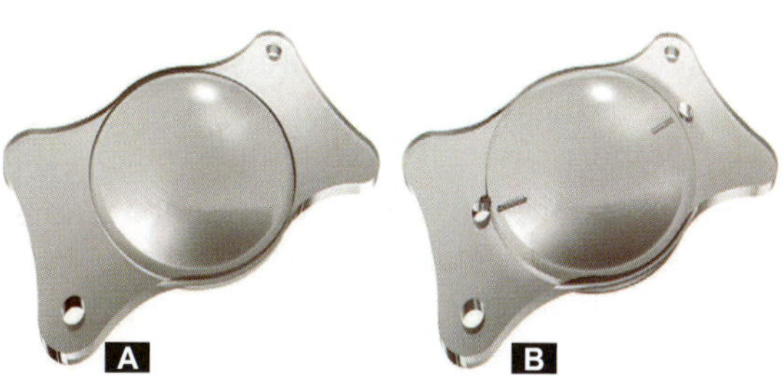

Fig. 11.15. *(A) Zeiss AT LISA tri 839MP; (B) Zeiss AT LISA tri toric 939 M/MP.*

halos as well as a reduced contrast sensitivity, but most patients after a certain adjustment period tolerate these well.

EXTENDED DEPTH-OF-FOCUS IOL

Until now, IOL correction for presbyopia was achieved through IOLs with different designs (bifocals, near segment sector-shaped, trifocals, etc.) that split the light in several focal areas or accommodative IOLs that change their shape and dioptric power when the ciliary muscles contract. Recently, a new optical technology for providing extended range of vision has been developed, i.e. TECNIS Symfony EDOF IOL ZXR00, which is different than the one used by current multifocal IOLs, for offering an extended range of vision.

Technology of EDOF IOL. Instead of several focus areas, Symfony IOL get one elongated focus area by implementing two technologies:

- Proprietary diffractive optic design that extends the length of focus and
- Achromatic technology that corrects chromatic aberration.

Because it tackles this chromatic aberration, this IOL is known as the EDOF IOL.

Features of EDOF IOL (Symfony IOL). It is made of UV blocking hydrophobic acrylic material with a biconvex, wavefront-designed anterior aspheric surface and a posterior achromatic diffractive surface with 6 mm optic diameter. It has a proTEC frosted, continuous 360-degree posterior square edge design of optic with C-loop haptics. The overall diameter of IOL is 13 mm with power varying from +5 to +34 D in 0.5 D increments.

Commonly available EDOF IOls are described below briefly.

1. TECNIS Symfony

The TECNIS Symfony IOL (Johnson & Johnson Vision) was the first EDOF IOL approved by the FDA for the treatment of presbyopia (Fig. 11.16).

Features of TECNIS Symfony Extended Range of Vision IOLs are as follows:

- The biconvex optic incorporates a proprietary wavefront-designed aspheric or toric-aspheric anterior optic, designed to compensate for corneal SA.

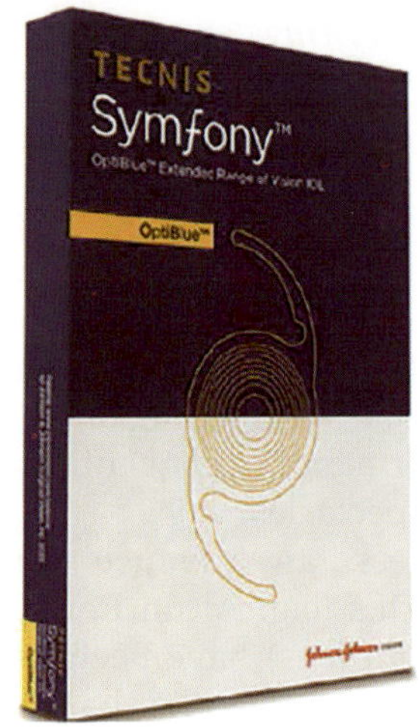

Fig. 11.16. *TECNIS Symfony IOL (Johnson & Johnson Vision).*

- The posterior optic has a proprietary achromatic diffractive surface designed to correct chromatic aberration and a unique echelette feature to extend the range of vision including far, intermediate, and near, while maintaining the corneal SA compensation.
- TECNIS Sym*f*ony IOLs are designed to have pupil-independent lens performance in any lighting condition.
- They correct spherical and chromatic aberration vision quality comparable to that of monofocal IOL. Compared to an aspheric monofocal IOL, the lens provides improved intermediate and near visual acuity, while maintaining comparable distance visual acuity.
- Has lower level of dysphotopsias than multi-focal IOLs.
- However, its new improvements, a violet light filter (OptiBlue) was added to lessen the severity of halos while still allowing the transmission of blue light, for scotopic vision and circadian rhythm entrainment. New design also has reduced light scatter to improve contrast and to reduce starburst symptoms with improvement in dysphotopsia symptoms.

1. AcrySof IQ Vivity

It is (Fig. 11.17) a non-diffractive EDOF lens. It has two transition zones that reshape the wavefront into a stretched wavefront (X-Wave technology). There is a 1 µm plateau located on

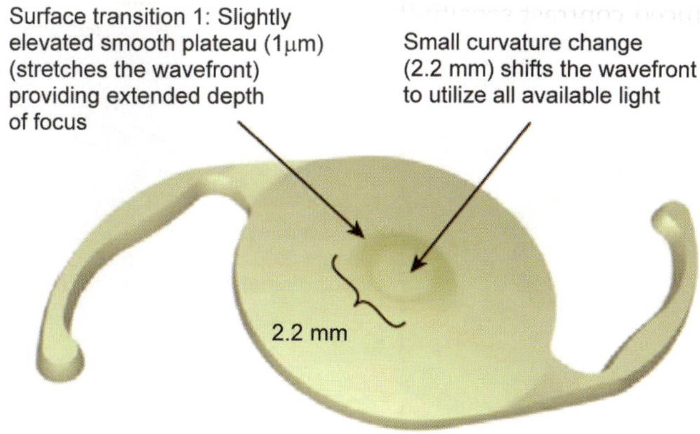

Fig. 11.17. *AcysofQ IQ Vivity IOL.*

the central 2.2 mm optic creates a transition that shapes and stretches the wavefront. Shifting the wavefront anterior to the retina provides intermediate vision at 66 cm and near vision at 44 cm. It provides good vision in both bright and dim environments because the X-Wave technology is not dependent on pupil size. The non-diffractive design is said to reduce the visual disturbances (dysphotopsias) compared to diffractive designs. This IOL is a good option for individuals who wish to be less dependent on glasses after cataract surgery but who are not good candidates for a multifocal lens because of mild glaucoma, higher-order aberrations after refractive surgery, or ocular surface disease; and those who may be bothered by dysphotopsias and have concerns about their quality of vision when driving at night. However, they may require glasses to read, very fine print.

2. TECNIS Synergy IOLs

TECNIS Synergy is a hybrid design that features both the echelette EDOF technology from the TECNIS Sym*f*ony IOL and combines it with diffractive multifocal (trifocal) optics for near vision (Fig. 11.18). It received FDA approval in April 2021. Both the non-toric, TECNIS Synergy (Johnson & Johnson Vision) IOLs and the toric, TECNIS Synergy Toric II (Johnson & Johnson Vision) IOLs are available.

The lens is designed to deliver a full range of vision with a peak at distance and with fewer so-called gaps in vision than trifocal lenses. The vision provided by this lens is less dependent on the pupil size than the case with trifocal IOLs.

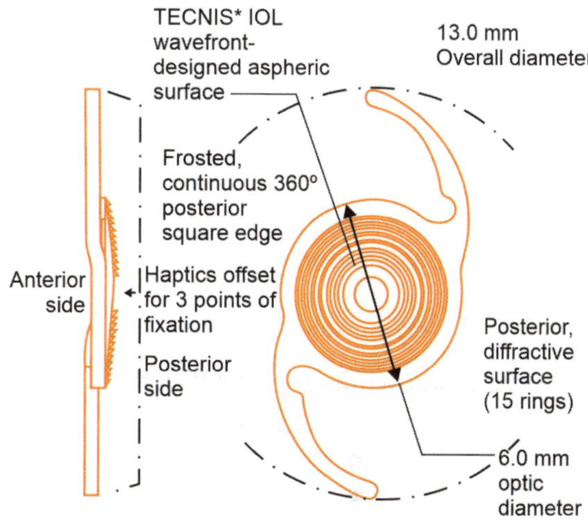

Fig. 11.18. *Non-toric, TECNIS Synergy (Johnson & Johnson Vision) IOL.*

IC-8, SMALL-APERTURE IOL

Small-aperture or pinhole optics increases the depth of focus and depth of field. Other EDOF IOL technologies use optical aberrations to flatten the depth of focus, but the IC-8 lens incorporates a pinhole to collimate light rays of light passing through an aberrated cornea to reach the retina through the central aperture. The small-aperture design blocks the peripheral defocused (and often aberrated) rays from disrupting the image and flattens the defocuscurve on both the myopic and hyperopic sides, providing EDOF in both slightly hyperopic and slightly myopic patients.

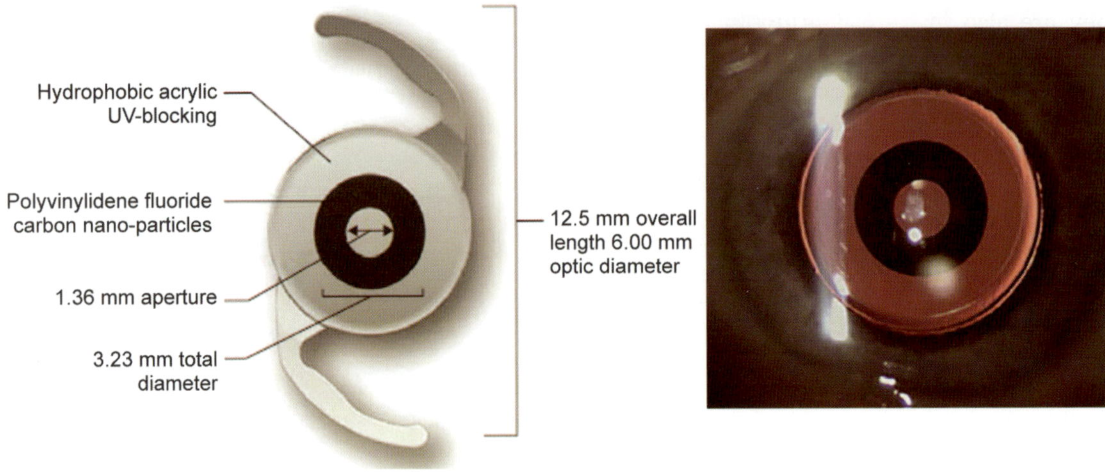

Fig. 11.19. *IC-9 small-aperture IOL.*

Therefore, such an IOL may benefit patients who have atypical corneas such as those with keratoconus, a history of radial keratotomy or corneal scarring. IC-8 IOL (AcuFocus) is a one-piece, aspheric, hydrophobic acrylic, monofocal lens with an embedded mask (Fig. 11.19). The IOL has a large landing zone for achieving an emmetropia result, and it eliminates much of the noise in the visual system from higher-order aberrations. The lens' wavefront-filtering design eliminates unfocused peripheral rays, so that only central-rays focus on the retina. Its small aperture provides an EDOF that makes the implant more tolerant of residual sphero-cylindrical refractive error than a multifocal IOL. IC-8 lens is implanted in the non-dominant eye of patients, and a standard monofocal lens is typically implanted in the dominant eye.

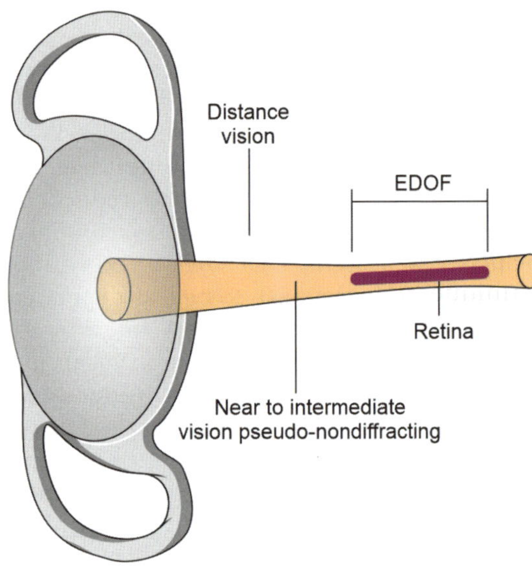

Fig. 11.20. *Swiss Advanced IOL.*

Swiss Advanced IOLs: Lucidis, Eden and Harmonis

All these three are EDOF lenses with their patented **Instant Focus Technology**.

The aspheric surface of the centre of the lens generates a peak of light through constructive light wave interference. The resulting beam of light is called pseudo-nondiffracting beam (PNDB) which enables to extend the depth of focus (Fig. 11.20):

- Lucidis integrates the EDOF technology **Instant Focus** built into its aspheric optical centre surrounded by its refractive outer surface.
- *Eden* integrates the EDOF technology **Instant Focus** built into its aspheric optical centre surrounded by its refractive–diffractive outer surface.
- *Harmonis* is a high--end customizable EDOF IOL. It offers patients the possibility to person-alize the lens using a dedicated online configurator. It integrates the EDOF technology **Instant Focus** built into its aspheric optical centre surrounded by its refractive–diffractive outer surface.

All three are available in power range of +5.0 to +30.0 D lens with 0.5 D increments. Lucidis and Eden offer an add/EDOF of +3.0 D and they are also in toric. Harmonis comes with add of +2.5 D to +3.5 D (by 0.25 D steps) and EDOF of 1.0 to 2.0 D (by 0.5 D steps).

Enhanced monofocal IOLs

Recently, a new generation of monofocal IOLs called enhanced monofocal IOLs has been introduced, with the aim of providing excellent visual acuity for distant (the same as conventional monofocal lenses) while improving intermediate distant performance, without the side effects traditionally caused by multifocality.

TECNIS Eyhance

TECNIS Eyhance and Eyhance Toric II IOLs (Fig. 11.21) (Johnson & Johnson Vision) were FDA approved in February 2021. The Eyhance is the first in a new class of monofocal IOLs that provides additional depth of focus without sacrificing the modulation transfer function or inducing dysphotopsias that are associated with multifocal and EDOF IOLs. The new lens is distinguished by a critical difference in design–namely, a continuous change in power from the periphery to the centre of the lens, creating a unique anterior surface that improves intermediate vision, maintains distance image quality comparable to aspheric monofocal IOLs.

RayOne EMV

The RayOne EMV (model 200E, Rayner) (Fig. 11.22) is a UV light–absorbing one-piece IOL intended for placement in the capsular bag using the RayOne injection system (Rayner). Antivaulting haptic technology allows the IOL to be implanted through a sub–2.2 mm corneal incision and promotes rapid centration and fixation in the capsular bag. The IOL is available in powers from 10.00 to 30.00 D in 0.50 D increments. The RayOne EMV is unique because it has positive SA at the centre of its optic and a blended edge region to maintain visual acuity

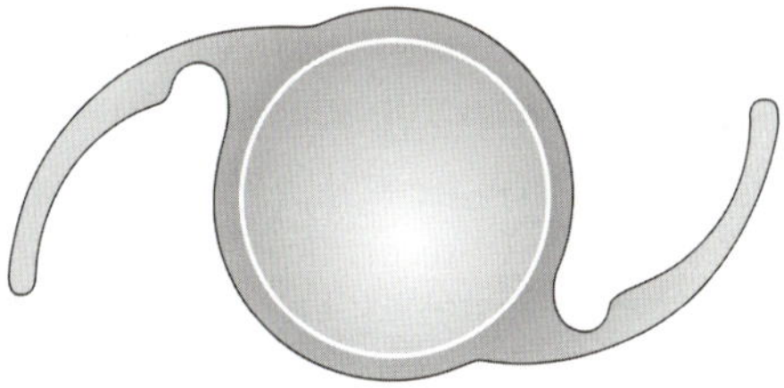

Fig. 11.21. *The Eyhance Toric II IOL.*

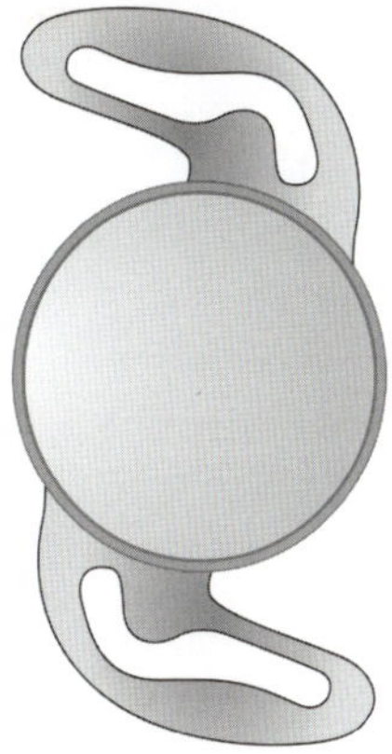

Fig. 11.22. *RayOne EMV IOL.*

and contrast sensitivity designed the IOL for patients who can tolerate defocus in the second eye or monovision. With a monovision strategy, elongated optical performance in the hyperopic direction allows the lens to maintain some distance vision in the patient's non-dominant eye.

Isopure PhysIOL

The PhysIOL ISOPURE Lens is a non-diffractive aspherical lens based on a poly-nomial technology. ISOPURE is designed to provide cataract patients high far vision quality, combined with functional intermediate vision by accentuating the EDOF effect without inducing photic phenomena. It has a larger depth of focus compared to a monofocal lens, low incidence of halos, glares or starbursts and comparable to a monofocal lens. Features include the following:

- Glistening-free hydrophobic acrylic IOL.
- 10–24.5 D: Overall diameter: 11 mm and optic diameter: 6 mm
- 25–30 D: 10.75 mm, optic diameter
- 25D–30 D: 5.75 mm optic polynomial surface design haptic design micro (four-closed loops) and posterior angulated haptic (Fig. 11.23).

ACCOMMODATIVE IOLs

Current commercially available accommodative IOLs are based on Helmholtz's theory of accommodation. These are IOLs which afford both distant and reasonable near visions as well with the help of haptics which can flex and also with the help of materials that expand and contract within the capsule bag along with

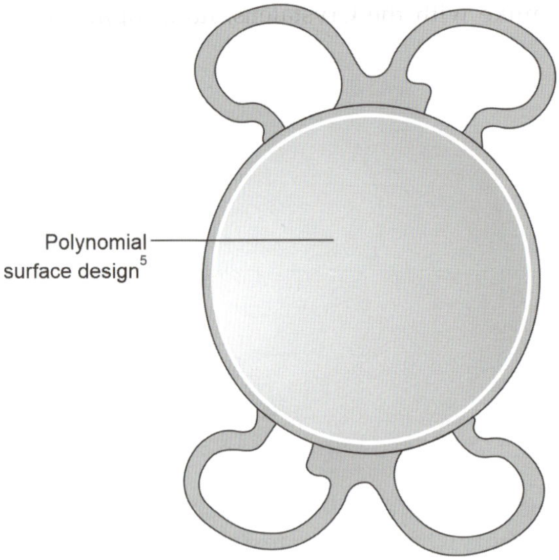

Fig. 11.23. *ISOPURE PhysIOL, four closed loops lens*

the ciliary body contraction and the to and fro piston like motion of the anterior vitreous.

Accommodative IOLs are designed in such a way that they exhibit anterior movement of the optic to improve near vision. As a result of anterior movement, these lenses give about 0.5–1.0 D of accommodative amplitude more than a standard monofocal IOL. With such lenses, about 90% of the patients achieve 6/9–6/12 and J_3 vision, which is adequate for driving and reading newspaper without correction. Furthermore, with accommodative lenses, the patients get same quality of distance vision that they get with monofocal lenses cf. multifocal lenses with which quality of distance vision is poor. In other words, with accommodative lenses, there is no loss of contrast sensitivity, no colour distortion and there are no halos at night. Because of these advantages, the implantation of accommodative lenses does make a sense.

A blended vision concept with accommodative IOLs is providing wonderful results. With blended vision, i.e. one eye slightly myopic and the other emmetropic, the patients are achieving good distance, intermediate (computer distance) and near vision, as well as good stereopsis at all distances, and no night vision syndrome.

Type of accommodative IOLs

The available models of accommodative lenses are divided into two main groups:

1. Single optic accommodative IOLs

These are designed to translate anteriorly with accommodative effort. This forward movement increases the effective lens power at the spectacle plane. The mechanism of action varies between the various single optic accommodative IOLs, and is dependent on ciliary muscle contraction either producing an increase in vitreous fluidic pressure (pushing the lens forward) or releasing the zonule tension and allowing the elastic capsular bag to press upon the IOL haptics. The accommodative amplitude of these IOLs is limited by the power of the IOL and can be reduced further with capsular opacification, as this reduces capsular bag elasticity. Roughly, the IOL movement of 0.6 mm causes 1 D of accommodation at the spectacle plane. The lenses based on the above mechanism are as follows:

- Crystalens,
- Medennium smart IOL and
- Kelman tetraflex IOL.

The Crystalens HD (Bausch & Lomb) is the most popular FDA-approved accommodative lens in use today. It is a 4.5 mm aspheric optic IOL with long hinged plate designed haptics with polyimide loops at their ends (Fig. 11.24). This hinged accommodative lens is designed to vault posteriorly against the capsular. This movement is dependent on positive vitreous pressure to shift the lens forward. These IOLs provide a 1.5 D add for near vision too. Being an aspheric monofocal optic, it provides clear distant vision without the associated halos and ghost images or loss of contrast sensitivity unlike the multifocal IOLs. The function of the accommodative IOL would greatly depend on the strength of ciliary muscle contraction, which may be waning off with age, so a few patients might still need reading glasses.

The Medennium smart IOL, (Medennium, Inc., Irvine, CA) may overcome many of the aforementioned obstacles. The lens is composed of a hydrophobic acrylic material with unique thermoplastic properties that permit a

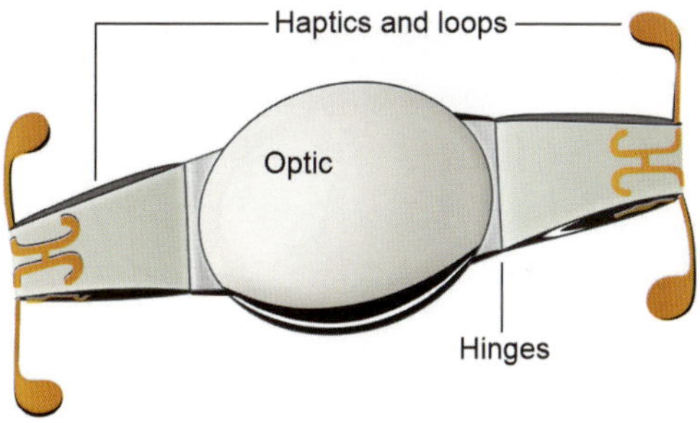

A

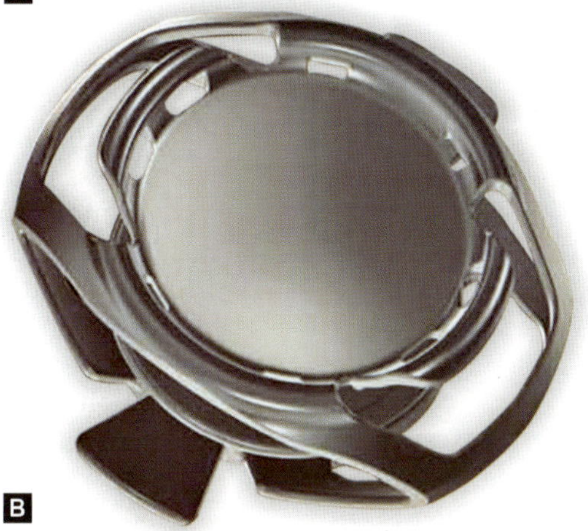

B

Fig. 11.24. *Accommodative IOLs: (A) Eyeonics crystalens (an accommodative lens with optic shift principle); (B) Synchrony dual optics IOL.*

temperature-induced change in its shape. Chemically, bonding wax to the acrylic polymer creates a 'smart' material, which remains in a solid state at room temperature. Since the wax component melts at body temperature, adjusting the percentage of wax content produces a semisoft gelatinous polymer once the lens is in the eye.

The Kelman tetraflex IOL features a square-edge design with a 5.75 mm optic, which may be inserted through a 2 mm incision. The lens is composed of PolyHEMA (hydroxyethyl methacrylate), a highly biocompatible material consisting of 26% water. The structural configuration of the tetraflex is entirely different from that of Crystalens. The tetraflex has no hinges and it is angulated forward (i.e. away from the capsular bag) and therefore, has a unique mechanism of accommodation independent of positive vitreous pressure. The haptic configuration of the tetraflex allows the lens to move with the entire capsular bag. Unlike with the Crystalens, no atropinization is necessary with the tetraflex IOL.

ii. Dual optics accommodative IOLs

In this type of lens, the optic consists of two lenses; a high plus anterior lens and a minus posterior lens, which are separated by spring-like haptics.

- *In the non-accommodative phase,* the tension in the capsular bag and zonules keeps the two optics in close proximity, whereas spring haptics are collapsed and exhibit potential energy.
- With accommodative effort, the zonules relax, the capsular bag expands and the springs exhibit kinetic energy. This change allows the optics to separate and the anterior plus lens moves forward, thus producing a higher optical power that yields accommodation. The lenses based on this principle include:
  - Synchrony dual optics IOL and
  - Sarfarazi elliptical accommodative IOL.

Synchrony Dual optics IOL (Visiogen, Inc., Irvine, CA, Fig. 11.24B) is the first dual-optic accommodating IOL to undergo clinical trials. It is designed to utilize the natural mechanism of accommodation according to the Helmholtz's theory. Made of the latest generation of silicone, the single-piece design is sized so as to distend and fill the capsular bag. With a relaxed ciliary muscle, the zonules become tense, and the taut capsular bag compresses two optics together. As the ciliary muscle contracts, the zonules and capsular bag relax. This relaxation permits the +34.00 D anterior optic to move forward. A small-diameter, 4.5 mm capsulorrhexis needed to confine the moving anterior optic (5 mm diameter) to the capsular bag. An injector system has been developed to deliver the lens through a 3.5 mm incision.

Note. Accommodative lenses that are currently available and those under investigation are effective in managing presbyopia. The available lenses are providing between 0.5 and 1.25 D of accommodation. The quality of retinal image provided by these lenses is superior to multifocal lenses. These favourable results open the door for more use of these lenses in future for presbyopia.

FUTURE IOL DESIGNS

Injectable gel IOLs

Femtosecond laser cataract surgery can create a controlled capsulorrhexis and can break up the lens into many pieces which means they can be removed through a small incision. The next step would be to introduce a lens into the eye through this small opening. This may be made possible using injectable gel IOLs, which are being researched in a project called Phaco-Ersatz which began in 1986 at the Bascom Palmer Eye Institute. Human trials will include a thorough antiposterior capsule opacification programme.

Similar to an accommodating IOL, this lens implantation will not be possible in case of posterior capsular rupture because of risk of extrusion into the vitreous cavity. Phaco-Ersatz is a very exciting and highly anticipated project. Injectable gel IOLs have the main advantage of restoring accommodation; but so far, this technology is not available commercially.

Electro-optic diffractive IOL

This lens which is under development has the following components:

- A static monofocal IOL
- A central aspheric modification for far and intermediate visions
- A smart electroactive diffractive liquid crystal lens for near
- Microsensors to detect physiological triggers for accommodation, and
- On-board processors and algorithms to control the power sequence.

Research in this IOL is being made by Elenza. While accommodation would induce an increase in power of 2–2.5 D, microsensors would sense a change in illumination with miosis and alter power using integrated circuits accordingly.

Light-adjustable IOL

Light-adjusted lenses (LALs) consist of a silicone matrix into which smaller, photosensitive molecules are embedded (Fig. 11.25). Two to four weeks after implantation of the lens, when the eye is healed, the refraction is measured and a low intensity beam of UV light is used

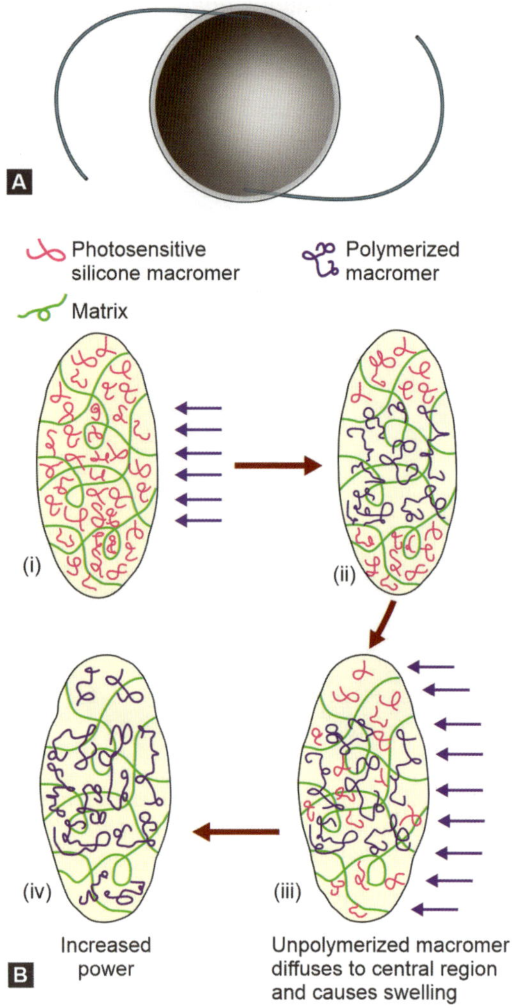

Fig. 11.25. *Light adjustable IOL (A) and its mechanism (B).*

to correct any residual error. This polymerizes the photosensitive molecules, which creates a concentration gradient between the irradiated region and the rest of the optic. Over a 12 h period, the photosensitive molecules migrate from untreated areas, down the concentration gradient, and into the irradiated region until there is no concentration gradient. This movement causes the irradiated region to swell and thereby increases the lens power, if centre of the lens is irradiated, and vice versa, if the periphery is irradiated. Even astigmatic errors and high-order aberrations can be corrected, if irradiation is done in a particular meridian. After verification of the new refraction, the surgeon 'locks in' the power by irradiating the

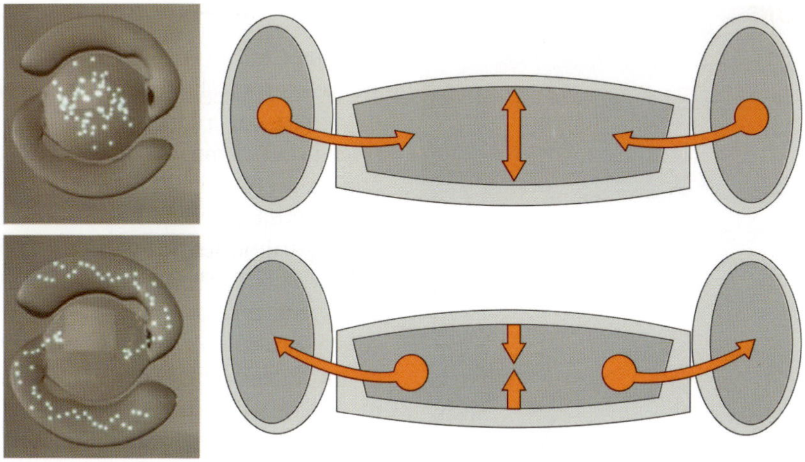

Fig. 11.26. *The FluidVision accommodating IOL in the accommodated (A) and unaccommodated (B) states*

entire lens optic, thereby achieving a stable power of the IOL. During the interval between the lens implantation and the light adjustment, patients need to wear sunglasses with UV absorbers while performing outside activities. This is necessary to avoid unwanted, non-controlled polymerization of the silicone macromers with unpredictable results regarding change in IOL power.

FUTURE ACCOMMODATING IOLs

All of the IOLs discussed here are currently under investigation.

Fluid vision

Design. The FluidVision lens (Alcon) is made of a flexible hydrophobic acrylic shell filled with index-matched silicone oil. The latest bench tests demonstrated that the IOL can be injected through a 3.2 mm incision with a new version of the PowerJect injection system (Alcon). A fluid-driven change in the shape of the IOL mimics the natural accommodation of the eye, creating a continuously variable monofocal lens. During accommodation, the capsular bag squeezes the fluid from the haptics into the centre, inflating the lens. In the unaccommodated state, the fluid moves the other way, deflating the lens (Fig. 11.26).

Juvene

Design. Juvene (LensGen) is a modular accommodating silicone IOL that is composed of two components—a base lens and a fluid lens (Fig. 11.27). The base lens is inserted first and fixated in the capsular bag. The fluid lens is then inserted and attached to the base lens. The dioptric power of the fluid lens changes in response to compressive forces from the capsular bag on the base lens.

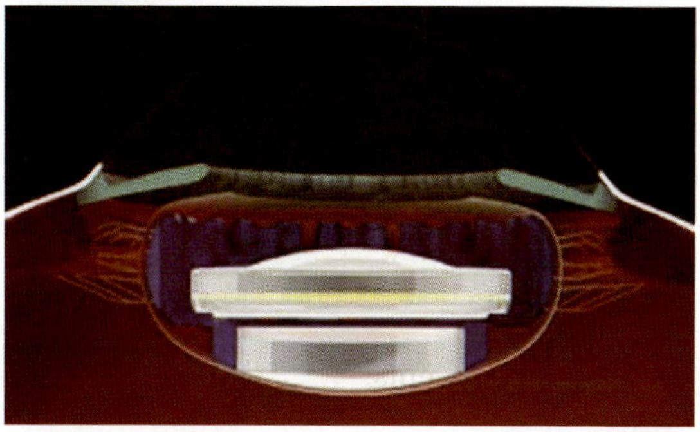

Fig. 11.27. *The Juvene accommodating IOL in the accommodated state*

Atia Vision

Design. The Atia Vision accommodating IOL (Atia Vision) is a modular system with two optical components (Fig. 11.28). The accommodating portion–the base–is in direct contact.

Lumina

Design. The Lumina (AkkoLens) is a hydrophilic acrylic lens designed for positioning at the sulcus plane (Fig. 11.29). The lens consists of two optical elements that each have an elastic omega-shaped loop with a spring function and

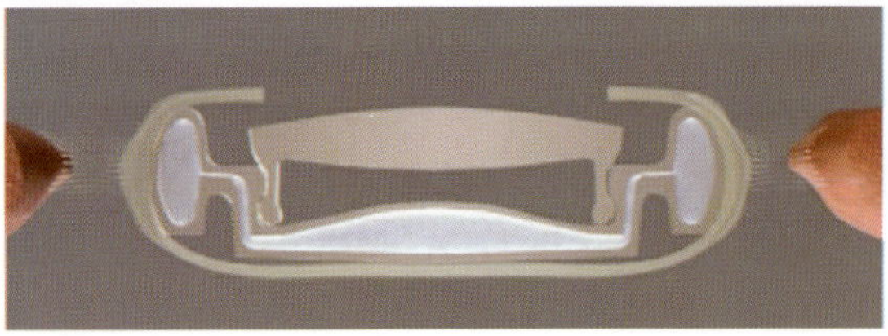

Fig. 11.28. *Schematic drawing showing the Atia Vision accommodating IOL in the accommodated state.*

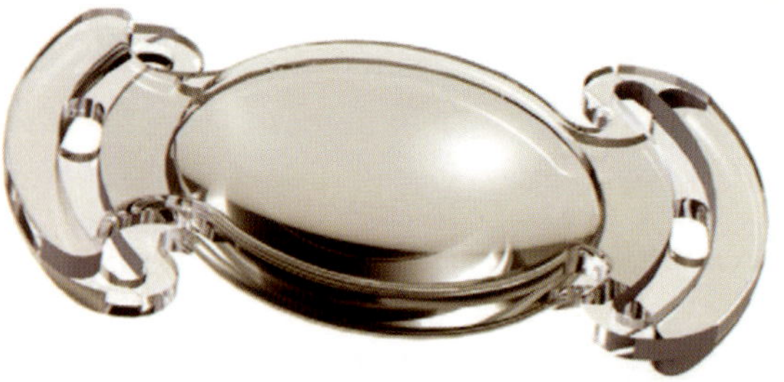

Fig. 11.29. *Schematic drawing of the Lumina accommodating IOL showing the overall design of the lens*

non-elastic connections to the main body of the lens. When the lens is positioned at the sulcus plane, the ciliary muscle contacts the body of the lens and drives accommodation directly.

In the unaccommodated state, the omega-shaped springs of the Lumina are relaxed, the optical elements overlap. When the eye accommodates, the ciliary muscle contracts and compresses the Lumina, resulting in a mutual shift of the optical elements. The optical power increases linearly with the shift, and the eye focuses at closer distances. The size of the Lumina is customized to each eye based on the measured sulcus-to-sulcus diameter.

Opira

Design. Opira (ForSight Vision6) is a dynamic, shape-changing lens made of silicone that is designed for placement in the sulcus plane (Fig. 11.30). This lens allows direct ciliary body engagement without zonular or capsular bag intermediaries. The haptics are fixated within the capsulorrhexis (Fig. 11.30A). The lens spans from the ciliary body on one side to the ciliary body on the other side. Contraction of the ciliary muscle compresses the peripheral aspect of the lens, which leads to a dynamic change in the shape of the anterior surface, thus changing the power of the IOL (Fig. 11.30B). The static posterior lens aspect could be used to correct regular astigmatism or for postoperative refractive adjustment.

SAV-IOL (Swiss Advanced Vision)–R-TASC

Real-Time Autofocus Servo Control (R-TASC) (Fig. 11.31) is an active IOL with real-time auto-focus and wireless connectivity system that detects the distance of objects.

The signals thus received trigger micro-pumps to move a liquid in and out of the optic, which causes the curvature of the optic to change, resulting in modification of the power of the lens in real time. The speed of this process is 0.2 s, equivalent to that of a healthy eye. Additionally, the lens is powered by solar energy in conjunction with induction.

R-TASC will be fitted alongside a monofocal lens (for distant vision) or added on patients who already have a monofocal lens but want to restore their visual accommodation. It will

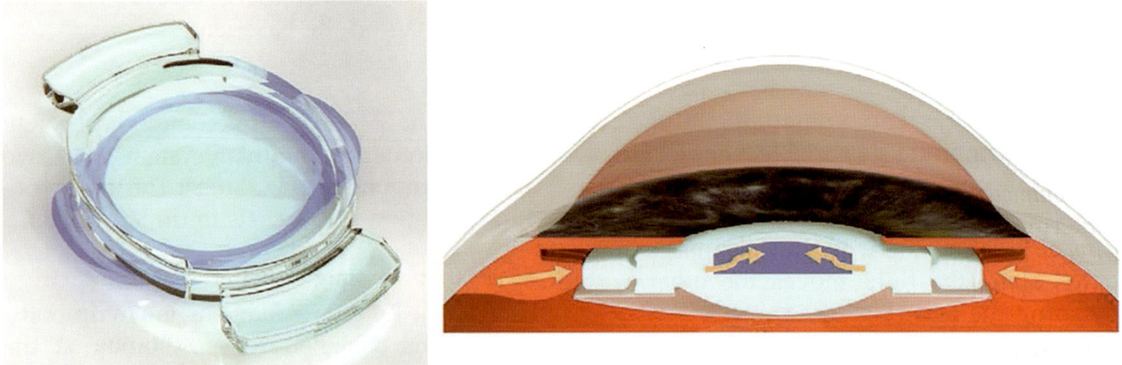

Fig. 11.30. *Overall design of the Opira accommodating IOL (A). Schematic drawing showing its site of fixation and mechanism of accommodation (B). Contraction of the ciliary muscle compresses the peripheral aspect of the lens, leading to a dynamic shape change of the anterior surface. (Courtesy: ForSight Vision6.)*

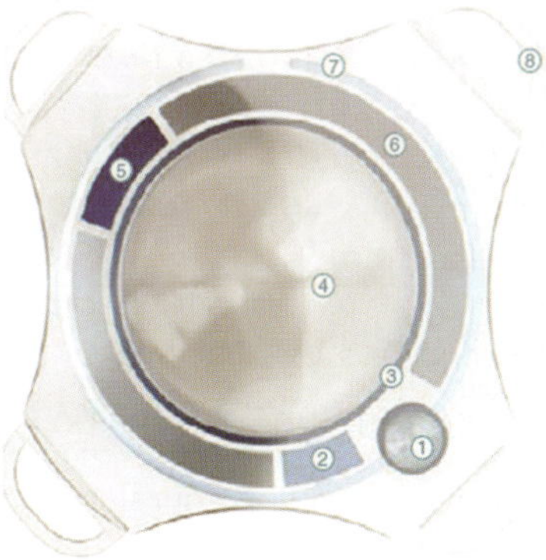

Fig. 11.31. SAV-IOL (Swiss Advanced Vision) – R-TASC

enable patients to retrieve a full and continuous visual accommodation range without any visual disturbances or loss of light. There is option of remote calibration of lens by the patient or surgeon for optimal vision at all times. The R-TASC platform is future proofed to incorporate interactive features such as augmented reality.

SUMMARY OF ADVANCES IN IOL FEATURES

Introduction of different IOLs have contributed towards improving the visual outcome following cataract surgery. The following changes have been incorporated to give better results:

- *Heparin-coated* IOLs to reduce anterior chamber inflammation.
- *Aspheric* IOLs to give better contrast acuity.
- *Toric IOLs* with a cylindrical component to correct astigmatism.
- *Multifocal IOLs* (diffractive and refractive types) to provide distant and near visions without need of glasses.
- *Multifocal toric IOLs* to correct both distance and near visions along with astigmatism.
- *Accommodative IOLs* which provide distance, intermediate and near visions.
- *Extended depth of focus IOL* provide distant, intermediate vision
- *Trifocal IOLs* allow good distant, intermediate and near vision
- *Application of laser* to alter the power or cylinder of IOLs after implantation is the new technology that is being explored.
- *Lens biomaterials* that would be flexible enough to change shape with accommodation are also being evaluated.

Concept of premium IOLs have been evolved with the introduction of multifocal, toric, accommodative, trifocal, EDOF and phakic refractive lenses.

BIBLIOGRAPHY

1. Alio JL, Julet EM, Ruiz-Moreno JM, et al. Intraocular telescopic lens evaluation in patients with age-related macular degeneration. J Cataract Refract Surg 2004;30:1177.
2. Apple DJ, Ram J, Foster A, Peng Q. Elimination of cataract blindness: A global perspective entering the new millennium. Surv Ophthalmol 45(Suppl 1):S1,2000.
3. Clayman HM. Ultraviolet-absorbing intraocular lenses. J Am Intraocul Implant Soc 1984;10:429.
4. Jaffe NS. Thirty years of intraocular lens implantation: The way it was and the way it is. J Cataract Refract Surg 1999;25:455.
5. Javitt J, Steinert R. Cataract extraction with multifocal intraocular lens implantation: A multinational clinical trial evaluating clinical, functional, and quality-of-life outcomes. Ophthalmology 2000;107:2040–2080.
6. Macsai M, Padnick-Silver L, Fontes B. Visual outcomes after accommodating intraocular lens implantation. J Cataract Refract Surg 2006;32: 628–633.
7. Oshika T, Suzuki Y, Kizaki H, Yaguchi S. Two years' clinical study of a soft acrylic intraocular lens. J Cataract Refract Surg 1996;22:104.
8. Rana A, Miller D, Magnante P. Understanding the accommodating intraocular lens. J Cataract Refract Surg 2003;29:2284–2287.
9. Steinert RS, Giamporcaro JE, Tasso VA. Clinical assessment of long-term safety and efficacy of a widely implanted silicone intraocular lens material. Am J Ophthalmol 1996;123:17.
10. Sun XY, Vicary D, Montgomery P, et al. Toric intraocular lenses for correcting astigmatism in 130 eyes. Ophthalmology 2000;107:1776.
11. Trivedi RH, Apple DJ, Pandey SK, et al. Sir Nicholas Harold Ridley. He changed the world, so that we might better see it. Indian J Ophthalmol 2003;51:211.
12. Werner L, Izak AM, Pandey SK, et al. Correlation between different measurements within the eye relative to phakic intraocular lens implantation. J Cataract Refract Surg 2004;30:1982.

CHAPTER 12

PREOPERATIVE WORKUP AND PREPARATION FOR CATARACT SURGERY

PREOPERATIVE EVALUATION AND PREPARATIONS

Review of general medical status of the patient

- Implications and considerations for the associated medical problems

Ocular evaluation

- Present and past ophthalmic history
- Ocular examination

PREOPERATIVE MEDICATION AND PREPARATION

- Consent
- Scrub bath, care of hair and marking of the eye
- Preoperative antibiotics and disinfectants
- IOP lowering
- Mydriasis

Preoperative check list

PREOPERATIVE EVALUATION AND PREPARATIONS

Once it has been decided to operate for cataract, a thorough preoperative evaluation should be carried out before contemplating surgery. This should include:

A. Review of general medical status of the patient.

B. Ocular evaluation

A. REVIEW OF GENERAL MEDICAL STATUS OF THE PATIENT

A general medical examination of the patient is recommended to:

- *Exclude the presence of systemic diseases* especially: diabetes mellitus; hypertension and cardiac problems; obstructive lung disorders, history of allergy to drugs, bleeding disorders, use of anticoagulants or immunosuppressants.
- *Presence of any musculoskeletal disorders* like kyphosis, scoliosis or excessive obesity, head tremors or nodding may pose difficulty during sleep.
- *Search for any potential source of infection* in the body such as septic gums, urinary tract infection, etc. should also be made.

Implications and considerations for the associated medical problems

1. Diabetes

It is a commonly found medical problem.

- *Diabetic retinopathy*, if detected, should be treated prior to cataract surgery, since proliferative diabetic retinopathy and macular oedema may develop or worsen following cataract surgery. Sometimes cataract surgery is recommended to improve visualization of the fundus for management of DR. Recommendation for such a situation is to perform a large capsulorhexis.
- *Other anticipated problems* in diabetics include smaller pupil, pigment dispersion, delayed wound healing, fibrinous uveitis and an increased risk of endophthalmitis.

Recommended protocol for a diabetic patient
Blood glucose is checked for everyone who undergoes a cataract surgery and this is rechecked on the day of surgery also for all known diabetics. It is necessary to maintain a special record for the monitoring of blood sugar and medications. The recommended values are: Fasting blood sugar (FBS) <140 mg% and Random blood sugar (RBS) <180 mg% on the day of surgery. Following FBS, patients should be advised to have their normal breakfast. If they are on oral anti-diabetic drugs, they should skip the morning dose of the medications only on the day of surgery. If on insulin, one-third of the dose should be administered in the morning. This is done to avoid hypoglycaemia during the preoperative period. The subsequent doses should be taken as per the routine of the individual patient.

2. Hypertension

Hypertension when associated, may rarely increase the risk of suprachoroidal (expulsive) haemorrhage.

Recommended protocol. Blood pressure (BP) is checked for everyone who undergoes a cataract surgery and this is rechacked on the day of surgery, irrespective of hypertensive status. It is necessary to maintain a special record for the monitoring of BP and the medications. *The recommended maximum blood pressure is 140/90 mmHg or less on the day of surgery. The following recommendations should be followed for all hypertensive patients.*

- The patient should take the prescribed antihypertensive medication on the day of surgery.
- Avoid adrenaline in local anaesthesia and phenylephrine eyedrops for dilation.

Use of sedatives a day before starting antihypertensive drug may work well in all outreach patients. It is prudent to check BP in the ward before sending them to the OR.

3. Cardiac artery disease

A detailed physician evaluation is required and his recommendations should be followed.

- Sugery may be done a minimum of *3–6 months after myocardial infarction.*
- *Oral antiplatelet need not be stopped for cataract surgery.*

Anticoagulant therapy needs special attention. Warfarin (INR should be less than 2.5) should be stopped at least 3 days prior to surgery in consultation with the haematologist. If required, injectable heparin may be started. If possible, topical anaesthesia should be used to decrease the risk of bleeding.

If on oral anticoagulants, check for prothrombin time (PT). *Surgey can be done, if PT is less than 18 seconds.*

- Continue routine medication on the day of surgery.
- *Phenylephrine should not be used* for pupillary dilation.
- Administer local anaesthesia *without adrenaline* in anaesthetic solution.
- Provide a stretcher or wheelchair to avoid exertions and stress.
- *Cautery should not be used in patients with pacemakers.*

It is preferable to have a *Stand by physician or anaesthetist* during the anaesthetic block and surgery for cardiac monitoring.

4. Asthmatics

Criteria for admission include:

- Asthma under control with drugs.
- Continue the medicines during hospital stay.
- Minimal or no wheeze before surgery and if *present to give IV bronchodilators* or steroids.
- *Avoid plastic drapes* and take *special care for ventilation* while draping for surgery.
- Use oxygen/nebulizer during surgery if the patient is uncomfortable.
- Inj. deriphylline/dexamethasone IV, SOS.
- Switch off the air-conditioner (optional).
- *Avoid NSAIDs.* If needed to use tablet nimusulide/paracetamol.

5. Renal failure/renal transplant

- A physician should certify fitness for surgery.
- Avoid tablet acetazolamide and NSAIDs. If pain killers are required, paracetamol is safer.
- Avoid systemic amino glycosides.
- If already on maintenance dose of oral steroids, double the dosage for a short interval (one to two weeks) following surgery.

6. Septic foci

- Check for dental infection, history of purulent discharge, skin infections, etc.
- Treat adequately before surgery.

Examination and advice of a physician is essential for the following:

- Uncontrolled diabetes mellitus and hypertension
  - If BP >170/100 mm Hg
  - RBS >200 mg%
- Known cardiac patients
- Recently diagnosed uncontrolled asthmatics
- Renal failure/transplants
- Liver disease
- Known bleeding disorders
- Obese or emaciated patients

B. OCULAR EVALUATION

Ocular evaluation before cataract surgery should include:

- Present and past ophthalmic history, and
- Ocular examination.

I. Present and past ophthalmic history

- ***Visual complaints.*** A cataract patient may be bothered by the glare, diplopia, polyopia or decreased contrast sensitivity apart from decreased visual acuity for near and/or distance.
- ***Patient's lifestyle*** may be compromised by the cataract. Therefore, cataract surgery should be planned on the basis of need, occupation and lifestyle of the patient.
- ***Past ophthalmic history*** should include enquiry about previous visual acuity, history of amblyopia, strabismus, previous surgery (especially refractive surgery), trauma and concurrent eye disease.
- ***Review the indications for surgery*** which include:

1. *Visual improvement.* This is by far the most common indication. When surgery should be advised for visual improvement varies from person to person depending upon the individual visual needs. So, an individual should be operated for cataract, when the visual handicap becomes a significant deterrent to the maintenance of his or her usual lifestyle including the profession.

2. *Medical indications.* Sometimes patients may be comfortable from the visual point (due to useful vision from the other eye or otherwise) but may be advised cataract surgery due to medical grounds such as:

- Lens-induced glaucoma,
- Phacoanaphylactic endophthalmitis, and
- Retinal diseases like diabetic retinopathy or retinal detachment, treatment of which is being hampered by the presence of lens opacities.

3. *Cosmetic indication.* Sometimes patient with mature cataract may insist on cataract extraction (even with no hope of getting useful vision), in order to obtain a black pupil.

II. Ocular examination

A thorough examination of the eyes including slit-lamp biomicroscopy is desirable in all cases. The following useful information is essential before the patient is considered for surgery.

1. *Assessment of visual status*

Visual status assessment should include:

- *Visual acuity* testing should be done unaided and best corrected and pinhole testing.
- *Perception of light* (PL) must be noted. Absence of PL indicates nil visual prognosis.
- *Projection of rays* (PR). Inaccurate PR may be due to old retinal detachment, visual pathway defects, advanced glaucoma, large area of chorioretinal atrophy and indicates poor visual prognosis. However, at times in dense cataracts, PR may be inaccurate with good visual prognosis.
- *Potential visual acuity tests* which may be required in the presence of opaque media include:
  - Laser interferometry (LI), and
  - Potential acuity meter (PAM) test.

2. *Examination of pupil*

Pupils should be examined to check for:

- Light reactions and RAPD, and
- Ability of the pupils to dilate adequately before surgery.

Small pupil may result in inadequate capsulorhexis, and uncomplete cortical cleanup. Small nuclear fragments may be left behind the iris because of poor visibility.

Management of small pupil should be planned preoperatively (*see* pages 287–290).

3. *Anterior segment evaluation*

Anterior segment evaluation by slit-lamp biomicroscopy is must before cataract surgery.

- *Cornea* should be examined to note any scarring, endothelial status (guttata). In patients with suspicion of endothelial dystrophy, *specular microscopy examination* should be carried out for endothelial cell count and morphology. Normal cell count in elderly patients is 2000–2500 cell/mm^2. Special care is needed in patients with cell counts below 1500 cells/mm^2.
- *Signs of uveitis. Keratic precipitates (KPs)* noted at the back of cornea suggest management of subtle uveitis before the cataract surgery. *Other signs of uveitis* which may be noted include pigment dispersal over the anterior lens capsule and presence of posterior synechiae.

Note. Ideally anterior chamber activity should be absent or minimal (+1 cells or less) for three months prior to surgery. In quiet eyes, topical steroids (prednisolone acetate 1% or dexamethasone 0.1%) are used six times a day, starting 1 week before surgery. A course of systemic steroids should also be considered.

- *Cataractous lens* should be evaluated for morphology and maturity of cataract and for grade of nuclear sclerosis (especially important for planning phacoemulsification surgery (pages 6 and 68).
- *Anterior chamber depth* assessment and detection of associated iridodonosis and pseudoexfoliation are very important.
  - *Shallow anterior chamber* is associated with reduction in safe zone for phacoemulsification. Therefore, protection of endothelium with OVD to create space is essential.
  - *Very deep anterior chamber* predisposes to difficulty in manipulation of nucleus.
  - *Pseudoexfoliation* is associated with poor pupillary dilation and weak zonules. Use of capsular tension ring (CTR) may minimize the risk of dropping the lens into the vitreous.

4. *Intraocular pressure*

Intraocular pressure (IOP) should be measured in each case, preferably by applanation tonometry. Presence of a raised IOP needs a priority management. The risk of postoperative steroid-induced rise in IOP especially in patients with POAG should also be kept in mind.

5. *Examination of lids, conjunctiva and lacrimal apparatus*

- *Search for local source of infection* should be made by ruling out conjunctival infections, meibomitis, blepharitis and lacrimal sac infection.
- *Conjunctival swab culture and sensitivity* should be carried out in following cases:
  - One-eyed patients
  - Prior dacryocystectomy (DCT)
  - History of chronic infection, e.g. blepharitis
  - Recently healed corneal ulcer
- *Lacrimal sac* should receive special attention. Lacrimal syringing should be carried out in a patient with history of watering from the eyes. In cases where chronic dacryocystitis is discovered, either DCR (dacryocystorhinostomy) or DCT (dacryocystectomy) operation should be performed, before the cataract surgery.
- *Trichiasis and entropion* should be looked for and corrected prior to cataract surgery.

6. *Posterior segment evaluation*

i. ***Fundus examination,*** wherever possible, should be carried out using direct ophthalmoscope and/or +90 D/+78 D lens, with special attention on the macula, to rule out other causes of decreased vision, especially age-related macular degeneration. Indirect ophthalmoscopy may be useful in hazy media.

ii. ***Macular function tests*** are important to predict the visual potential in patients with very dense cataracts where fundus examination is not possible. A few simple macular functions tests are as below:

- *Projection of rays (PR).* It is a crude but an important and easy test for function of the peripheral retina. It is tested in a semi-dark room with the opposite eye covered. A thin beam of light is thrown in the patient's eye from four directions (up, down, medial and lateral) and the patient is asked to look straight ahead and point out the direction from which the light seems to come.

- *Two-light discrimination test.* The patient is asked to look through an opaque disc perforated with two pinholes behind which a light is held. The holes are 2 inches apart and kept about 2 feet away from the eye. If the patient can perceive two lights, it indicates normal macular function.
- *Maddox rod test.* The patient is asked to look at a distant bright light through a Maddox rod. An accurate perception of red line indicates normal function.
- *Colour perception.* It indicates that some macular function is present and optic nerve is relatively normal.
- *Entoptic visualization.* It is evaluated by rubbing a point source of light (such as bare-lighted bulb of torch) against the closed eyelids. If the patient perceives the retinal vascular pattern in black outline, it is favourable indication of retinal function. Being subjective in nature, the importance of negative test can be considered if the patient can perceive the pattern with the opposite eye.
- *Potential acuity meter (PAM) test.* It is a subjective method to determine the potential of vision in patients with hazy media. This test is performed with dilated pupil, with the help of PAM devise attached to the slit-lamp. This device projects the image of Snellen's acuity chart to the macula of the patient, who is asked to read the chart. A reasonably accurate assessment of potential visual acuity may be made with this test.
- *Laser interferometry (LI).* Like PAM test, LI is also a subjective test for estimating visual acuity in patients with mild to moderate hazy media. It utilizes the principle of light interference. The interference fringes generated by a Helium-Neon laser are focused on the eye from two sources, which overlap behind the lens. By changing size of the fringes, visual acuity can be ascertained. This test is not possible in patients with very dense cataracts.

iii. *Objective tests for evaluating retina* are required, if some retinal pathology is suspected. These tests include ultrasonic evaluation of posterior segment of the eye; electrophysiological studies such as ERG (electroretinogram), EOG (electro-oculogram) and VER (visually-evoked response).

7. Keratometry and biometry

Keratometry and biometry to calculate power of the intraocular lens (IOL) to be implanted are performed in each case to be taken up for cataract surgery (For details *see*, Chapter 9 pages 109–118).

PREOPERATIVE MEDICATION AND PREPARATION

1. Consent

Consent with detailed information about the procedure, risks involved and outcome expected, should be obtained from each patient. (Annexure I).

2. Hygiene (scrub bath, care of hair and marking of the eye)

- Each patient should be instructed to have a scrub bath including face and hair wash with soap and water.
- Male patients must get their beard cleaned and hair trimmed.
- Female patients should comb their hair properly.
- Eye to be operated should be marked.
- Change of street clothes to operating room clothes is mandatory on the day of surgery.

3. Preoperative antibiotics and disinfectants

These are required to prevent postoperative endophthalmitis:

- *Topical antibiotics* such as fourth-generation fluoroquinolone (0.3% moxifloxacin or 0.3% gatifloxacin) may be used QID for 3 days before surgery and every 15 min 4–6 times just before surgery to eradicate conjunctival bacterial flora.
- *Povidone-iodine (10%) solution* should be used to paint the lids, brow region, and facial skin 3 hours before surgery.

- *Povidone-iodine (5%) solution* should be used to irrigate the conjunctival sac 5 minutes before surgery. It is the most important preoperative measure.

4. IOP lowering

IOP lowering is must for conventional extracapsular cataract extraction (ECCE). A few surgeons also prefer to lower IOP in manual small incision cataract surgery (SICS) and phacoemulsification. It can be accomplished by mechanical pressure (digital massage or Honan balloon) and/or by IOP lowering drugs (IV mannitol or acetazolamide).

5. Mydriasis

Mydriasis, sustained throughout the procedure is essentially required. It can be obtained by:

- *Topical tropicamide* 1% (or cyclopentolate) + phenylephrine 2.5% instilled every 15 minutes 4 times before surgery.
- *Topical cyclo-oxygenase inhibitor,* e.g. flurbiprofen 0.3% or, ketorolac 0.5%, or diclofenac 0.1% instilled 3 times, a day before the surgery and every 15 minutes, 4 times immediately before the surgery helps in maintaining mydriasis during the procedure.

PREOPERATIVE CHECK LIST

It is always advisable for the ward nurse to prepare a preoperative check list to varify whether the preoperative preparation has been done properly (Annexure II).

ANNEXURE I

Sample of consent form for cataract surgery

Name of the patient ....

Father's name ....

Address ....

Date of birth ....

Sex: M ( ) F ( ) I( )

A. Interpreter needs

An interpreter service is required? Yes ( ) No ( )

B. Condition and treatment

The doctor has explained that you have the following condition: (Doctor to document in patient's own words) ....

....

This condition requires the following procedure. (Doctor to document include site and/or side where relevant to the procedure)

....

....

Left eye ( ) Right eye ( )

The following will be performed:

The cataract is surgically removed. The lens in the eye is replaced by an artificial lens or what is commonly known as an implant.

C. Risks of this procedure

There are risks and complications with this procedure. They include but are not limited to the following:

General risks

- Infection can occur, requiring antibiotics and further treatment.
- Bleeding could occur and may require a return to the operating room. Bleeding is more common, if you have been taking blood thinning drugs such as warfarin, asprin, clopidogrel or dipyridamole.
- Small areas of the lung can collapse, increasing the risk of chest infection. This may need antibiotics and physiotherapy.
- Increased risk in obese people of wound infection, chest infection, heart and lung complications, and thrombosis.
- Heart attack or stroke could occur due to the strain on the heart.
- Blood clot in the leg (DVT) causing pain and swelling. In rare cases, part of the clot may break off and go to the lungs.
- Death as a result of this procedure is possible.

Specific risks

- A cloudy cornea which may or may not settle. This may require further surgery.
- An acute inflammatory reaction causing pain. This may need further treatment.
- A fragment of the cataract may fall into the back of the eye. This may require further surgery.
- Infection of the eye which could cause loss of vision or loss of the eye.
- Glaucoma (eye disease). This may need further treatment.
- Macular oedema (collection of fluid); and retinal haemorrhage (bleed). This usually settles with time.

- Retinal detachment may occur. This will require further treatment.
- Any of these complications may occur but these complications are now rare.
- Any of these complications may permanently damage sight.
- Any of these complications may involve a second operation being necessary.

D. Significant risks and procedure options

(Doctor to document in space provided. Continue in Medical Record, if necessary)

....

....

....

E. Risks of not having this procedure

(Doctor to document in space provided. Continue in Medical Record, if necessary)

....

....

....

F. Anaesthetic

This procedure may require an anaesthetic. (Doctor to document type of anaesthetic discussed)

....

....

G. Patient consent

I acknowledge that the doctor has explained;

- My medical condition and the proposed procedure, including additional treatment, if the doctor finds something unexpected. I understand the risks, including the risks that are specific to me.
- The anaesthetic required for this procedure. I understand the risks, including the risks that are specific to me.
- Other relevant procedure/treatment options and their associated risks.
- My prognosis and the risks of not having the procedure.
- That no guarantee has been made that the procedure will improve my condition even though it has been carried out with due professional care.
- The procedure may include a blood transfusion.
- Tissues and blood may be removed and could be used for diagnosis or management of my condition, stored and disposed of sensitively by the hospital.
- If immediate life-threatening events happen during the procedure, they will be treated based on my discussions with the doctor or my Acute Resuscitation Plan.
- A doctor other than the Consultant may conduct the procedure. I understand this could be a doctor undergoing further training.

I have been given the following Patient Information Sheet/s:

( ) Anaesthetic Eye Operation

( ) Cataract Surgery

- I was able to ask questions and raise concerns with the doctor about my condition, the proposed procedure and its risks, and my treatment options. My questions and concerns have been discussed and answered to my satisfaction.
- I understand I have the right to change my mind at any time, including after I have signed this form but, preferably following a discussion with my doctor.
- I understand that image/s or video footage may be recorded as part of and during my procedure and that these image/s or video/s will assist the doctor to provide appropriate treatment.

On the basis of the above statements,

I request to have the procedure

Name of Patient ....

Signature ....

Date ....

Patients who lack capacity to provide consent

Consent must be obtained from a substitute decision maker/s.

Name of Substitute Decision Maker/s ....

Signature ....

Relationship to patient ....

Date ....

Ph No ....

H. Doctor's statement

I have explained to the patient all the above points under the Patient Consent section (G) and I am of the opinion that the patient/substitute decision-maker has understood the information.

Name of Doctor: ....

Designation:...

Signature: ....

Date:..............................

I. Interpreter's statement

I have given a sight translation in .... (state the patient's language here) of the consent form and assisted in the provision of any verbal and written information given to the patient/parent or guardian/substitute decision-maker by the doctor.

Name of Interpreter ....

Signature ....

Date ....

Annexure II

Preoperative check list

Name of Patient...

Medical Record no...

1. Investigation

Hb (if under GA)......... Blood sugar.......... BP ......

Weight .... Others ....

2. Eye examination: Eye ....

Vision .... Sac ....

Xylocaine sensitivity ....

IOP .... IOL power ....

3. Obtained written consent? Y......... , N ....

Attached GVP consent form?

4. Does the patient have DM? Y......... , N ....

5. Does the patient have hypertension?
   Y......... , N ....

6. Eye prepared for operation? Y......... , N ....

7. Eyebrows and eyelashes painted with povidone iodine. Y......... , N ....

8. Eye dilated for operation? Y......... , N ....
   Dilated adequately?

9. Is it cataract (IOL) surgery? Y......... , N ....
   IOL brought as per No.?

10. Did medical officer examine?
    Y......... , N ....

11. Examination by anaesthetist ....

12. Did patient have a bath/wash face? (Comment on patient hygiene)

....

....

Suggestion of Doctor

....

....

Date ....

Signature of ward Nurse ....

BIBLIOGRAPHY

1. American Academy of Ophthalmology (2008–2009). Basic and Clinical Science Course: Lens and Cataract, San Francisco.
2. Becker D. Preoperative Medical Evaluation: Part 1: General Principles and Cardiovascular Considerations. Anesthesia Progress 56(3): 92–103, 2009.
3. Fischer S, Bader A, Sweitzer B. Preoperative Evaluation, In Anesthesia, Miller R, 1001–1066, 2010. Churchill Livingstone, ISBN 978-0-443-06959-8, Philadelphia.
4. Fleisher L. Routine Laboratory Testing in the Elderly: Is it indicated? Anesthesia and Analgesia, 93:249–50;2001.
5. Fong K, Malhotra R (2008). Assessment of the patient with cataract, In: Cataract (eye essentials*)*, Malhotra R, 18–32, Elsevier, ISBN 978-0-08-044977-7, USA. Gwinnut, C (2004). Clinical Anaesthesia (2nd ed), Blackwell, ISBN 978-1-4051-1552-0, Massachusetts.
6. Hata T, Moyers J. Preoperative patient assessment and management, In: Clinical Anesthesia, Barash P, pp 569–597, 2009. Lippincott Williams & Wilkins, ISBN 978-0-7817-8763-5, Philadelphia.
7. Hepner D. The role of testing in the preoperative evaluation. *Cleveland* Clinic Journal of Medicine, 76(4): S22–S27, 2009.
8. Ismael S, Mowafi H. Melatonin provides anxiolysis, enhances analgesia, decreases intraocular pressure, and promotes better operating conditions during cataract surgery under topical anaesthesia. Anaesthesia and Analgesia 108(4):1058–1061, 2009.
9. Kubitz J, Motsch J. Eye surgery in the elderly. Best Practice and Research clinical Anaesthesiology 17(2): 245–257, 2003.
10. Lichtor J. Ambulatory Anesthesia, In: Clinical Anaesthesia, Barash P, 833–46, Lippincott Williams & Wilkins, ISBN 978-0-7817-8763-5, Philadelphia, 2009.

CHAPTER 13

INTRACAPSULAR AND CONVENTIONAL EXTRACAPSULAR CATARACT EXTRACTION

TYPES AND CHOICE OF SURGICAL TECHNIQUES

ICCE VERSUS ECCE

Intracapsular cataract extraction (ICCE)

In this technique, the entire cataractous lens along with the intact capsule is removed. Therefore, weak and degenerated zonules are a prerequisite for this method.

Indications. ICCE has stood the test of time and had been widely employed for about 100 years over the world. Now (for the last 40 years) it has been almost entirely replaced by modern extracapsular techniques. At present the only indication of ICCE is markedly subluxated and dislocated lens.

Extracapsular cataract extraction (ECCE) techniques

In these techniques, major portion of anterior capsule with epithelium, nucleus and cortex are removed; leaving behind intact posterior capsule.

Indications. Presently, extracapsular cataract extraction techniques are the surgery of choice for almost all types of childhood as well as adulthood cataracts unless contraindicated.

Contraindications. The only absolute contra-indication for ECCE is markedly subluxated or dislocated lens.

Different techniques of planned extracapsular cataract extraction

The surgical techniques of ECCE presently in vogue are: Planned modular extracapsular cataract extraction (ECCE), manual small incision cataract surgery (SICS), and phacoemulsification.

Advantages of ECCE techniques over ICCE

1. ECCE is a universal operation and can be performed at all ages, except when zonules are not intact; whereas ICCE cannot be performed below 40 years of age.
2. Posterior chamber IOL can be implanted after ECCE, while it cannot be implanted after ICCE.

3. Postoperative vitreous-related problems (such as herniation in anterior chamber, pupillary block and vitreous touch syndrome) associated with ICCE are not seen after ECCE.
4. Incidence of postoperative complications such as endophthalmitis, cystoid macular oedema and retinal detachment is much less after ECCE as compared to that after ICCE.
5. Postoperative astigmatism is less with ECCE techniques, as the incision is smaller.
6. Prognosis for subsequent glaucoma filtering or corneal transplantation (if required) is much improved with ECCE.
7. Incidence of secondary rubeosis in diabetics is reduced after ECCE.

PLANNED MODERN ECCE VERSUS SICS

Planned large incision (8 mm) ECCE, though still being performed by many surgeons, is being largely replaced by small incision cataract surgery (SICS) and phacoemulsification techniques.

Merits of planned modern ECCE over SICS

The only merit of conventional ECCE over SICS is that it is a simple technique to master with short learning curve.

Demerits of planned modern ECCE over SICS

- Long incision (8–10 mm).
- Multiple sutures are required.
- Open chamber surgery with high risk of vitreous prolapse, operative hard eye and expulsive choroidal haemorrhage.
- High incidence of postoperative astigmatism.
- Postoperative suture-related problems like irritation and suture abscess, etc.
- Postoperative wound-related problems such as wound leak, shallowing of anterior chamber and iris prolapse.
- Needs suture removal, during which infection may occur.

SICS VERSUS PHACOEMULSIFICATION

Merits of manual SICS over phacoemulsification

1. *Universal applicability,* i.e. all types of cataracts including hard cataracts (grades IV and V) can be operated by this technique.
2. *Learning curve.* This procedure is much easier to learn as compared to phacoemulsification.
3. *Not machine dependent.* The biggest advantage of manual SICS is that it is not machine dependent and thus can be practised anywhere.
4. *Less surgical complications.* Disastrous complication like nuclear drop into vitreous cavity is much less than phacoemulsification technique.
5. *Operating time* in manual SICS is less than that of phocoemulsification, especially in hard cataract. Therefore, it is ideal for mass surgery.
6. *Cost-effective.* With manual SICS, the expenses are vastly reduced as compared to considerable expenses in acquiring and maintaining phaco machine. There is no need to spend on consumable items like the phaco tip, sleeves, tubing and probe. Further, in SICS always PMMA IOLs are used which are much cheeper than foldable IOLs.

Demerits of manual SICS over phacoemulsification

1. *Conjunctival congestion* persists for 5–7 days at the site of conjunctival flap.
2. *Mild tenderness* sometime may be present owing to scleral incision.
3. *Postoperative hyphaema* may be noted sometime.
4. *Surgical induced astigmatism* is more as the incision in SICS is large (about 6 mm) as compared to phacoemulsification (about 3.2 mm).

Merits of phacoemulsification over manual SICS

1. *Topical anaesthesia* may be sufficient for phacoemulsification in expert hands.
2. *Postoperative congestion* is minimal after phacoemulsification, as phaco is usually performed through a clear corneal incision.
3. *Small incision.* The chief advantage of phacoemulsification over manual SICS is that it can be performed through a smaller (3.2 mm) incision.
4. *Less corneal complications.* Phacoemulsification can be performed in the posterior chamber without prolapsing the nucleus into the anterior chamber, thereby minimising the risk of corneal complications.

5. *Visual rehabilitation* is comparetively quicker in phacoemulsification as compared to manual SICS.
6. *Postoperative astigmatism* is comparatively less when foldable IOLs are implanted through a smaller incision (3.2 mm).

Demerits of phacoemulsification vis-á-vis manual SICS

1. *Learning curve* for phacoemulsification is more painful both for the surgeons and patients.
2. *Complications* encountered during phacoemulsification like nuclear drop are unforgiving.
3. *Machine dependent.* This procedure is solely machine dependent and in the event of an unfortunate machine failure in the middle of surgery one has to shift to conventional ECCE.
4. *High cost.* Cost of this technique is very high because of expensive machine, accessories and maintenance.
5. *Limitations.* It is very difficult to deal with hard cataracts (grades IV and V) with this technique, and also there is high risk of serious corneal complications due to more use of phaco energy in such cases.

Conclusion

In spite of the demerits listed above, the phacoemulsification has become the preferred method of cataract extraction worldwide because the complication rate in the expert hands is minimal and the technique provides an almost quiet eye early postoperatively and an early visual rehabilitation. However, for the masses, especially in developing countries, the manual SICS offers the advantages of sutureless cataract surgery as a low cost alternative to phacoemulsification with the added advantages of having wider applicability and an easier learning curve.

INTRACAPSULAR CATARACT EXTRACTION

Presently, the technique of intracapsular cataract extraction (ICCE) is obsolete and sparingly performed worldwide. However, the surgical steps are described here as a mark of respect to the technique which has been widely employed for about 100 years over the world and is an important landmark in the history of cataract surgery.

PREPARATION OF THE PATIENT

Preparation of the patient is described in Chapter 12 on pages 176–183. Essential points to be revised for ICCE are as below:

- *Pupil* should be fully dilated.
- *Peribulbar block anaesthesia* needs to be administered.
- *Intraocular pressure (IOP)* should be lowered.

CLEANSING AND DRAPING OF THE EYE

Once anaesthesia is achieved, the skin of the lids and the surrounding area should be prepared by cleansing with 10% povidone-iodine solution. The area is then wiped dry with a cotton swab. After thorough cleansing, the drapes are applied. Use of an eye patch with a bag to collect the fluid is quite hygienic.

SURGICAL STEPS OF ICCE

Surgical steps of the ICCE technique are as follows:

1. ***Exposing the eye.*** The eye to be operated is exposed by the insertion of a lid speculum.

2. ***Superior rectus (bridle) suture*** is passed to fix the eye in downward gaze (Fig. 13.1A).

3. ***Conjunctival flap*** (fornix-based) is prepared to expose the limbus (Fig. 13.1B) and *haemostasis* is achieved by wet field or heat cautery. All surgeons do not make conjunctival flap.

4. ***Partial thickness groove or gutter*** is made through about two-thirds depth of anterior limbal area from 9.30 to 2.30 o'clock (150°) with the help of a razor blade knife (Fig. 13.1C).

5. ***Corneoscleral section.*** The anterior chamber is opened with the razor blade knife or with 3.2 mm keratome and section is completed using sclerocorneal scissors (Fig. 13.1D).

6. ***Iridectomy*** (Fig. 13.1E). A peripheral iridectomy may be performed by using iris forceps and de Wecker's scissors to prevent postoperative pupil block glaucoma.

7. ***Delivery of lens*** (Fig. 13.1F). In ICCE, the lens can be delivered by any of the methods described below:

i. *Smith Indian method.* Here the lens is delivered with tumbling technique by

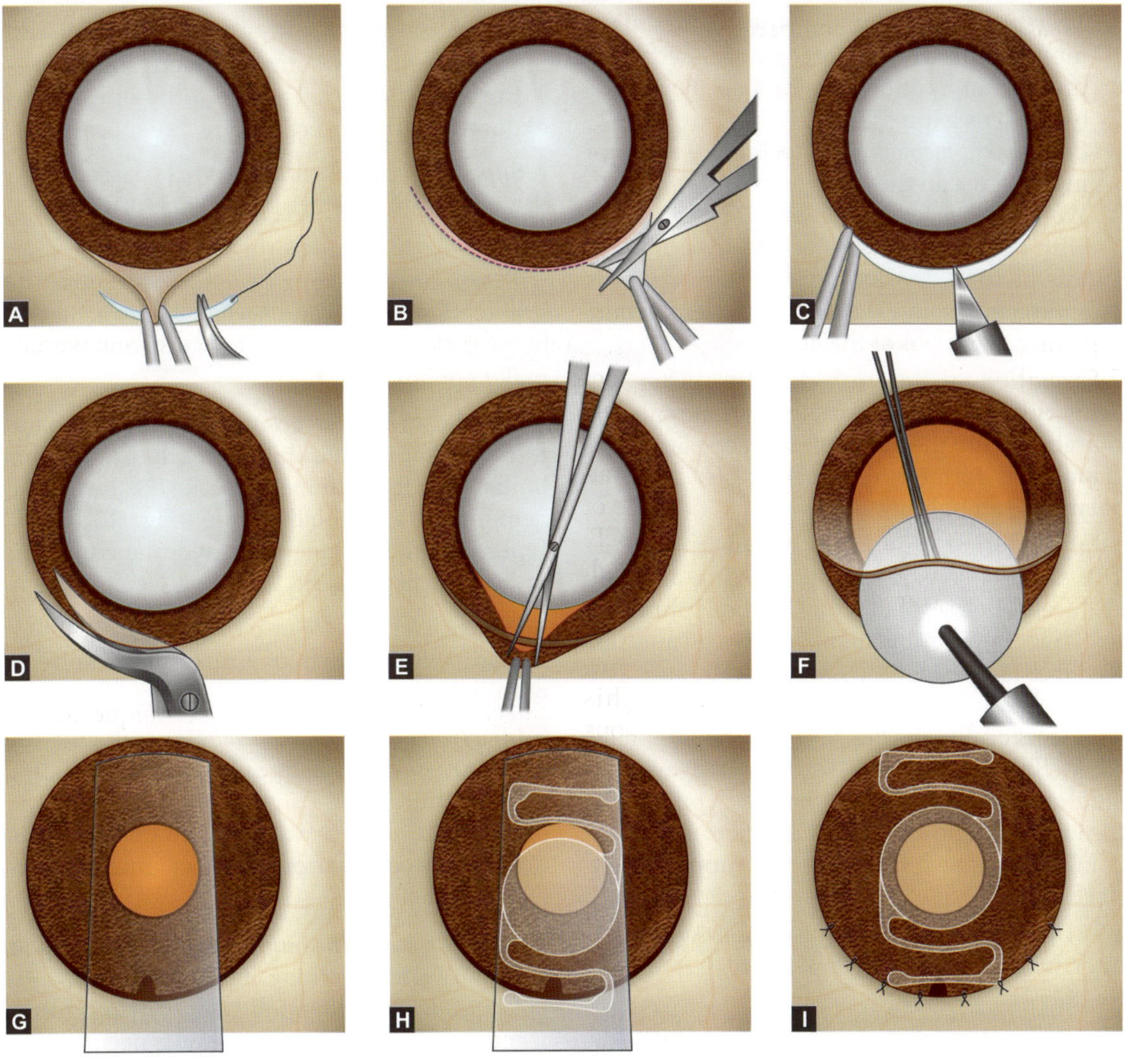

Fig. 13.1. *Surgical steps of intracapsular cataract extraction (ICCE) with anterior chamber intraocular lens implantation: **(A)** Passing of superior rectus suture; **(B)** Fornix-based conjunctival flap; **(C)** Partial thickness groove; **(D)** Completion of corneoscleral section; **(E)** Peripheral iridectomy; **(F)** Cryolens extraction; **(G)** Insertion of acrylic glide sheat, **(H)** Insertion of Kelman multiflex intraocular lens in the anterior chamber; **(I)** Corneoscleral suturing.*

applying pressure on limbus at 6 o'clock position with lens expressor and counter-pressure at 12 o'clock with the lens spatula. With this method, lower pole is delivered first.

ii. *Cryoextraction.* In this technique, cornea is lifted up, lens surface is dried with a swab, iris is retracted up and tip of the cryoprobe is applied on the anterior surface of the lens in the upper quadrant. Freezing is activated (–40°C) to create adhesions between the lens and the probe. The zonules are ruptured by gentle rotatory movements and the lens is then extracted out by sliding movements. In this technique, upper pole of the lens is delivered first (Fig. 13.1F).

iii. *Capsule forceps method.* The Arruga's capsule holding forceps is introduced close into the anterior chamber and the anterior capsule of the lens is caught at 6 o'clock position. The lens is lifted slightly and its zonules are ruptured by gentle sideways movements.

Then the lens is extracted with gentle sliding movements by the forceps assisted by a pressure at 6 o'clock position on the limbus by the lens expressor.

iv. *Erysiphakee method.* This technique was not in much use in the later years.

v. *Wire vectis method.* It is employed in cases with subluxated or dislocated lens only. In this method, the loop of the wire vectis is slide gently below the subluxated lens, which is then lifted out of the eye.

8. ***Formation of anterior chamber.*** After the delivery of lens, iris is reposited into the anterior chamber with the help of iris repositor and chamber is formed by injecting sterile air or balanced salt solution.

9. ***Implantation of anterior chamber (ACIOL)*** The pupil is constricted by injecting a miotic (1% acetylcholine, pilocarpine without preservative) into the anterior chamber between anterior chamber is filled with 2% methylcellulase. The acrylic glide sheat in child in the anterior chamber (optional) (Fig. 13.1G). The IOL, held by McPherson forceps, is gently slid into the anterior chamber. Inferior haptic is pushed in the inferior angle at 6 o'clock position and upper haptic is pushed to engage in upper angle (Fig. 13.1H)

10. ***Closure of incision*** is done with 5–7 interrupted sutures (8-0, 9-0 or 10-0 nylon) (Fig. 13.1I).

11. ***Conjunctival flap*** is reposited and secured by wet-field cautery.

12. ***Subconjunctival injection*** of dexamethasone 0.25 ml and gentamicin 0.5 ml is given.

13. ***Patching of eye*** is done with a pad and sticking plaster or a bandage is applied.

PLANNED MODERN EXTRACAPSULAR CATARACT EXTRACTION

PREPARATION, CLEANSING AND DRAPING

Preparation, cleansing and draping of the eye is similar to ICCE, except that neither ocular massage nor hyperosmotic agents are used by most of the surgeons to lower IOP. Maintenance of pupillary dilation is critical for the success of ECCE.

SURGICAL STEPS

Surgical steps of planned modern ECCE are:

1. ***Exposing the eye.*** The eye to be operated is exposed by the insertion of a lid speculum.

2. ***Superior rectus (bridle) suture*** is passed to fix the eye in downward gaze (Fig. 13.1A).

3. ***Conjunctival flap*** (fornix-based) is prepared with conjunctival spring scissors to expose the limbus (Fig. 13.1B) and *haemostasis* is achieved by wet field cautery. Many surgeons do not make conjunctival flap.

4. ***Partial thickness groove or gutter*** is made through about two-thirds depth of anterior limbal area from 10 to 2 o'clock (120°) with the help of a razor blade knife (Fig. 13.1C). It represents the first step of a two-plane incision to be completed later.

5. ***Corneoscleral entry into the anterior chamber*** is made with the help of a razor blade knife or with 3.2 mm keratome.

6. ***Injection of viscoelastic substance in anterior chamber.*** A viscoelastic substance such as 2% methylcellulose or 1% sodium hyaluronate is injected into the anterior chamber. This maintains the anterior chamber and protects the endothelium.

7. ***Anterior capsulotomy.*** It can be performed by any of the following methods:

i. *Can-opener technique.* In it, an irrigating cystitome (or simply a 26 gauge needle, bent at its tip) is introduced into the anterior chamber and multiple small radial cuts are made in the anterior capsule for 360° (Fig. 13.2A).

ii. *Linear capsulotomy* (envelope technique). Here a straight incision is made in the anterior capsule (in the upper part) from 2–10 o'clock position. The rest of the capsulotomy is completed in the end after removal of nucleus and cortex.

iii. *Continuous circular capsulorhexis* (CCC). Recently, this is the most commonly performed procedure. In this, the anterior capsule is torn in a circular fashion either with the help of an irrigating bent-needle cystitome or with a capsulorhexis forceps (Fig. 13.2B). For details *see* pages 201–203.

8. ***Removal of anterior capsule.*** It is removed with the help of a Kelman-McPherson forceps (Fig. 13.2B) or by injecting viscoelastic material behind the free capsule flap.

9. ***Completion of corneoscleral section.*** The second step of two-plane incision is completed from 10 to 2 o′ clock position either with the help of corneoscleral section enlarging scissors or 5.2 mm blunt keratome (Fig. 13.2C). This two-plane incision facilitates better apposition of the wound edges, thereby improving wound closure and reducing postoperative astigmatism induced by the sutures.

10. ***Hydrodissection.*** After the anterior capsulotomy, the balanced salt solution (BSS) is injected under the peripheral part of the anterior capsule. This manoeuvre separates the corticonuclear mass from the capsule. For details *see* page 203.

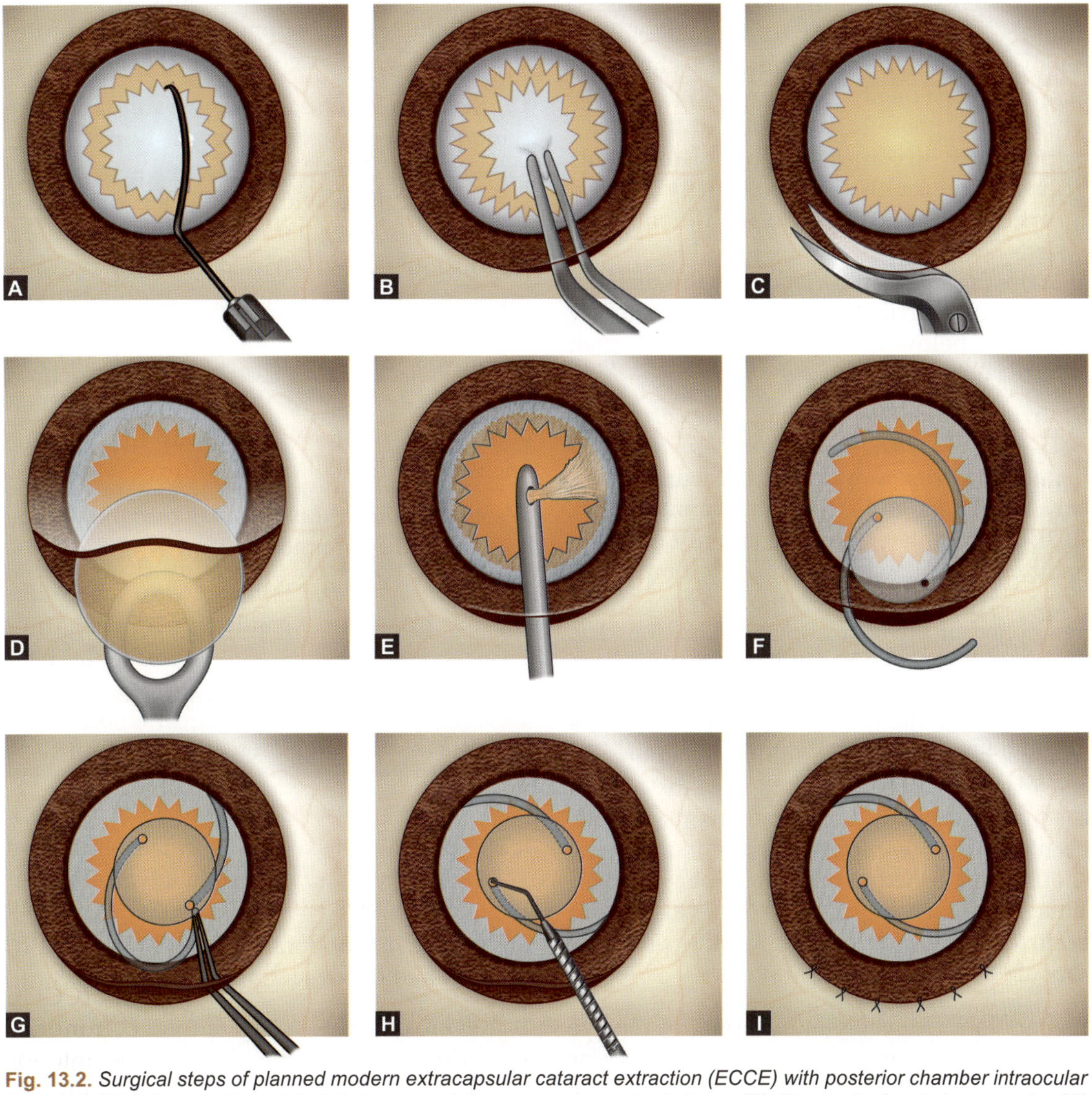

Fig. 13.2. *Surgical steps of planned modern extracapsular cataract extraction (ECCE) with posterior chamber intraocular lens (PC IOL) implantation:* ***(A)*** *Anterior capsulotomy can-opener technique;* ***(B)*** *Removal of anterior capsule;* ***(C)*** *Completion of corneoscleral section;* ***(D)*** *Removal of nucleus (pressure and counter-pressure method);* ***(E)*** *Aspiration of cortex;* ***(F)*** *Insertion of inferior haptic of posterior chamber IOL;* ***(G)*** *Insertion of superior haptic of PC IOL by flexing technique;* ***(H)*** *Dialling of the IOL;* ***(I)*** *Corneoscleral suturing.*

11. ***Removal of nucleus.*** After hydrodissection, the nucleus is prolapsed into the anterior chamber either by rotating with the same hydrodissection cannula or with the help of a Sinskey hook after injecting viscoelastic material in the anterior chamber. Expression of the nucleus should never be attempted while the nucleus is still inside the capsular bag because zonular rupture may occur necessitating the continuation of the surgery as an unplanned intracapsular cataract extraction. Therefore, once it is ensured that the nucleus has passed into the anterior chamber, then it can be removed by any of the following techniques:

i. *Pressure and counter-pressure method.* In it, the posterior pressure is applied at 12 o'clock position with corneal forceps or lens spatula and the nucleus is expressed out by counter-pressure exerted at 6 o'clock position with a lens hook (Fig. 13.2D).

ii. *Irrigating wire vectis technique.* In this method, loop of an irrigating wire vectis is gently passed below the nucleus, which is then lifted out of the eye.

12. ***Irrigation and aspiration of the cortex and polishing of the posterior capsule.*** The remaining cortex is aspirated out using a two-way irrigation and aspiration cannula (Fig. 13.2E). To maintain adequate anterior chamber depth during irrigation and aspiration of the cortex, a nylon 10-0 cross-suture may preferably be applied in the central part of incision. The height of BSS bottle should be adjusted from 40–80 cm to increase or reduce the irrigation in relation to the depth of anterior chamber. The residual cortex from the subincisional area of capsular bag can be aspirated with the help of a J-shaped cannula. Once the lens matter has been removed completely, the posterior capsule should be polished with the help of a polisher. This manoeuvre prevents or delays the occurrence of opacification of the posterior capsule.

13. ***Implantation of IOL.*** The PMMA posterior chamber IOL is implanted in the capsular bag after inflating the bag with viscoelastic substance and removing the central stay suture, if used.

Note. The PMMA PCIOL is in graphed by the optic with the help of IOL holding forceps. The inferior haptic and optic of IOL is gently inserted into the capsular bag behind the iris at 6 o' clock position (Fig. 13.2F). The superior haptic is then grasped by its tip, and is gently pushed down and then released to slide in the upper part of the capsular bag behind the risk (Fig. 13.2G). The IOL is then dialled into the horizontal position (Fig. 13.2H). In the absence of intact capsular bag, the IOL can be implanted in the ciliary sulcus.

14. ***Closure of the incision*** is done by a total of 5–7 interrupted or continuous 10-0 nylon sutures applied in a shoe-lace pattern (Fig. 13.2I).

15. ***Removal of viscoelastic substance.*** Before tying the last suture, the viscoelastic material is aspirated out with 2-way cannula and anterior chamber is filled with BSS. When the IOL is implanted in the ciliary sulcus, preferably the pupil should be constricted to 4 mm by using intracameral preservative free 2% pilocarpine or 1% acetylcholine.

16. ***Conjunctival flap*** is reposited and secured by wet field cautery. Alternatively, the two extremities of the conjunctival flap can be anchored with 10-0 nylon sutures.

17. ***Subconjunctival injection*** of dexamethasone 0.25 ml and gentamicin 0.5 ml is given.

18. ***Patching of eye*** is done with a pad and sticking plaster or a bandage is applied.

POSTOPERATIVE MANAGEMENT AFTER ICCE AND ECCE

Postoperative care and medication

1. The patient is asked to lie quietly upon the back for about 2–3 hours and advised to take nil orally.
2. For mild to moderate postoperative pain, injection diclofenac sodium may be given.
3. Next morning, bandage/eye patch is removed and eye is inspected for any postoperative complication.
4. Antibiotic-steroid eyedrops are used for four times, three times, two times and then once a day for 2 weeks each.

Suture removal

After 6–8 weeks of operation, corneoscleral sutures are removed (when applied). *Nowadays most surgeons are doing sutureless cataract surgery.*

Spectacle prescription

Final spectacles are prescribed after about 8 weeks of operation.

BIBLIOGRAPHY

1. Brown, Nicholas Phelps. "Medical Treatment of Cataract." *Optometry Today* 28–32;November 30, 2001.
2. Grinbaum, A., M. Blumenthal, and E. Assia. "Comparison of Intraocular Pressure Profiles During Cataract Surgery by Phacoemulsification and Extracapsular Cataract Extraction." *Ophthalmic Surgery, Lasers and Imaging* 34:182–186;May–June 2003.
3. Kalpadakis P, et al. "A Comparison of Endophthalmitis After Phacoemulsification or Extracapsular Cataract Extraction in a Socio-Economically Deprived Environment: A Retrospective Analysis of 2,446 Patients." *European Journal of Ophthalmology* 12:395–400; September-October 2002.
4. Minassian, D. C., et al. "Extracapsular Cataract Extraction Compared with Small Incision Surgery by Phacoemulsification: A Randomised Trial." *British Journal of Ophthalmology* 85: 822–829; July 2001.
5. Pesudovs, Konrad, and David B. Elliott. "The Evolution of Cataract Surgery." *Optometry Today*: 30–32;October 19, 2001.
6. Rowden, A., and R. Krishna. "Resident Cataract Surgical Training in United States Residency Programs." *Journal of Cataract and Refractive Surgery* 28:2202–2205; December 2002.

ICCE

1. Arch. of Ophthal., Vol. IX, No. 6, p. 912.
2. Arch. of Ophthal., Vol. II, No. 1, p. 108.
3. Duke-Elder.-Recent Advances in Ophthalmology, 3rd Edition, p. 379.
4. Trans. Ophthal. Soc. U.K., Vol. LII, 1932.
5. Arch. of Ophthal., Vol. X, No. 1, p. 10.
6. Arch. of Ophthal., Vol. XII, No. 1, p. 128, et seq.
7. Arch of Ophthal., Vol. X, No. 1, p. 7.
8. Thomson.-Trans. Ophthal. Soc. U.K., Vol. XLV, p. 151.

CHAPTER 14

MANUAL SMALL INCISION CATARACT SURGERY

INTRODUCTION

Undoubtedly, the present day ideal technique of cataract surgery is phacoemulsification. However, the manual small incision cataract surgery (M-SICS) is a good alternative technique which complements the surgeons armamentarium. Since its introduction in late 1980s, the M-SICS has become popular because of its merits over planned extracapsular cataract extraction (ECCE) as well as phacoemulsification technique highlighted below. In this technique, ECCE with posterior chamber intraocular lens implantation is performed through a sutureless self-sealing corneoscleral valvular tunnel incision.

MANUAL SMALL INCISION CATARACT SURGERY (SICS) VERSUS PLANNED EXTRACAPSULAR CATARACT EXTRACTION (ECCE)

Planned conventional large incision extracapsular cataract extraction (ECCE), though still being performed by some surgeons, is being largely replaced by small incision cataract surgery (SICS) and phacoemulsification techniques.

Merits of planned ECCE over SICS

The only merit of planned ECCE over SICS is that it is a simple technique to master with short learning curve.

Demerits of planned ECCE over SICS

- Long incision (10–12 mm).
- Multiple sutures are required.
- Open chamber surgery with high risk of vitreous prolapse, operative hard eye and expulsive choroidal haemorrhage.
- High incidence of postoperative astigmatism.
- Postoperative suture-related problems like irritation and suture abscess, etc.
- Postoperative wound-related problems such as wound leak, shallowing of anterior chamber and iris prolapse.
- Needs suture removal, during which infection may occur.

MANUAL SICS VERSUS PHACOEMULSIFICATION

Merits of manual SICS over phacoemulsification

1. *Easy to learn.* The SICS is much easier to learn as compared to phacoemulsification because of the following reasons:
   - Manoeuvrability through larger incision is easy.
   - Can be completed even if capsulorhexis is not intact. The procedure can be done even with a can-opener technique of anterior capsulotomy, which is much easier.
   - Hand and foot co-ordination and ambidexterity, which are essential for phacoemulsification, are not necessary in manual SICS.

   Note. Once the technique of manual SICS is mastered, it becomes easy for the surgeon to learn the technique of phacoemulsification.

2. *Universal applicability.* The manual SICS can be performed in all types of cataracts and prevailing ocular conditions as below:
   - Nuclei with all grades of hardness including grades IV and V can be easily managed by slightly increasing the incision size.
   - The procedures can be safely performed in eyes having undergone retinal detachment surgery, vitrectomy or having traumatic cataracts.
   - Can be easily combined with trabeculectomy operation in patients having co-existing glaucoma requiring surgery.
3. *Not machine dependent.* The biggest advantage of manual SICS is that it is not machine dependant and thus can be practised anywhere with the basic instrument set.
4. *Less surgical complications* are encountered vis-à-vis phacoemulsification:
   - *Disastrous complications* like nucleus drop into the vitreous cavity is much less common.
   - *Phaco machine-related complications* such as corneal burn due to excessive heat generated by probe and iris chaffing are not encountered in manual SICS.
5. *Operating time* in manual SICS is less than that of phacoemulsification especially in hard cataracts. Therefore, it is ideal for mass surgery.
6. *Cost-effective* as compared to phacoemulsification.
7. *Useful in conversion during phacoemulsification.* If the surgeon is trained in SICS, it is very useful when the conversion is required due to machine failure during phaco surgery.
8. *Ideal for mass surgery.* The manual SICS is ideal for mass surgeries in eye camps and in high volume setups for eradication of cataract blindness in developing countries with a large cataract backlog, because of the above advantages, i.e.
   - Not machine dependent
   - Much cheaper
   - Less time consuming
   - Less surgical complications
   - Universal applicability.

Demerits of manual SICS over phacoemulsification

1. *Conjunctival congestion* persists for 5–7 days at the site of conjunctival flap.
2. *Mild tenderness* sometime may be present owing to scleral incision.
3. *Postoperative hyphaema* may be noted sometimes.
4. *Surgical induced astigmatism* is more as the incision in SICS is large (about 6 mm) as compared to phacoemulsification (about 3.2 mm).

Merits of phacoemulsification over manual SICS

1. *Topical anaesthesia* may be sufficient for phacoemulsification in expert hands.
2. *Postoperative congestion* is minimal after phacoemulsification, as phaco is usually performed through a clear corneal incision.
3. *Small incision.* The chief advantage of phacoemulsification over manual SICS is that it can be performed through a smaller (3.2 mm) incision.
4. *Less corneal complications.* Phacoemulsification can be performed in the posterior chamber without prolapsing the nucleus into the anterior chamber, thereby minimising the risk of corneal complications.
5. *Visual rehabilitation* is comparetively quicker in phacoemulsification as compared to manual SICS.

6. *Postoperative astigmatism* is comparatively less when foldable IOLs are implanted through a smaller incision (3.2 mm).

Conclusion

Inspite of the long list of merits of SICS over phacoemulsification, the later technique has become the preferred method of cataract extraction worldwide because the complication rate in the expert hands is minimal and the technique provides an almost quiet eye early postoperatively and an early visual rehabilitation. However, for the masses, especially in developing countries, the manual SICS offers the advantages of sutureless cataract surgery as a low cost alternative to phacoemulsification with the added advantages of having wider applicability and an easier learning curve.

INDICATIONS AND CONTRAINDICATIONS OF SICS

Indications

From the above discussion, it is quite clear that manual SICS is a very good alternative for phacoemulsification which is a present day ideal. Therefore, it is indicated in situations where phacoemulsification cannot be performed as below:

- *Mass surgeries in high volume setups* to reduce cost and time of surgery, to cope up with the problem of cataract backlog.
- *Non-availability of phacoemulsification,* i.e. when surgeon is untrained or patient cannot afford or phaco machine is out of order.
- *Contraindications to phacoemulsification,* e.g. patients with ultra-hard cataract, borderline corneal endothelial status.

Contraindications for manual SICS

1. *Crystalline lens conditions,* such as dislocated and subluxated lens with inadequate zonular support.
2. *Corneal conditions,* such as microcornea, peripheral corneal thinning, endothelial dystrophy and conditions with low endothelial cell count.
3. *Scleral conditions* such as *scleritis* or past history of scleritis with associated scleral ectasia and/or ciliary staphyloma.
4. *Conjunctival conditions,* e.g. inflammatory conjunctival scarring disorders.
5. *Bleeding disorders* to avoid hyphaema. Under such circumstances, clear corneal tunnel is better than sclerocorneal tunnel.
6. *Skill and experience* of the surgeon, when lacking, are the major limiting factors.

SURGICAL TECHNIQUE OF MANUAL SICS

Surgical steps of manual small incision cataract surgery (SICS) depicted at a glance in Fig. 14.1 are as below.

BRIDLE SUTURE

Superior rectus bridle suture is passed to fix the eyeball in downward gaze. To place the bridle suture, the conjunctiva along with underlying Tenon's capsule and superior rectus tendon is grasped with the help of a strong tooth forceps about 10 mm away from the superior limbus at 12 o' clock point and a 3-0 silk suture is passed below it with the help of a half-curved cutting needle (Fig. 14.1A).

Note

- Placement of bridle suture is especially important in manual SICS, where in addition to fixation of the globe, it also provides a countertraction force during delivery of the nucleus and epinucleus.
- When SICS is performed by the temporal approach, the bridle suture is placed below the tendon of lateral rectus muscle and all the next steps of surgery are performed in the temporal quadrant.

CONJUNCTIVAL FLAP, EXPOSURE OF SCLERA AND HAEMOSTASIS

A small fornix-based conjunctival flap (Fig. 14.1B) is made with the help of sharp-tipped scissors along the limbus from 10 to 2 o'clock positions. Conjunctiva and the Tenon's capsule are dissected, separated from the underlying sclera and retracted to expose about 4 mm strip of sclera along the entire incision length. *Haemostasis* is achieved by applying gentle and just adequate wet field cautery.

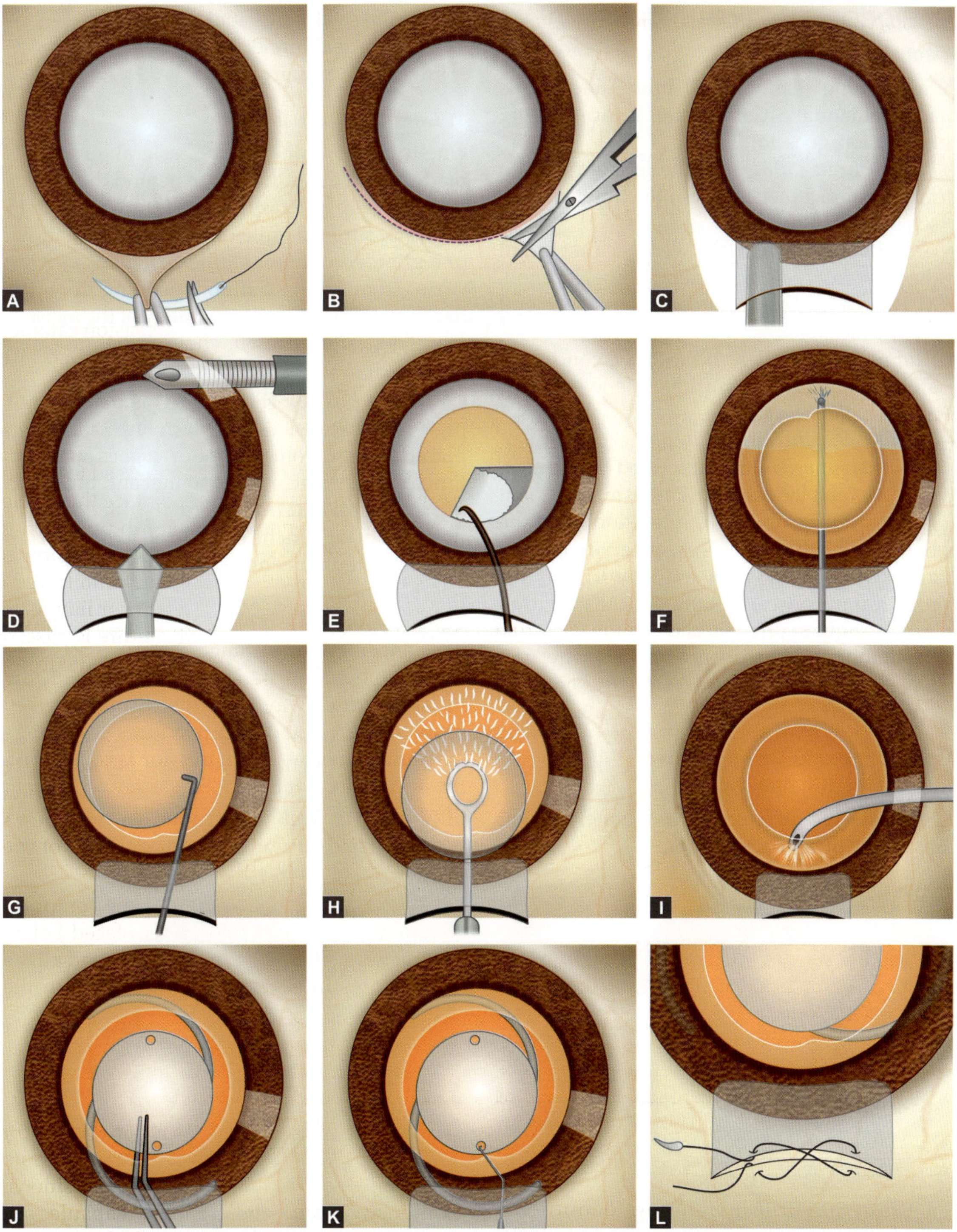

Fig. 14.1. ***(A)*** *Superior rectus bridle suture;* ***(B)*** *Conjunctival flap and exposure of the sclera;* ***(C)*** *Sclerocorneal tunneling with crescent knife;* ***(D)*** *Making internal corneal with 3.2 mm keratome;* ***(E)*** *Continuous curvilinear capsulorhexis with cystitome;* ***(F)*** *Hydrodissection;* ***(G)*** *Prolapse of nucleus in the anterior chamber with Sinskey hook;* ***(H)*** *Nucleus extraction with irrigating wire vectis;* ***(I)*** *Aspiration of cortex;* ***(J)*** *Insertion of inferior haptic and optic of IOL with McPherson or IOL holding forceps;* ***(K)*** *Insertion of superior haptic of IOL by dialling technique;* ***(L)*** *Wound closure with infinity suture (when required).*

SCLEROCORNEAL TUNNEL INCISION

Historical review

A self-sealing sclerocorneal tunnel incision is made in manual SICS. The credit for evolving this incision goes to:

- *Richard Kratz (1982)* was the first surgeon to move cataract incision from the limbus to the sclera.
- *Girard and Hoffman (1984)* were the first to call the posterior incision a scleral tunnel incision.
- *McFarland (1989)* introduced two-plane scleral tunnel incision.
- *Paul Ernest (1990)* introduced the concept of an internal corneal lip (three plane incision) acting as one way valve.
- *Paul Koch,* who postulated the concept of *incisional funnel,* which described the interaction between induced astigmatism, incisional length and distance of the incision from the limbus. This funnel represents an imaginary area where incisions made will, for all practical purposes, be astigmatically neutral. Accordingly shorter incision made closer to the limbus and longer ones further away, will have an equivalent effect on the corneal curvature (Fig. 14.2).

Architecture and Components of Sclerocorneal Tunnel Incision

The architecture of sclerocorneal tunnel incision consists of three components:

- External scleral incision
- Sclerocorneal tunnel
- Internal corneal incision.

1. *External scleral incision*

One-third to half *thickness* scleral groove is made *located* about 1.5–2 mm behind the limbus with the help of a razor blade fragment, or a 15 or 11 no. surgical knife on Bard Parker handle, or a guarded diamond knife. *Length* of incision varies from 5.5 to 7.5 mm depending upon the hardness of nucleus. *Configuration* of the incision may be straight, frown, chevron or trapezoid (Fig. 14.3).

i. *Straight incision* (Fig. 14.3A) is usually not preferred, because as shown in Fig. 14.2, when placed at 2 mm from the limbus, it goes out of the limit of astigmatic neutral funnel and produces more of astigmatism, and if placed quite posteriorly to fit in the funnel, the manoeuvring of instruments becomes difficult in the long scleral tunnel.

ii. *Frown incision,* also called as antismile incision, described by Singer is curved opposite to the limbus (Fig. 14.3B). As the ends of this incision curve away from the cornea, it gives more stable wound and produces less astigmatism. Therefore, frown incision is considered the best option for SICS.

iii. *Chevron incision,* also called as reverse V-incision (Fig. 14.3C), described by Gills, has the

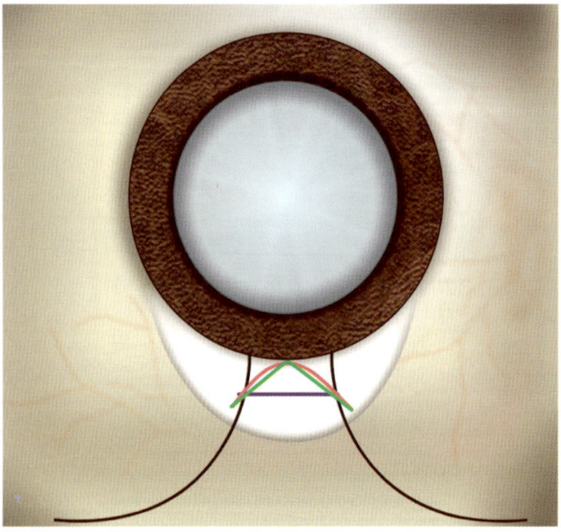

Fig. 14.2. *Koch's astigmatic neutral incisional funnel, and various configurations of the external scleral incision.*

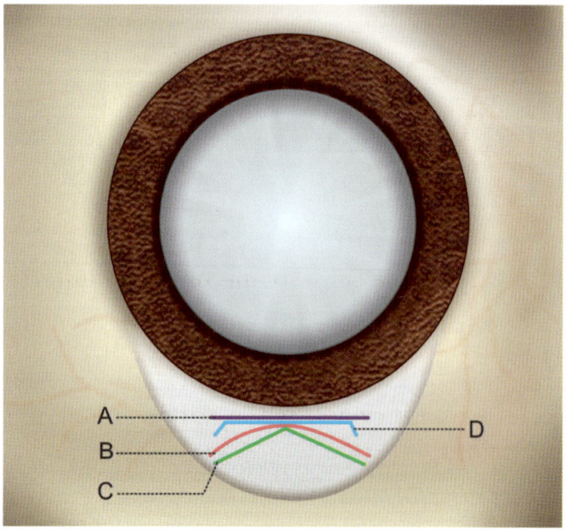

Fig. 14.3. *Types of scleral incisions: **(A)** Straight; **(B)** Frown; **(C)** Chevron (V-shaped); **(D)** Trapezoid.*

same effect on wound stability and astigmatism as frown incision.

iv. *Trapezoid incision* (Fig. 14.3D) consists of a central straight part of incision with radiating cuts at both the ends. This incision is particularly useful for a bigger nucleus.

2. *Sclerocorneal tunnel*

It is made with the help of a 2.8 mm crescent knife and should extend anteriorly 1–1.5 mm into the clear cornea (Fig. 14.4). The scleral tunnel should neither be superficial (blade of crescent knife very clearly visible through the sclera), nor deep (blade barely visible) but should be of optimum depth (blade just visible). A superficial flap is complicated by button holing and deep by premature entry into the anterior chamber. Further, the flap should be of uniform thickness, i.e. the dissection should be in the same plane. Since the cornea is more curved than the sclera, so while tunnelling near the limbus, the tip should be lifted up and heel depressed to avoid premature entry into the anterior chamber.

Scleral pockets (Fig. 14.4C) may be dissected on either side to accommodate the nucleus in cases with hard and big nucleus. Scleral pockets are like pleats of trousers and are not necessary in cases with soft nuclei. To dissect the scleral pockets, the side edge of the crescent blade is advanced laterally with a tilt confirming to the contour of corneal curvature.

3. *Internal corneal incision*

Internal corneal incision is made with the help of a sharp 2.8 or 3.2 mm angled keratome (Fig. 14.5). The heel of the keratome is raised until the blade becomes parallel to the iris plane resulting in a dimple of the corneal surface. The keratome is then advanced anteriorly in the same plane until the anterior chamber is entered and the internal wound is visualized as a straight line. During extension, care should be taken to keep it in the same plane. Any tilt or too much backward cutting may result in a smiling, frown-shaped or S-shaped incision which may not be self-sealing. Therefore, it is desirable to cut while moving forward so that the cuts in the Descemet's membrane are uniform and in one line.

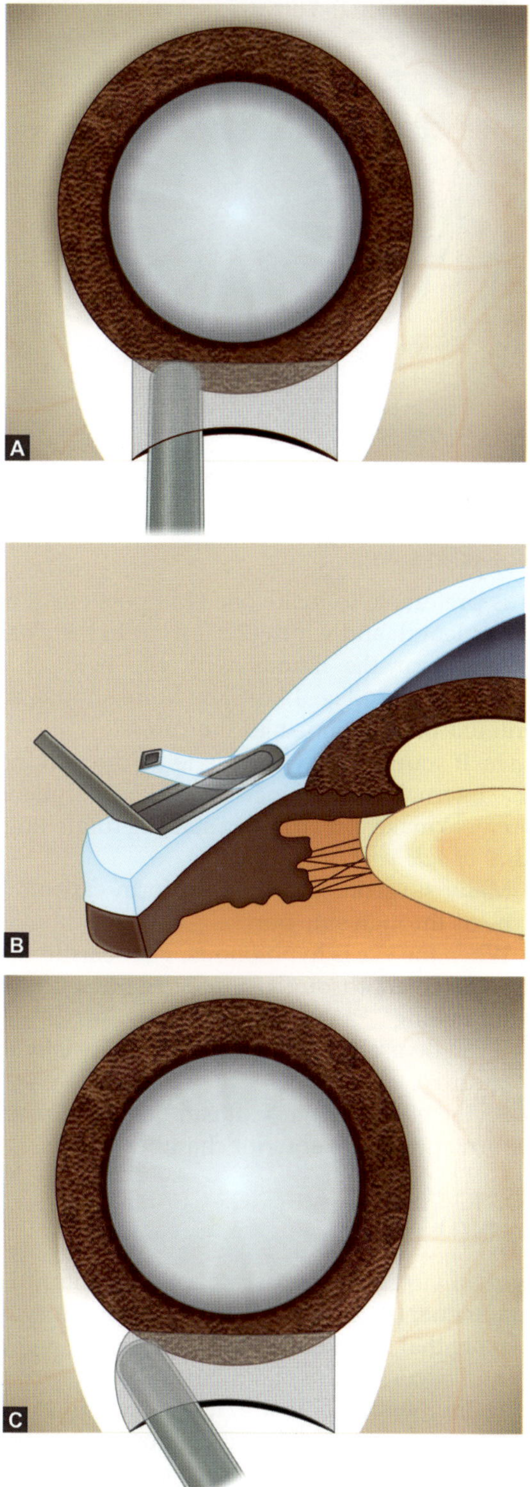

Fig. 14.4. *Sclerocorneal tunnelling with crescent knife: **(A)** Surgeon's view; **(B)** Cut section showing movement of crescent along the dome of cornea; **(C)** Dissection of the side pockets.*

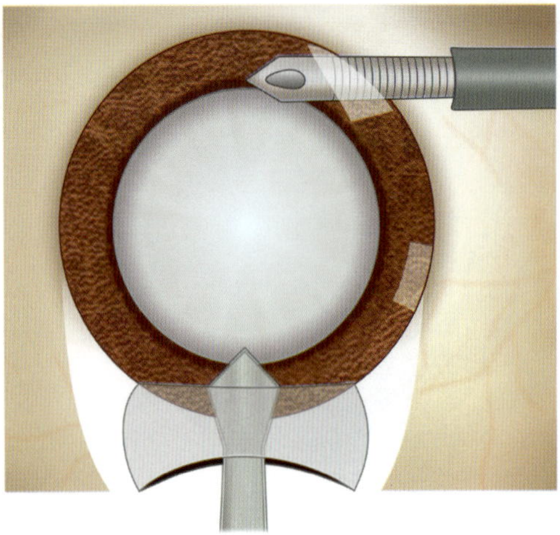

Fig. 14.5. *Making internal corneal incision with sharp pointed keratome.*

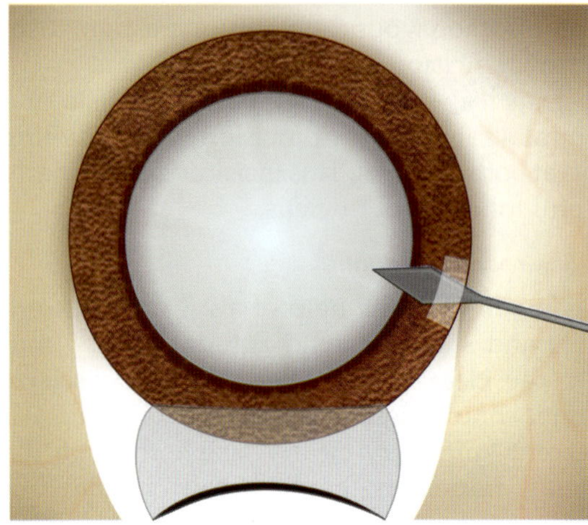

Fig. 14.6. *Side port entry.*

SIDE PORT ENTRY

It is preferable to make one side port enrty of 2 mm length and width (2 × 2 mm) in the clear cornea near the limbus with the help of a 15°MVR knife (Fig. 14.6). The knife should be entered perpendicular to the tunnel.

Note. It should always be made before making the internal corneal incision. Some surgeons prefer to make it even before starting tunnelling.

Uses of side port include:

- Many surgeons prefer to perform capsulorhexis through side port.
- When the eye is hypotonous, viscoelastic can be injected through side port for smooth tunnelling.
- It can be used for aspiration of subincisional cortex.
- At the end of surgery, it can be used for reformation of the anterior chamber.

FIXING THE ACM (ANTERIOR CHAMBER MAINTAINER)

Not all surgeons are using anterior chamber maintainer (ACM). Use of ACM is mandatory in Blumenthal technique of nucleus management. When used ACM is fixed before the internal corneal incision is made, i.e. before anterior chamber is entered from the main incision. Capsulorhexis may be performed through the side port entry before or after fixing the ACM.

For fixing ACM, a 1.5 mm long bevelled entry is made at 6 o'clock parallel to the limbus, away from the vascular arcade of cornea. The ACM is a hollow tube with a 0.9 mm outer and 0.65 mm interior diameter. It is screwed entered with bevel up and then screwed (fixed) with bevel turned downwards, i.e. facing iris. The ACM is always entered from the temporal side (Fig. 14.7). The silicone tubing of the ACM is attached to the bottle of BSS suspended at a height of 50–60 cm from the patient's eye.

ANTERIOR CAPSULOTOMY

Instrumentation

Anterior capsulotomy can be performed by using a cystitome, or capsulorhexis forceps or combination of both.

Cystitome. Prefabricated cystitomes are also available but most surgeons make it from 26 gauge needle by bending it twice. During first bend, about one-third of the needle bevel is turned out making an obtuse angle of about 110° (Fig. 14.8A). The second bend is made about 2 mm from the needle hub making an angle of about 100° (Fig. 14.8A).

Capsulorhexis forceps (Utrata's forceps). A good Utrata's forceps (Fig. 14.8B) is an essential instrument for making capsulorhexis, but McPherson's capsule may also be used.

Dyes in anterior capsulotomy

Trypan blue dye is used to stain the anterior capsule for identification especially in cases with no red reflex, i.e. mature and hypermature

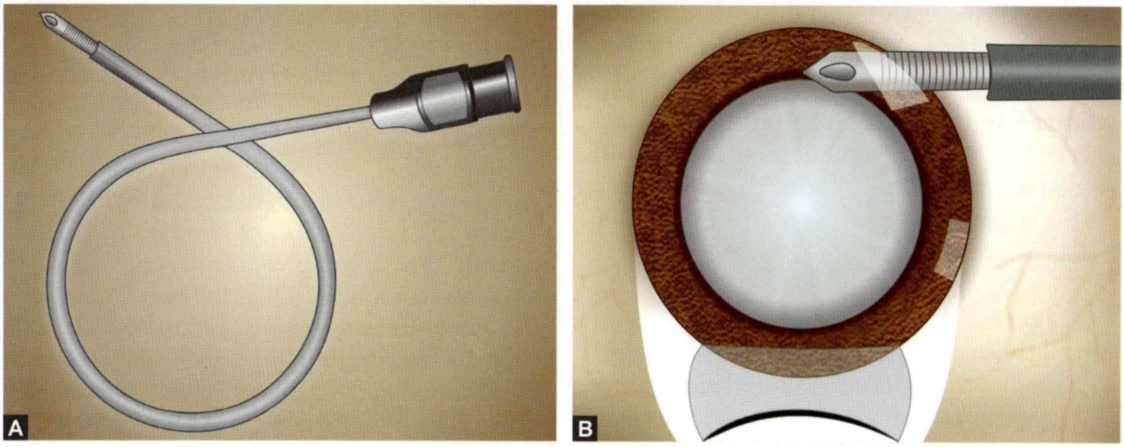

Fig. 14.7. *Anterior chamber maintainer (ACM)* ***(A)*** *as fixed from the temporal side* ***(B)****.*

cataracts. Some surgeons feel more comfortable with the use of dye even in immature cataracts with good red reflex. The use of tryphan blue dye is safe without any side effects. Indocyanine green (ICG) dye can also be used, but is comparatively expensive.

Method of use. A moderate size air bubble is placed in the anterior chamber (to prevent corneal endothelium from staining) and a small amount of dye is injected below the air-bubble using a 26 gauge cannula. Soon it is washed by injecting sufficient amount of BSS in the anterior chamber. The anterior chamber is then filled with viscoelastic substance and the air is removed completely.

Techniques of anterior capsulotomy

Though a large continuous curvilinear capsulorhexis (CCC) technique of anterior capsulotomy is preferred; but SICS can also be performed by can-opener capsulotomy, or linear capsulotomy (envelop technique).

1. *Can-opener capsulotomy*

Can-opener technique (Fig. 14.9A) of capsulotomy, though not much popular, can be used successfully in manual SICS under following situations:

- By the beginners who are yet mastering the technique of capsulorhexis.

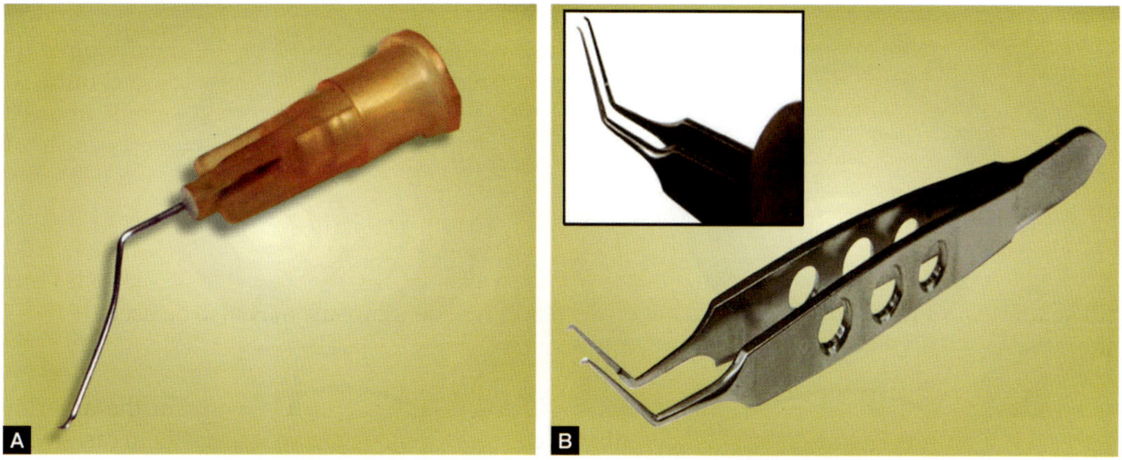

Fig. 14.8. *Instruments used for anterior capsulorhexis:* ***(A)*** *Cystitome;* ***(B)*** *Utrata's forceps.*

- When unsuccessful in completing capsulor-hexis. Conversion to a can-opener can be made at any time.
- Some surgeons prefer can-opener technique in certain difficult situations such as mature cataract, narrow pupil, calcified of fibrosed anterior capsule, and grade IV nuclear sclerosis.

Procedure. After pressurizing the anterior capsule with a viscoelastic device, a sharp 26 G bent needle is introduced in the anterior chamber and either small multiple radial cuts (as is made while opening a can) or multiple punctures (as in postage stamp) are made for 360° (restricting the size of capsulotomy to 6.5 mm and avoiding damage to the zonular attachments).

Drawbacks of this technique include:
- Inadvertent damage to the zonules
- Extension of radial tears to the posterior capsule.

2. *Linear capsulotomy (envelope technique)*

In this method (Fig. 14.9B), a straight cut is made in the upper part of anterior capsule either with a keratome or 26 G bent needle. The rest of capsulotomy is completed in the end of surgery after implantation of IOL in the bag. To complete the capsulotomy, a vertical cut is made with Vanna's scissors either on one or both the ends of the initial linear cut and the capsule is teared off with the help of capsulor-hexis forceps. This technique is popular with the surgeons managing the nucleus with fish hook technique and is useful in patients with hypermature Morgagnian cataract.

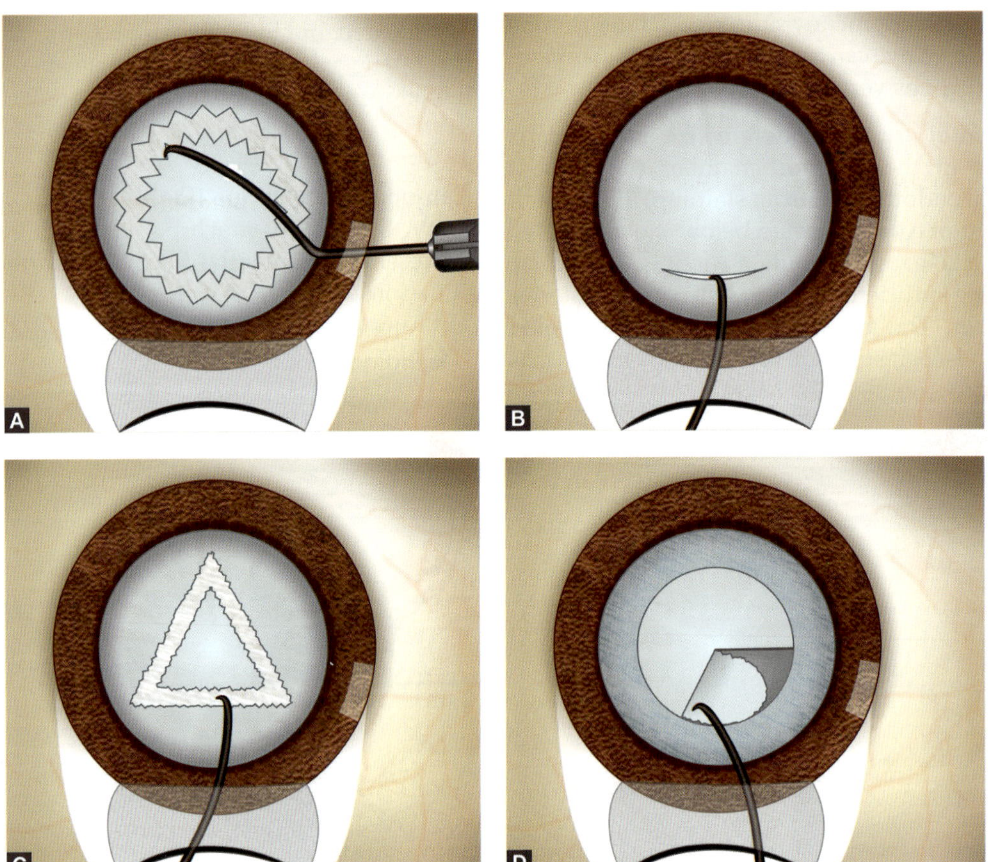

Fig. 14.9. *Techniques of anterior capsulotomy: **(A)** Can-opener capsulotomy; **(B)** Linear capsulotomy (envelop technique); **(C)** Christmas tree technique; **(D)** Continuous curvilinear capsulorhexis (CCC).*

3. Christmas tree capsulotomy

Christmas tree capsulotomy, introduced by Kelman, did not become much popular. In this technique, a triangular piece of anterior capsule (with apex towards 6 o'clock position) was removed by making zig-zag incision with the help of a 26 G bent needle (Fig. 14.9C). The main disadvantages of this technique are damage to the zonules and tendencies for radial extension.

4. Continuous curvilinear capsulorhexis

Continuous curvilinear capsulorhexis (CCC) (Fig. 14.9D), as described by Horward Gimble and Thomas Neuhann, is the ideal and most preferred technique of capsulotomy. Pre-requisites for good CCC include good akinesia, moderate preoperative hypotony, good red reflex. In this technique, a circular disc of anterior capsule about 6–6.5 mm diameter is torn out either with the help of a cystitome, Utrata's capsulorhexis forceps or both as described below.

i. Cystitome method of CCC

Pressurize the eyeball with viscoelastic till the lens-iris diaphragm moves backwards and the anterior capsule becomes flat. The CCC can be performed from the side port entry or from the main port. With side port approach, there is less manoeuvrability but chamber is better maintained as there is no leakage of viscoelastic. On the other hand, the mainport approach provides better manoeuvrability but there is more leakage of viscoelastic and there is need to reform the chamber.

After introducing the cystitome in the anterior chamber, an initial puncture is made in the centre of capsule with the tip of the bent needle and the cut is extended horizontally to the right (Fig. 14.10A). Then a flap is created by lifting the cut edge of the capsule at the level of medial two-thirds and lateral one-third of the cut. As soon as the flap is lifted, the force with the needle tip should be directed downward to make at least 1 mm curvilinear extension (Fig. 14.10B). Once a flap is created, the capsulor-

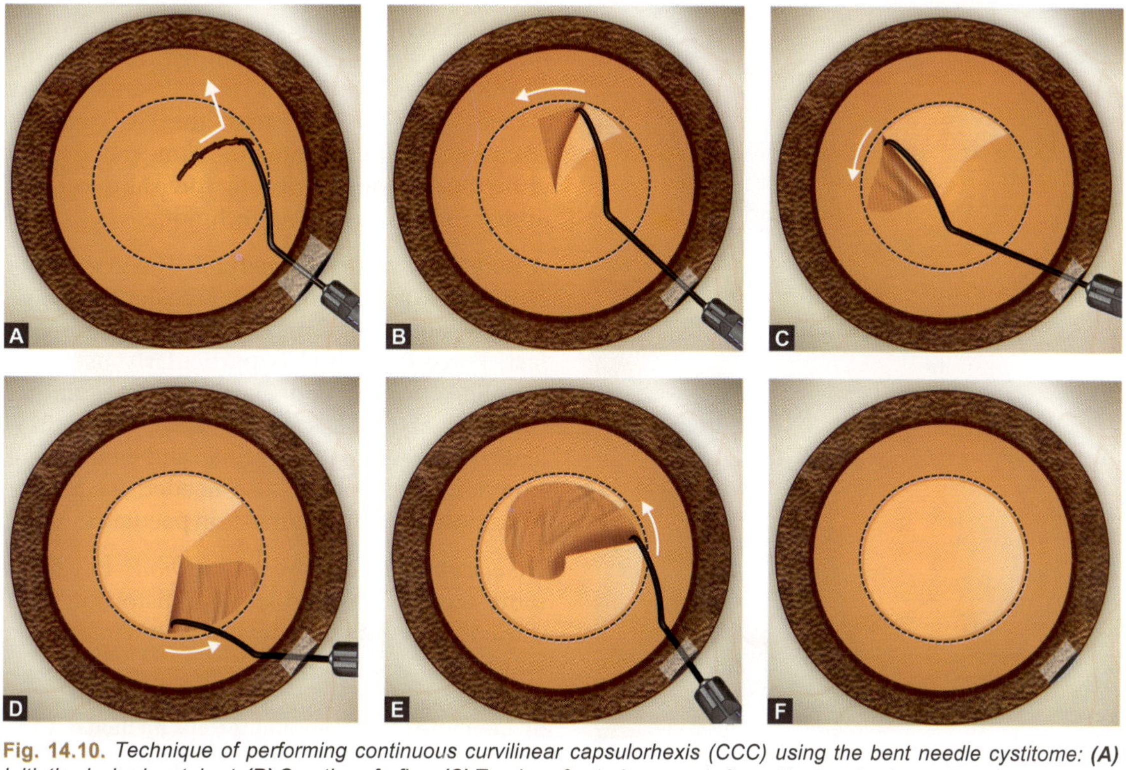

Fig. 14.10. *Technique of performing continuous curvilinear capsulorhexis (CCC) using the bent needle cystitome:* **(A)** *Initiation by horizontal cut;* **(B)** *Creation of a flap;* **(C)** *Tearing of anterior capsule flap with shearing force;* **(D to F)** *Completion of flap by slow movement with shearing force.*

hexis can be completed in two ways, i.e. either tearing the capsule with shearing force or by ripping.

Tearing with shearing force (Fig. 14.11A). The flap is folded over the intact capsule and capsulorhexis is completed by exerting gentle pushing traction with the needle tip at the junction of flat and intact capsule. Throughout the procedure, the direction of the tear should be controlled by directing the tip concentric to pupil and applying the force centripetally. In order to better control, the diameter and the regularity of the capsulorhexis, it is better to stop the manoeuvre after achieving every 2–3 clock hours of CCC; injecting viscoelastic if needed to flatten the flap and regrasping it close to the tear (Fig. 14.10). It may need over 5–10 strokes for completion of CCC.

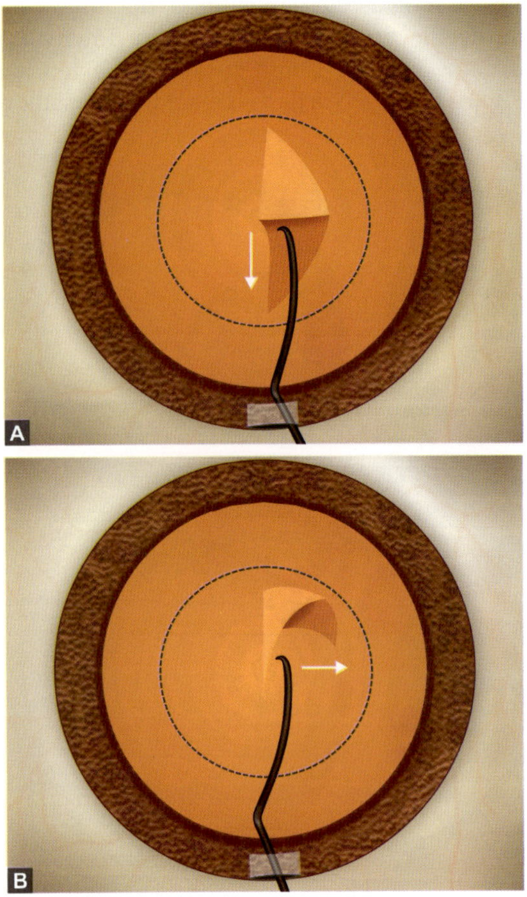

Fig. 14.11. *Techniques of tearing the capsule using:* ***(A)*** *Shearing force;* ***(B)*** *Ripping force.*

Since in the shearing technique, the vector force is in the same direction as tearing of capsule (Fig. 14.10C to E), so there is better control on the direction of the tear. Thus shearing movement is safer, but it is slow. Therefore, when the tear is close to the zonular attachments, the ripping force will redirect the tear more effectively.

Tearing with ripping force. The flap is engaged with the tip of needle close to the origin of the tear and pulling force is applied perpendicular to the direction of tear (Fig. 14.11B). The tear has to be directed through continuous pull-release-pull movements changing direction of pulling according to the direction of tear.

Since in this technique, the pulling force is applied perpendicular to the direction of tear, there are more chances of the tear going haywire and extending to the periphery towards zonular attachment and even resulting radial tears to the equator or up to the posterior capsule.

ii. Forceps method of CCC

After pressurizing the eyeball with viscoelastic, the tip of Utrata's capsulorhexis forceps is introduced in the anterior chamber and a flap is created by grasping and lifting up the capsule in the centre (Fig. 14.12).

Once the flap is created, the CCC can be completed by performing the same manoeuvre either by shearing or ripping force as described above for the cystitome technique.

Advantages of forceps method. The grip of the flap is very good and also it is easier to change the direction of the flap. Thus it is comparatively fast. Forceps method is particularly useful in fibrotic, atrophic and elastic (i.e. paediatric) capsules and soft cataract with high intra-lenticular pressure (Morgagnian and intumescent cataracts). Forceps are also needed for performing posterior capsulorhexis in paediatric cases.

Disadvantages of forceps method. It causes more wound leak and corneal distortion. It is difficult to use it with low viscosity viscoelastic substance.

iii. Combined cystitome and forceps method of CCC

In this technique, the flap is created and the initial quadrant CCC is performed with the

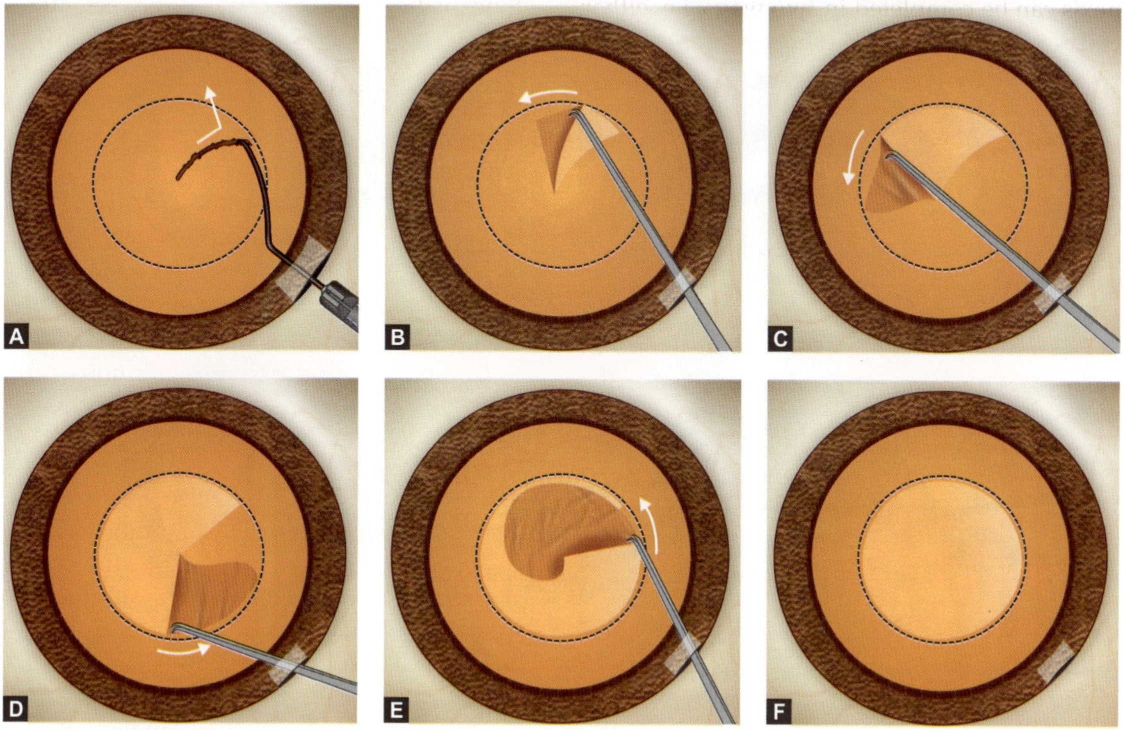

Fig. 14.12. *Technique of CCC using Utrata forceps:* ***(A)*** *Initiation with cystitome;* ***(B to F)*** *Completion of CCC by slow movement with Utrata's forceps.*

help of cystitome. The rest of CCC up to the subincisional area is then performed with the help of forceps. Again cystitome is used to complete the CCC.

HYDROPROCEDURES

The hydroprocedures include hydrodissection and hydrodelineation.

Hydrodissection

Hydroprocedures were first described by Blumenthal but the term hydrodissection was coined by *Faust*.

Definition. Hydrodissection refers to the separation of corticonuclear mass from the capsule with the help of a mechanical fluid wave. In addition, the procedure facilitates nuclear rotation and hydrates the peripheral cortex, making it easier to aspirate.

Procedure. After completion of CCC, the viscoelastic substance in the anterior chamber is replaced with BSS. This step is important to prevent posterior capsular rupture and nucleus drop occurring during hydrodissection. For the same reason, the hydrodissection should always be done from the main port rather than the side port entry.

To perform hydrodissection, the fluid is injected below the anterior capsule with a bent cannula (25–30 G) connected to a 2 cc syringe loaded with 1cc BSS. Before injecting the fluid, it must be ensured that the tip of cannula passes at least 1 mm beneath the capsular rim and the capsule is lifted (Fig. 14.13A and B). Otherwise the fluid will flow out without dissecting the cortex.

The gentle continuous injection of fluid results in a wave that passes circumferentially under the capsule, clearing it from the cortex lying over it (Fig. 14.13C and D). The fluid wave is not seen in patients with mature cataract, i.e. cases with no red reflex. When the fluid wave has passed around the posterior aspect of lens, the entire lens bulges forward because of the fluid trapped and the anterior chamber becomes shallow. After this, the procedure of further

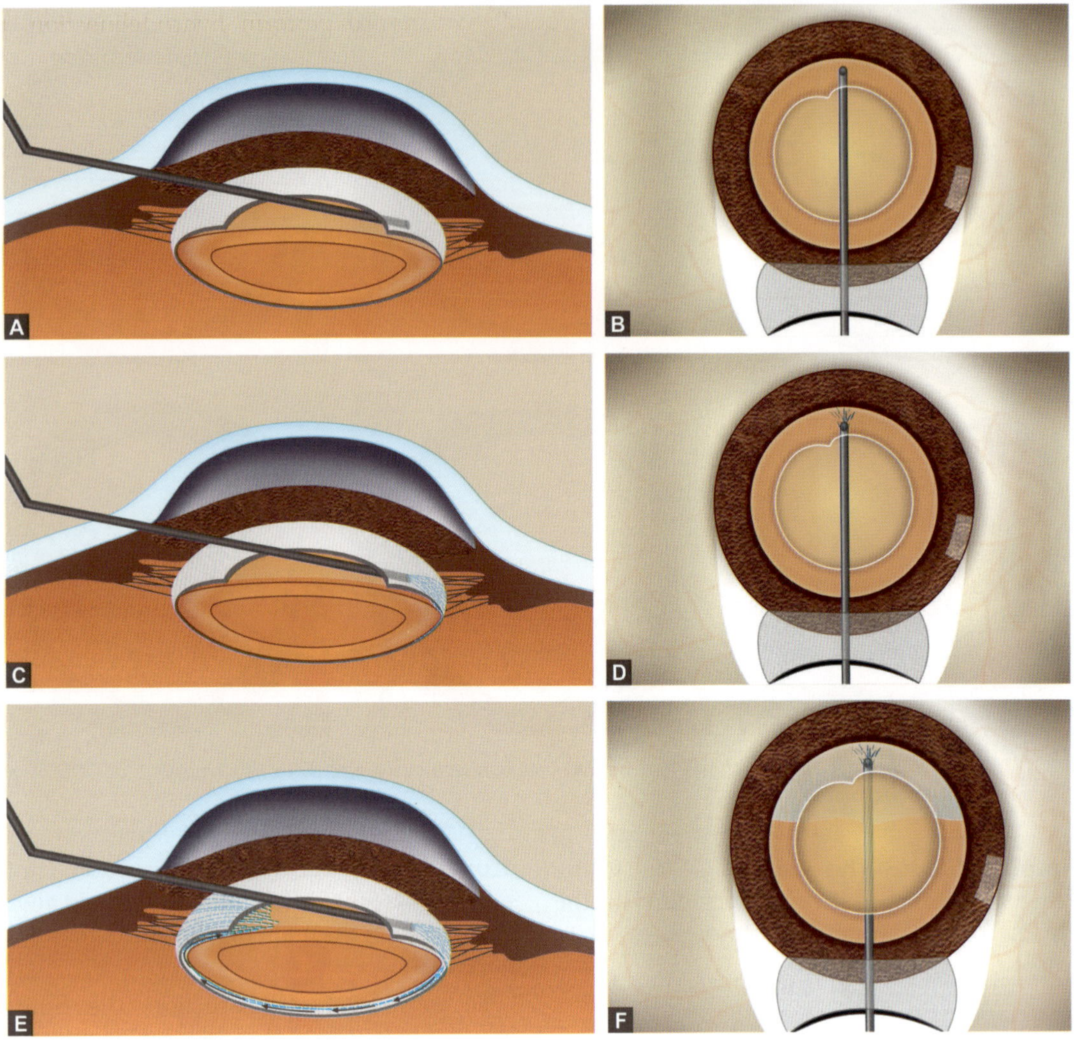

Fig. 14.13. *Hydrodissection:* ***(A and B)*** *Proper placement of tip of cannula under CCC margin by 1 to 1.5 mm;* ***(C to F)*** *Note the wave of fluid (created by gentle continuous injection) that passes circumferentially under the capsule.*

continuation of hydrodissection slightly differs for SICS and phacoemulsification as below.

For SICS, good hydrodissection should end in hydroprolapse of nucleus out of the capsular bag. So at this juncture, the nucleus should be pressed down while gently injecting the fluid with the cannula. This combination of mechanical and hydrostatic forces causes the opposite pole of the nucleus to pop out of the capsulorhexis margin. The rest of the nucleus then should be dialled out with continued mechanical rotation with cannula combined with injection of the fluid below it.

For phacoemulsification, once the lens bulges forward the fluid injection should be stopped here and the capsular bag should be decompressed by gently depressing the central portion of the lens with the side of the cannula in a way that forces the fluid to come around the lens equator from behind. Once the capsular bag is decompressed, the process of hydrodissection may be repeated in different quadrants till all the corticocapsular connection are broken and corticonuclear mass can be easily rotated by the cannula inside the bag.

Sometimes, one pole of the nucleus prolapses into the anterior chamber, it can be reposited into the bag with viscoelastic material and application of slight pressure posteriorly on the nucleus.

HYDRODELINEATION

Definition. The term hydrodelineation, coined by Anis, refers to the separation of the outer epinuclear shell or multiple shells from the central compact mass the endonucleus, by forceful injection of BSS into the substance of the nucleus.

Note. Not all surgeons perform hydrodelineation in SICS as well as phacoemulsification. When performed, the epinuclear mass separated behind from the endonucleus acts as a cushion to protect the underlying posterior capsule from the inadvertent trauma during nucleotomy. However, per se it may create difficulty in aspirating it out. In SICS, hydrodelineation is indicated only when the incision is kept 5 mm or less and nucleus is to be divided in pieces. Hydrodelineation is not effective in white or densely brunescent cataracts.

Procedure. To perform hydrodelineation, the cannula is placed on the nucleus off centre to either side and is passed in the lens substance until it meets the resistance from endonucleus. The cannula is then moved to and fro to create a tract in the nucleus. The cannula is then pulled back halfway in the track and the fluid is injected by a gentle but steady pressure. In immature cataracts, a fluid wave can be seen to separate the endonucleus from the epinucleus and produce the typical *'golden ring sign'* (Fig. 14.14). The procedure may be repeated at different depths.

NUCLEAR MANAGEMENT

Nuclear management involves two manoeuvres:

- Prolapse of the nucleus out of the capsular bag into the anterior chamber
- Delivery of the nucleus outside the eye through corneoscleral tunnel.

PROLAPSE OF THE NUCLEUS OUT OF THE CAPSULAR BAG INTO THE ANTERIOR CHAMBER

i. ***Hydroprolapsing method.*** As described above during hydrodissection, the efforts should be

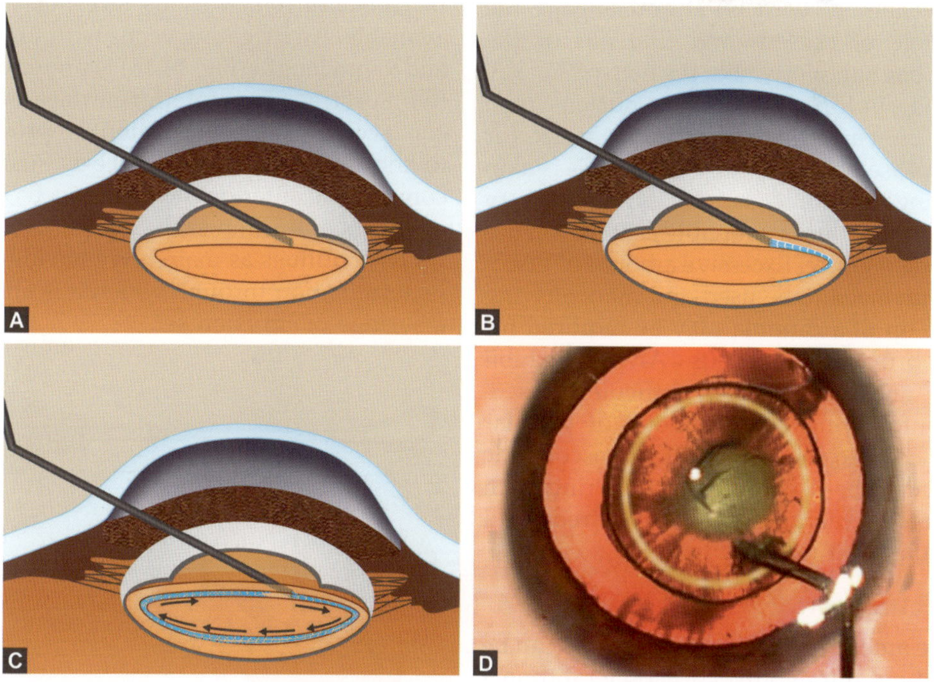

Fig. 14.14. *Hydrodelineation:* ***(A to C)*** *Separation of epinucleus from endonucleus by fluid wave, diagrammatic;* ***(D)*** *Golden ring sign of hydrodelineation seen in immature cataract.*

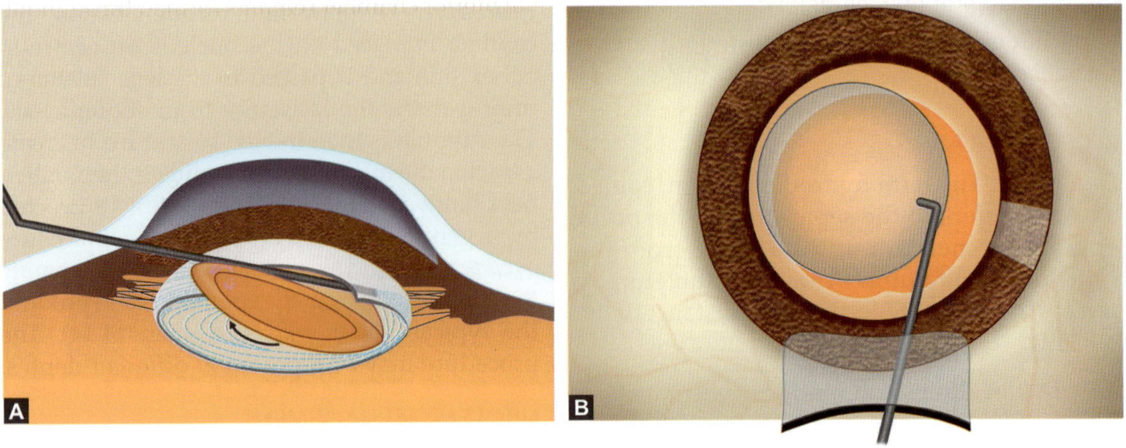

Fig. 14.15. *Prolapse of nucleus:* ***(A)*** *Hydroprolapse;* ***(B)*** *Prolapse with Sinskey's hook.*

made to prolapse the nucleus out of the bag. The good hydroprolapse occurs (Fig. 14.15A), if the fluid injection is combined with pressing downwards of the nucleus (*see* page 204).

ii. ***Nuclear prolapsing with Sinskey hook.*** This method is used when hydroprolapsing is not possible and that the size of rhexis is adequate (more than 6 mm). If rhexis is small, it is better to give relaxing incision. Then pressurize the anterior chamber with OVD and engage the upper pole of nucleus and dial out of the capsular bag superiorly with the help of Sinskey hook (Fig. 14.15B). Rest of the nucleus then should be cartwheeled out clockwise or anticlockwise with a Sinskey hook. This is akin to bringing out a tube from the tyre. Never try to prolapse the nucleus forcibly as it may cause zonular dehiscence. Excessive amount of viscoelastic may need to be used and manoeuvring with the tip of a cannula may be required for a large brunescent nucleus. Always exhibit patience and gentleness in difficult cases to avoid unforgiving complications of zonular dehiscence. Excessive amount of viscoelastic may need to be used and manoeuvring with the tip of the cannula may be required for a large brunescent nucleus.

Nucleus extraction

From the anterior chamber, the nucleus can be extracted out through the corneoscleral tunnel by any of the following methods:

- Irrigating vectis method
- Blumenthal's technique
- Phacosandwich technique
- Fish-hook technique
- Phacosection technique

1. Nucleus extraction with an irrigating vectis

This technique, first described by Steinert, is a very simple and the most commonly used one. It is time tested and gives excellent results.

Instrumentation. Various sizes of vectis are available. An irrigating vectis with 4 mm width and 9 mm length (Fig. 14.16) is preferred. It has two surfaces. The anterior surface is slightly concave and has got serrations to provide grip to the lens. Posterior surface is smooth and convex. The anterior end of the vectis has three openings of 0.3 mm each. The posterior end of vectis continues as main body having a hub at its termination through which it is attached to a syringe or infusion set.

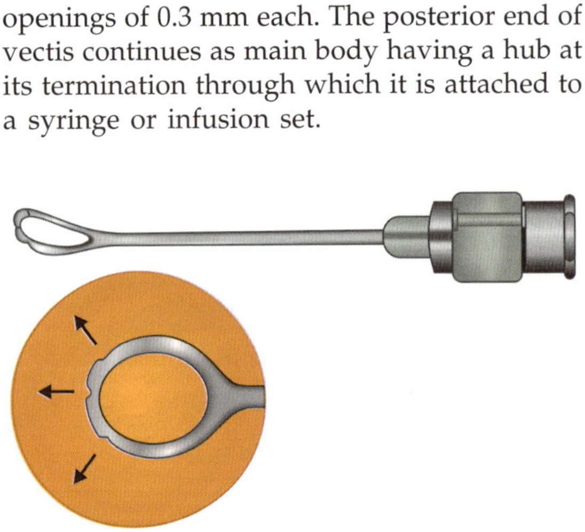

Fig. 14.16. *Irrigating vectis*

Surgical technique is as below:

- *Injection of OVD in the AC.* Once the nucleus is prolapsed in the anterior chamber, copious amounts of OVD should be injected both in front (to protect endothelium) and behind the nucleus (to push the posterior capsule and iris diaphragm posteriorly).
- *Insertion of vectis in the AC.* After holding the superior rectus bridle suture loosely in the left hand, the vectis should be gently insinuated behind the nucleus (after testing its patency outside).
- *Manoeuvre to extract nucleus.* Once the vectis is positioned propely (Fig. 14.17), the following manoeuvre should be made in synchrony. The superior rectus should be pulled tight and with the globe thus fixed, the irrigating vectis should be withdrawn slowly without irrigation till the superior of the nucleus is engaged in the tunnel. At this juncture, the fluid is injected (when using syringe) or irrigation is started and the vectis is slowly and gently withdrawn while pressing down the scleral lip. The force of irrigation should be reduced once the maximum diameter of the nucleus clears the tunnel, so as to prevent forceful extrusion of the nucleus and the consequential sudden decompression and shallowing of the anterior chamber.
- *Injection of OVD in the AC* should be made immediately after the delivery of the nucleus.

Advantages of vectis method are:

- Only single instrument is used inside the anterior chamber.
- Anterior chamber remains formed throughout the procedure.
- Delivery of the nucleus is fast and easy.
- Brunt of the nucleus is taken up by the walls of the tunnel sparing the corneal endothelium.
- Especially useful in cases with premature entry in the anterior chamber and superior zonular dehiscence.

Disadvantages of vectis method are:

- Iris trauma or iris stretching or *iridodialysis* may occur during insuniation of the vectis (at 12 o'clock) or due to entrapment of iris between vectis and the nucleus, especially at 6 o' clock position.
- *Posterior capsular rent* with vitreous loss may occur due to sharp edge of the vectis or forceful extrusion of the nucleus.
- *Corneal endothelial damage* may occur due to misjudged nuclear size, inadequate use of viscoelastic or inadvertently lifting the vectis rather than pressing the posterior lip of sclera while extracting out the nucleus.

2. Blumenthal mini-nucleus technique

Blumenthal's mini-nucleus technique is the second most popular technique after irrigating vectis method of delivering the nucleus in SICS. In this technique, the nucleus is delivered with hydropressure and so the technique is also known as *hydroexpression of nucleus.* The technique is based on the modern clinical anatomy of the lens which divides it into three parts: soft *superficial cortex* which can be aspirated easily, the intermediate *epinucleus* (semisoft

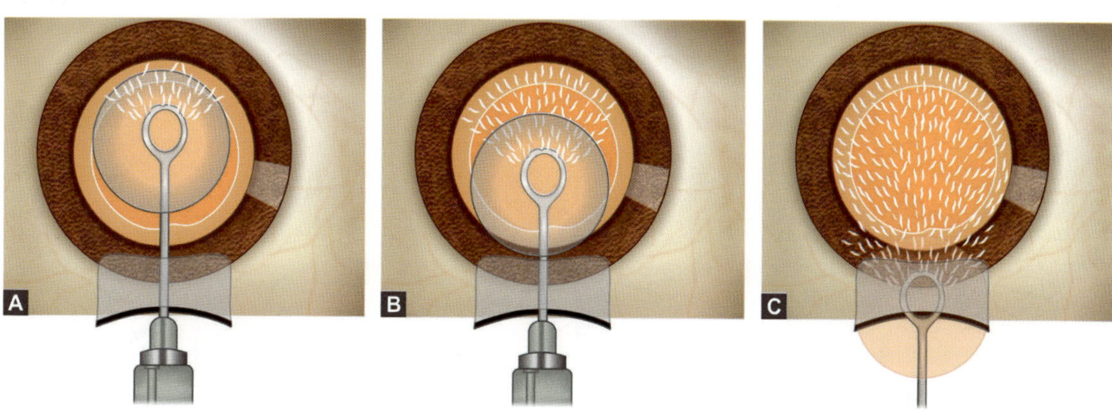

Fig. 14.17. *Steps of nucleus extraction with an irrigating vectis.*

material that can be expressed or even aspirated), and the hardcore *endonucleus* which can be expressed or fractured. In Blumenthal's technique, the endonucleus is expressed so it is also called *mini-nucleus technique*.

Surgical steps specific to this technique include:

• ***Anterior chamber maintainer (ACM) system*** is the main principle on which this technique of hydroexpression of the nucleus is based. Method of fixing ACM has been described on page 198.

• ***Manoeuvres to hydroexpress the nucleus*** are as below: After the prolapse of nucleus in the AC, a *plastic lens glide* (3–4 mm wide, 0.3 mm thick and 3 cm long) or simply an iris repositor is inserted under the nucleus at 12 o' clock position (Fig. 14.18A). Care should be taken to avoid injury to the iris and capsular bag. Once the lens glide is positioned properly; the AC maintainer flow is switched on fully with the bottle height already maintained at 50–60 cm from the table. With the flow of fluid and slight pressure applied on the lens glide with the tip of closed forceps, the nucleus is soon lodged in the tunnel (Fig. 14.18B). At this juncture, a few intermittent taps on the lens glide result in delivery of the hard core nucleus (shedding and leaving behind the epinucleus). A few more taps will allow hydroexpression of the epinucleus and most of the cortex.

• ***Assisted delivery*** may be required in some cases. When the nucleus is stuck up in the section, the BSS bottle height should be raised by 10–15 cm in order to increase the IOP which may facilitate hydroexpression. If the nucleus is still stuck up, the efforts should be made to cartwheel out the nucleus with the help of a 23 gauge needle held in left hand (Fig. 14.18C). In case the nucleus is too large to be expressed, an attempt should be made to chip the exposed part of the nucleus, making its smallest diameter small enough to allow expression. Failing this, the inner lip or even outer lip of the incision should be enlarged using the same out to in movements.

After the delivery of the nucleus, AC maintainer should be removed and the cortex aspirated by Simcoe's cannula (*see* page 214).

3. *Fish-hook technique*

Fish-hook technique, popularized by Albrecht Hennig working at Lahan Hospital, Nepal, since 2000, and is also known as 'Hennig technique or *Lahan technique*'. In this technique, capsulorhexis or envelop technique of anterior capsulotomy may be used.

Instrumentation. In this technique, the nucleus is extracted out with the help of a hook (Fig. 14.19) made from a 30 G ½" needle by bending in a hook shape near the tip (which will insert into the central nucleus) and a slight bend between the tip and plastic mount to give concavity to assure an easy insertion between the lower part of capsule and the posterior capsule.

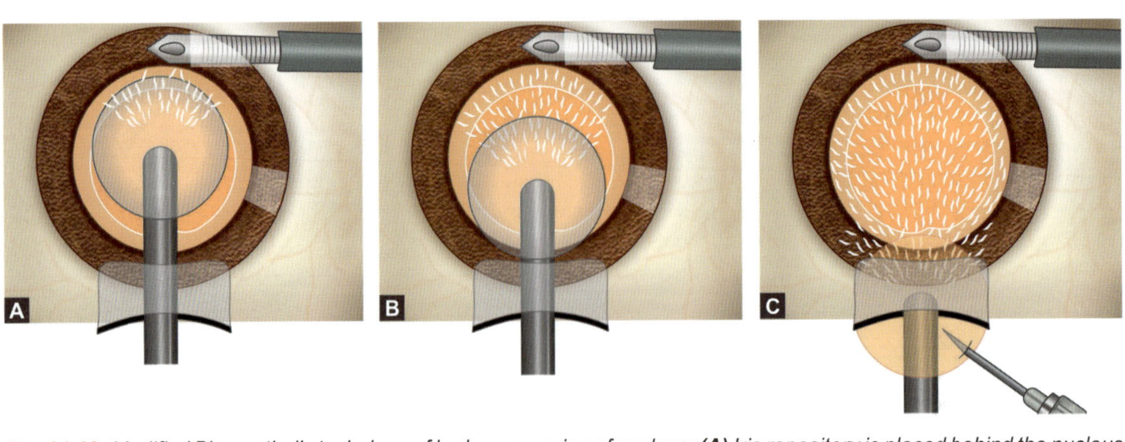

Fig. 14.18. *Modified Blumenthal's technique of hydroexpression of nucleus:* ***(A)*** *Iris repository is placed behind the nucleus and ACM is turned on;* ***(B)*** *Nucleus engaged in the tunnel;* ***(C)*** *Assisted nucleus delivery using 23 G needle.*

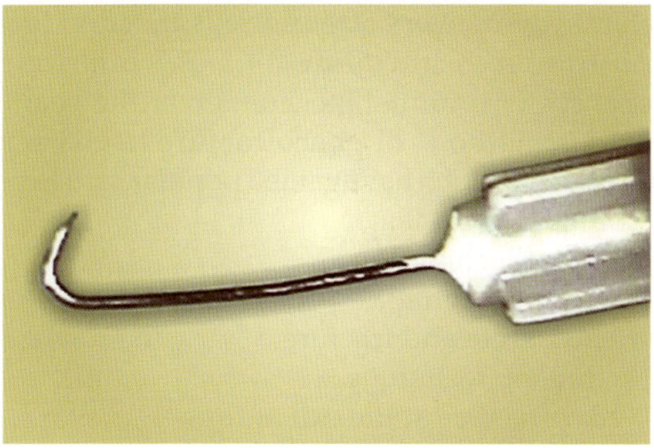

Fig. 14.19. *Fish-hook made from 30 G $^1/_2$" needle.*

Technique of nucleus hook extraction. In this technique, there is need to prolapse the superior pole of the nucleus in the anterior chamber.

- After injecting the OVD between nucleus and posterior capsule and into the anterior chamber, the 'needle hook' is inserted between the nucleus and the posterior capsule with the sharp needle tip pointing to the right (Fig. 14.20A).
- Then the hook is turned and slightly pulled back, so that the needle tip is engaged into the central lower portion of the nucleus (Fig. 14.20B).
- Once the nucleus is hooked, it is pulled out of the capsular bag and through the tunnel with slight pressure by the fish-hook on the posterior lip of the tunnel (Fig. 14.20C).
- Thus, the nucleus is delivered without performing extensive manoeuvres in the anterior chamber.

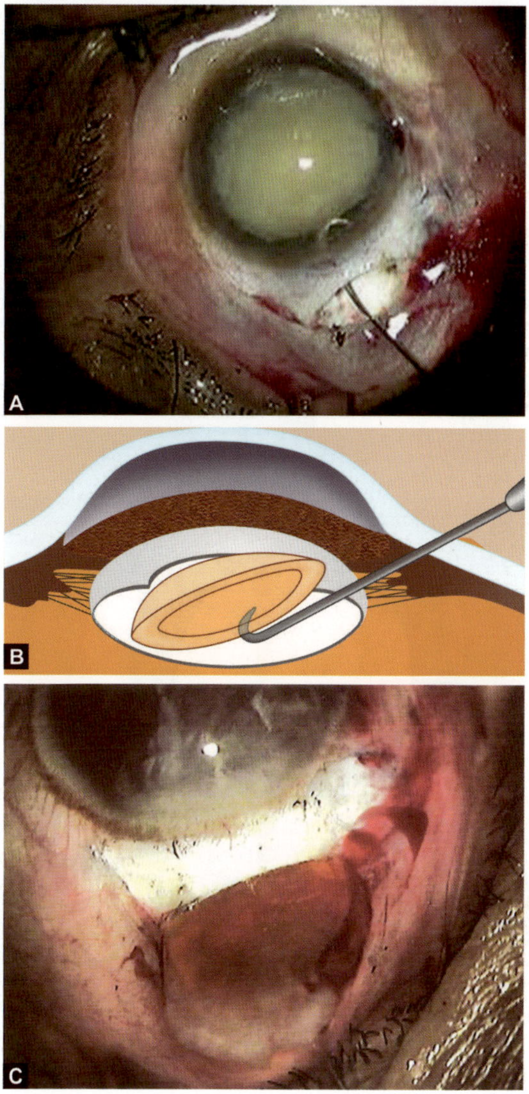

Fig. 14.20. *Fish-hook technique of nucleus extraction:* ***(A)*** *Insertion of fish hook;* ***(B)*** *Hook tip engaged into central lower portion of the nucleus;* ***(C)*** *Extraction of the nucleus.*

4. *Phacosandwich technique*

Introduced initially by Luther L. Fry in 1985, the phacosandwich technique has been greatly modified by many workers.

Surgical technique. After prolapsing the nucleus in the AC, copious amount of OVD is injected both in front and behind the nucleus to create sufficient space. The irrigating vectis 4 × 9 mm is introduced underneath the nucleus and is held in the left hand. Then a Sinskey hook is carefully placed on top of the nucleus with the help of right hand, sandwiching it in between the vectis and Sinskey hook (Fig. 14.21A). The sandwiched nucleus is then extracted out using both hands (Fig. 14.21B). During the manoeuvre, the assistant is asked to pull the superior rectus bridle suture to facilitate the delivery of the nucleus. Alternatively, instead of the Sinskey hook, the cannula of viscoelastic syringe may be used as second instrument. In this technique, viscoelastic is also injected while extracting out the nucleus.

5. *Phacosection/phacofracture techniques*

Phacosection, also known as phacofracture technique, first introduced by Peter Kansas,

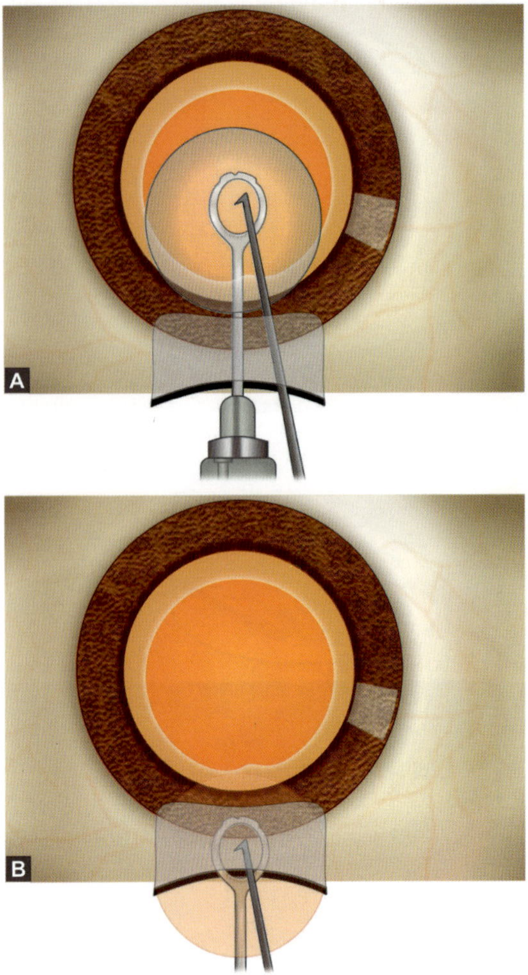

Fig. 14.21. *Phacosandwich technique of nucleus extraction.*

refers to the delivery of the nucleus after dividing it into pieces, through a 4.5–5.5 mm long corneoscleral tunnel incision. Over the years, various methods of phacofracture have been introduced which have gained popularity. These techniques include:

- Bisector technique
- Trisector technique
- Phacosalute and fracture
- Wire loop technique
- Phacofracture at the exit of tunnel
- Phacofragmentation by slider pincer technique
- Quarter's extraction technique
- Chop-section technique
- Prechop manual phacofragmentation

i. ***Bisector technique.*** After injecting the visco-elastic material in front and behind the nucleus, a solid vectis (Kansas vectis or cutting board) 3 × 9 mm in size is introduced below the nucleus. The nucleotome is positioned on the anterior surface of nucleus and the two instruments are manoeuvred towards each other and the nucleus is divided into two halves.

In an alternative technique, irrigating vectis replaces the solid vectis and Sinskey hook replaces the nucleotome (Fig. 14.22A and B). Each half is then removed with the help of Kansas fragment forceps or by phacosandwich technique (Fig. 14.22C and D).

ii. ***Trisector technique.*** In this technique, the nucleus is divided into three pieces using a solid vectis and a trisector (Fig. 14.23) by a similar manoeuvre as described above in bisector technique.

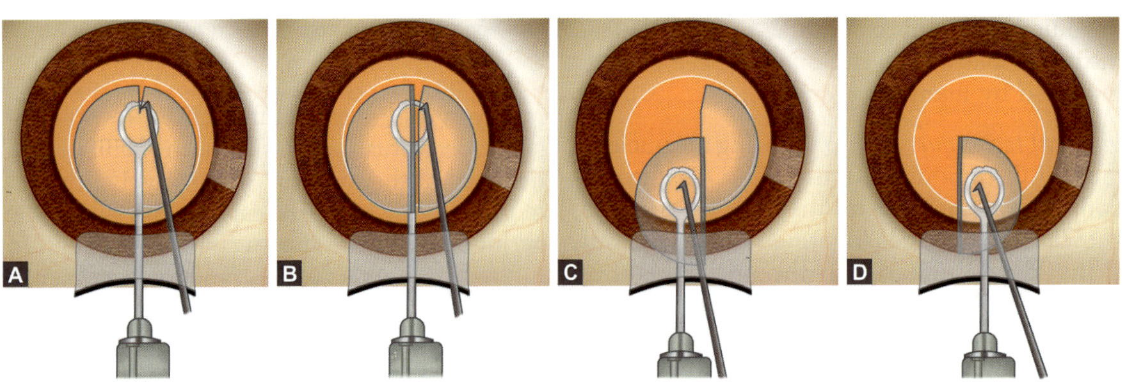

Fig. 14.22. *Phacofracture with microvectis and Sinskey's hook* ***(A and B)*** *and removal of each half of the nucleus by phacosandwich technique* ***(C and D)****.*

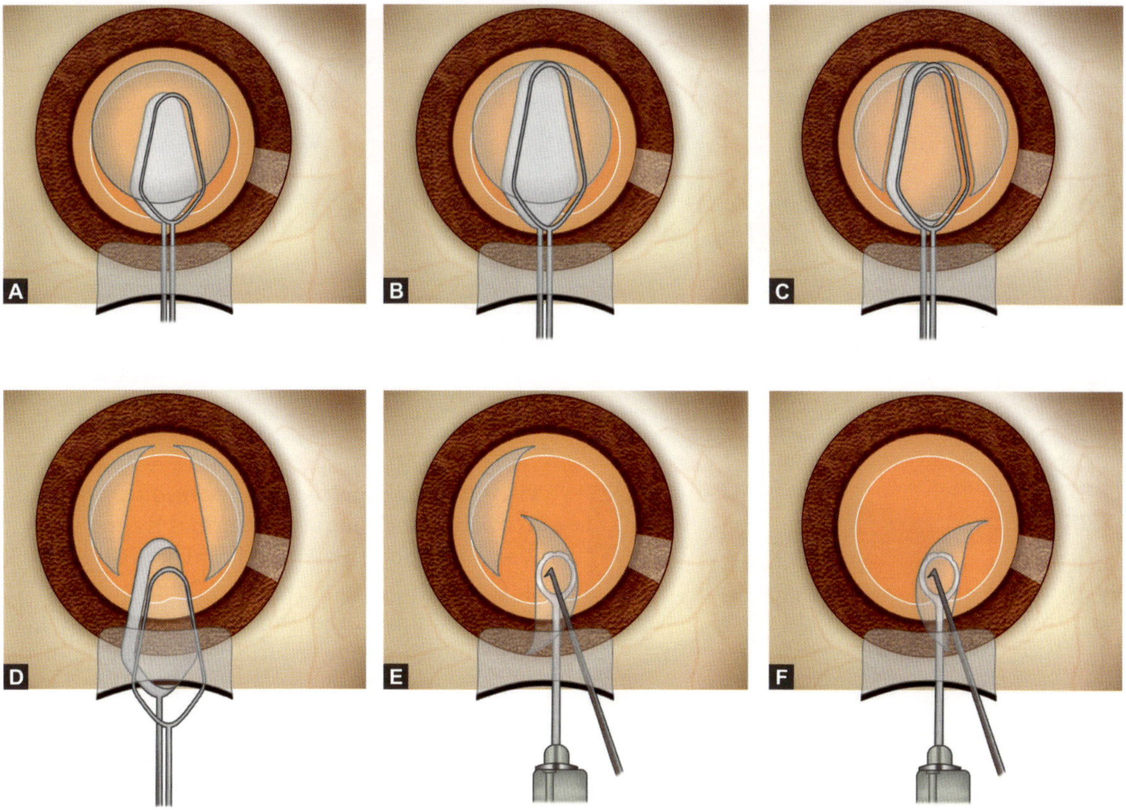

Fig. 14.23. *Phacofracture with a trisector: **(A)** Placement of trisector around the nucleus; **(B and C)** Fracture of nucleus into three parts; **(D to F)** Removal of three parts of nucleus one by one by phacosandwich technique.*

iii. ***Phacosalute and fracture.*** In this technique, the nucleus is prolapsed out of the bag at either 3 or 9 o'clock position and is then aligned vertically in the 6–12 o'clock meridian. The part of the nucleus lies in the bag and part of it in the anterior chamber. The superior half of the nucleus is then amputated and pinched off using a capsule forceps (Fig. 14.24) and is then expressed out using irrigating wire vectis. Main disadvantage of this technique is high risk of damage to corneal endothelium. So this technique is not popular at all.

iv. ***Phacofracture with a wire loop.*** This technique introduced by Gerald Keener, has not gained popularity. In this technique, nucleus is cheese wired into two halves with the help of a nuclear snare similar to tonsilar snare (Fig. 14.25).

v. ***Phacofracture at the exit of tunnel.*** In this technique, a small portion of the nucleus exiting out of the tunnel is fractured when it is being delivered with irrigating vectis. The process is repeated many a times till the remaining nucleus can be delivered out of the tunnel (Fig. 14.26).

vi. ***Phacofragmentation by slider pincer technique.*** In this technique, introduced by Dr. Keiki Mehta from India, the nucleus is divided into fragments using the slider pincer instrument (Fig. 14.27A). After the nucleus is prolapsed in the anterior chamber, the slider-pincer instrument is introduced into the anterior chamber in its closed form, and is then gradually opened up to encompass the width of the nucleus. Once it is properly positioned the jaws are closed which automatically sections the nucleus into two parts (Fig. 14.27B). In hard nucleus, more than two pieces can be made. Each piece of the nucleus is then removed using specially designed forceps.

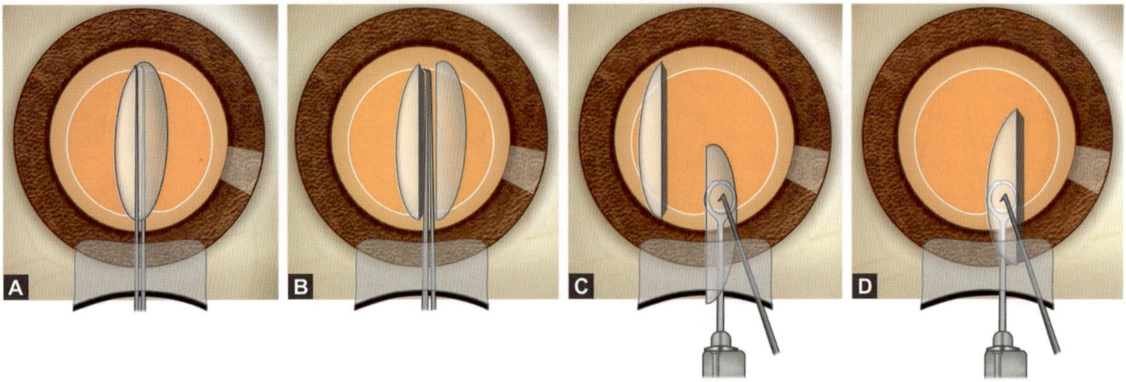

Fig. 14.24. *Phacosalute and fracture: **(A)** Vertical placement of nucleus; **(B)** Vertical fracture of nucleus into two parts; **(C and D)** Removal of each half of the nucleus.*

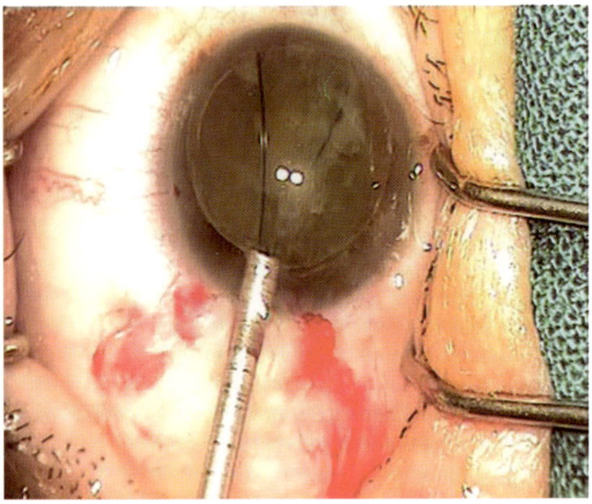

Fig. 14.25. *Phacofracture with a wire loop.*

vii. *Quarter's extraction technique.* Quarter's extraction technique for manual fragmentation was introduced by Akura J et al. in the year 2000 (J. Cataract Refract Surgery, 200;26:1281–7). In this technique, after prolapsing the nucleus in the anterior chamber, the front quarter of the nucleus is cut using nucleus puncher (Fig. 14.28A and B). The remaining three quarters of nucleus is extracted via the 4.5–5 mm wound using Akura's irrigating claw vectis (Fig. 14.28C) while rotating the nucleus along its radius in the wound (Fig. 14.28D).

viii. *Chop-section technique.* Chop-section technique of manual phaco fragmentation was

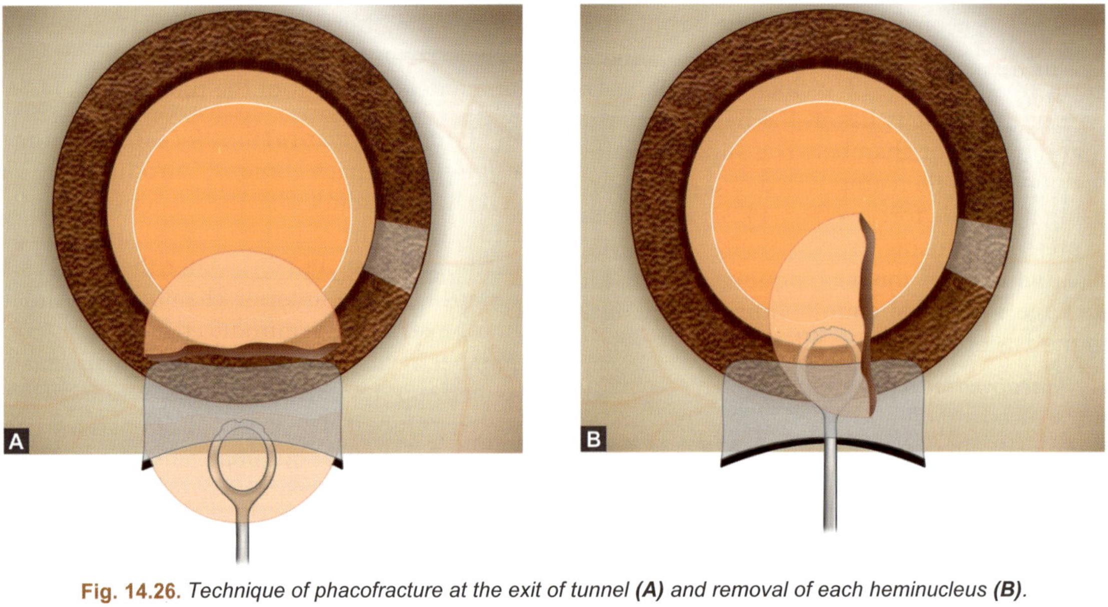

Fig. 14.26. *Technique of phacofracture at the exit of tunnel **(A)** and removal of each heminucleus **(B)**.*

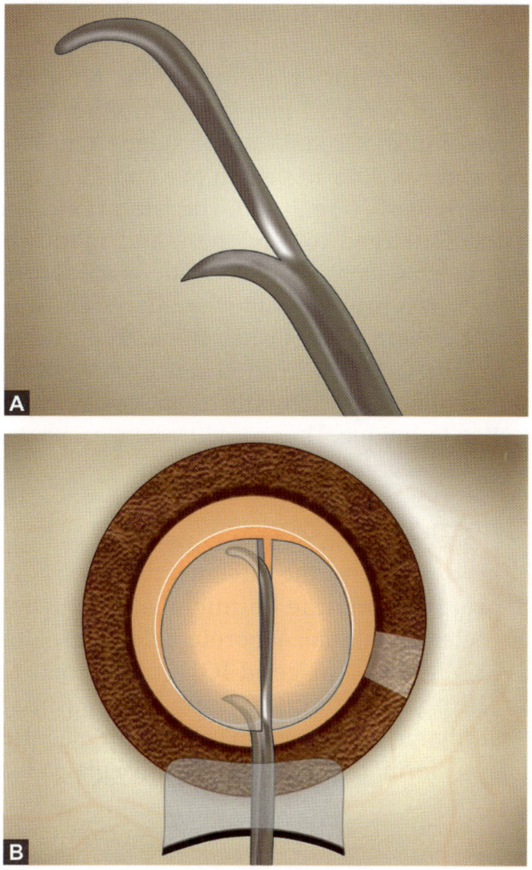

Fig. 14.27. *The slider pincer instrument* ***(A)*** *and technique of phacofragmentation* ***(B)****.*

introduced by Jorge Alvarez Marin et al in 1996. In this technique, the nucleus is divided into two (chop-bisection), or three (chop-trisection) or more fragments (chop-multi-section) depending on the hardness of nucleus, simply with the help of a spatula (Barraquer vitreous spatula) and a chopper (e.g. Nagahara chopper).

Surgical technique. After the nucleus is prolapsed into the anterior chamber, the copious viscoelastic material is put in front and posterior to the nucleus. Then, the spatula is introduced below and a chopper in front of the nucleus (Fig. 14.29). The nucleus is bisected or trisected or multisected with a cutting manoeuvre by the chopper from 6 to 12 o'clock position, and a counterpressure created by the spatula. The nuclear pieces depending upon the hardness

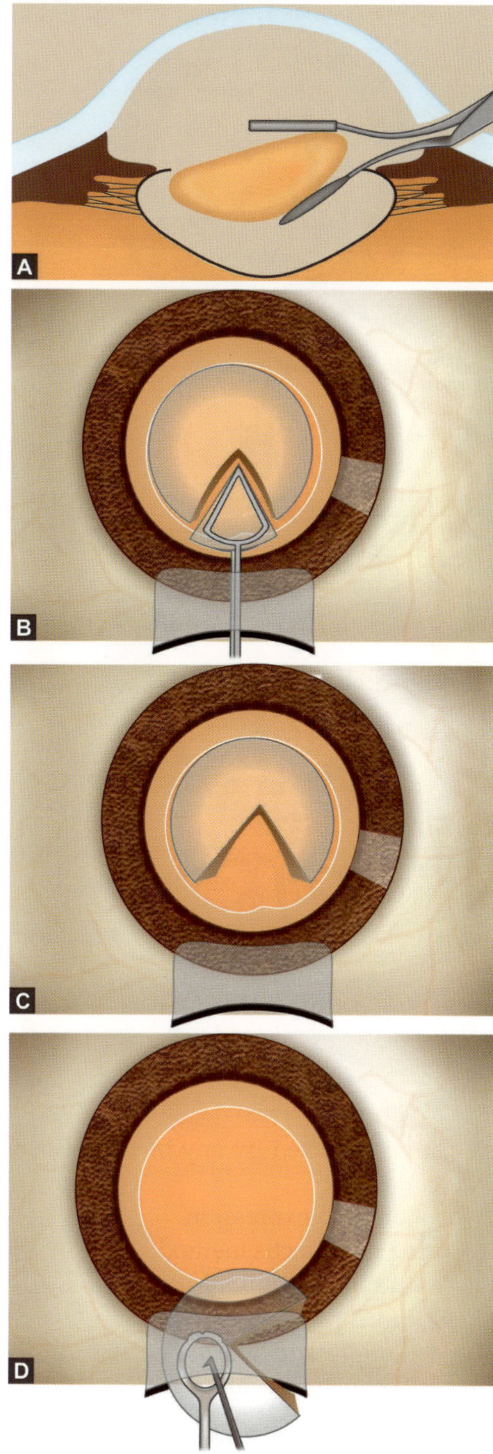

Fig. 14.28. *The quarter extraction technique:* ***(A to C)*** *The front quarter of the nucleus is cut using nucleus puncher;* ***(D)*** *The remaining three quarters of nucleus is extracted using Akura's irrigating claw vectis.*

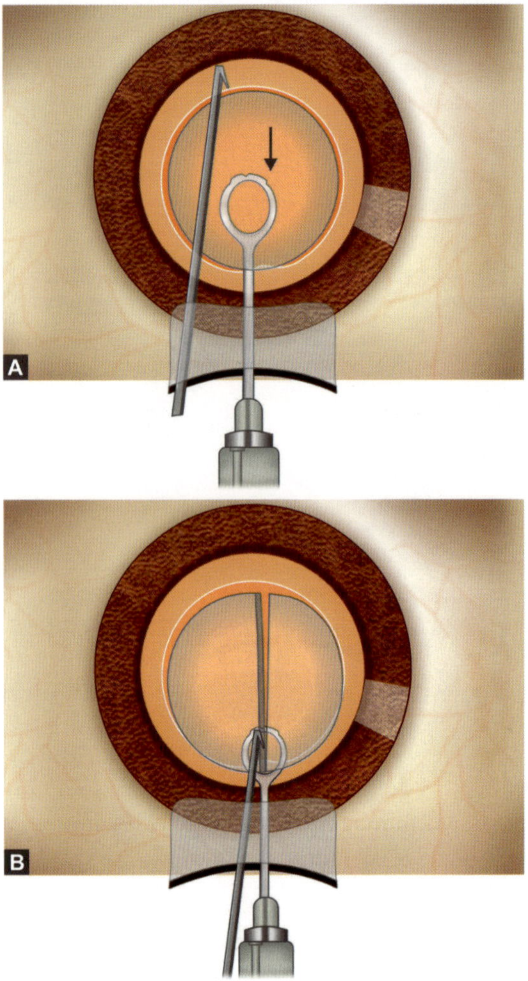

Fig. 14.29. *Chop-section technique: **(A and B)** Note chopper sliding direction and angulation between the chopper and the spatula.*

then can be extracted by any of the following methods:

- Hydro- or visco-expression
- Irrigating mini-vectis method
- Phacosandwich technique
- Nuclear forceps
- Using chopper and spatula by the so-called Chinese chopstick technique.

ix. ***Prechop manual phacofragmentation.*** Prechop manual phacofragmentation technique was described by Wiriyaluppa and Kongsap (Ocular Surgery News Internated, 2003:21(20):48–49). In this technique, after hydrodissection and hydro-delineation, the nucleus is divided into two fragments in the bag using prechopper forceps introduced through the temporal cataract incision 3.2 mm in size and a nuclear chopper introduced through a sideport incision mode at 5 o'clock in the left eye and 11 o'clock in the right eye (Fig. 14.30). The cataract incision is then enlarged to 5–5.5 mm, and filling the anterior chamber with viscoelastic, one fragment of nucleus is prolapsed into the anterior chamber with the help of a Sinskey hook. The nuclear fragment is then extracted out by any of the above methods mentioned above in chop-section technique. The procedure is then repeated with the second nuclear fragment.

ASPIRATION OF CORTEX

After delivery of the nucleus, the remaining debris may include epinucleus, cortex and viscoelastic material. A thorough clean-up of this debris is must for good IOL centration and avoiding the complications such as post-operative iritis, cystoid macular oedema, after cataract formation and postoperative glaucoma.

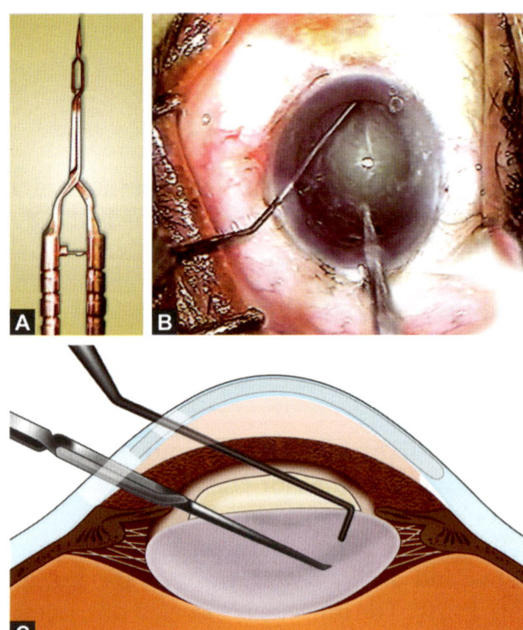

Fig. 14.30. *Prechopper technique of phacofracture: **(A)** Prechopper; **(B and C)** Manual phacofragmentation using a prechopper forceps and nucleus chopper.*

Prerequisites for good cortical clean up

Prerequisites for good cortical clean up include:
Capsulorhexis, instead of can opener capsulotomy.
Hydrodissection, performed gently and thoroughly.
Simcoe cannula should be of good quality.
Golden rules to be followed while aspirating, the cortex are:

- Never to aspirate blindly
- To discourage aspiration at the periphery
- To keep balance between aspiration and irrigation to avoid collapsing of anterior chamber
- To keep an eagles eye watch on accidental engagement of posterior capsule (seen as the radiating folds of the capsule or the so-called spider formation).

*Learning to tackle the special situations,*which include:

- Tackling intact epinucleus
- Managing 12 o'clock cortex
- Cortex aspiration in small pupil
- Managing cortex in the event of posterior capsule rupture.

Cortical aspiration in the presence of AC maintainer (Blumenthal technique)

In the presence of AC maintainer, the cortical debris and the epinucleus can be easily expressed out by the increased pressure from the fluid coming through the AC maintainer, by simply pressing the posterior scleral lip. The intact epinucleus, left in the bag need to be manipulated as described below.

Management of intact epinucleus in the bag can be done by following methods:

- *Flipping technique.* By insinuating the cannula under the anterior capsular rim, the epinucleus can be lifted into the anterior chamber.
- *Viscodissection technique.* Viscoelastic material is injected under the capsular rim, between the capsule and cortex and lifted out of the bag into the anterior chamber (Fig. 14.31) and extracted through the tunnel thereafter. The remaining cortex can be aspirated with the help of Simcoe's cannula.

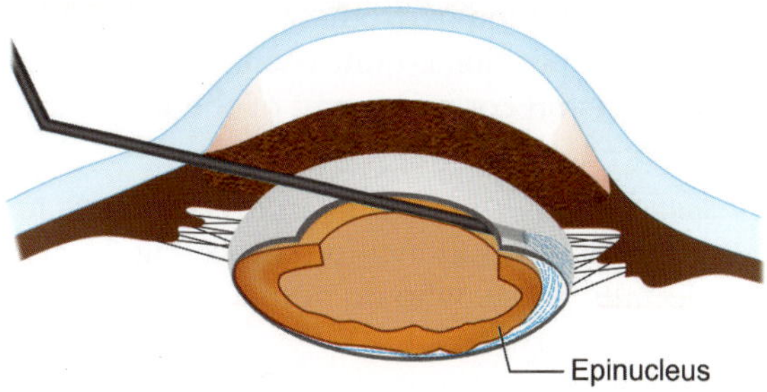

Fig. 14.31. *Technique of lifting epinucleus out of the bag by injecting BSS or viscoelastic material below the anterior capsular rim.*

Cortical aspiration in the absence of AC maintainer

When AC maintainer is not used, i.e. in the techniques other than Blumenthal, the remaining epinucleus and cortex is removed by Simcoe's cannula, which is attached to the BSS bottle. To begin with, cannula is opened with full flow and taken to 6 o'clock position and with slight depression of posterior wall of tunnel. Alternatively, the epinucleus can be extracted with the help of irrigating vectis. The intact epinucleus in the bag is managed into the anterior chamber as described above in the Blumenthal technique. Along with epinucleus, part of cortex is also extracted out. The remaining cortex can be aspirated out with the help of Simcoe's cannula. While performing irrigation–aspiration, the tip of cannula should be placed close to the rhexis margin, cortex should be engaged and dragged to the centre from the periphery and then aspirated. At times, in immature cataract, a thin transparent sheet of cortex may remain adherent to the capsule, especially when hydrodissection is not proper. The edge of such a sheet can be lifted by a gentle stroke with a capsule polisher, iris repositor, or even the tip of Simcoe cannula; and then aspirated out.

Management of 12 o'clock cortex

The aspiration of 12 o'clock cortex with Simcoe cannula is difficult through the main incision because of restricted approachability caused by:

- Long sclerocorneal tunnel
- Capsulorhexis.

Technique. A good hydrodissection performed at 12 o' clock position is quite useful in managing the subincision cortex by any of the following methods:

- *J-shaped cannula* is used by many surgeons to aspirate out the sub-incision cortex (Fig. 14.32), especially those, who do not want to make a sideport entry.
- *Side-port entry* made between 9 and 10 o'clock position is quite useful in aspirating the sub-incisional cortex. It is the technique of choice using Simcoe's cannula (Fig. 14.33).

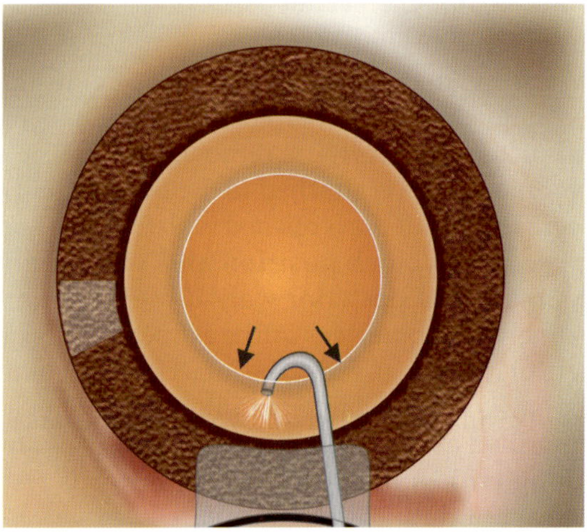

Fig. 14.32. *Aspiration of the sub-incisional cortex using J-shaped cannula.*

- *Bimanual irrigation and aspiration* through two side-port entries made at 10 and 2 o'clock positions, is also a good technique (Fig. 14.34).
- *Displacing the cortex* by dialling the IOL in the bag is also used by some surgeons. Many a times, it may not be possible to dislodge the cortex completely by this method.

Cortex aspiration in small pupil

Cortex aspiration in small pupil needs patience and gentleness. It can be accomplished by any of the following techniques:

- Aspiration through side-port entry
- Bimanual irrigation–aspiration.

Managing cortex in the event of posterior capsular rupture

Once the posterior capsular rupture occurs, immediately stop the irrigation to prevent hydration of the vitreous, and managed as below:

- *Dry aspiration.* When posterior capsular rupture is not associated with vitreous disturbance, it should be sealed by injecting visco-cohesive OVD and the remaining cortex should be removed by gentle dry aspiration, i.e. either without or with minimal irrigation. The peeling of the cortex should be done from the equator towards the rent.
- *Anterior vitrectomy,* preferably by bimanual technique (i.e. introducing irrigation through one port and aspiration and vitrectomy

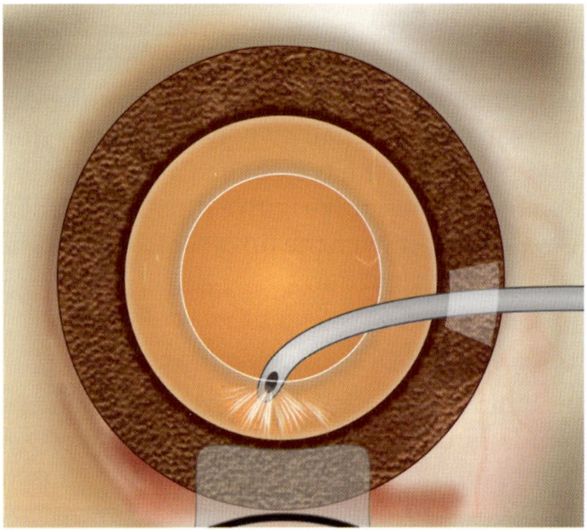

Fig. 14.33. *Aspiration of the sub-incisional cortex through a side-port incision.*

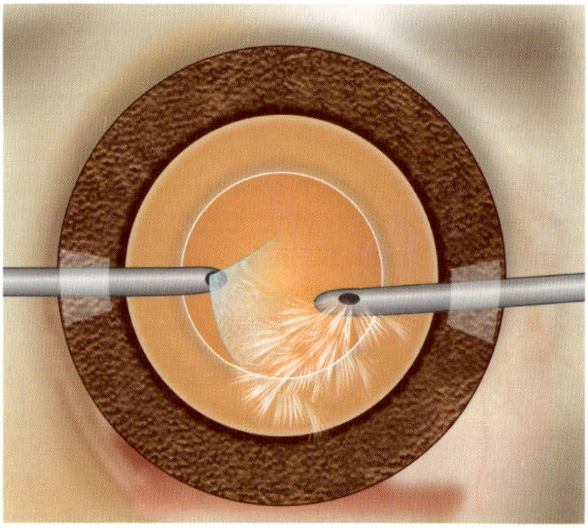

Fig. 14.34. *Technique of bimanual aspiration of the cortex.*

through the other) should be done, if posterior capsular tear is associated with vitreous disturbance. Immediately after capsular rupture, the tamponade with air or healon should be done. Efforts should be made to conserve as much capsule as possible. The residual cortex should be aspirated with minimal irrigation.

IOL IMPLANTATION

Choice of IOL

Mainly choice of IOL depends upon the incision size:

- *PMMA IOL with 6 mm optic size* is choosen mostly, since the incision size is between 6 and 7 mm.
- *Phacoprofile PMMA IOL*with 5 or 5.25 mm optic size is used when incision size can be reduced to 5.5 mm in soft cataracts or when using phacofracture techniques of nucleus extrction.
- *Foldable IOL* is used where incision is less than 5 mm (in phacofragmentation technique). Some surgeons routinely use square edge foldable IOLs in all cases of SICS, irrespective of incision size, because of the advantages of such IOLs such as decreased incidence of posterior capsular opacification.

Techniques of implanting rigid PMMA IOL

After thorough cortical clean up, the capsular bag is inflated and anterior chamber is filled with viscoelastic material. The PMMA IOL can be implanted in the bag by any of the following two techniques:

i. ***Dialling technique.*** The PCIOL is grasped by the optic with the help of an IOL holding forceps or McPherson's forceps and the inferior haptic and optic of IOL is gently inserted within the capsular bag behind the iris at 6 o'clock position (Fig. 14.35A). Then a hole or optic-haptic junction is engaged by a Sinskey or Lester hook, the IOL is pushed inferiorly and posteriorly and is dialled clockwise till the superior haptic completely goes into the bag (Fig. 14.35B and C). The IOL is then positioned horizontally.

ii. ***Flexing or looping technique.*** In this technique, after inserting the inferior haptic in the bag at 6 o'clock position, the tip of superior haptic is grasped with the McPherson's forceps and is flexed or looped until its highest convexity comes underneath the upper capsular margin. The superior haptic is then released slowly to slide it into the upper part of the capsular bag behind the iris (Fig. 14.36A). The IOL is then dialled into the horizontal position (Fig. 14.36B).

Ciliary sulcus fixation of IOL

Ciliary sulcus fixation of IOL may have to be done when it is not possible to fix the IOL in the capsular bag under following circumstances:

- Big tear in the posterior capsule with intact anterior capsulorhexis.
- When anterior capsular flaps left are very small.
- After can-opener capsulotomy with small flaps.
- Secondary IOL implantation with obliterated capsular fornices.

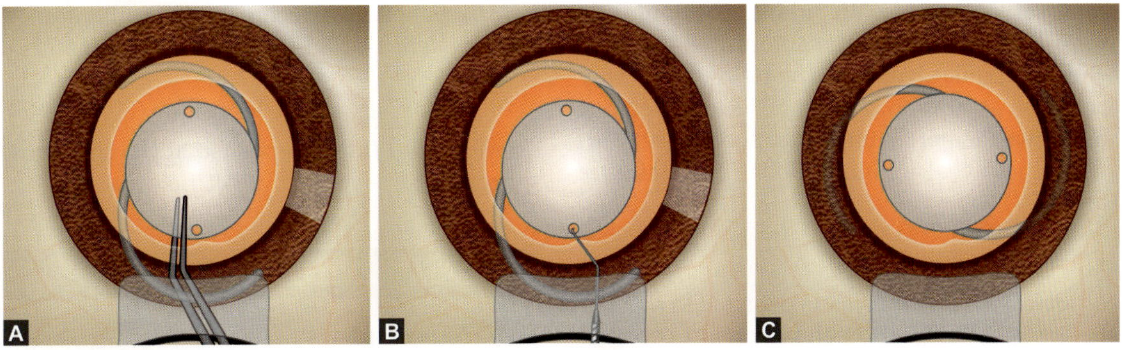

Fig. 14.35. *Dialling technique of PMMA IOL implantation:* ***(A)*** *Insertion of inferior haptic with the help of McPherson's forceps;* ***(B and C)*** *Insertion of superior haptic by dialling technique.*

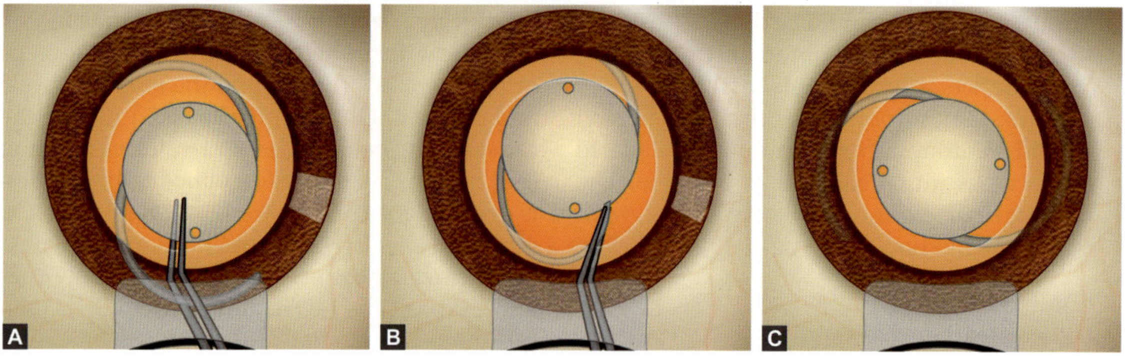

Fig. 14.36. *Flexing or looping technique of PMMA IOL implantation. For explanation see text.*

Scleral fixation of posterior chamber IOL

Scleral fixation of posterior chamber IOL is indicated in the absence of adequate capsular support or after accidental ICCE or secondary IOL implantation in an aphakic eye (with old ICCE done). Scleral fixation of PCIOL is preferred over anterior chamber (AC)IOL implantation. In this technique, PCIOL is fixed to the sclera in the ciliary sulcus region with the help of sutures or a biological glue (glued IOLs). For details *see* pages 338–344.

Implantation of foldable IOL

Implantation of foldable IOL is usually required when the nucleus is removed by phacofracture technique through a 4–4.5 mm under tunnel incision. Implantation, if foldable IOL is made either with the help of holder-folder forceps or the foldable IOL injector (more popular nowadays). For details *see* page 274.

REMOVAL OF VISCOELASTIC MATERIAL

Removal of viscoelastic material should be done thoroughly from the anterior chamber as well as capsular bag with the help of two-way irrigation aspiration cannula. Excessive left out viscoelastic material may cause secondary glaucoma and uveal inflammation (for details *see* page 137).

WOUND CLOSURE

Sutureless wound closure is possible in most of the cases. The anterior chamber is deepened with balanced salt solution injected through the side-port entry. This leads to self-sealing of the sclerocorneal tunnel incision due to valve effect.

Wound closure with sutures is required in following cases:

- Large scleral tunnel (> 6.5 mm), to avoid against the rule astigmatism
- A leaking tunnel
- Premature entry in the anterior chamber
- Cases with combined SICS and trabeculectomy surgery, done for co-existing cataract and glaucoma
- Paediatric cataract (due to thin sclera).

Suturing techniques used for the scleral tunnel in SICS include:

- *Vertical sutures* in the form of radial or cross sutures can be used (Fig. 14.37). These sutures appose the external lip, but result in internal separation of corneal lips.
- *Horizontal sutures* are preferred over the radial sutures, as the former flattens the scleral tunnel, makes it watertight and produces comparatively less astigmatism. Two types of horizontal suture techniques popular are:
  - *Shepherd's* single horizontal suture (Fig. 14.38A)
  - *Fine's infinity* suture technique (Fig. 14.38B).

Conjunctival flap is reposited at the end of the surgery and secured by wet field cautery.

ASTIGMATISM CONTROL IN SICS

The uncorrected visual acuity (UCVA) can be markedly improved by becoming astigmatism conscious during SICS.

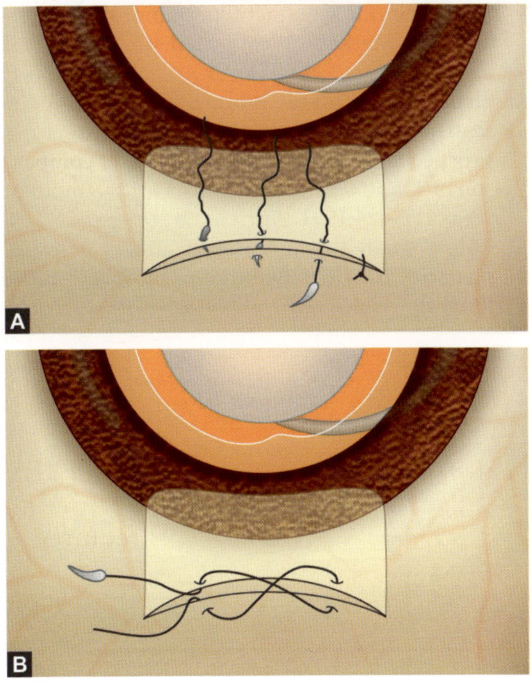

Fig. 14.37. *Technique of vertical suturing: **(A)** Radial sutures; **(B)** Cross-suture (infinity suture).*

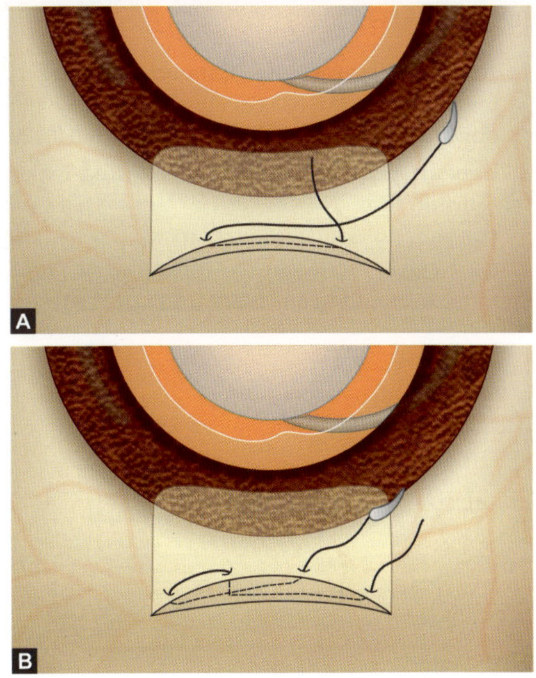

Fig. 14.38. *Technique of horizontal suturing: **(A)** Shephard's single horizontal suture; **(B)** Fine's infinity suture.*

Basic principles and modalities

Basic principles of managing astigmatism are similar to that for phacoemulsification technique *see* page 330).

Modalities for control of astigmatism in SICS include:

- Cataract incision on deep axis
- Relaxing incisions
- Toxic IOLs
- Postoperative corneal laser ablation procedures.

Cataract incision and OCCI: protocols for management of astigmatism in SICS

For details *see* page 330.

SICS IN SPECIAL SITUATIONS

During small incision cataract surgery (SICS), certain special considerations are required in special situations given below:

I. *SICS in difficult situations*
  - Posterior polar cataract
  - Small pupil
  - Traumatic cataract
  - Complicated cataract
  - Subluxated cataract

II. *SICS in paediatric cataract*

III. *SICS in cataract associated with glaucoma*

Note. Special considerations for some of the above situations have been described in Chapter 16, on 'Cataract Surgery in Special Situation' (*see* pages 287–305).

COMPLICATIONS OF SICS

Complications of small incision cataract surgery (SICS) can be discussed under following headings:

- Postoperative complications.

  For details *see* Chapter 20, pages 345 to 361.
- Preoperative complications
- Peroperative complications

BIBLIOGRAPHY

1. Allen D; Vasavada A. "Cataract and surgery for cataract.". *BMJ* 333 (7559): 128–32, (Jul 2006). doi:10.1136/bmj.333.7559.128. PMID 16840470.
2. Clinical Ophthalmology by Kanski, 7th ed, Expert Consult Title.
3. Duker, Jay S.; Myron Yanoff MD; Yanoff, Myron; Jay S. Duker MD (2009). *Ophthalmology*. St. Louis, Mo: Mosby/Elsevier. ISBN 0-323-04332-1.
4. Small Incision Cataract Operation. R H Keates and K H Merkley. West J Med. 157(4):453;1992 October.
5. Steinert RF, Brint SF, White SM, Fine IH. Astigmatism after small incision cataract surgery. A prospective, randomized, multicenter comparison of 4- and 6.5 mm incisions. Ophthalmology. 98(4):417–424,1991 Apr.
6. Role of small incision cataract surgery in Indian scenario. Indian J Ophthalmol. 57(1):1–2;2009 Jan–Feb.

PHACOEMULSIFICATION AND MICROINCISION CATARACT SURGERY

15 CHAPTER

15.1 HISTORICAL OVERVIEW

CONCEPT OF PHACOEMULSIFICATION

Concept of phacoemulsification was introduced by *Charles D Kelman* (Fig. 15.1.1) as early as 1948, but it was accepted after 1967. Charles Kelman garnered the idea, reportedly, after a visit to the dentist, where he found an ultrasonic device being used to help remove plaque and debris from there. The phacoemulsification basically acts through a hollow 1 mm titanium needle which vibrates by piezoelectric crystal at an ultrasonic speed of 40,000 times a second, and fragments the nucleus of the cataractous lens and then emulsifies these fragments. The technique also uses a surgeon-controlled automated irrigation and aspiration system to aspirate the emulsified nucleus and cortical matter.

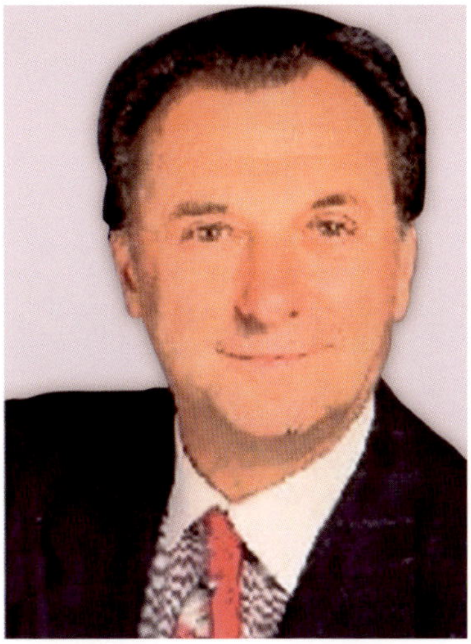

Fig. 15.1.1. *Charles D Kelman.*

EARLY RELUCTANCE TO ACCEPT PHACOEMULSIFICATION

Early reluctance to accept phacoemulsification was mainly due to:

- *Higher risk of complications,* especially posterior capsular ruptures and damage to corneal endothelium due to proximity to the phaco-needle.
- *Necessity to enlarge the incision* after completion of the procedure to accommodate the large sized PMMA intraocular lens implant.

SUCCESSFUL ACCEPTANCE OF PHACOEMULSIFICATION

Successful acceptance of phacoemulsification in 1980s was possible due to following landmark developments:

- *Ophthalmic viscoelastic devices (OVDs),* which have revolutionized the cataract surgery, were first used in 1979. The first commercial OVD used to protect the endothelium was 'Healon' a preparation of sodium hyaluronate. Subsequently many OVDs have been developed (*see* Chapter 10, pages 132–138).
- *Foldable intraocular lenses,* which could be introduced through a 3 mm incision, is the major landmark for the acceptance of phacoemulsification. In 1980, Thomas Mazzocco developed and implanted the first foldable IOL design manufactured from hydrophobic and hydrophilic acrylics as well as silicone biomaterials have been developed (*see* pages 153–155).
- *Introduction of technique of continuous curvilinear capsulorhexis (CCC)* independently by *Neuhann* from Germany and *Gimbel* from Canada, in 1986, has gone a long way in refining the technique of phacoemulsification and reducing the complications.
- *Refinements in the quality of phacoemulsification machines,* especially the solid state electronic control mechanism, making them surgeon friendly, have encouraged even the average surgeon to shift to phacoemulsification.

LANDMARKS IN THE DEVELOPMENT OF NUCLEOTOMY IN PHACOEMULSIFICATION

Landmarks in the development of nucleotomy techniques in phacoemulsification, which need to be reviewed for the historical perspective are as below:

- *Anterior chamber phacoemulsification* is the original technique described by Kelman in 1967. Kelman's first operation using phaco on a human eye took 3 hours and 5 litres of fluid. At that time patients were left aphakic or the incision needed considerable enlargement to implant non-foldable 6 mm IOLs.
- *Posterior chamber phacoemulsification* was first of all introduced by Sinskey in 1970. Many advances have occurred in posterior chamber and endocapsular phacoemulsification over the years. For details *see* pages 256–258.

15.2 PHACO MACHINE

- Introduction
- Console
- Handpiece
- Foot pedal

INTRODUCTION

Phaco machine has undergone a sea of change since its introduction by Charles D Kelman in 1967. The original phaco machine known as Cavitron–Kelman Phacoemulsifier Mark I was an equipment almost of the size of a household refrigerator (Fig. 15.2.1). The modern machines are highly sophisticated with portable models now being available. Though, there are many variations in these models, basically each machine functions on the same principle and consists of three base parts (Fig. 15.2.2):

- Console
- Handpiece
- Foot pedal and their connections.

CONSOLE

The console houses a computer that controls all the functions of the machine which include:

- Phaco power delivery system
- Irrigation and aspiration system.

The modern microprocessor control with software enhancements allows sophisticated

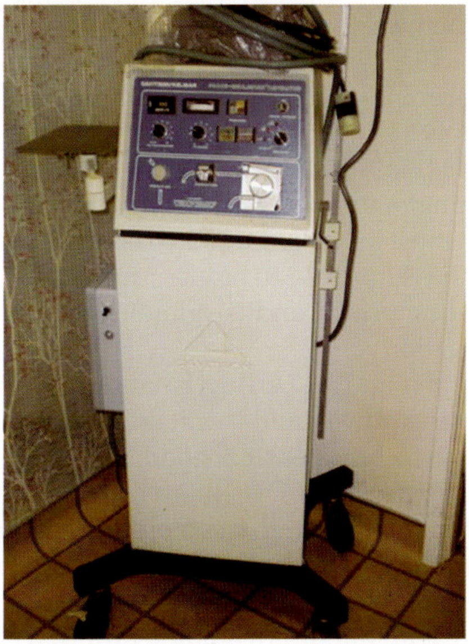

Fig. 15.2.1. *The Cavitron–Kelman phacoemulsifier.*

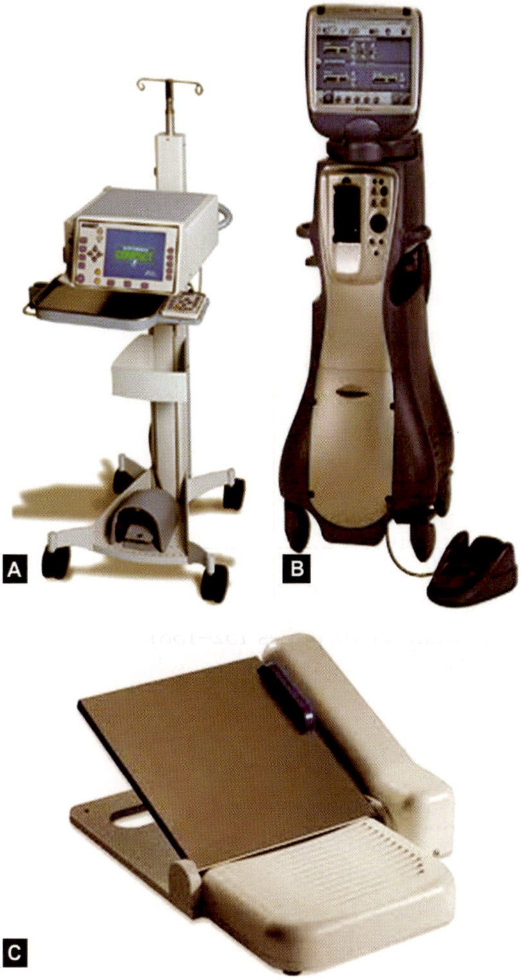

Fig. 15.2.2. ***(A and B)*** *Modern phacoemulsification machines;* ***(C)*** *Foot pedal.*

adjustment of various parameters in the most modern machines.

Display panel of the machine allows manipulation of the settings for the various parameters such as power, vacuum, flow rate, etc. The modern machines have a multimode panel, where multiple settings of all variables as required by different surgeons can be fed.

HANDPIECE

Each machine is provided with two types of handpieces: phaco handpiece and irrigation-aspiration handpiece.

PHACO HANDPIECE

Phaco handpiece (Fig. 15.2.3), also known as *ultrasonic handpiece*, has been likened to a jackhammer vacuum/garden hose instrument that allows breaking the nucleus of the crystalline lens into fragments and aspirating them from the eye. Thus, the phaco handpiece through its tip at the distal end allows:

- Delivery of power system
- Irrigation
- Aspiration control system.

For these functions, the proximal end of the handpiece is connected to the console with an electric cord, with irrigation tubing and with aspiration tubing (Fig. 15.2.3).

Power generating system

Phaco power or the so-called ultrasonic power is produced by the *piezoelectric crystal* present in the handpiece. The piezoelectric crystal converts electric energy into mechanical vibrations which are transmitted to the phaco tip.

Phaco tip

Phaco tip is a hollow titanium needle which oscillates to and fro at ultrasonic frequency that is preset for each machine between 27,000 hertz (Hz) and 60,000 Hz. Its distal opening functions as the aspirating port. The phaco tip is covered by a silicone sleeve. The irrigation fluid flows through two ports located 180° apart on the silicone sleeve. The irrigation fluid cools the handpiece and also keeps the anterior chamber formed.

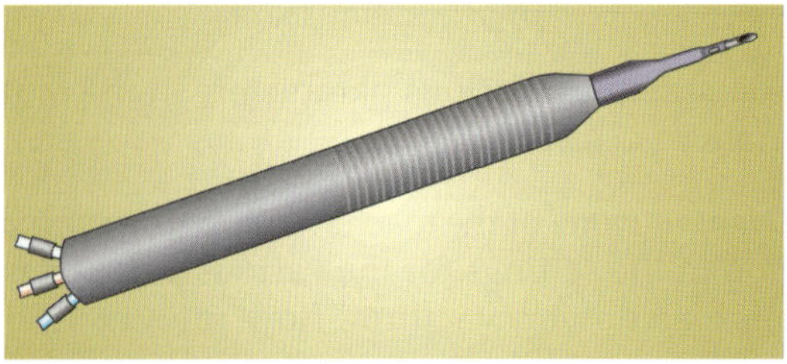

Fig. 15.2.3. *Phaco handpiece. Note the proximal end of the handpiece which is to be connected to the console with an electric code, irrigation tubing and aspiration tubing.*

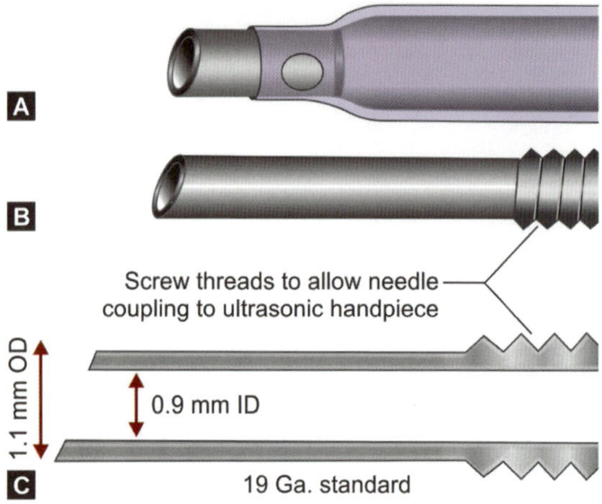

Fig. 15.2.4. *A standard phacotip: **(A)** With sleeve; **(B)** Bare needle without sleeve; **(C)** Cut section. OD: outer diameter; ID: inner diameter*

Types of phaco tips. Presently available phaco tips are standard phaco tips, e.g. Kelman phaco tip, micro phaco tip, Mackool phaco tip, flared ABS tip, micro flow tip, cobra tips, diaphragm tips, and turbosonics.

Standard phaco tips. Standard phaco tip is a straight shaft 19 G bore needle with outer diameter of 1.1 mm and inner diameter of 0.9 mm (Fig. 15.2.4). It is a commonly used tip in phacoemulsification.

According to the angle of the tip bevel and size of lumen, various types of phaco tips available are 0°, 15°, 30°, 45° and 60° and combined 30°/60°(turbo) (Fig. 15.2.5). Their characteristics are as below:

- *0° tip* (Fig. 15.2.5A) is a flat tip with minimum cutting power but very strong holding power. It is most suitable for phaco chop techniques.
- *15° tip* (Fig. 15.2.5B) has less cutting and more holding power and is suitable for improving flowability.
- *30° tip* (Fig. 15.2.5C) has balanced cutting and holding power, and is suitable for most of the phaco techniques. It is good for beginners.
- *45° tip* (Fig. 15.2.5D) is sharp cutting with good cutting ability and less holding power. It is used mainly for sculpting.
- *60° tip* (Fig. 15.2.5E) has a very sharp cutting edge with minimum holding power. It is being sparingly used these days.

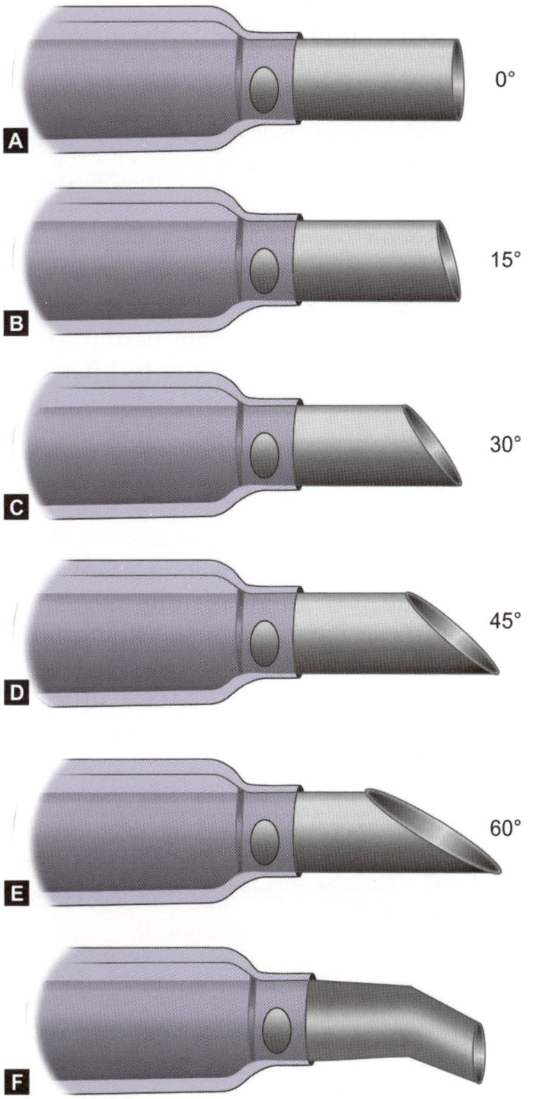

Fig. 15.2.5. *Phaco tips: **(A)** 0°; **(B)** 15°; **(C)** 30°; **(D)** 45°; **(E)** 60°; **(F)** Kelman bent tip.*

Kelman (bent) tip. It differs from the standard tip by the fact that its distal end is bent (Fig. 15.2.5F). The distal bend adds a non-axial vibration to the primary longitudinal vibration; which increases total cavitation at the tip relative to a standard tip with the same amount of ultrasound energy input. The non-axial vibration further augments the axial vibration by producing an elliptical motion at the cutting tip which enhances mechanical breakdown of nuclear material and is thus more effective in

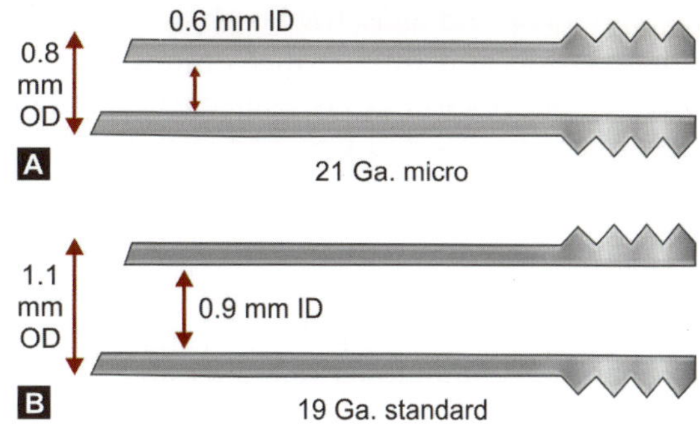

Fig. 15.2.6. *Diameter of micro-tip **(A)** as compared to standard tip **(B)**.*

cutting hard (grade 4) nuclei. Further, because of the downward curve, it is more ergonomic providing lesser stress on the wound by keeping the handpiece more aligned to the incision.

Micro-tip. A micro-tip is straight shaft 21G bore needle with outer diameter of 0.8 mm and inner diameter of 0.6 mm (Fig. 15.2.6).

Advantages of micro-tip include:

- Needs smaller incision
- Increased visibility and manoeuvrability
- Provides precise cutting for the lower average ultrasonic power used
- Provides enhanced surge protection because of smaller internal lumen.

Mackool tips. Mackool tips contain a thin polyimide insulation tubing which separates the metallic shaft of the tip from the infusion sleeve (Fig. 15.2.7). Dr. Richard Mackool's microseal

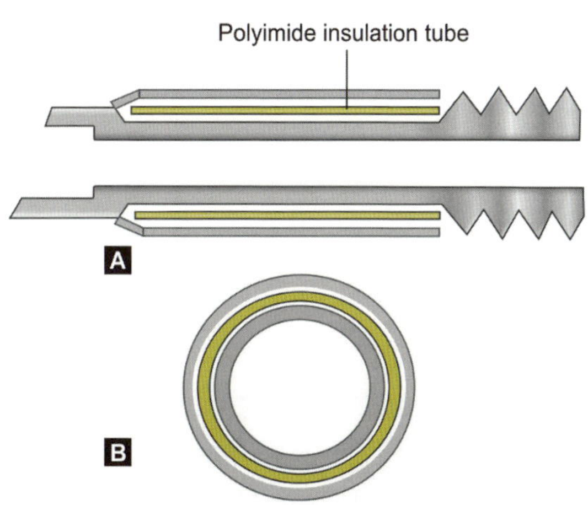

Fig. 15.2.7. *Cut sections of Mackool tip (Alcon and Bausch and Lomb microseal tips) showing polyimide insulation tube: **(A)** Longitudinal section; **(B)** Transverse section.*

design (Alcon and Bausch & Lomb) reduces heat transmission and thus reduces thermal burn. *Mackool's microseal design* is available in standard tips, micro-tips, flared tips, and ABS tips.

Flared tips. Flared tips provide advantages of both micro-tip and standard tip. The proximal part of the flared tips have an internal diameter of 0.6 mm like micro-tip, but the distal end is enlarged to 0.9 mm inner diameter and 1.1 mm outer diameter similar to a standard tip. Therefore, these tips provide better holding power when occluded and due to smaller diameter proximal shaft provides fluidic resistance similar to micro-tips. This resistance is an advantage (especially with vacuum pumps) for the surgeons who desire a high vacuum level for nuclear manipulation and chopping but do not want the attendant dangerously high flow levels which would be present with an unoccluded standard tip. Another advantage of the bigger diameter of the distal end is that more volume of nuclear material can be engaged and aspirated per unit time of ultrasound power application. Flared tips are available with Mackool micro-seal design and ABS system (described below).

Aspiration bypass system (ABS) tip. Aspiration Bypass System (ABS) refers to a small hole 0.18 mm in diameter at the distal end of the phaco tip (Fig. 15.2.8). This extra opening provides continuous outflow throughout nucleus emulsification, even during occlusion.

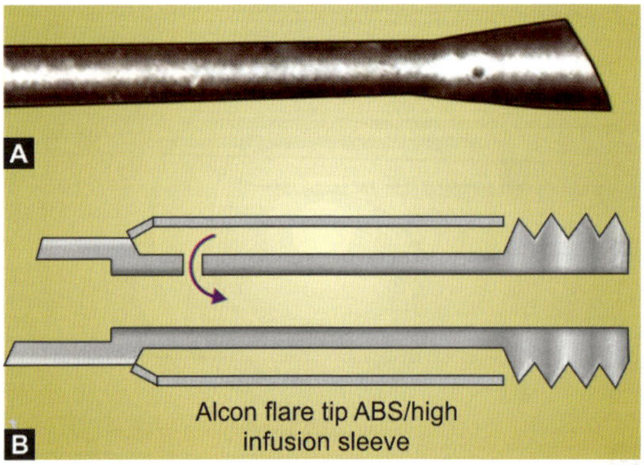

Fig. 15.2.8. *Flared ABS tip:* ***(A)*** *Photograph of naked tip. (Note the hole);* ***(B)*** *Diagrammatic cut section.*

Advantages of the ABS tip are:

- *Cools down* the phaco needle, the incision site, and the entire anterior chamber by replacing the fluid continuously.
- *Decreases the chances of surge* after the occlusion breaks.

Aspiration bypass system is available with Mackool's microseal design, standard tip, flared tip, and micro-tip.

Micro-flow tips. Micro-flow tip (Bausch and Lomb) is designed by Grham Barrett, so also called Barrett's micro-flow tip. It differs from a standard tip in having external longitudinal gooves and thus decreased inner diameter (Fig. 15.2.9).

Advantages of micro-flow tip:

- *Provide continuous cooling irrigation* fluid, even when the silicone sleeve is compressed against the needle by incision pressure.
- *Smaller inner diameter* provides fluidic benefit of surge resistance.

Cobra tips. The cobra tips have increased width at their distal extremity. These tips have an increased tendency to heat up.

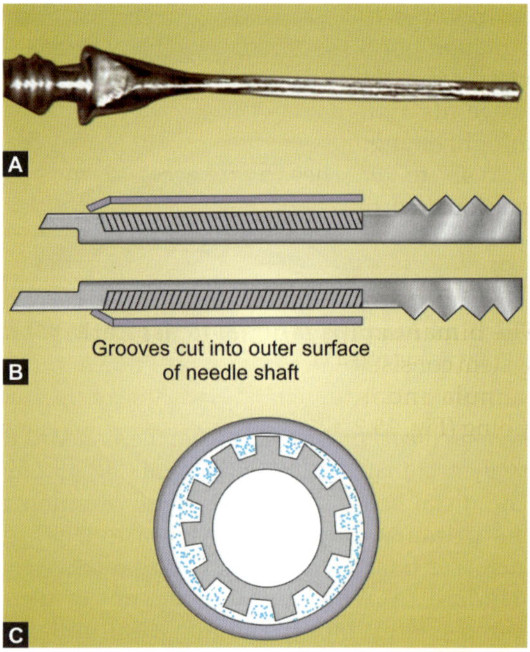

Fig. 15.2.9. *Micro-flow tips:* ***(A)*** *Photograph showing external grooves;* ***(B)*** *Diagrammatic longitudinal cut section to show grooves;* ***(C)*** *Transverse cut section to demonstrate irrigation fluid in the grooves.*

Diaphragm tips. Diaphragm tips have a constriction of the internal lumen at the distal end which acts like a diaphragm giving less surge on break of the occlusion. Thus, these tips can be used with vacuum settings.

Turbosonics tip. Turbosonics refers to the series 20000 ultrasonic tip design (Fig. 15.2.10), characterized by following features:

- Specially hydrodynamically tapered hub design, and
- Harmonically balanced to the ultrasonic handpiece.

Phaco power delivery mechanism

Phaco power delivery mechanism is discussed in phaco dynamics (*see* pages 236–240).

CO-AXIAL IRRIGATION ASPIRATION HANDPIECE

The co-axial irrigation and aspiration (I/A) handpiece (Fig. 15.2.11) has a smooth and rounded tip with single aspiration port on the side of the tip. The size of aspiration port varies from 0.2–0.7 mm, the 0.3 mm being the most commonly used. The smaller port has better vacuum seal but prolonged aspiration time and the reverse is true for the large port. The irrigation ports are placed most commonly 90° away from the aspirating port. The silicone sleeve fits around the I/A tip. The tip may be straight or angulated. The angulation may vary from 45° to 90°. These allow access to the sub-incisional cortical matter.

BIMANUAL IRRIGATION AND ASPIRATION HANDPIECES

The bimanual irrigation and aspiration (IA) system consists of two cannulae—the aspiration cannula and infusion cannula with attached tubing (Fig. 15.2.12).

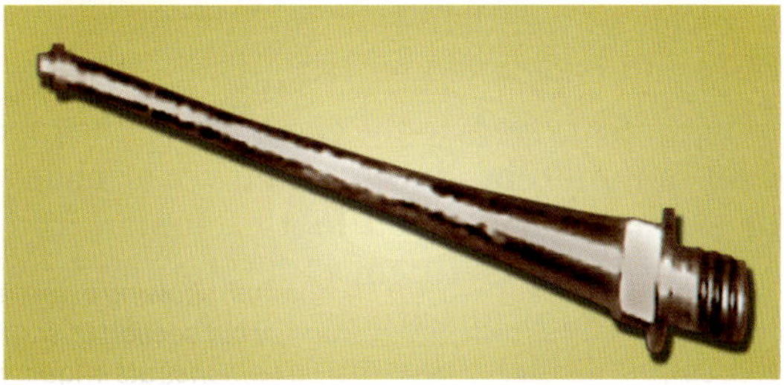

Fig. 15.2.10. *Turbosonics tip.*

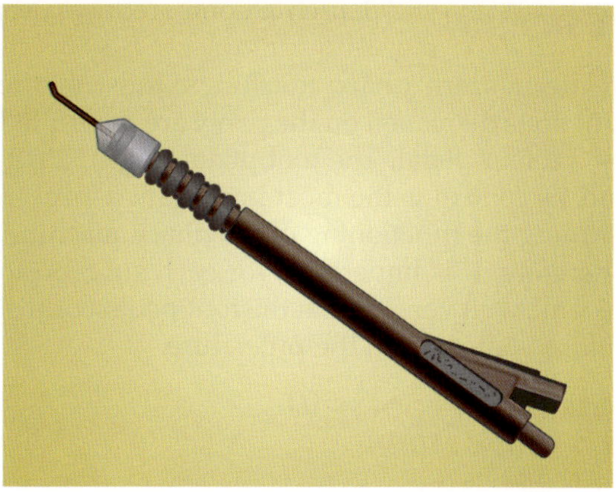

Fig. 15.2.11. *Co-axial irrigation-aspiration handpiece.*

1. ***Aspiration handpiece*** **(Fig. 15.2.12A).** It is usually curved having a rounded tip and a port 1 mm away from the tip. The port size may vary from 0.2 to 0.7 mm, 0.3 mm being the one most commonly used. The tubing attached to it is connected with the aspiration line of the phaco machine.

2. ***Infusion/irrigation handpiece*** **(Fig. 15.2.12B).** It may be straight or curved having a port at the tip or away from the tip. The 80 mm infusion cannula has two ports on either side (each 0.5 mm in size). The tubing attached to it is connected with the infusion line.

Irrigation-aspiration function occurs through a vacuum mechanism operated by pump system built in the console of the phaco machine. Its details are given in phacodynamics (*see* pages 230–236).

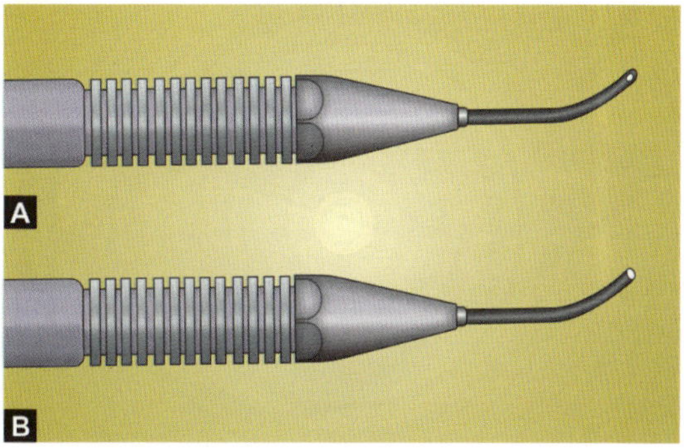

Fig. 15.2.12. *Bimanual irrigation-aspiration handpieces: **(A)** Aspiration handpiece; **(B)** Irrigation handpiece.*

FOOT PEDAL

In the modern phaco machines, most of the functions displayed on the panel are controlled by the foot pedal. The foot pedal (Fig. 15.2.13) and its control is the most important aspect in learning the functioning of the phaco machine. Therefore, it is imperative for each surgeon to become well versed with the foot pedal control before venturing in the procedure.

POSITIONS OF FOOT PEDAL AND FOOT GRADIENT

The foot pedal has four positions which can be achieved by pressing the pedal down. The different positions achieved by pressing the pedal can be identified with the feel of deviations of the pedal (*tactile feedback*) and the different sounds the machine makes (*auditory feedback*). These positions are as below (Fig. 15.2.14):

Position 0. It is the resting position with the foot pedal being at fully upright position (Fig. 15.2.14A). In this position, no function (P_0) of the phaco machine is performed.

Position 1 (irrigation mode). It is achieved by pressing the pedal up to the feel of the first excursion (Fig. 15.2.14B). In this position (P_1), the plunger slides away from the tubing and irrigation becomes on. There is no gradient in this step and the irrigation is either switched fully on or off.

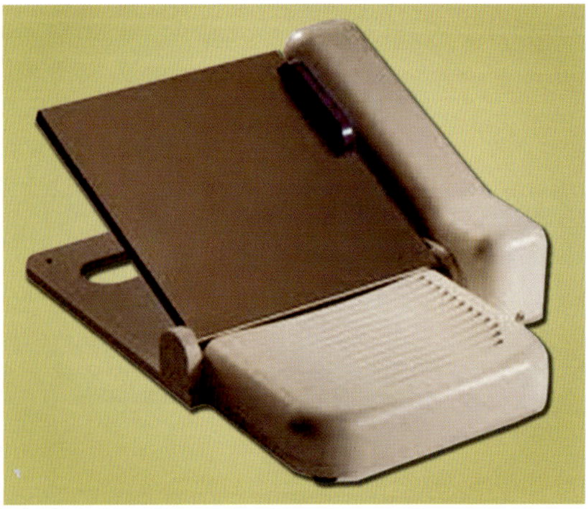

Fig. 15.2.13. *Foot pedal of a modern phacoemulsification machine.*

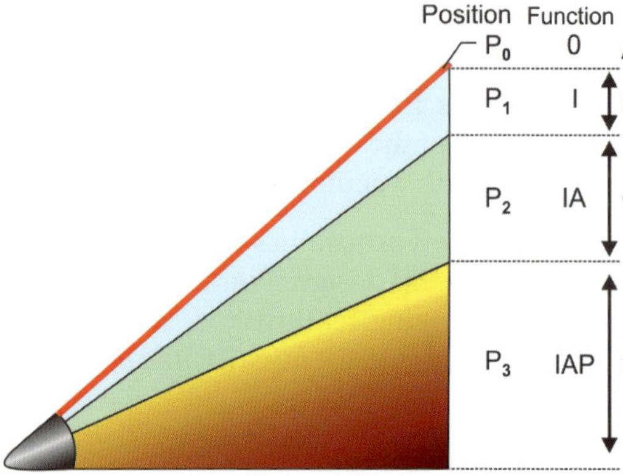

Fig. 15.2.14. *Positions of foot pedal:* ***(A)*** *P_0 – no function;* ***(B)*** *P_1 – only irrigation (I);* ***(C)*** *P_2 – irrigation and aspiration (IA);* ***(D)*** *P_3 – irrigation, aspiration and power (IAP).*

Position 2 (irrigation-aspiration (IA) mode). This position remains during the excursion of pedal between the dentation 1–2 (Fig. 15.2.14C). As the position 2 (P_2) is entered after the first dentation, the pump head begins to rotate and irrigation and aspiration (IA) occurs simultaneously. In IA excursion, the irrigation is fully on and the amount of aspiration keeps on increasing with the excursion till the full preset value is achieved.

Position 3 [irrigation-aspiration phaco (IAP) mode]. The excursion after second dentation is considered position 3. The start of position 3 of the foot pedal represents the point at which in addition to irrigation and aspiration, the ultrasonic (phaco) power becomes active (Fig. 15.2.14D). Therefore, the position 3 (P_3) is called irrigation-aspiration phaco (IAP) mode. In the IAP excursion, the irrigation is fully on, the aspiration is at the maximum preset, and the phaco power keeps on increasing with the excursion in position 3. Just before the beginning of position 3, the phaco power is zero and is denoted as IAP_0 and at maximum excursion in position 3, the phaco power delivered is at the maximum preset and is denoted by IAP_{max}.

Foot gradient refers to the excursion of the foot pedal in mm to produce unit power of phaco. For example, if the total foot excursion from IAP_0 to IAP_{max} is 10 cm (100 mm) and the maximum preset phaco power is 100%, then the foot gradient (FG) = 100 mm/100 = 1 unit power per mm of excursion. If the maximum preset phaco power is changed to 50%, then FG = 100 mm/50 = 1 unit power per 2 mm of excursion; and at 25% maximum preset power the FG = 100 mm/25 = 1 unit power per 4 mm excursion (Fig. 15.2.15).

Pedal set up for IAP mode versus IA mode. As described above in IAP mode, there are 3 positions (1, 2 and 3) with two dentation (D_1 and D_2). Some phaco machines have similar pedal set up for IA mode also; while others continue the travel of position 2 and 3 into a single longer excursion for position 2 in the I/A mode with only one dentation (Fig. 15.2.16).

SIDE KICK MOVEMENT FUNCTION OF FOOT PEDAL

In addition to the irrigation (I), aspiration (A), and phaco (P) being controlled by the downward excursion of the foot pedal; the other functions are also controlled by the side kick movement of the pedal as below.

1. ***Foot pedal reflux control.*** It is present in most of the modern phaco machines. On kicking the side switch, aspiration flow rate is inverted and the fluid is pushed from the aspiration line to the anterior chamber to push back the engaged iris or capsule. Since it is not a continuous function, for further reflux, the switch needs to be kicked again.

2. ***Continuous infusion mode (CIM).*** It is present in most of the modern phaco machines. It is started by kicking the side switch and remains on till it is switched off by again kicking the side switch. In this mode, the infusion remains on in all the four positions of the foot pedal (0–3). Therefore, in this mode, the eye remains pressurized even when the pedal is released. The CIM is particularly useful for the beginners.

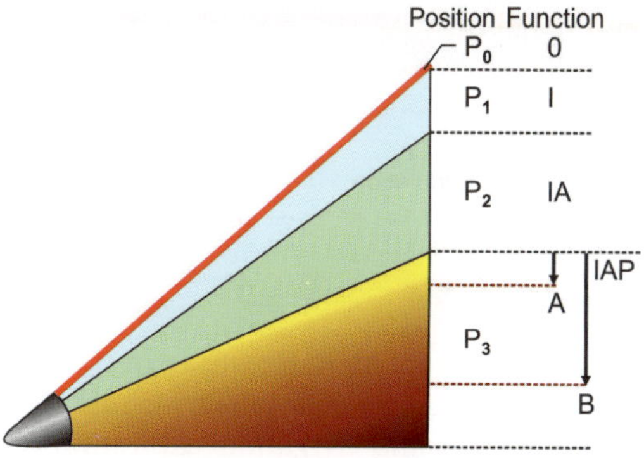

Fig. 15.2.15. *Foot gradient. Note, when maximum power set is 100% then 1 unit foot pedal excursion produces 1% power **(A)**, and when P_{max} is 25% the 1% power is produced by 4 units of excursion **(B)**.*

OTHER FUNCTIONS OF FOOT PEDAL

Other functions of the foot pedal which are present in the newer models of phaco machines include:

- Pulse on-off function
- Bottle height adjustments
- Multimode panel
- Dual linear control, i.e. separate linear control is present for fluidic and ultrasound into two planes of pedal movement, viz. pitch (up and down movement) and yaw (side to side movement). This function is present in 'Bausch and Lomb's Surgical Millennium' mode of phaco machine.

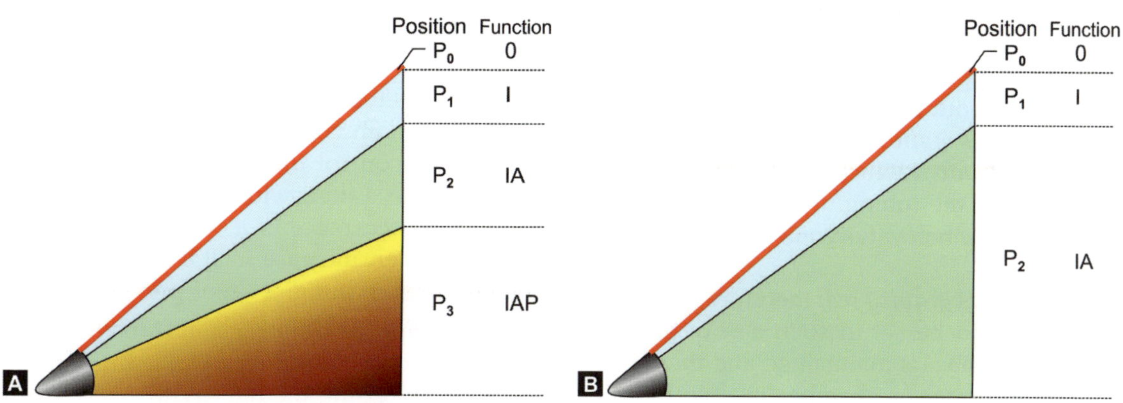

Fig. 15.2.16. *Foot pedal setting for IAP mode **(A)** versus IA mode **(B)**. (0–no function; I–irrigation; IA–irrigation and aspiration, IAP–irrigation, aspiration and power).*

15.3 PHACODYNAMICS

- Introduction
- Fluidics
- Phaco power modulation
- Surge
- Salient phacodynamic features of some phaco machines
- Phacodynaimc features of an ideal phaco machine

INTRODUCTION

Phacodynamics refers to the study of the main functions of phaco machine which include phaco power delivery and irrigation–aspiration and their inter-relationship. The phacodynamics can be studied under the following headings:

- Fluidics
- Phaco power modulation
- Surge and its prevention.

Note. Phacodynamics of conventional as well as microincision phaco are discussed simultaneously.

FLUIDICS

Fluidics refers to irrigation–aspiration system and the parameters on which it depends. Fluidics is of paramount importance in the performance of modern phaco machines. The two components of fluidics which need to be understood thoroughly are:

- Irrigation system
- Aspiration system.

IRRIGATION (INFUSION) SYSTEM

IRRIGATION IN CONVENTIONAL PHACO

- ***The irrigation and aspiration are arranged co-axially*** on a single handpiece which enters the eye through a 3 mm incision. The irrigation occurs through an irrigating silicone sleeve, delivering about 80–85 cc of fluid/minute.
- ***Irrigation is mainly determined by the height of irrigation bottle*** which provides the gradient for flow and the tubing, which runs from the bottle to the pinch valve controlled by the foot pedal.
- ***Irrigation is gravity fed;*** therefore, the bottle height should be set in such a way that the anterior chamber is maintained and there is no collapse of anterior chamber in case there is surge. At the same time, IOP should also be maintained at a safe level without putting a stress on zonules and the lens-iris diaphragm. A bottle height of 3 ± 1ft maintains a safe IOP with sufficient fluid entering the eye. Though, if the wound is water-tight, at 3 ft bottle height, the IOP should be about 16 mm Hg (3 ft = 900 mm water column; so pressure will be equal to 900/13.6 = about 66 mm Hg). However, since the wound and side-port are leaking, a safe IOP is maintained.

IRRIGATION IN MICRO-PHACO

While in microincision phaco (micro-phaco), the aspiration occurs through the phaco tip and the irrigation occurs through an irrigating chopper, each introduced through a separate incision (1.2–1.5 mm in width). In micro-phaco, hardly 40–45 cc of fluid is delivered per second to the eye. This is not enough, so there is need to increase irrigation through the irrigating chopper.

Methods to increase irrigation through the irrigating chopper

1. ***Increasing bottle height*** by 12 inches from the conventional (about 30 inches) helps in increasing the irrigation due to the effect of atmospheric pressure.

2. ***Use of atmospheric pressure pump,*** such as *fish pond pump* (pioneered and popularized by Dr. Amar Aggarwal), to infuse air into the BSS bottle, causes the fluid to gush out and prevent surge. The main concern of the system is the inability to control the pressure of the fluid entering the eye along with extremely high IOP. Therefore, occurrence of a vascular occlusion due to sudden increase in IOP, though rare, must be kept in mind.

3. ***Use of anterior chamber maintainer (ACM)*** through an extra port increases the fluid in the AC without raising the IOP. With ACM, even capsulorhexis can be performed without viscoelastics.

4. ***Use of pressurized bottle*** has been suggested by some surgeons to increase the irrigation by micro-phaco especially during nucleus removal with the phaco tip. The irrigation bottle of one litre is pressurized by injecting about 50 cc of sterile air. The airway needle should be removed after injecting the air. This pressurized bottle allows for about 85 cc/min of fluid to enter the eye. During cortex removal with IA tip, less flow is required, so the 20 G airway needle should be inserted in the bottle at this stage to allow the bottle to be gravity fed rather than pressurized.

5. ***Mechanized pressure infusion*** provided by the combination anterior-posterior machines such as the Accurus (Alcon) and Millennium (Bausch and Lomb) are very effective.

6. ***Pressurized plastic bottle*** using BP cuff has also been reported to enhance the irrigation. Here a normal sphygmomanometer cuff is wrapped around a plastic BSS bottle and is inflated in order to achieve the desired pressure.

ASPIRATION SYSTEM

FUNCTIONS OF ASPIRATION SYSTEM

The two main functions of the aspiration system are:

- *Lavage of anterior chamber* (outflow) which is governed by the flow rate
- *Creation of hold* for emulsification/crushing of the nucleus, which is controlled by the vacuum generated by the system.

ASPIRATION SYSTEM TERMINOLOGIES

Before discussing the dynamics of aspiration system and to understand concepts related to the removal of nuclear and cortical material, it will be worth-while to be familiar with the following terms:

Aspiration refers to withdrawal of fluid and lens material from the eye. It begins by pressing the foot pedal to position 2 and continues in position 3.

Aspiration flow rate (AFR) refers to the volume of fluid in ml/min removed from the eye. Some facts about AFR are as follows:

- *In a peristaltic system,* the AFR is determined by the speed of the pump. Other factors that influence the AFR are compliance, venting and tubing.
- *For a greater AFR,* the bottle must be adjusted to a higher position to compensate for increased fluid loss.
- *High AFR* results in attraction of lens material toward the phaco tip like a magnet with faster vacuum build up and swifter removal of the lens matter but with less power.
- *Low AFR* should be used when working near the capsule.
- *In the segment removal mode,* changes in the AFR influence the speed of surgery, and it is recommended to tweak these settings before modifying power or vacuum.

Vacuum refers to the amount of negative pressure (suction) created in the tubing. It is measured in mm Hg or inches of water. Some important facts about vacuum are as follows:

- ***Vacuum is generated*** during occlusion when the peristaltic pump is trying to aspirate fluid.
- ***Rise time*** (RT) refers to the time taken from occlusion of phaco tip to reach the maximum preset vacuum (Fig. 15.3.1).
  - *In venturi system,* the RT is fast, linear and dependent on the highest preset vacuum (Fig. 15.3.1V).
  - *In a peristaltic pump,* the RT depends on the AFR setting, which is related to the pump speed. The faster the AFR, the faster the RT. However, the relation is not absolutely linear (Fig. 15.3.1 P_1 and P_2).

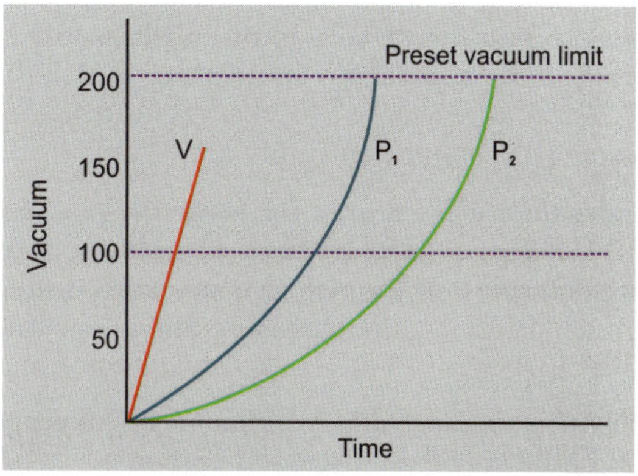

Fig. 15.3.1. *Rise time (RT), i.e. time taken from occlusion of phaco tip to reach the maximum preset in a venturi system (V), is fast and linear, as compared to peristaltic system. In peristaltic system, RT is faster with higher flow rate (P_1 with AFR of 30 ml/min and P_2 with 20 ml/min.).*

- RT is also influenced by the bore size of the phaco tip, smaller the bore, faster the RT.

Occlusion refers to the obstruction of the aspiration port or the aspiration tubing. When the lens matter occludes the tip, vacuum builds until the material is evacuated.

Vacuum helps to hold nuclear material and provides the ability to manipulate lens fragments. High vacuum also decreases the need of total pressure required to remove the lens.

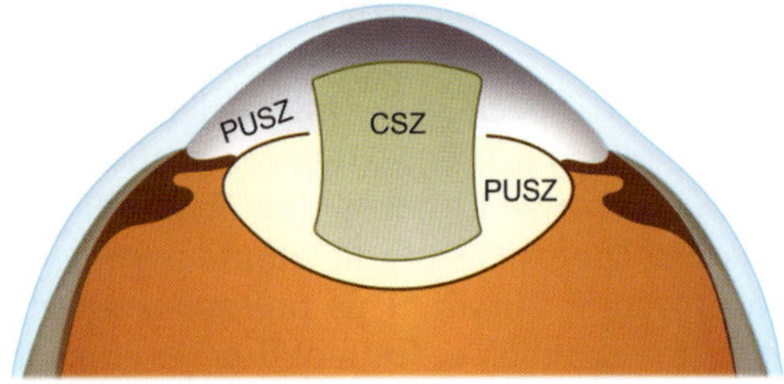

Fig. 15.3.2: *Concept of central safe zone (CSZ) (represented by the shaded area) and peripheral unsafe zone (PUSZ) represented by the remaining peripheral part of the anterior chamber and capsular fornices.*

ZONES OF ASPIRATION

For the purpose of safe aspiration, the concept of central safe zone and peripheral unsafe zone has been floated.

Central safe zone (CSZ) refers to the central area within the capsulorhexis margin (Fig. 15.3.2). Aspiration of the lens matter should be done in this zone only. In hypermetropia, patients with narrow pupil, and small CCC, the CSZ is smaller. Conversely in myopes, zonular stress syndromes and vitrectomized eyes, the CSZ is larger.

Peripheral unsafe zone (PUSZ) includes the capsular fornices and the region of angle of anterior chamber (Fig. 15.3.2). It is dangerous to do phacoaspiration in PUSZ, since the vital structures are extremely close.

FLOWABILITY

Flowability refers to the ability of the fluidic system to attract and hold nuclear or cortical material on the distal end of an ultrasonic or irrigation/aspiration handpiece until the material is evacuated by the vacuum forces. Some facts about flowability are as below:

Flowability is created by pressure gradient of the tip, which in turn is achieved by the interplay of the positive pressure due to infusion and negative pressure due to vacuum (Fig. 15.3.3).

Positive pressure due to infusion is governed by bottle height as discussed earlier.

Negative pressure is regulated by the aspiration pump. Venturi pump is more efficient than peristaltic pump in creating negative pressure, so flowability is good in the venturi system.

Flowability is more for smaller pieces of nucleus, highlighting the importance of mechanical crushing of pieces to increase the flowability.

Zones of flowability. When the aspiration tip is placed in the central safe zone (CSZ), then depending on the flowability, the area can be divided into three zones:

- *Zone of good flowability.* It is the area around the phaco tip (Fig. 15.3.4A). All fragments in this area are attracted towards the tip.
- *Zone of poor flowability.* These are peripheral areas such as near the angle of anterior chamber and the capsular fornices (Fig. 15.3.4B). Fragments located in these areas do not get aspirated easily. Flowability in these areas can be increased by moving the probe closer to the fragments avoiding holding the iris and bringing the piece quickly to the central safe zone before aspiration.
- *Zone of no flowability.* It is the area of anterior chamber from where the fluid is spontaneously leaking out, i.e. the area around the main wound and the sideport incision (Fig. 15.3.4C). Another area of no flowability is near the dome of cornea. Fragments in these areas do not come into the tip at all, and need to be brought mechanically in front of the aspiration tip.

TYPES OF ASPIRATION SYSTEMS

The aspiration system basically consists of an aspiration pump housed in the console. Broadly, the aspiration pumps are of following types:

A. ***Flow pumps,*** in which vacuum is indirectly controlled, include:

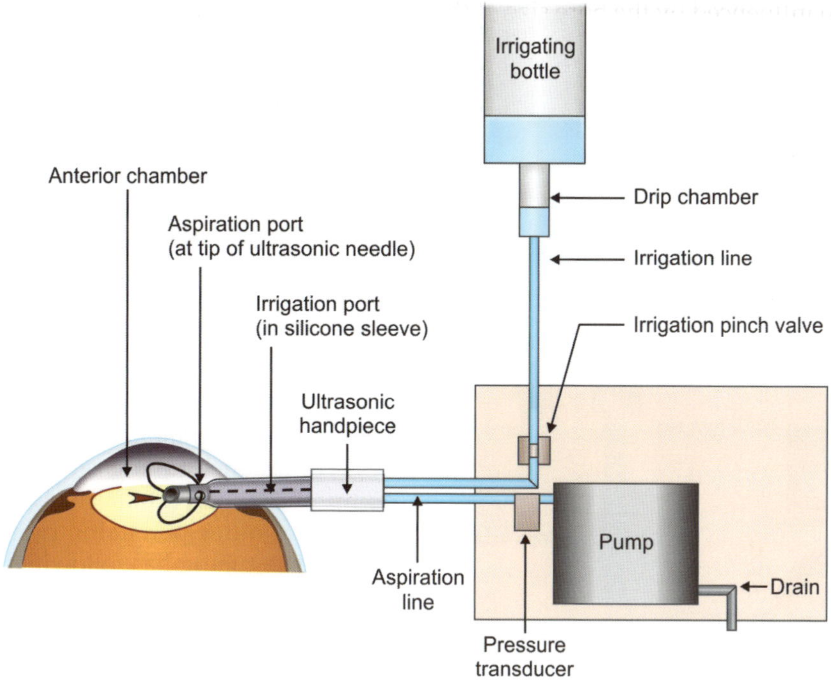

Fig. 15.3.3. *The line diagram depicting irrigation and aspiration systems of phacoemulsification. The gradient created at the phaco handpiece tip due to negative pressure of aspiration system and positive pressure of infusion system creates flowability.*

- Peristaltic pumps
- Scroll pumps.

B. ***Vacuum pumps,*** in which aspiration flow rate (AFR) is indirectly controlled, include:

- Venturi pumps
- Diaphragmatic pumps
- Rotary vane pumps.

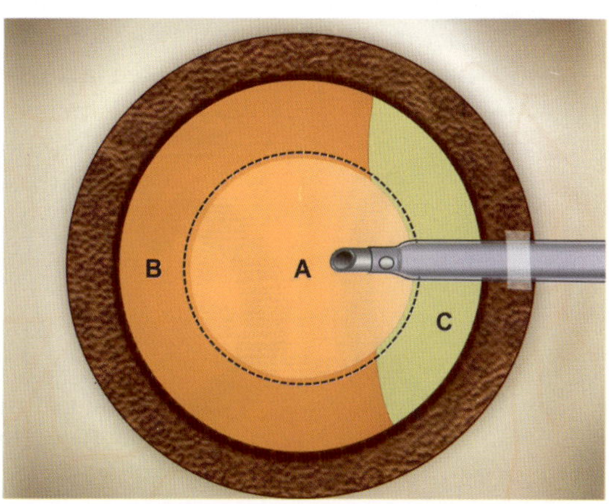

Fig. 15.3.4. *Zones of flowability:* ***(A)*** *Zone of good flowability;* ***(B)*** *Zone of poor flowability;* ***(C)*** *Zone of no flowability.*

A. FLOW PUMPS

1. Peristaltic pumps

Peristaltic pump is a simple design popularized by heart-lung machines used in open heart surgey. In it, as the pump head rotates, rollers engage the stationary aspiration tubing and collapse it at each point of roller contact. With continued rotation, bolluses of fluid are created between the rollers and are propagated in a peristaltic fashion in the direction of rotation as indicated by the arrows (Fig. 15.3.5). The faster the rollers rotate, more the fluid is withdrawn and therefore, higher is the flow rate. This fluid flow creates a pressure differential at the beginning of pump head and as the aspirating port is occluded by the nucleus, vacuum is created in the aspirating tubing. At higher flow rates, vacuum is produced in the lining even without an occlusion of the aspirating port.

Salient features of peristaltic pump are as below:

- *Slow vacuum build up* is seen in the peristaltic pump as compared to the rapid rise in the venturi pump.

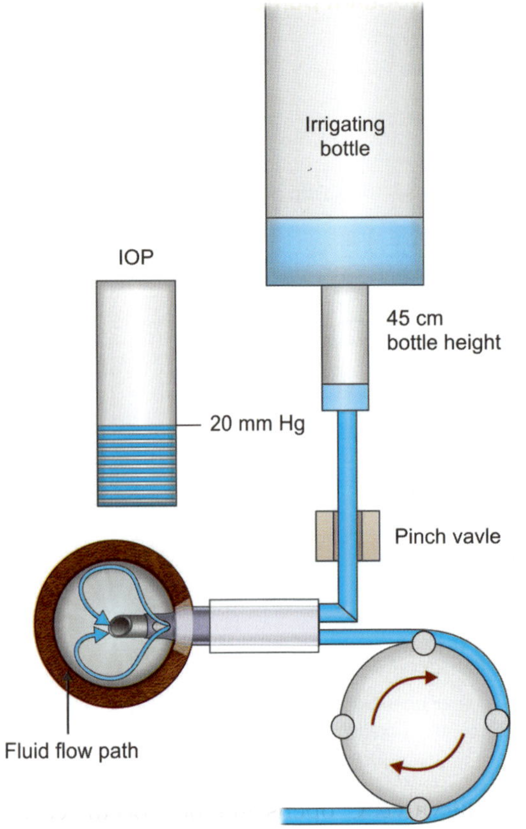

Fig. 15.3.5. *Mechanism of peristaltic pump with rotating rollers and tubing.*

- *Nuclear fragments need to be approached* in the peristaltic system to produce occlusion and then vacuum will rise. While in venturi pump, rapid rise in vacuum occurs spontaneously which pulls the nuclear fragments towards the phaco tip on pressing the foot pedal.
- *Higher safety margin* in peristaltic pump makes it user friendly, especially for the beginners.
- *Aspiration flow rate (AFR) and vacuum* can be set independently in a peristaltic system. The AFR is commanded whereas the vacuum varies with the degree of tip occlusion up to the preset vacuum limit.

Disadvantages of peristaltic pumps due to highly compliant tubing include:
- Potential surge problem
- Pump leakage (poor volumetric efficiency).

Recent advances in peristaltic pump design made to overcome the above problems include the following:
- Use of biocompliant tube (*see* page 244)
- Use of sealed rigid cassettes (*see* page 244)
- Use of software control algorithms to compensate for the leakage (*see* page 244).

2. Scroll pump

Scroll pump (concentric system) comprises of a rigid, orbitally rotating pump element placed directly within the fluidic circuit. As shown in Fig. 15.3.6, the scroll element and pump housing are fixed between the two rigid flat plates to confine the fluid into the scroll channels.

Advantages of scroll pump over conventional peristaltic flow pump are as below:
Less compliance tubing works well in scroll pump, as compared to fairly compliant tubing needed in older peristaltic pumps. The less compliance tubing has following advantages:
- *Surge problem* is comparatively decreased, and
- *Pump leakage* is decreased due to tighter tolerance. This makes the scroll pump suitable for being used in vacuum emulation mode.

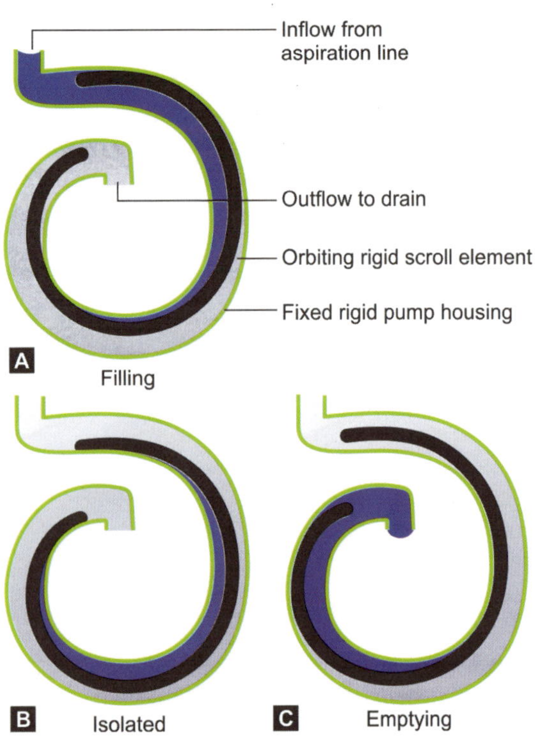

Fig. 15.3.6. *Scroll pump (concentric system) comprising of a rigid, orbitally rotating pump element:* ***(A)*** *Filling;* ***(B)*** *Isolated;* ***(C)*** *Emptying stage.*

B. VACUUM PUMPS

Salient features of vacuum pumps

1. ***Vacuum level,*** preset in the machine, is instantaneously achieved on pressing the foot pedal. Therefore, in such a pump, the surgeon directly commands the actual vacuum level and not just a vacuum limit in mm Hg.

2. ***Aspiration flow rate*** (AFR) is directly controlled and cannot be commanded. Therefore, in vacuum pump phaco machines, the flow rate is not depicted on their display. AFR in such pumps is governed by:
   - Level of preset vacuum
   - Aspiration port size
   - Degree of occlusion of aspiration port
   - Viscosity of the aspiration fluid.

3. ***Vacuum pumps are indirectly linked*** to the fluid in the aspiration line via the air in their drainage cassettes.

4. ***Rigid drainage cassette or panel,*** which does not collapse with the applied commanded vacuum, is used in the vacuum pumps in contrast to the flexible drainage pouch used in the flow pumps.

5. ***Good flowability*** to the lens matter is provided by the rapid rise in vacuum.

6. ***Increased risk of posterior capsular rupture,*** and iris trauma (particularly by the beginners) are encountered due to rapid rise in vacuum with these pumps.

Types of vacuum pumps

1. *Venturi pump*

- Venturi pump is the most commonly used vacuum pump in the phaco machines.
- *Driven by the compressed gas* (nitrogen or air) which generates vacuum.
- *Production of vacuum* is related to the flow of gas in the pump chamber (B in Fig. 15.3.7) which is regulated by varying the size of opening (A in Fig.15.3.7) by a valve. The pressure differential created between the rigid drainage cassette (D in Fig. 15.3.7) and the chamber B due to venturi effect of the gas flow over the opening C, creates a vacuum in the rigid drainage cassette D which pulls fluid in from the aspiration tubing.

2. *Diaphragmatic pump*

As shown in Fig. 15.3.8, in the diaphragmatic pump, the vacuum is generated by in and out movements of a flexible diaphragm 'A' caused by a rod connected to the rotating electric motor as indicated.

- ***When diaphragm 'A' is pulled out,*** (Fig. 15.3.8X) due to negative pressure created in the chamber 'B', the valve 'C' opens and there occurs corresponding movement of the air from drainage cassette 'E' to chamber 'B'. The vacuum created in cassette E pulls the fluid from the aspiration tubing.

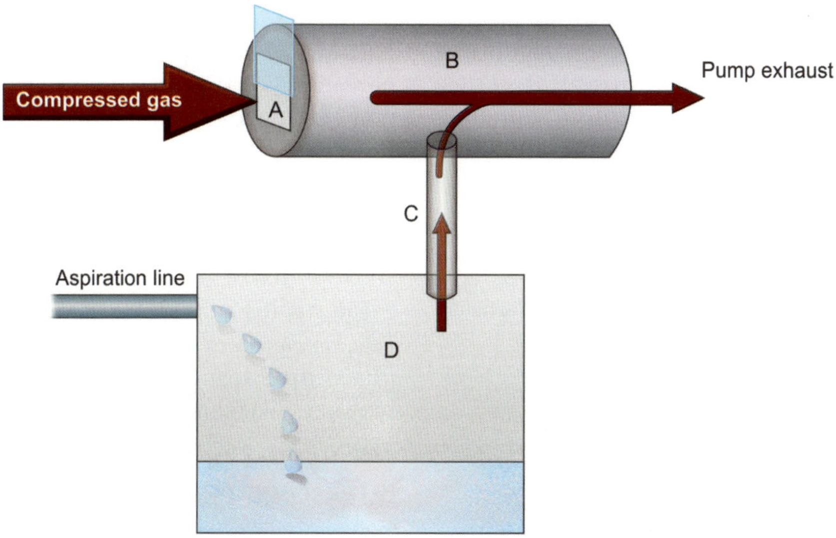

Fig. 15.3.7. *Mechanism of venturi pump driven by the compressed gas.*

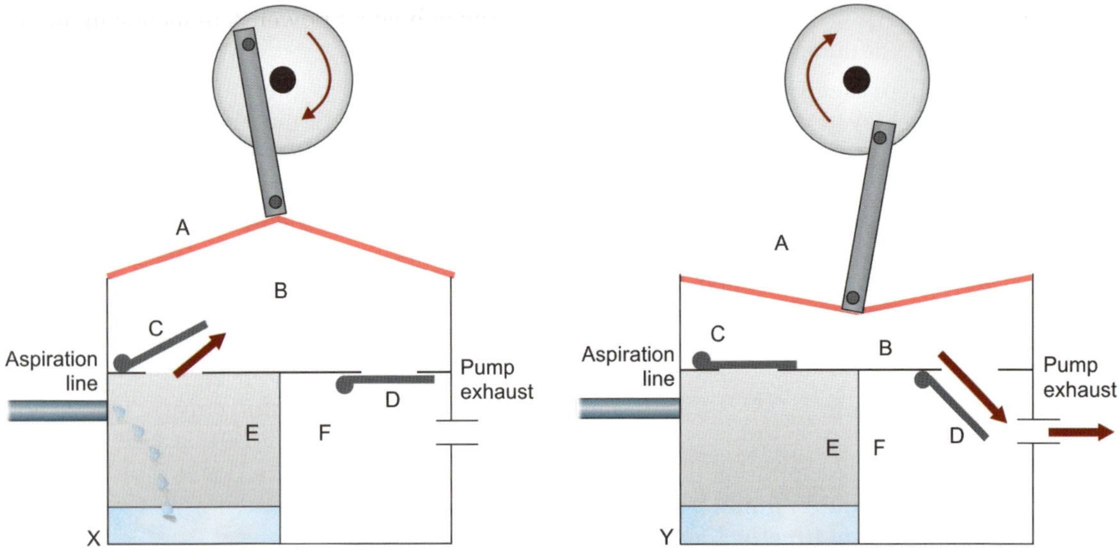

Fig. 15.3.8. *Mechanism of operation of the diaphragmatic pump: Pulled out position of the diaphragm **(X)**; and Pushed in position of the diaphragm **(Y)**. For explanation, see text.*

- ***When diaphragm 'A' is pushed in*** Fig. 15.3.8Y due to positive pressure created in chamber 'B' the valve 'C' closes and the valve 'D' opens and exhausts out the air pulled in from the cassette 'E'. Thus, the amount of vacuum created is directly proportional to the pump motor speed.

Note. Diaphragmatic pump is similar to venturi pump in sharing both relatively fast aspiration flow rate (AFR) and rapid rise in vacuum.

3. *Rotary vane pump*

As shown in Fig. 15.3.9, in this pump, the vacuum is created by the motor driven movements of a rotor containing freely sliding flat vanes, mounted eccentrically in the pump housing. Similar to diaphragmatic pump, the amount of vacuum created in rotary vane pump is directly proportional to the pump motor speed.

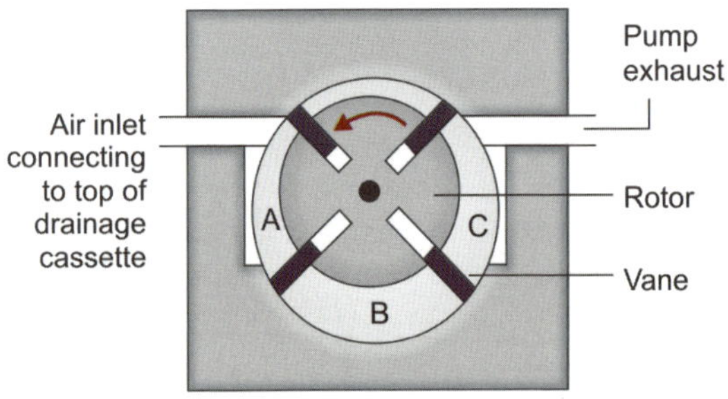

Fig. 15.3.9. *The rotary vane pump.*

PHACO POWER MODULATION

PRODUCTION OF PHACO POWER

Phaco or the so-called ultrasonic power is produced by the piezoelectric crystal present in the handpiece. The piezoelectric crystal converts electrical energy into mechanical vibrations which are transmitted to the phaco tip. Phaco power is produced when the foot pedal is depressed to position 3.

Phaco power refers to the ability of the phaco needle to vibrate and cavitate the adjacent lens material. Phaco power is noted as a linear percentage of the maximum stroke length of which the needle is capable.

Stroke refers to the magnitude of tip movement which occurs at each excursion. Power varies depending upon the stroke length, i.e. to and for movement of the tip which varies from 2/100 to 6/100 of an inch. More the stroke length, greater is the power.

Frequency refers to the rate of movement of the phaco tip. Most handpieces have a frequency between 27,000 and 60,000 Hz.

MECHANISM OF ACTION OF ULTRASONIC PHACO POWER

The ultrasonic phacoemulsification is thought to be combined effect of the following mechanisms:

1. ***Direct impact***. The direct impact or the bombarding action of the tip is also called the *Jackhammer* effect (Fig. 15.3.10A and B).

- Direct impact depends upon the stroke length and frequency of vibration. A higher frequency is thought to cut more smoothly with less repulsion via the Jackhammer effect.
- For Jackhammer effect, the nucleus needs to be fixed, as during trenching and nuclear fragment held by vacuum, during fragment eating.
- ***Chatter*** refers to the repulsion of the nuclear fragments from the ultrasonic tip occurring as a result of the Jackhammer effect. The chatter occurs when the ultrasonic stroke overcomes the vacuum or holding power. A reduction in phaco power can diminish chatter by decreasing the stroke length, thereby reducing forces pushing the fragment away from the tip.

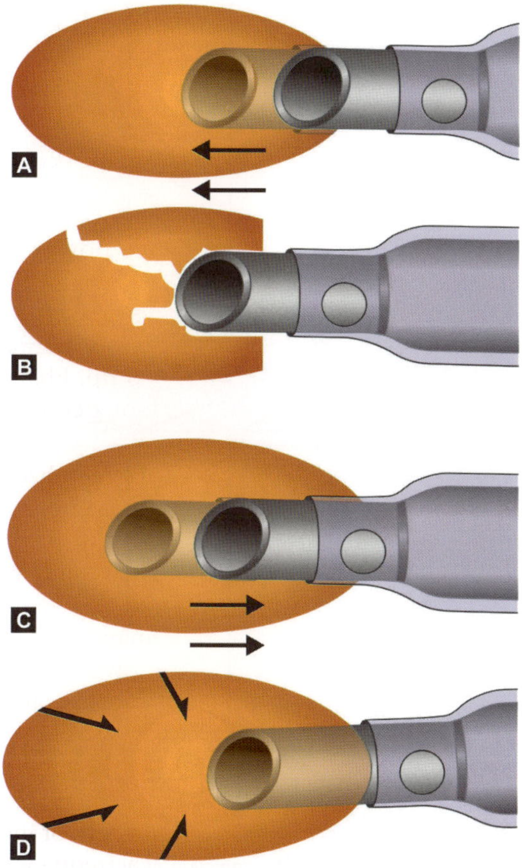

Fig. 15.3.10. *Mechanism of action of ultrasonic phaco power: **(A** and **B)**, Direct effect (Jackhammer effect) occurs where to and fro movements of the tip bombards the tissue in front **(A)** and disintegrates it **(B)**; **(C and D)** Cavitation effect is produced when swift backward movement of the tip **(C)**; results in a cavitation phenomenon causing an implosion of surrounding tissue **(D)**.*

2. ***Cavitation effect.*** Cavitation refers to formation of gas bubbles from the fluid in response to pressure changes at the phaco tip occurring due to swift movement of solid in a liquid. At the end of each oscillation backstroke, the tip retracts and creates a vacuum which causes cavitation bubbles (Fig. 15.3.10C and D). The implosion of these bubbles produces brief instances of intense heat and pressure which are thought to intensify adjacent lens matter. A lower frequency (28 Hz) is thought to produce more cavitation effect.

3. ***Acoustic wave effect.*** It is thought that sonic wave propagation through the fluid results in acoustic breakdown of the lenticular material. The disadvantage of this sonic wave is that it may push lenticular pieces away, if the hold is not good and thus decrease the Jackhammer effect.

CONTROL AND DELIVERY OF PHACO POWER

The *fixed panel control of continuous ultrasound* developed by Charles Kelman, persisted as such for about 20 years. However, over the years various efforts have been made to modulate phaco power delivery in order to reduce phaco time, reduce the risk of thermal burns and increase the efficiency.

MODES OF PHACO POWER DELIVERY

The basic modes of phaco power delivery developed include:

- Continuous mode
- Pulse mode
- Burst mode
- HyperPulse mode.

1. Continuous mode

Continuous power settings allow constant delivery of the phaco power when the machine is in position 3. The continuous power delivery can be controlled either by the panel (panel control mode) or the surgeon (surgeon/linear control mode).

Fixed panel control mode allows the power to be set from 0–100%; and the set level of power is delivered and there is no variation in the power when the foot pedal is depressed throughout the position 3 excursion (Fig. 15.3.11). *Panel mode is not preferred* in general, except in very hard cataracts where the nucleus is uniformly hard, requiring uniformly high power for emulsification.

Surgeon/linear control mode allows a variable power delivery from '0' to maximum that one sets on the panel. Thus, the surgeon controls the amount of phaco power delivered by varying the excursion of the foot pedal which is in position 3. Since the power delivered increases linearly with the depression of foot pedal in position 3 (Fig. 15.3.12). It is also called *linear control* of continuous ultrasound power.

Preferably, the maximum preset power should be based on the density of the nucleus to be emulsified.

Indications. Continuous phaco power delivery with surgeon control is best suited for sculpting deep grooves in the lens nucleus (e.g. for 'divide and conquer' or phaco 'stop and chop' technique).

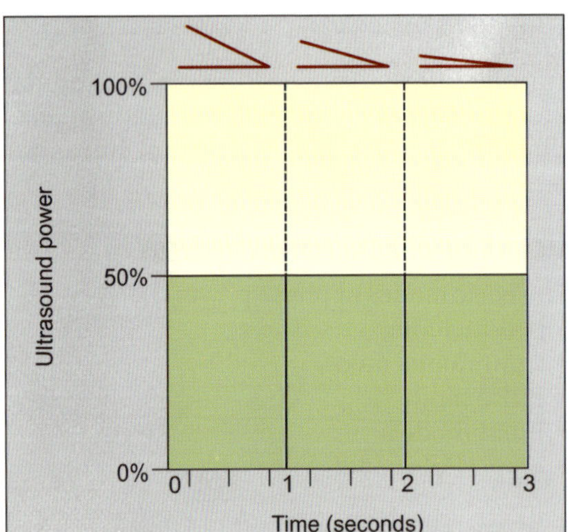

Fig. 15.3.11. *Diagrammatic depiction of power delivery in fixed continuous ultrasound power on panel control mode. Note that in this mode with fixed settings of 50%, the same power level is obtained at each of three foot pedal positions during 1st second (1/3rd depressed pedal); 2nd second (2/3rds depressed pedal); and 3rd second (fully depressed pedal).*

2. Pulse mode

In pulse mode, the power delivery is modulated to turn 'on' and 'off' a certain number of time per second; i.e. power is delivered in pulse per second (pps). In pulse mode, there is linear power delivery but at fixed intervals, e.g. 2, 3 or 4 pulses per second (Fig. 15.3.13).

- ***Pulse*** consists of an 'on' and 'off' period. For example, if set at 4 pulses per second (pps) then each pulse will be of 250 milliseconds out of which 125 milliseconds will be power on and

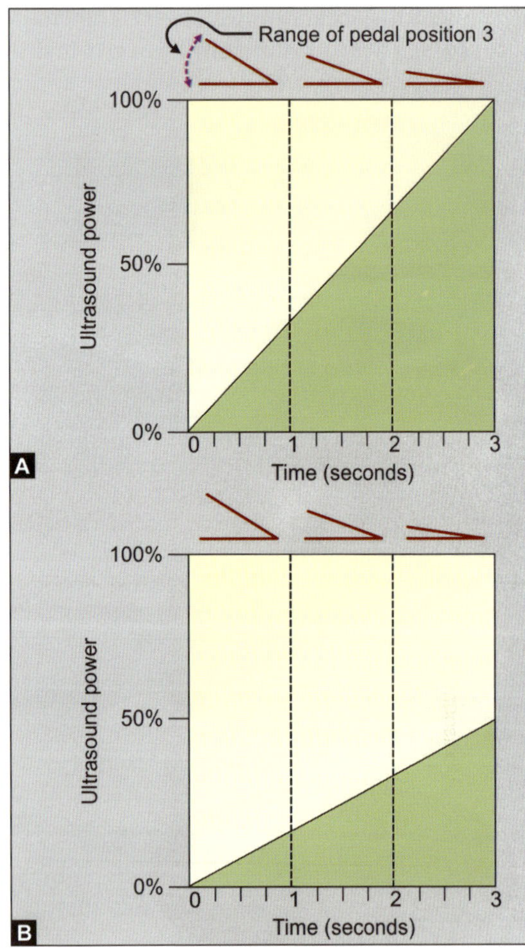

Fig. 15.3.12. *Diagrammatic depiction of phaco delivery in surgeon/linear control mode of phaco power:* ***(A)*** *When the maximum preset power is 100%; and* ***(B)*** *When the maximum preset power is 50%. Note that when the foot pedal is progressively depressed from top of position 3 to the bottom of position 3 over a 3 second time interval, there occurs a correspondingly continuous rise in ultrasound power over that time.*

next 125 milliseconds, power shall be off (Fig. 15.3.13B). Most machines have facility for 0 to 12 pulses per second. Average performance in 3–4 cycle time refers to the total time of each pulse, i.e. Duty cycle = on time/on + off time. Thus in continuous mode, duty cycle is 100% because phaco power is always on; while in pulse mode, duty cycle is always 50%.

Duty cycle (expressed as a percentage) is the preposition of the 'on' period relative to the cycle time (on + off time).

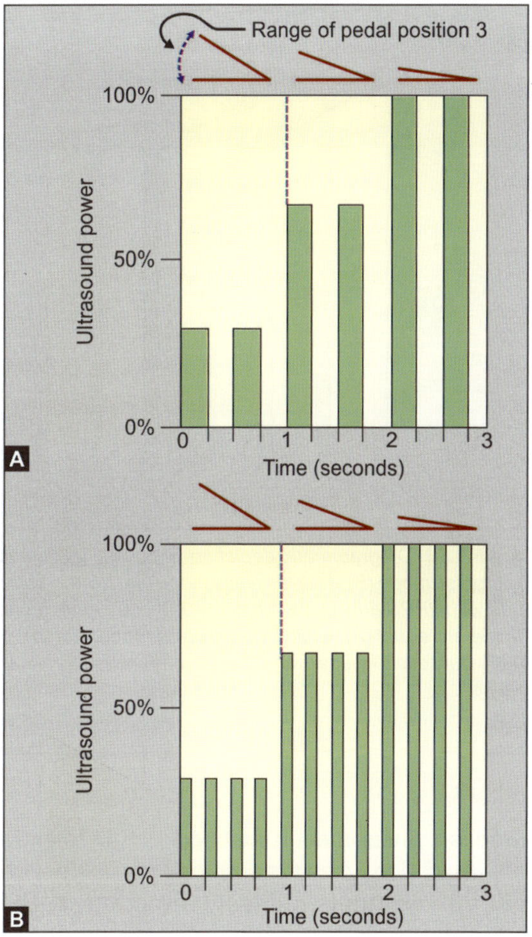

Fig. 15.3.13. *Diagrammatic depiction of power delivery in pulse mode:* ***(A)*** *When set at 2 PPS, each pulse is of 500 millliseconds of which 250 milliseconds the power is on and next 250 milliseconds the power is off;* ***(B)*** *When set at 4 PPS, each pulse is of 250 milliseconds, out of which 125 milliseconds is power on and next 125 milliseconds power is off. Note that when foot pedal is sequentially depressed to three positions within position 3, the power goes on increasing but the pulse duration and frequency remains the same.*

Advantages of pulse mode are as below:
- Phaco-power delivery is reduced by 50% and a stable anterior chamber is maintained.
- Allows firmer grasp on the lens material and decreases the chatter at the tip because vacuum builds between each pulse.
- Allows more flowability and swifter emulsification.

3. Burst mode

Burst mode facility is available in the higher end (third generation) machines. In burst mode, the maximum per-set power is delivered with each burst, but the interval between each burst decreases as the foot pedal is depressed (Fig. 15.3.14). Therefore, in contrast to pulse mode, which uses pedal movement within position 3's excursion to modulate phaco power with a fixed number of pulses per second (Fig. 15.3.14A), the burst mode uses the pedal movements to modulate the interval between bursts (i.e. there is linear control of number of bursts per second) while phaco power remains fixed at the machine panel setting (Fig. 15.3.14B). Note that unlike pulse mode which has always 50% duty cycle, the burst mode allows duty cycles that are shorter than 50% (i.e. off time is longer than on time). At the end of position 3 excursion, the power is no longer delivered in bursts, but becomes continuous.

Advantages of burst mode. Burst mode is particularly helpful for hard, brunescent cataracts, making the initial vertical chop and while impaling nuclear fragments. It uses much less ultrasound energy in any grade of cataract, than the pulse mode.

4. HyperPulse technology

HyperPulse is modification of the pulse mode. In it, like pulse mode, there is linear control of phaco power delivery; and as advantage over pulse mode the 'off' time in each pulse is more than 'on' time (Fig. 15.3.15). Thus, in the hyper-Pulse technology, the duty cycle (on time/off time) is less than 50%. Furthermore, in comparison to the 15–20 maximum PPS of traditional pulse mode, the hyperPulse technology allows up to 100 PPS with adjustable pulse duration as short as 5 msec (micropulse/sec). The term *HyperPulse* is used in Alcon Infinity machine,

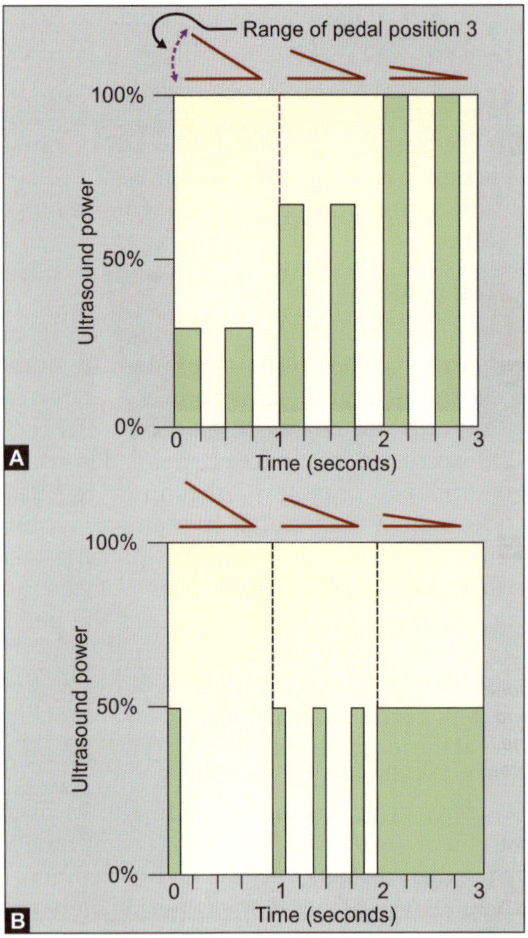

Fig. 15.3.14. *Diagrammatic depiction of power delivery in burst mode (B) as compared to pulse mode **(A)**. Note that in burst mode **(B)**, when the foot pedal is sequentially depressed to three positions within the foot pedal position 3, a fixed amount of the power is delivered in every position, but the number of bursts increase with the increasing level of depression of foot pedal.*

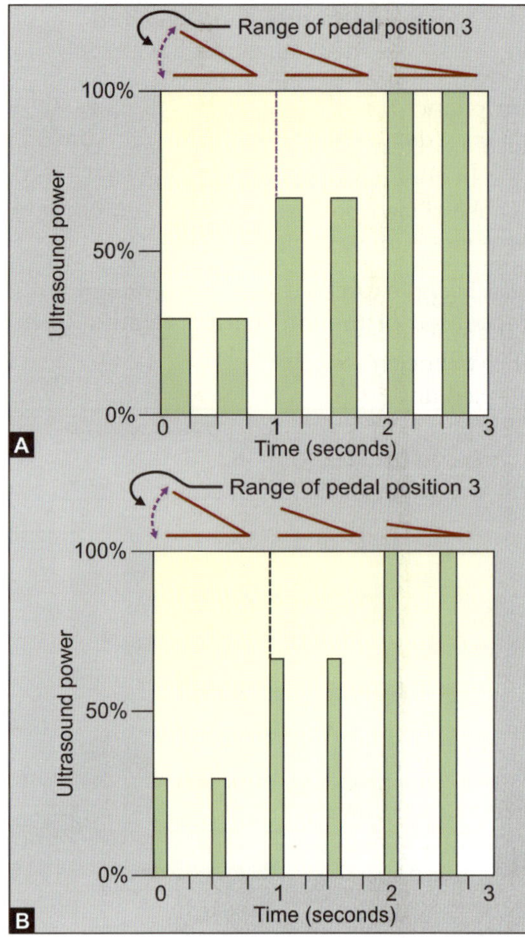

Fig. 15.3.15. *Diagrammatic depiction of power delivery in Hyperpulse mode (B) vis-à-vis pulse mode **(A)**. Note in pulse mode with 2PPS duty cycle is always 50%, i.e. on-time and off-time are equal (A), while in hyperpulse mode with 2PPS **(B)** the duty cycle is less than 50%, i.e. off-time is more than on-time.*

while in the AMO Sovereign machine the term used is *Whitestar technology*.

Advantages of HyperPulse technology are as below:

- *Ultrasound energy delivered* is low due to brief duration pulses.
- *Thermal protection against corneal burns* is most, as the increased 'off' times decrease heat built up on the vibrating phaco tip. Because of this, the HyperPulse or Whitestar technology is also termed *'cold phaco'*.
- *Flowability is increased and chatter is decreased* lending to swifter emulsification.

SURGE

Surge is a phenomenon that occurs due to extra fluid aspiration when the occluded phaco tip with built up vacuum is suddenly disoccluded. The extra fluid aspiration, obviously, results due to rush of fluid from the higher (positive) pressure anterior chamber to the lower (negative) pressure phaco tip.

Effects of surge. When the negative surge exceeds the inflow capability of the irrigation line, anterior chamber collapse may occur causing damage to the iris, cornea, and/or capsular rupture.

FACTORS CONTRIBUTING TO SURGE

1. Compliance of the tube

Compliance refers to the property of tubing to collapse (deform under pressure). A collapsing tube is an important contributing factor. As shown in Fig. 15.3.16A, when rollers are rotating and there is no occlusion, and so no collapse of tubing. When occlusion occurs, vacuum builds up and rollers stop; negative pressure is created in the system and tubing collapse (Fig. 15.3.16B). Once the occlusion breaks, negative pressure is released and tubing re-expands to the original size. The extra fluid flows from the anterior chamber to the tubing to fill up this extra volume and this causes surge (Fig. 15.3.16C).

2. Vacuum and aspiration flow rate

- *High vacuum level* will cause more collapse of tubing on occlusion and so more surge when occlusion is broken (Fig. 15.3.17).
- *High aspiration flow rate (AFR)* (more than critical limit) is associated with proportionate higher risk of surge.
- *Critical limit* is the upper limit of AFR at which the anterior chamber remains stable for a fixed bottle height and fluid leakage. Then at critical level, the AFR plus wound leakage is equal to the infusion and thus maintains a constant volume and IOP of the anterior chamber. At AFR higher than critical limit, the anterior chamber is unstable. Lower the AFR than the critical limit, more is the safety margin.

Relationship between vacuum, surge and aspiration flow rate

Relationship between vacuum, surge and aspiration flow rate (AFR) can be studied by a hypothetical situation of various parameters as given:

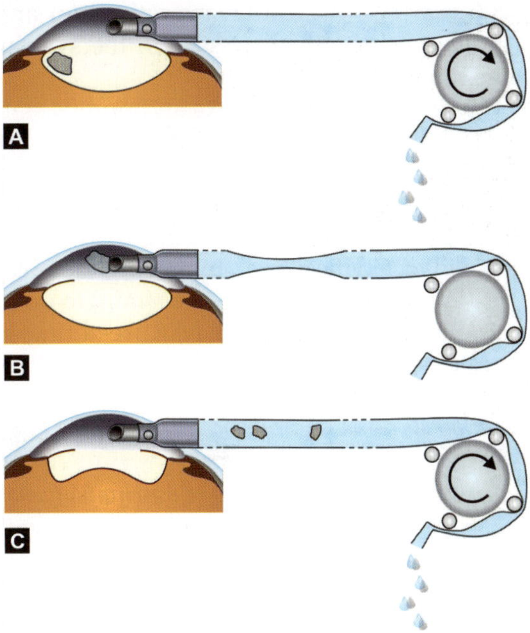

Fig. 15.3.16. *Effect of compliance of the tube in a peristaltic pump: **(A)** No collapse of tubing, when rollers are ratating and there is no occlusion of tip; **(B)** Tubing collapses when the tip is occluded and rollers stop; **(C)** When the occlusion breaks there occurs surge. For explanation, see text.*

- Critical limit of AFR: 35 cc/min setting
- Aspiration flow rate (AFR): 30 cc/min
- Vacuum setting: 200 mm Hg.

Result: Surge beyond acceptable limit.

Action for surge: Either one may reduce AFR or the vacuum. The dynamics of parameters under these situations is graphically represented in Fig. 15.3.18 and explained below:

- *From point X to Y* in the graph (Fig. 15.3.18A) is the time of no occlusion, during which AFR is in the safe limit (25 cc/min).
- *At point Y*, there occurs occlusion and AFR becomes '0'(zero), the vacuum builds up to

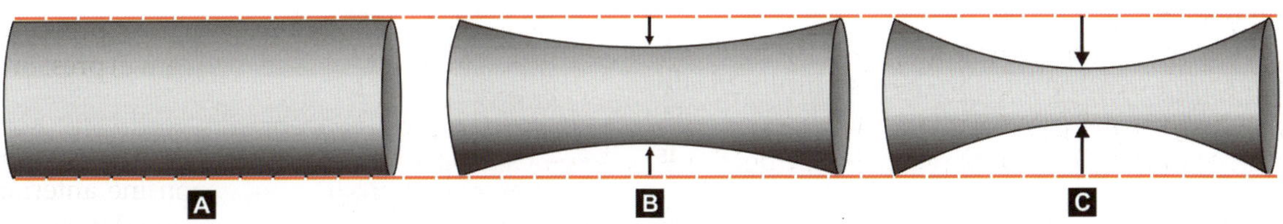

Fig. 15.3.17. *Depicting more collapse of tubing **(A)** as compared to vacuum level of 100 mm Hg **(B)** at vacuum level of 200 mm Hg **(C)**.*

200 mm Hg (maximum preset value) and because of negative pressure in the system, the tubing is collapsed.

- *At point Z,* occlusion breaks and pumps start withdrawing fluid. At the same time, due to release of negative pressure, the tubing re-expands to the original size and momentarily due to withdrawl of extra fluid, the AFR exceeds the critical limit, bypassing the point 'T' (level of preset AFR of 25 cc/min) to point of 'O' (level of increased AFR) resulting in surge (represent of triangle of surge—TOS).

Effect on surge of decreasing AFR at constant vacuum

Figure 15.3.18B is the graphical representation when AFR is lowered from 25 cc/min to 12 cc/min to cope up with surge, with preset vacuum of 200 mm Hg. The graph can be explained as below:

- *From point X to Y,* is the time of no occlusion during which the ARF is 12 cc/min, much below the critical limit.
- *At point Y,* occlusion occurs, AFR becomes zero, vacuum builds up to 200 mm Hg (maximum preset) and tubing collapse by same amount as in the situation in Fig. 15.3.18A.
- *At point Z,* occlusion breaks and AFR increases and bypasses the preset value (12 cc/min) by similar amount as in the situation shown in Fig. 15.3.18A. The triangle of surge (TOS) is of the same size as in situation A due to similar amount of tubing collapse. But as still, the AFR remains below the critical limit and so surge is not encountered in situation B.

Effect on surge of decreasing the vacuum at constant AFR

Figure 15.3.18C is the graphical representa-tion, where vacuum is decreased from 200 to 100 mm Hg, but keeping the AFR 25 cc/min (same as in situation A). The interpretation of graph is as below:

- *From point X to Y,* is the time of no occlusion, during which AFR is in the safe limit (25 cc/min).
- *At point Y,* occlusion occurs, AFR becomes zero, vacuum builds up to 100 mm Hg (maximum preset value), tubing is collapsed but less than as occurs in situation A.

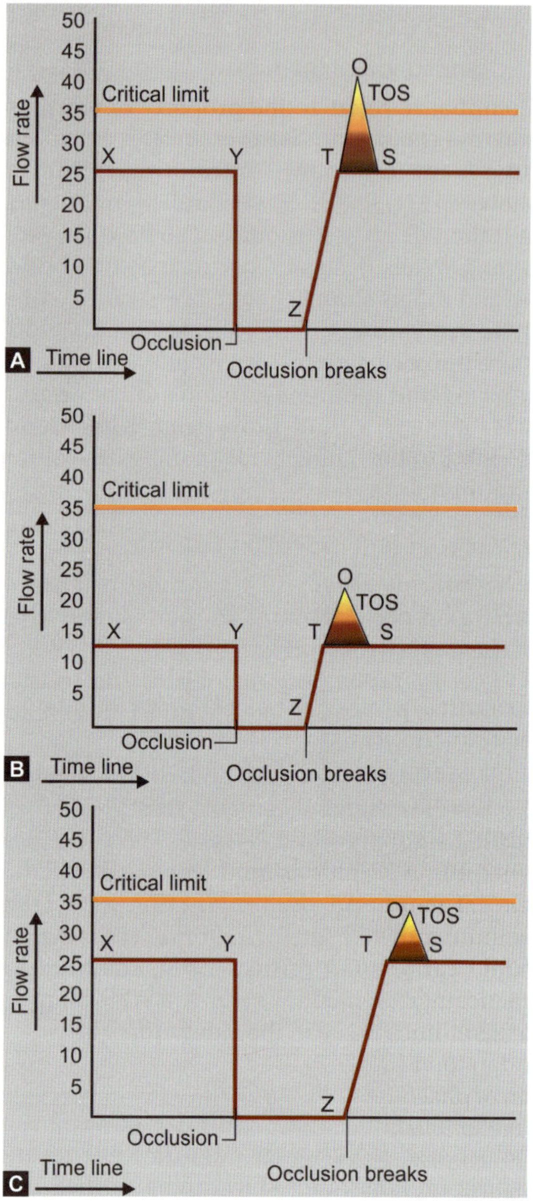

Fig. 15.3.18. *Graphic representation of relationship between vacuum, surge and aspiration flow rate:* ***(A)*** *Surge, equal to the triangle of surge (TOS), occurs at the break of occlusion;* ***(B)*** *Effect on surge of decreasing AFR at constant vacuum;* ***(C)*** *Effect on surge of decreasing the vacuum at constant AFR. For explanation see text.*

- *At point Z,* occlusion breaks, and AFR bypasses the preset value (25 cc/min) but is still near to critical limit; as the triangle of surge (TOS) is smaller due to comparatively lesser collapse of tubing in situation C as compared to situation A. Since AFR remains near the critical limit, surge is not encountered.

Conclusion

From the above graphical representation, it is quite clear that the surge encountered in situation A can be decreased by decreasing AFR (situation B) as well as by decreasing vacuum (situation C).

- *Decreasing AFR, decreases the surge,* but at the same time increases the rise time and makes the procedure slow. It will be logical to reduce the surge by decreasing AFR and not vacuum where holding power is required as in chopping and phacoaspiration of hard cataract.
- *Vacuum can be decreased to control the surge without decreasing AFR* in situations where firm hold is not required as in divide and conquer technique, phacoaspiration of soft cataract and removal of epinuclear plate.

3. Peristaltic versus venturi pump and surge

Peristaltic pump can independently control vacuum and AFR, and, therefore, theoretically should carry a lower risk of surge. However, this theoretical advantage of a flow pump is offset by the need of more compliant tubing than is required by a vacuum pump.

Venturi pump cannot independently control vacuum and AFR and, therefore, theoretically should carry a higher risk of surge. However, practically it is not so, and in a venturi system surge is encountered less often. This can be understood from the diagrammatic representation of phacodynamics of venturi pump as below (Fig. 15.3.19):

- *When foot pedal is at rest* in a venturi pump machine, i.e. when machine is off, the walls of the tubing are in their normal position (Fig. 15.3.19).
- *When foot pedal is pressed to position 2, and the tip is not occluded,* even at this stage, the maximum vacuum is built and there occurs some amount of collapse of tubing (say by amount M, Fig. 15.3.19B), as the negative pressure in the venturi is transmitted into the system without occlusion.
- *When foot pedal is in position 2, and the tip is occluded,* the vacuum will rise to maximum preset and an increased collapse of tubing to say up to amount N will take place (Fig. 15.3.19C).
- *When occlusion breaks,* the tubing will expand, but will still remain collapsed by an amount X as the machine is still on with negative pressure in the system as shown in Fig. 15.3.19B. Thus, on break of occlusion, only a small amount of fluid is aspirated, with triangle of surge (TOS) being small and AFR still remaining below the critical limit (Fig. 15.3.20A).
- *Surge in venturi system can be controlled by foot pedal.* As shown in Fig. 15.3.20B, when the foot pedal is kept between positions 1 and 2, i.e. at half way of the maximum vacuum preset, the AFR is markedly decreased (as AFR is indirectly controlled by vacuum in a venturi system) and thereby surge is decreased.

CONTROL OF SURGE

Someone has rightly said, ***"If there was no surge, anyone could have mastered the technique of phacoemulsification".*** Therefore, efforts are

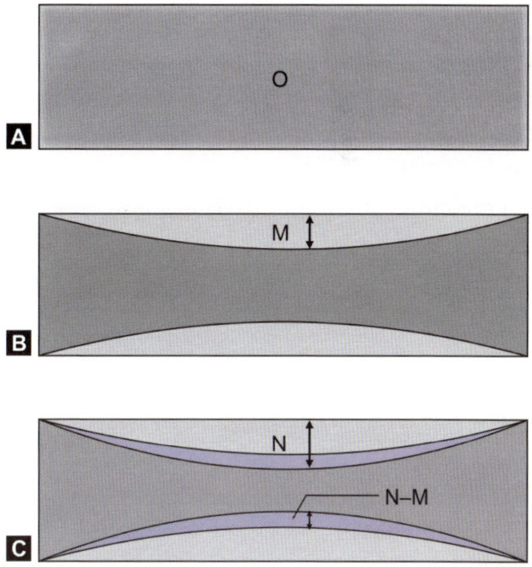

Fig. 15.3.19. *Effect of vacuum on tubing in a venturi pump: **(A)** Foot pedal position '0' – no vacuum and no collapse of tubing; **(B)** Foot pedal position 2–vacuum on without occlusion, collapse of tubing occurs up to 'M', as the negative pressure in venturi is transmitted into the system even without occlusion; **(C)** Foot pedal position 2 –vacuum rises to maximum preset with occlusion of tip and causes an increased collapse of tubing up to N.*

being made by the manufacturers of the machines to incorporate measures to control surge. Further, the measures are also suggested for the surgeons to learn, master and apply during the procedure.

A. Improvisation in the phaco machine to control surge

1. ***Efforts to reduce compliance in peristaltic pump machines.*** Advances in the peristaltic pump machines made to overcome the problem of compliance include the following:

i. *Use of biocompliant tubing,* i.e. a hybrid aspiration line tubing for example in Alcon Legacy and AMO machines), more compliant tubing is used only at the point of pump rollers and less compliant (more rigid) tubing is used over the much greater length between the pump and the handpiece to reduce potential surge problem.

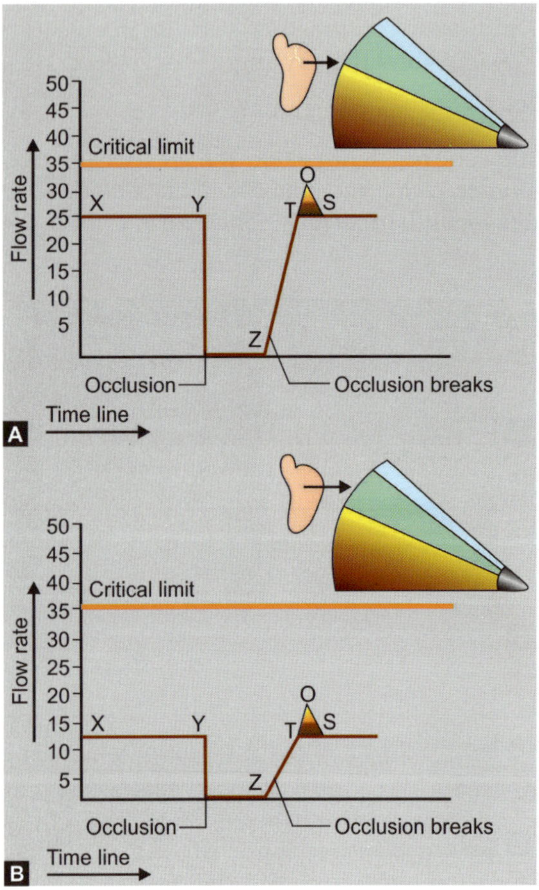

Fig. 15.3.20. *Graphic representation of relationship between vacuum, surge and aspiration flow rate (AFR) in a venturi pump: **(A)** Note the smaller triangle of surge (TOS) in a venturi pump on break of occlusion; **(B)** By decreasing vacuum; the AFR is indirectly decreased in a venturi pump which remains below the critical limit and thus there is no surge.*

ii. *Use of sealed rigid cassettes* with a stiff polymer membrane (over which the pump head rollers traverse, in place of tubing over rollers as in *Alcon's infiniti machines*), minimizes the compliance and maximizes the responsiveness.

iii. *Use of software control algorithms to compensate for leakage* increase volumetric efficiency (as in Bausch and Lomb's Advanced Flow System). Control over volumetric efficiency allows a greater ability to alter the character of machine from slow and gentle to fast and more aggressive, depending on surgeon's preference.

2. ***Efforts to increase inflow*** have also been made to control the surge. These include:

i. *High infusion phaco sleeve introduced by Alcon* which reduces surge by providing more inflow potential to keep the anterior chamber formed.

ii. *Second irrigation bottle* is used in the *Surgical Design* machine to control the surge.

3. ***Use of pressure transducer and logarithmically control of pump.*** Most modern peristaltic pumps logarithmically decrease the pump speed as the actual vacuum approaches the maximum vacuum preset. When the pressure transducer senses an occlusion break, there is delay in starting the pump by a second or so, as the speed is increased again logarithmically rather than abruptly. Since on break of occlusion, immediately pump is not working, so AFR is actually zero. Start of the pump is delayed till the expansion of the tubing is complete. This ensures that the fluid withdrawn by the re-expanding tubes is not added to the aspiration flow rate and thus remains within the safe limit.

The pressure transducer and related circuitry create a *model eye* that mirrors IOP and, therefore, chamber stability; the machines respond to inputs from their feedback mechanism in order to limit anterior chamber irritability during the procedure.

4. ***Venting.*** Venting mechanisms function by neutralizing the aspiration line vacuum between the pump (either peristaltic or venturi) and the occlusion at the aspiration tip (Fig. 15.3.21). Immediately after the occlusion breaks, the vent valve opens and the volume of the re-expanding collapsed tubing is filled either with air (*air-venting)* or fluid (*fluid-venting*), (Fig. 15.3.21C) thereby preventing the extra fluid being withdrawn from the anterior chamber and thus controlling the surge.

Note. Fluid-venting is superior to air-venting, since air is compressible and if it remains in the system, it increases the compliance of tubing and thus increases surge.

5. ***Smaller diameter tubings and phaco tips.*** Flared phaco tips and micro-flow 20 G phaco tips have an internal bore of 0.6 mm (Fig. 15.3.22A) as compared to 0.9 mm in the conventional tips (Fig. 15.3.22B). This restricts the flow and then prevents surge. The flared tip has a 19 G opening for a better grip with 20 G shaft for controlling the surge.

6. ***ABS tip (Alcon).*** This has a small bore in the side of the phaco tip shaft, which allows the

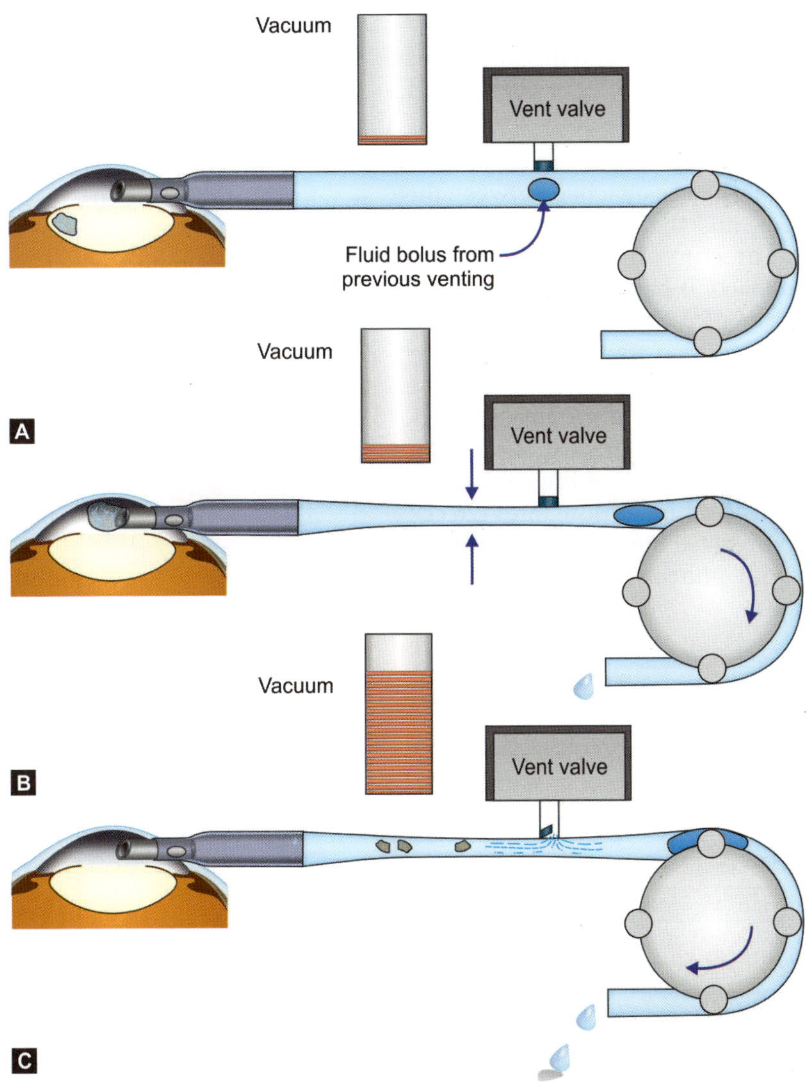

Fig. 15.3.21. *Venting (air or fluid) to prevent surge:* ***(A)*** *No occlusion, vent valve is closed, tubing normal, pump is rotating;* ***(B)*** *On occlusion, the vent valve remains closed, vacuum builds up and tubing is collapsed;* ***(C)*** *When occlusion breaks, the vent valve opens and the volume of re-expanding collapsed tubing is filled with air or fluid from the vent valve preventing withdrawal of fluid from the anterior chamber and thus preventing surge.*

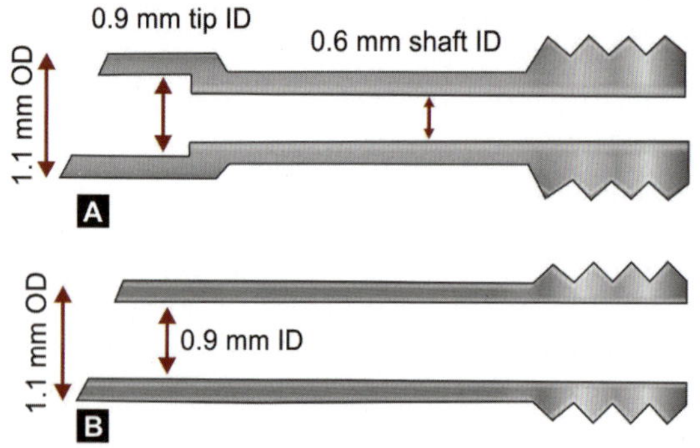

Fig. 15.3.22. *Internal bore of phaco tip: **(A)** Alcon flare tip (0.6 mm); **(B)** Standard 19 G phaco-tip (0.9 mm).*

irrigation fluid to be sucked into the shaft, thus preventing the surge (Fig. 15.3.23). The ABS tip cannot be used in micro-phako.

7. *Cruise control.* Cruise control is a disposable flow restrictor that can be attached between the phaco handpiece and the aspiration tubing. It can be used for conventional as well as microincision phaco. It has a flow restrictor of internal diameter of 0.3 mm which is placed behind a mesh filter that traps all the nucleus emulsified (Fig. 15.3.24). This prevents the narrow 0.3 mm lumen from getting clogged. This reduces surge, allowing the use of a regular phaco tip (maintaining the holding power). It also allows the use of higher flow rates (26 cc/min) and vacuums (400 mm Hg) as one would use with coaxial phaco. At 400 mm Hg of vacuum on occlusion break, momentary surges can reach between 200 and 300 cc/min. This device has practically no effect of surge on regular aspiration flow rates below 50 cc/min, making it an extremely useful tool in microincision phaco.

8. *Differential AFR and vacuum settings before and after occlusion.* Some machines have facilities for differential AFR and vacuum settings. Immediately after the occlusion breaks, the AFR and vacuum are decreased for a short period to prevent the surge. After the nuclear piece has been aspirated, the settings revert back to higher values to allow a better grip of the next nuclear piece.

B. Surgeon's measures to control surge

Undoubtedly, the various advances in the machines described above are helpful, it is ultimately up to the surgeon to take measures and to set parameters which optimizes a given machine for a given patient with regard to surge prevention.

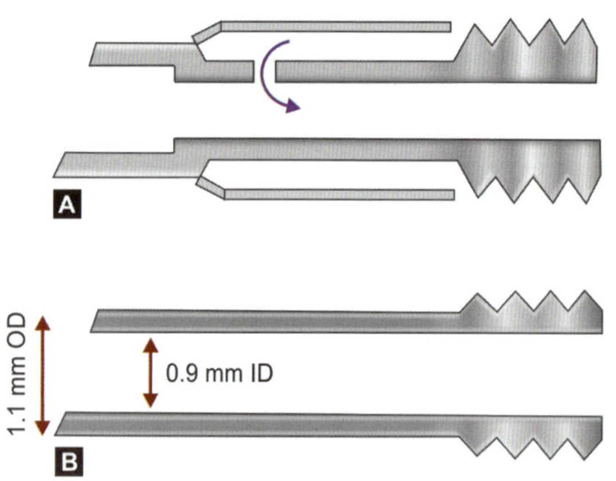

Fig. 15.3.23. *Alcon ABS tip vis-à-vis standard phaco tip: Note the bore in the side of ABS phacotip shaft which allows the irrigation fluid to be sucked into the shaft, thus preventing the surge **(A)** as compared to standard phaco tip with no side bone **(B).***

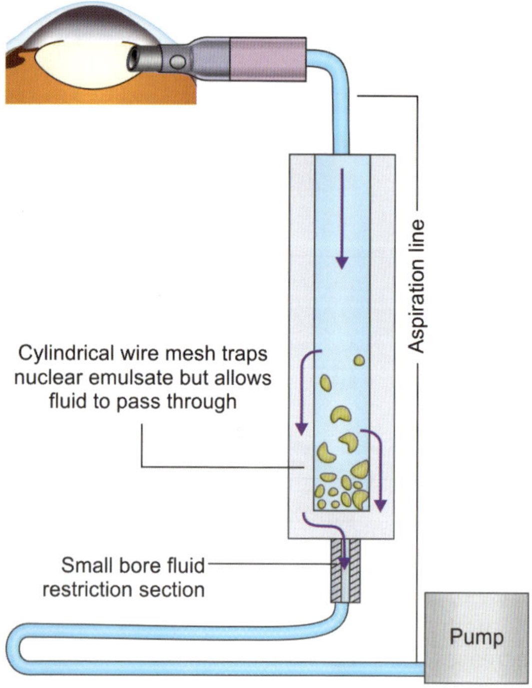

Fig. 15.3.24. *Cruise control attached between the phaco handpiece and the aspiration tubing to prevent surge. For mechanism of reducing surge, see text.*

1. ***Choices of hardware before starting surgery*** include:

i. *More resisitive phaco needle* (e.g. Bausch and Lomb Microflow or Alcon Flare tip)

ii. *More resistive tubing set* (e.g. Alcon Max Vac)

iii. *Inflow can be augmented* by using:
- Alcon high infusion sleeves
- Anterior chamber maintainer (ACM).

2. ***Proper wound construction*** by the surgeon is an essential step. Both the leaky or too tight wound can increase the surge. The optimum size of wound is 2.8–3 mm.

- *Leaky wound* disturbs the equilibrium of anterior chamber and a very small amount of fluid withdrawn on break of occlusion can cause surge.
- *Tight wound or long tunnel* reduces inflow and disturbs equilibrium of inflow versus outflow, leading to surge.

3. ***Manipulation of bottle height, and settings for AFR and vacuum.*** When the surgeon observes surge during nucleus emulsification, he may immediately take following steps:

- Raise the bottle height
- Lower the vacuum setting
- Decrease the AFR, as per requirement.

4. ***Partial occlusion of the tip*** with another nuclear fragment, before the occlusion breaks and the occluding piece is aspirated, is a smart step by the surgeon to ensure that any surge that occurs is used to draw the next piece to occlude the tip. Such manoeuvres are learned by experience.

5. ***Good foot control*** of the pedal by the surgeon is most important for controlling surge. Each surgeon should learn to swiftly lift the foot to bring the foot pedal at 1A position immediately before the occlusion is about to break. This will ensure that the handpiece goes on its own momentum without producing any surge, as the AFR is markedly decreased.

6. ***Use of viscoelastic substances (VES)*** such as 2% methylcellulose during fragment removal decreases the surge by decreasing the effective flow rate, as the viscous fluid increases the resistance and does not flow out easily. It is particularly useful to inflate the bag with VES when the last piece is being phaco aspirated.

SALIENT PHACODYNAMIC FEATURES OF SOME PHACO MACHINES

FEATURES OF ALCON INFINITI

Alcon has developed new features:

- ***NeoSonix technology.*** Standard ultrasonic phacoemulsification produces longitudinal forward to and fro movements. The NeoSonix technology produces rotational oscillations (clockwise-counterclockwise rotations) up to 2° at 120 Hz. A software upgrade for the Legacy phacoemulsification machine (Alcon) permits the use of NeoSonix technology without purchase of additional hardware.
- *Ozil torsional technology,* which incorporates a new handpiece capable of creating rotatory ultrasound movements of the phaco needle at 32 kilohertz (KHz) and longitudinal movements at 44 KHz is the most current upgrade. When combined with an angled phaco needle, these torsional movements create a side-to-side motion at the tip, enhancing the needle's cutting effectiveness with significantly reduced thermal energy generation. The to and fro movement at the tip allows emulsification on both excursions, with reduced repulsion of fragments, in contrast to longitudinal phacoemulsification.
- *More efficient use of power* results in less delivered energy and less heat, 2 of the goals of the new systems.

FEATURES OF BAUSCH AND LOMB MILLENNIUM

- *Unique foot pedal* of this machine features dual-linear independent control of both aspiration and phaco power.
- *High vacuum without commensurate phaco power* permits chopping, with reduced total phaco power delivered.
- *Custom control software (CCS)* allows a choice of 5 ultrasound modes (continuous, pulse, single-burst, fixed-burst, and multiple-burst). In pulse mode, up to 120 pulses per second (PPS) are possible.
- *Multiple burst setting* is capable of microburst [minimum 4 milliseconds (msec)], with a duty cycle limit that can be set to prevent continuous ultrasound even at full depression of the foot

pedal. These features have allowed this platform to be used for bimanual microphacoemulsification.

FEATURES OF SONIC WAVE PHACOEMULSIFICATION MACHINE (STAAR SURGICAL)

- *Sonic technology*, introduced by STAAR Surgical, operates at sonic frequency (40–400 Hz) as compared to standard ultrasonic frequency which is much higher (100–1000 times more). Sonic frequency produces less heat and tip does not produce cavitation effect.
- *High vacuum*, up to 650 mm Hg, is provided by *SuperVac tubing*. Higher vacuum permits nuclear dismantling with less power delivered during mechanical techniques such as chopping.
- *Auto-correlation mode*, i.e. ability to adjust vacuum as a function of ultrasound power is unique feature of this machine.
- *Surge control* is provided by the coiled SuperVac tubing. Continuous change in direction of flow through the coiled tubing increases resistance through the tubing at high flow rates such as upon clearance of occlusion of the tip. This effect only takes place at high flow rates (>50 cc/min). The fluid resistance of the SuperVac tubing increases as a function of flow and unoccluded flow is not restricted.
- *Cruise control chamber* allows sequestration of nuclear material from the aspiration line and reduces post-occlusion surge.

FEATURES OF SOVEREIGN (ALLERGAN) PHACOEMULSIFICATION MACHINE

Its features are:

- *WhiteStar ICE* (increased control and efficiency) is a new power modulation within ultrasonic phacoemulsification that virtually eliminates the production of thermal energy. Its main concept is to deliver a punch of higher phaco energy in the initial part of pulse. 'Punch' physically separates nuclear material from the phaco tip and allows for the creation of a 'microvoid' between the occluded tip and the nuclear material. The 'microvoid' allows fresh BSS to get between the phaco tip and the nuclear material. The fresh BSS interacts with the ultrasonic power to accelerate cavitational emulsification. Thus the efficiency of ultrasonic power is increased.
- *Digital ultrapulsing of ultrasound energy* feature of this machine allows the surgeon to select a duty cycle that allows sensitive control over the delivery of phaco power. By reducing the interval of phaco power delivery (micropulsing), the machine reduces total expanded energy and heat reduction.
- *WhiteStar CASE* (chamber stabilization environment) is another new advance in fluidics that dynamically enables surgeons to optimize fluidics by anticipating occlusion breaks. It proactively adjusts vacuum before occlusion break by reversing the pump to actively to step down vacuum. It reacts in as little as 26 milliseconds and significantly reduces chamber shallowing.
- *Marked reduction in heat* in this machine makes it useful for bimanual micro-phacoemulsification, which is an advanced technology in which the surgery is performed through a less than 2 mm incision.

PHACODYNAMIC FEATURES OF AN IDEAL PHACO MACHINE

I. Parameters

- It should have preset linear and pulse modes in phaco mode.
- It should have facility for preset vacuum and flow rate.
- A minimum vacuum range, between 0 and 201 mm Hg (desirable 0–400 mm Hg in the ultrasonic mode (US mode) to provide sufficient vacuum for phaco chop techniques).

II. Monitor display features

- The monitor should be provided with a panel display of parameters such as a phaco power, irrigation, aspiration, I/A minimum, I/A maximum, vacuum, flow rate, bottle height, etc.
- The monitor should display total phaco power and effective phaco power used to emulsify cataract.
- Monitor should display the error or any fault arising in the phaco machine.

III. Accessories

- Phaco machine should ideally have accessories for wet field diathermy and anterior vitrectomy.
- The machine should have the scope for re-usable tubing and cassettes.

IV. Facilities

- It should have a multifunction foot switch.
- Reflux facility should be present in the foot pedal to disengage capsule or iris from the aspiration tubing.
- The surgeon should be able to feed the memory with the parameters of at least phaco power, vacuum and flow rate to emulsify different density of cataracts.
- It is desirable to have an auditory feedback in a phaco machine. It can indicate different functions by auditory clues.
- It is desirable to have a remote control which can be kept in a sterile area to change the parameter during phacoemulsification.

15.4 PHACOEMULSIFICATION—SURGICAL STEPS

- Cleaning, draping and exposing the eye
- Side port incision
- Phaco wound construction
- Capsulorhexis
- Hydroprocedures
- Nucleotomy and phacoaspiration
- Epinuclear plate removal
- Cortical aspiration
- IOL implantation

CLEANING, DRAPING AND EXPOSING THE EYE

After thoroughly cleaning the lids with 10% povidone iodine and irrigating the conjunctival sac with 5% povidone iodine solution, the eye to be operated is meticulously draped with sterile disposable drape and is exposed by applying the universal eye speculum.

SIDE PORT INCISION

Purposes of making side port incision include:

- *Injection of viscoelastic* to maintain and pressurize the anterior chamber.
- Performing capsulorhexis with the help of a cystitome or fine capsulorhexis forceps.
- *Stabilisation of globe* during surgery.
- *Introduction of chopper/Sinskey hook* for chopping and for manipulation of nucleus.
- *Introduction of second instrument* (round iris repositor/Sinskey hook) to protect the posterior capsule during phacoemulsification.
- *Irrigation and aspiration* of cortical matter.

Location of side port incision, on left side of main incision for right handed surgeon, varies depending on the technique of nucleotomy to be performed as below.

- *For divide and conquer and central chop,* the side port incision should preferably be made 3 o' clock away from the main incision.
- *For peripheral chop,* the preferred position should be 2 o' clock hours away from the main incision. However, this position makes removal of subincisional cortex tougher through side port incision.
- *Two side port incisions,* when made the second should be 180° apart from the first, which is about 2–3 o'clock hours to the left of main incision.

Advantages of two side ports are as below:

- *Good anterior chamber stability* with a few capsular folds and less risk of tear.
- *Easier to grasp cortical matter* in a formed capsular bag.
- *Less risk of iris touch* during manipulation.
- *Ability to crush the epinucleus and small nuclear fragments* between the two instruments.
- *Capsular polishing* becomes safe and easy.

Size of side port incision is usually equal to 1 to 1.5 mm square tunnel. If using bimanual irrigation/aspiration (I/A), the incision should be less in width.

- *An optimal size tunnel* allows a free instrument movement with minimal leak.
- *A tight tunnel* makes entry of instrument difficult and there occurs localised corneal whitening or oedema.
- *A large tunnel* results in iris prolapse and unstable chamber.

Technique. The side port incision is made with the help of a sharp pointed (always check the tip) 15° blade/MVR blade. The incision should be made inside the clear cornea, parallel to the iris surface (Fig. 15.4.1). A counterpressure may be applied with the help of a 270° fixation ring or a toothed forceps/chopper. Under topical anaesthesia, the muscle tone obviates the need for stabilisation of the globe.

Note. Some surgeons prefer to make side port incision after making the main phaco wound.

PHACO WOUND CONSTRUCTION

'Well begin is half done'—is very true for phacoemulsification. Phaco wounds in vouge are of three types:

1. Sclerocorneal tunnel incision,
2. Limbal-corneal tunnel incision
3. Clear corneal tunnel incision.

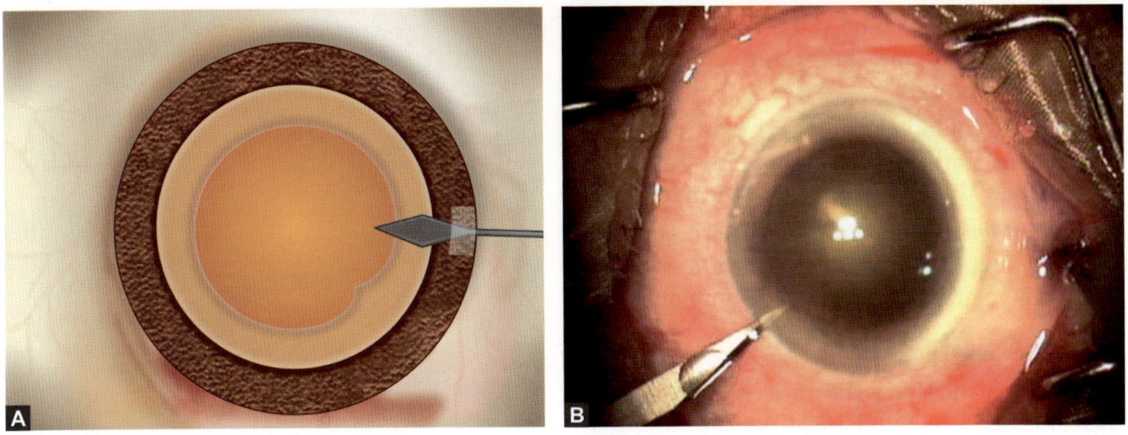

Fig. 15.4.1. Techniques of making side port incision.

SCLEROCORNEAL TUNNEL INCISION

Sclerocorneal tunnel incision is usually preferred when non-foldable (PMMA) IOL is to be implanted. Width of incision about 3–3.5 mm (1.5 mm scleral part + 1.5–2 mm corneal part) and the length need to be enlarged to 5.5 mm before IOL implantation. Some surgeons still prefer sclerocorneal tunnel (3.5 mm × 3.5 mm in size) even for foldable IOL.

Technique of making sclerocorneal tunnel incision is the same as described for SICS (*see* pages 196–197 and Figs 14.3, 14.4 and 14.7).

Advantages of sclerocorneal incision include:

- Less astigmatism
- Less chances of infection due to wound being covered by conjunctiva
- Early healing and stabilisation of wound due to vascular scleral part of the incision.

Disadvantages include:

- Cannot be performed under topical anaesthesia.
- Longer time and greater precision are required.
- Bleeding may be troublesome sometimes.
- Instrumental manipulation is difficult due to wider tunnel.
- Iris prolapse may occur during instrumental manipulation.

LIMBAL TUNNEL INCISION

***Technique of limbal tunnel incision involves three steps** (Fig. 15.4.2):*

- *An external vertical groove* about 3.2 mm in length is made in the anterior limbal area about 0.5 mm behind the edge of the vascular arcade with the help of a razor blade or no. 11 or no. 15 blade.
- *Limbal–corneal tunnel* of about 2–2.5 mm width is then dissected with the help of a crescent blade.

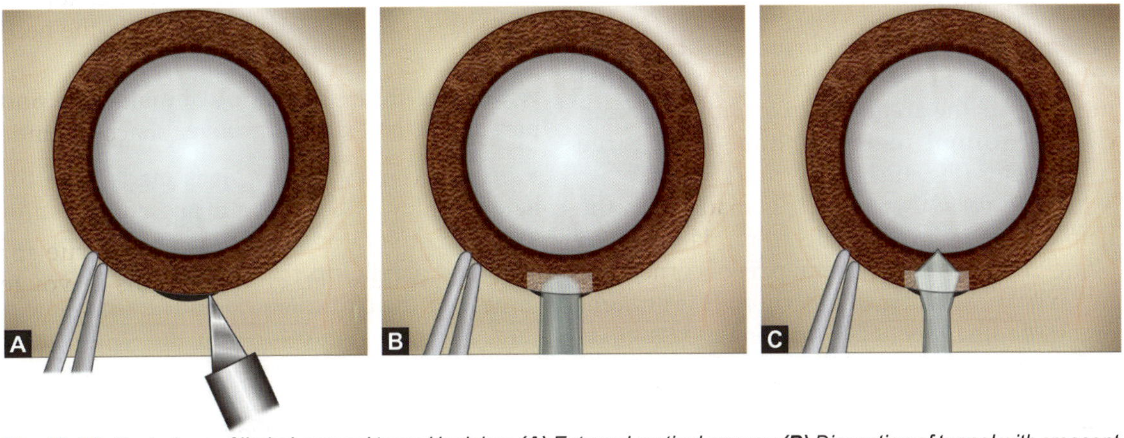

Fig. 15.4.2. Technique of limbal-corneal tunnel incision: **(A)** External vertical groove; **(B)** Dissection of tunnel with crescent blade; **(C)** Internal corneal wound with sharp-tipped keratome.

- *Internal corneal incision* is then made with the help of 2.8–3.2 mm keratome, entering the anterior chamber.

Advantages include less astigmatism and early healing, as limbal incision provides a wider tunnel and valve than the clear corneal incision.

Disadvantages include ballooning of conjunctiva and bleeding into the anterior chamber when incision is enlarged prior to the IOL implantation.

CLEAR CORNEAL INCISION

Clear corneal incision is the most commonly used incision for phacoemulsification with foldable IOL implantation because of following advantages.

Advantages

- No need of conjunctival flap.
- No need of cautery and no bleeding while extending the incision.
- Can be performed under topical anaesthesia and takes less time.
- Instrumental manipulation is easy.
- No distortion of cornea with phaco handpiece and no compromisation in the view of intraocular structures.

Technique

Clean corneal incisions are of three types (Fig. 15.4.3):

- Triplanar clear corneal incision
- Biplanar clear corneal incision
- Uniplanar clear corneal incision.

Triplanar clear corneal incision

Technique for triplanar clear corneal incision (Fig. 15.4.3A) is similar to triplanar limbal incision, i.e. the architecture of triplanar clean corneal tunnel incision consists of three components (Fig. 15.4.2):

- *External vertical groove.* It is made with the help of either a razor blade, or no. 11 or no. 15 blade in the most peripheral part of cornea just in front of conjunctival insertion. It is straight and its depth is about 500 microns and length is 3–3.5 mm.
- *Corneal tunnel.* It is made with the help of a crescent knife and should be about 1.75 mm in width. Its inner lip should be straight and parallel to the external groove.

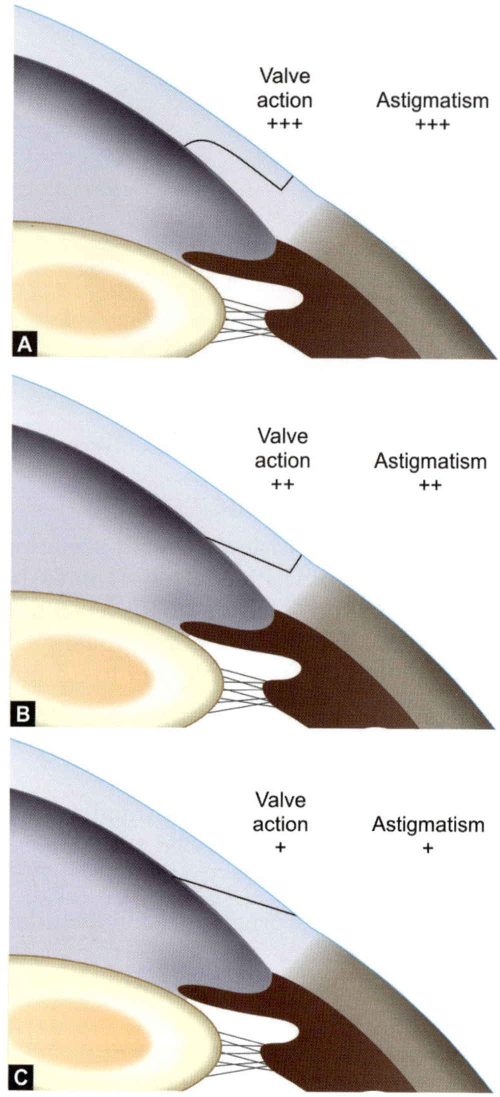

Fig. 15.4.3. *Types of corneal incisions:* ***(A)*** *Triplanar;* ***(B)*** *Biplanar;* ***(C)*** *Uniplanar.*

- *Internal corneal incision.* It is made with the help of a sharp 2.8 or 3.2 mm angled keratome. The heel of keratome is raised until the blades becomes parallel to the iris plane resulting in dimple of the corneal surface. The keratome is then advanced anteriorly in the same plane untill the anterior chamber is entered and the internal wound is visualised as a straight line parallel to the external groove. During extension, care should be taken to keep it in the same plane. Any tilt or too much backward cutting may result in a smiling, frown-shaped or S-shaped incision which may not be self-sealing. Therefore, it is desirable to cut while moving forward so that the cuts in the Descemet's membrane are uniform and in one line.

Advantages of triplanar are that it is well controlled with an exellent self-sealing valve.

Disadvantages are that it takes sligtly more time to make and requires additional instru-ments (crescent knife and razor blade.)

Biplanar incision

Technique. For biplanar clear corneal incision (Fig. 15.4.3B), after making the initial external groove, with the help of a razor blade, a 1.75 mm corneal tunnel and internal corneal incision are made with the help of 2.8 or 3.2 mm keratome (crescent knife is not used).

Advantage is that valve action is as effective as triplanar and additional instrument (crescent knife) is not required.

Disadvantages are that chances of premature entry and torn edges are more.

Uniplanar or single plane valvular stab corneal incision (Fig. 15.4.3C)

It should be avoided by beginners. In fact, it is recommended for expert hands only.

Technique. A direct valvular corneal stab incision is made with the help of 2.8 or 3.2 mm keratome. The external incision should be at the most peripheral part of cornea and the internal corneal incision about 1.75–2 mm internal and parallel to external corneal incision.

Modified triplanar or three step corneal incision

It is nowadays more popular (Fig. 15.4.4).

Technique. It is made with the help of a very sharp steel keratome or diamond knife 2.8–3.2 mm in size as below:

- *Vertical stab* in the cornea, at the site of external incision, is made with keratome keeping it perpendicular to the cornea (Fig. 15.4.4A).
- *Corneal tunnel* (about 1.75 mm in width) is then made with the same keratome by rotating it horizontally and keeping parallel to the corneal lamellae (Fig. 15.4.4B).
- *Internal corneal incision* is also made with the same keratome by rotating it vertically to make it parallel to the iris plane resulting in a dimple of the corneal surface (Fig. 15.4.4C). The keratome is then advanced anteriorly in the same plane until the anterior chamber is entered and the internal wound is visualised as a straight line (Fig. 15.4.4D).

Note. It is best to make external groove incision with razor blade and then complete the corneal tunnel and internal incision as described above.

SUPERIOR VERSUS TEMPORAL INCISION

Superior incision

Advantages

- Surgeon's hand can rest on patients's forehead.
- Incision is underneath the upper lid and causes less discomfort.

Disadvantages

- Orbital edge impairs access for the surgical field, specially so in deep set eyes.
- More surgically induce astigmatism.

Temporal incision

More advantages than disadvantages have made the temporal incision a preference for phacoemulsification.

Advantages

- *Less induced astigmatism,* as the distance of temporal corneal periphery from the visual axis is longest, so flattening around the incision is less likely to cause flattening at the visual axis. Further, pre-existing against-the-rule astigmatism is more common in elderly patients.
- *Access to surgical field is good,* as the superior orbital margin and eyebrows do not hinder surgery specially so in deep set eyes.
- *Bell's phenomenon* does not pose problem, under topical anaesthesia.
- *Glaucoma filtration bleb* or future trabeculectomy site is not compromised.
- *Natural drainage of irrigating fluid,* as the lateral canthel angle is directly behind the incision.
- *Less chances of locking of instruments* in the temporal approach.

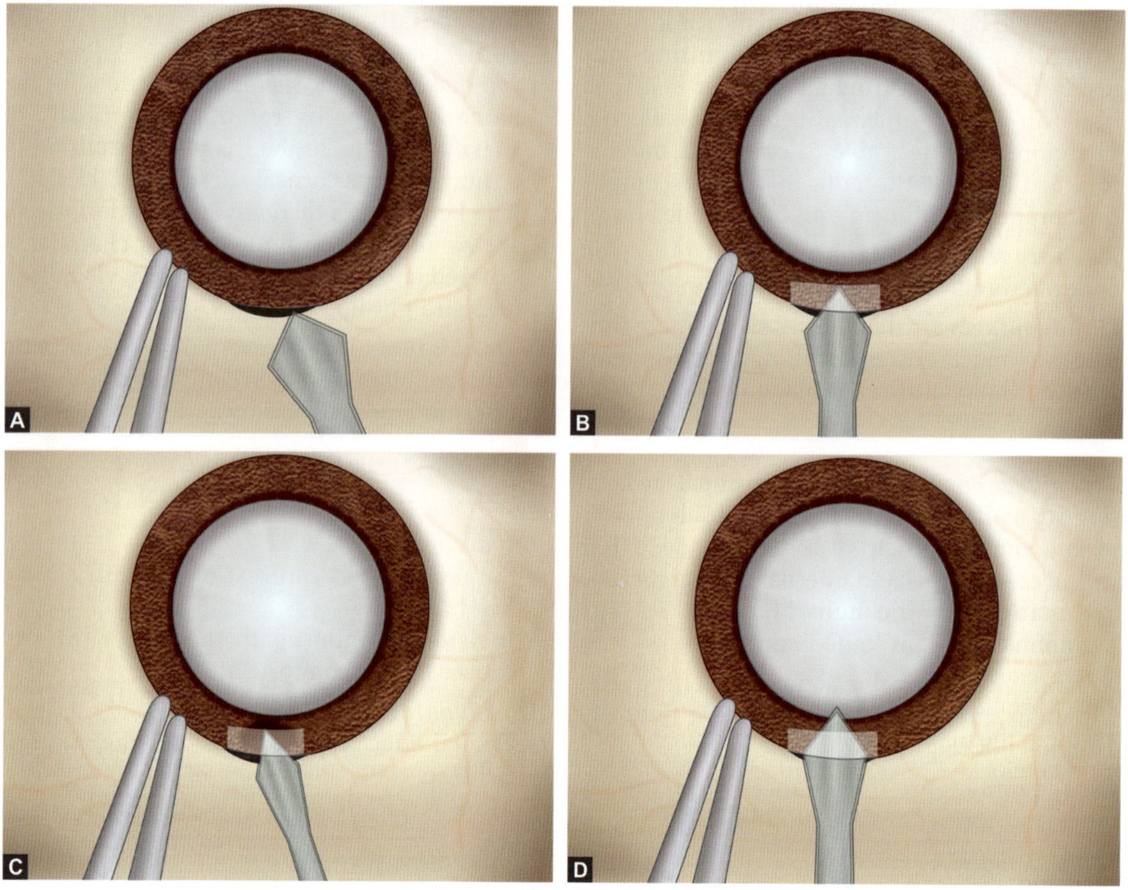

Fig. 15.4.4. *Technique of making modified triplanar or three step corneal incision:* ***(A)*** *Vertical cut in cornea about 300–500 μ deep with 3.2 keratome;* ***(B)*** *Corneal tunnel with the same 3.2 keratome;* ***(C)*** *Vertical rotation of same keratome at the site of internal corneal wound (note the dimple on the corneal surface);* ***(D)*** *Internal corneal incision with the same keratome.*

- *Red reflex* is comparatively better in temporal approach.

Disadvantages

- Tendency of the patient for turning the head away from the surgeon.
- Tendency for the eye to roll nasally by the phaco handpiece.
- Frequent change in the set up for the right and left eyes of the patients.
- Theoretically more chances of discomfort and infection than superior incision which is protected underneath the upper eyelid.

CAPSULORHEXIS

ADVANTAGES

A continuous curvilinear capsulorhexis (CCC) placed in the centre of the anterior capsule is a most important step in the phacoemulsifi-cation because of the following advantages:

- *Ensures safe endocapsular surgery and hydrodissection,* as the rhexis is strong and resistant to stretching.
- *Permits insertion of posterior chamber IOL,* even in the event of posterior capsule tear and vitreous loss.
- *Allows quick removal of cortical lens matter* as there are no flaps.
- *Helps to centralize the IOL properly.*
- *Eliminates complications* like uveitis–glaucoma–hyphema (UGH) syndrome and pigment dispersal.

TECHNIQUE OF CCC

Technique of CCC is described in the Chapter 14 on 'Manual Small Incision Cataract Surgery', pages 210–203.

Size of CCC in phacoemulsification varies between 5 and 6 mm. Ideally, the CCC should cover the optic of the IOL by 0.25 mm circumferentially. This presses IOL optic against the posterior capsule and this reduces chances of opacification of posterior capsule and keeps the IOL well centred. Harder cataracts would require larger rhexis opening.

HYDROPROCEDURES AND NUCLEAR ROTATION

HYDROPROCEDURES

See pages 203–205.

NUCLEAR ROTATION

Technique. After cortical cleaning hydrodissection, it becomes easy to rotate the nucleus. For nucleus rotation, anterior chamber is pressurised with OVD and rotation can be done by one-hand or two-hand technique.

- *One-hand technique.* With the help of a Sinskey hook, applied near the margin of capsulorhexis through the main incision, the nucleus is gently rotated clockwise or anticlockwise (Fig. 15.4.5). A rotation by 2–3 o'clock hours is sufficient to ensure free mobility.
- *Two-hand technique* allows more controlled rotation with comparatively less risk of zonular dehiscence. The two Sinskey hooks or a hook and a chopper or a hook and phaco tip can be used for bimanual rotation. The two instruments should be applied (through two paracentesis or a paracentesis and a main incision) and should be pushed towards each other to get a grip on the nucleus. To rotate the nucleus, the two instruments should be moved in opposite direction taking counterpressure from each other (Fig. 15.4.6).

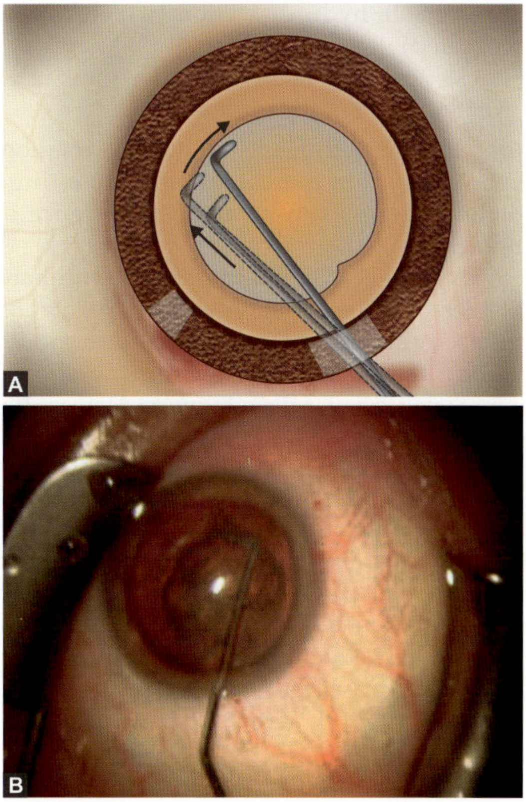

Fig. 15.4.5. *One-hand technique of nucleus rotation.*

Difficulty in rotation of the nucleus may occur due to:

- Soft nucleus (where rotation is not essential)

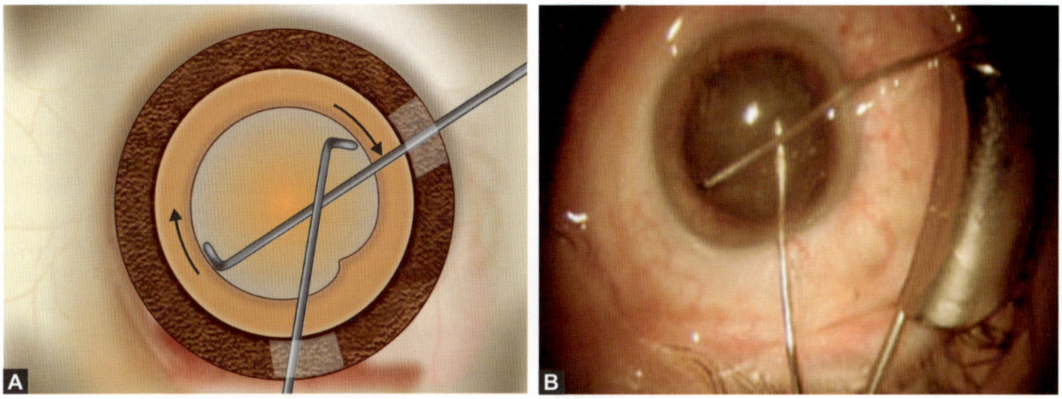

Fig. 15.4.6. *Two-hand technique of nuclear rotation.*

- Inadequate hydrodissection (which can be repeated)
- Loose zonules which can cause the bag to rotate instead of the nucleus.

Note. In case of difficulty in nucleus rotation, always look for the cause, never continue rotation aggressively to avoid dehiscence of zonules.

- *Special care* is required in patients with hard cataract, pseudoexfoliation, and where rotation has been difficult. In such cases, one should perform the rotation very gently and should immediately reverse the rotation to decrease the torsional stretch on the zonules.

NUCLEOTOMY

Aim of nucleotomy and phacoemulsification is to remove the lens (9–10 mm diameter) through a small incision (2.8–3 mm) without damaging the adjacent structures. The technique and parameters vary according to the density of the nucleus.

TERMINOLOGY OF CERTAIN MANOEUVRES DURING NUCLEOTOMY

Certain surgical manoeuvres, which are common in different procedures of nucleotomy, are described briefly.

Sculpting

Sculpting refers to the process of debulking the cataractous nucleus. It is accomplished by shaving action of the phaco tip, which is never occluded during the manoeuvre.

Indications. Sculpting manoeuvre is required during following steps of nucleotomy:

- *Trenching,* i.e. formation of deep groove in the centre of nucleus.
- *Crater formation,* i.e. debulking of the most of the anterior part of the central nucleus, forming a remaining bowel of posterior part of nucleus with a peripheral nuclear rim.

Nucleofractis

Nucleofractis, the term coined by Howard V. Gimbel in 1985, refers to divide and fragment the dense nucleus rim after sculpting all that can be safely sculpted. The nucleofractis, also known as *fracturing* or *cracking* the nucleus, is being used in many different techniques of phacoemulsification.

Phaco chop

Phaco chop refers to technique of splitting the nucleus into pieces with the help of the instrument called chopper, after impaling the nucleus with phaco tip.

EVOLUTION OF TECHNIQUES OF NUCLEOTOMY (PHACOEMULSIFICATION)

Since the introduction of phacoemulsification by Kelman in 1967, the procedure has been modified over the years by the masters in the field. Virtually at present there are as many techniques as the masters in the field. Many of the older techniques are not being used nowadays. However, for a broader prospective, it will be worthwhile to review the various techniques evolved over the time, which can be grouped as below:

- Anterior chamber phacoemulsification
- Pupillary plane phacoemulsification
- Supracapsular phacoemulsification
- Posterior chamber phacoemulsification
- Endocapsular or in the bag phacoemulsification.

Note. The above classifications and their discription given below are just of historical interest to know the evolution of techniques of phacoemulsification. All present day techniques are endocapsular and other techniques are obsolete; ***so, presently the term phacoemulsification is synonymous with endocapsular techniques.***

I. ANTERIOR CHAMBER PHACOEMULSIFICATION (KELMAN'S TECHNIQUE, 1970)

Kelman's original technique consisted of prolapsing the nucleus into anterior chamber with the help of irrigating cystitome after performing wide anterior christmas tree capsulotomy. The nucleus then was emulsified starting from superior pole, i.e. at 12 o'clock position. Therefore, it was also called ***single-handed phacoemulsification*** technique. However, several factors (mainly being the damage to corneal endothelium) limited the universal application of Kelman phacoemulsification as the procedure of choice for cataract extraction. Anyhow, Kelman had set the stage for further refinement of his invention.

II. PUPILLARY PLANE PHACOEMULSIFICATION (LITTLE'S TECHNIQUE, 1975)

This technique, initiated by Little in 1975 and Kartz in 1976, was adapted and popularized by Malony who taught it to many surgeons. In this technique, emulsification occurs halfway between corneal endothelium and the posterior capsule, there by reducing the risk of damage to other structures. This technique involves use of both hands and so began the era of ***two-handed technique of nuclear disassembly***—the concept which still continues.

Salient features of the Little's technique

Phaco handpiece is introduced through the main incision and a spatula through the side port incision made 3 o'clock hours to the left of main incision. This technique consists of four basic stages:

- *Central sculpting in situ.* After making a wide anterior capsulotomy, the central nucleus is not mobilised, i.e. remains connected to the cortex, then part of the nucleus is emulsified leaving behind a thin saucer-shaped nuclear plate.
- *Subluxation of the nucleus on the pupillary plane, i.e. separation of nuclear plate* from the cortex is than done with the help of the cyclodialysis spatula and the equator of nuclear plate is lifted up to the pupillary plane.
- *Equatorial fragmentation* is then completed with phaco tip by rotating the nuclear plate in the pupillary plane.
- *Fragmentation of the central remaining nucleus* is then carried out.

III. SUPRACAPSULAR PHACOEMULSIFICATION

This technique involves prolapse of nucleus after anterior capsulotomy and then repositing the nucleus on the top of anterior capsule remanants (as suggested by Malony) or leaving a pole anterior to the iris (as recommended by David Browr). Theoretically, this approach was supposed to reduce the stress on the zonules during nuclear manipulation. The nucleus was managed by 'two-handed technique'. This technique involved greater chances of aspirating and damaging the iris in the phaco tip.

IV. POSTERIOR CHAMBER PHACOEMULSIFICATION (MALONEY'S TECHNIQUE, 1988)

Though numerous workers had contributed to this technique, but it was Maloney who popularised it in 1988.

Salient features of Maloney's technique

In this technique, most of the nucleus is emulsified in the posterior chamber. This technique involved following steps:

- Preliminary steps
- Central sculpting with ultrasonic power
- Mobilisation of the nucleus
- Emulsification of the residual plate

Preliminary steps included:

- Conjunctival flap and haemostasis
- Sclerocorneal tunnel incision
- Can-opener anterior capsulotomy.

Central sculpting of about 70% of the nuclear mass was then performed with phacoemulsification using 30° tip, converting the nucleus into a deep and wide bowel.

Mobilisation of the nucleus. The remaining bowel of the nucleus was then mobilised mechanically using the phaco tip and a cyclodialysis spatula.

Phacoemulsification of the residual nucleus. The equatorial part of the nucleus was then emulsified by simultaneously rotating the nucleus. Once the equatorial part was emulsified, the central remaining plate of the nucleus was then emulsified in the posterior chamber.

Note. The above technique represents the end of evolution of traditional phacoemulsification associated with traditional anterior capsulotomy.

V. ENDOCAPSULAR PHACOEMULSIFICATION TECHNIQUE

This technique became popular in late 1980s and early 1990s. The success of the technique involved technological advances in the phacoemulsification machines as well as few other simultaneous surgical innovations such as:

- Self-sealing corneal incision
- Capsulorhexis
- Hydrodissection
- Implantation of the foldable IOLs.

Endocapsular phacoemulsification became popular because of reduced risk of damage to the corneal endothelium as well as the iris tissue.

Classification of the endocapsular techniques

Various endocapsular techniques evolved over the period can be classified as below.

A. *Endocapsular techniques without nucleofracture*

1. One-handed endocapsular phacoemulsification (Shepherd's technique)
2. Intercapsular technique

3. Two-handed endocapsular phacoemulsification (cut and suck technique)
4. Chip and flip technique.

B. *Endocapsular techniques with mixed nuclear fracture (cracking)*
1. Divide and conquer technique
   - Crater divide and conquer (CDC)
   - Trench divide and conquer (TDC)
   - Trench divide and conquer with down slop sculpting
2. Shepherd's in situ fracture
3. Maloney and Dillman's fractional 2:4 phacoemulsification
4. Crack and flip technique

C. *Endocapsular techniques with pure nucleofracture*
1. Phaco chop
2. Lens quake
3. Pre-chopping

SURGICAL TECHNIQUES OF PHACOEMULSIFICATION

From the discription of evolution of phacoemulsification, it is quite clear that all present day techniques are endocapsular phacoemulsification. Therefore, in further discussion, the term phacoemulsification will be used as synonymous with endocapsular phacoemulsification. Present day techniques of phacoemulsification are described below.

A. PHACOEMULSIFICATION TECHNIQUES WITHOUT NUCLEOFRACTURE

All these techniques involve emulsification of the nucleus while working entirely within the capsular bag without performing nucleofracture. ***These techniques are not used presently*** but are described briefly below as apart of the evolution of phacoemulsification technique.

1. One-handed endocapsular phacoemulsification (Shepherd's technique)

This technique suites soft to moderately hard cataracts and involves:
- *Central sculpting* in the capsular bag after hydrodissection.
- *Emulsification of equatorial nucleus* is then carried out by freely rotating the nucleus. The peripheral part of nucleus is captured in occlusion at 6 o'clock position and gently pulled towards centre and emulsified. The same procedure is repeated by further rotating the nucleus till all the peripheral part of the nucleus is emulsified.
- *Removal of the residual nuclear plate* is then carried out at the centre of capsular bag.

2. Intercapsular phacoemulsification (Michelsiar and Kara technique)

In this technique, emulsification of nucleus is carried out through a very small capsulorhexis which is just big enough to comfortably accommodate the tip of phacoemulsifier. It is suited for nucleus of grade I and grade II hardness.

3. Two-handed endocapsular phacoemulsification (Cut and Suck technique)

Salient features of this technique are:
- *Distal central sculpting* is performed after CCC and hydrodissection.
- *Peripheral part (equator of nucleus)* is then emulsified after rotating the nucleus.
- *Residual nuclear plate* is than emulsified by bringing the piece towards tip with spatula in the second hand.

4. Chip and flip technique

The technique introduced by Dr. Howard Fine was considered ideal for cataracts of medium-low hardness (grades II–III). After CCC (Fig. 15.4.7A), hydroidssection (Fig. 15.4.7B) and hydrodelineation, the nucleus is managed as below:
- *Central sculpting* is carried out to remove about 70% of the central nucleus mass (Fig. 15.4.7C).
- *Equatorial nucleus* is then emulsified at 6 o'clock position by slowly rotating the nucleus clockwise (Fig. 15.4.7D). In this way by trimming the peripheral rim, the inner nuclear bowl is converted into a 'chip'.
- *Separation of nuclear chip* from the epinucleus is then carried out with the help of spatula and the chip is elevated into the centre of capsular bag, (Fig. 15.4.7E) and is then emulsified (Fig. 15.4.7F).
- *Flipping and removal of epinucleus.* The epinuclear bowl is then displaced from the capsular fornix at 5–6 o'clock using the phaco tip, in aspiration mode only. The epinuclear bowl is loosened by pulling the rim at 5–6

o'clock towards 12 o'clock and pushing with the second instrument in the bottom of epinuclear bowl towards 5–6 o'clock in an attempt to tumble the soft centre nuclear bowl (Fig. 15.4.7G and H). By *flipping the bowl* away from the posterior capsule, it can be removed softly either with aspiration or low power of emulsification.

B. PHACOEMULSIFICATION TECHNIQUES WITH MIXED NUCLEAR FRACTURE

All mixed techniques of nuclear fracture include the following steps:

- Creation of a groove with sculpting
- Nucleofracture mechanically
- Capture, emulsification phacoaspiration of the fragments.

Mixed techniques of nucleofracture include:

- Divide and conquer method which may be:
  - Trench divide and conquer
  - Crater divide and conquer
  - Trench divide and conquer with down slop sculpting
- Shepherd in situ fracture
- Maloney and Dillman's fractional 2:4 phacoemulsification
- Crack and flip technique.

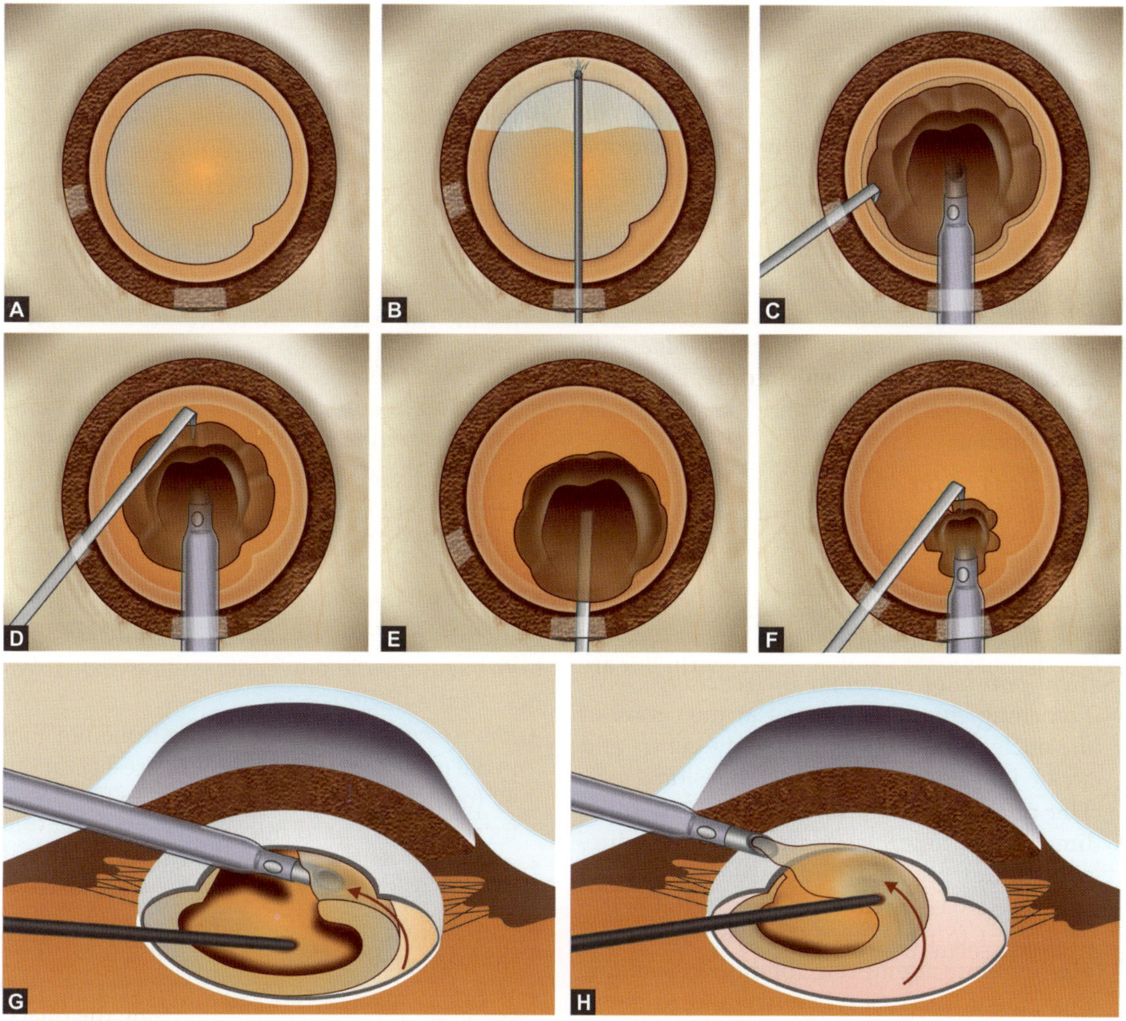

Fig. 15.4.7. *Chip and flip technique of phacoemulsification:* ***(A)*** *Capsulorhexis;* ***(B)*** *Hydrodissection;* ***(C)*** *Central sculpting;* ***(D)*** *Phacoemulsification of equatorial nucleus at 6 o'clock position by slow rotation;* ***(E)*** *Separation of nuclear chip from the epinucleus;* ***(F)*** *Slow emulsification of nuclear chip;* ***(G)*** *Flipping of epinucleus;* ***(H)*** *Phacoaspiration of flipped epinucleus.*

DIVIDE AND CONQUER NUCLEOFRACTURE TECHNIQUE

This technique, introduced by Howard V. Gimbel in 1986, includes two variations to deal with different types of cataracts:

- *Trench divide and conquer* for soft to moderately hard nucleus
- *Crater divide and conquer* for moderattly hard to very hard and even dense brunescent nucleus.

Trench divide and conquer technique

Steps of nucleus management with this technique include:

- Deep maltease cross-trenching,
- Fracture of the nucleus in four quadrants, and
- Phacoemulsification of each quadrant.

1. *Trenching*

A deep malteese cross-trench is made in the capsulorhexis zone of the nucleus (Fig. 15.4.8A to D).

Machine parameters recommended are as below:

- *Vacuum (low):* 25 ± 5 mm Hg
- *Flow rate:* 24–26 cc/min
- *Power depending upon the grade of hardness:* 40 for grade I, add 10 for each grade, i.e. 50 for grade II, 60 for grade III, and 70 for grade IV hard nucleus.

Dimensions of the trench should be:

- *Length:* 4–5 mm in the zone of capsulorhexis.
- *Width:* 2 tip diameter to accommodate the sleeve.
- *Depth:* Sculpting should be continued till red glow is visible in the trench.

Salient points of technique of trenching

- Trenching should be started at the centre of the nucleus or just proximal to the centre and created up to CCC in the cross-incisional axis. The nucleus should than be rotated three times, every time 90° and the same procedure should be repeated to complete the deep malteese cross-trench (Fig. 15.4.8A to D). It is important to pressurize the eye with visco-elastic before attempting rotation to facilitate movement, increase visibility and to avoid damage to the zonules.
- 30° U/S tip should be preferred for trenching, and the sculpting should be done by a shaving action movement without occluding the tip. On the return stroke, the foot pedal should be at position 1 (only irrigation). In systems with continuous irrigation mode (CIM), one can in fact take the foot off the pedal.
- End point of trenching is just visibility of the red reflex.

2. *Splitting of nucleus (nucleofracture)*

The splitting (fracture) of nucleus first into two parts and then each half into two quadrants each can be done by using two instruments (either the phacoprobe and a chopper or two choppers Sinskey hooks).

Salient features of technique of nucleofracture

- The two instruments used for splitting should be kept as deep as possible in the trench (Fig. 15.4.9A and B) and not superficially, which is wrong position (Fig. 15.4.9C and D).
- The two instruments must be kept very close to each other both vertically as well as horizontally (Fig. 15.4.9A and B).
- The split should be initiated in the periphery by applying opposing forces and then moving the instruments toward the centre to complete the split (Fig. 15.4.8E to H).

3. *Phacoemulsification of nuclear fragments (quadrants)*

After the nucleus is divided into four quadrants, each fragment is then removed by phacoemulsification (Fig. 15.4.8I to L).

Machine parameters

General principle is to have high flow rate and high vacuum, and power depending upon hardness of the nucleus.

- *Phaco power* required can be controlled by foot pedal excursion. The maximum preset is about 40 for grade I and II, 50 for grade III and 60 for a grade IV hard nucleus.
- *Aspiration flow rate* should be about 25–30 cc/sec.
- *Bottle height* should be about 03 to 04 feet from the eye level.
- *Vacuum should be* 100–280 mm Hg depending upon the hardness of the nucleus.
- *Mode.* Pulse mode is recommended with 2–6 pulses (average 3 pulses)/second.

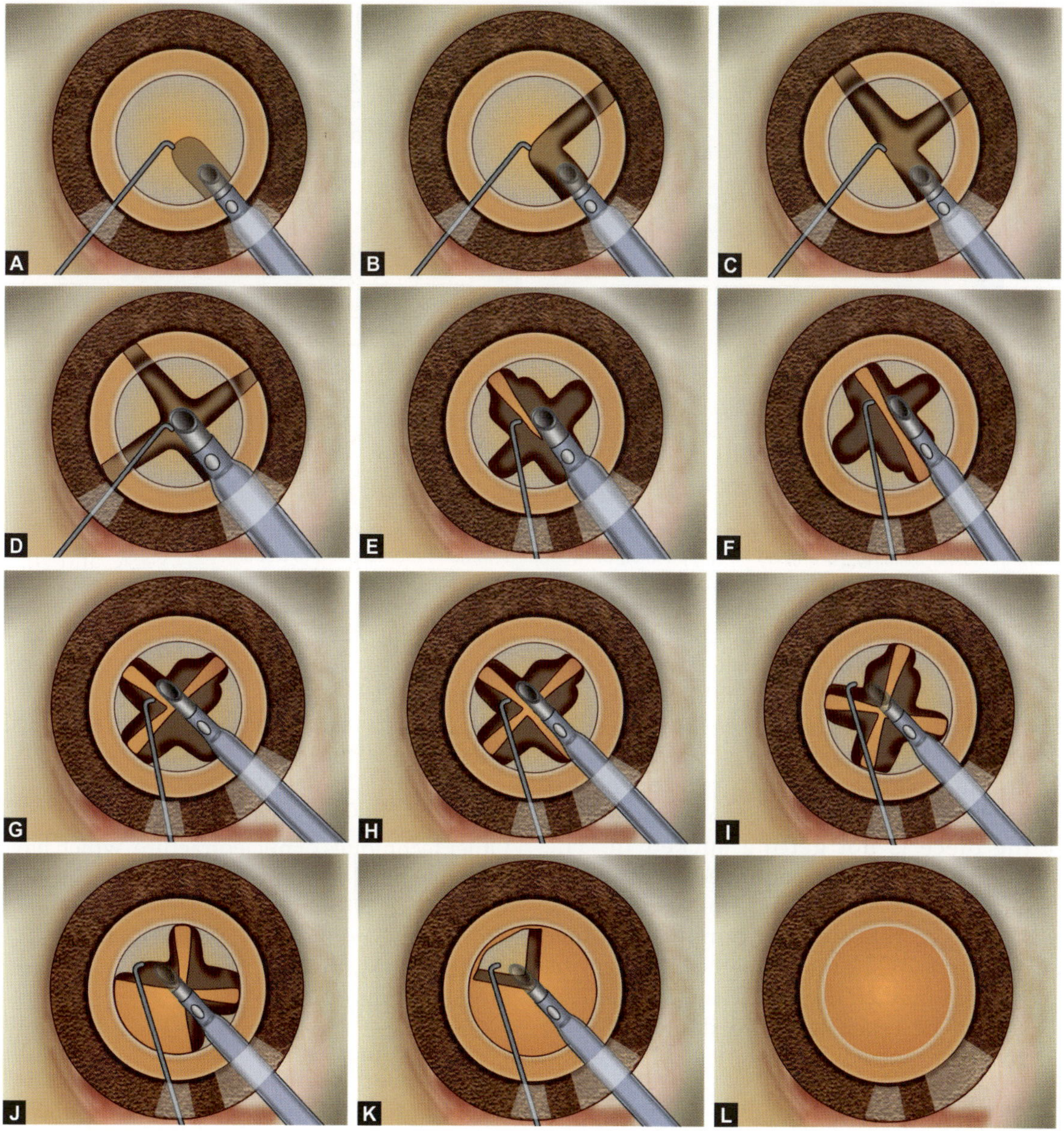

Fig. 15.4.8. *Divide and conquer nucleofracture technique:* ***(A to D)*** *Trenching to make a deep malteese cross;* ***(E to H)*** *Splitting of nucleus (nucleofracture) into four fragments;* ***(I to K)*** *Quadrant removal by phacoemulsification;* ***(L)*** *Complication of quadrant removal.*

Salient points of technique of lens fragment phacoemulsification

Aim. Should be to use minimum phaco power, more aspiration and the procedure should be done in the central safe zone (CSF) to avoid damage to corneal endothelium as well as to the posterior capsule.

Manoeuvres involved include holding each quadrant with phaco tip, pulling the quadrant in the CSF and phacoaspirating the lens fragment.

- *Holding of nucleus quadrant and pulling in CSF.* To hold the quadrant, the phaco tip should be brought near the body of the fragment and embedded in it with a hold to build up vacuum and then pull the fragment out of capsular fornix into the CSF.
- *Phacoaspiration of the quadrant.* After the quadrant is pulled in the CSF, with continued

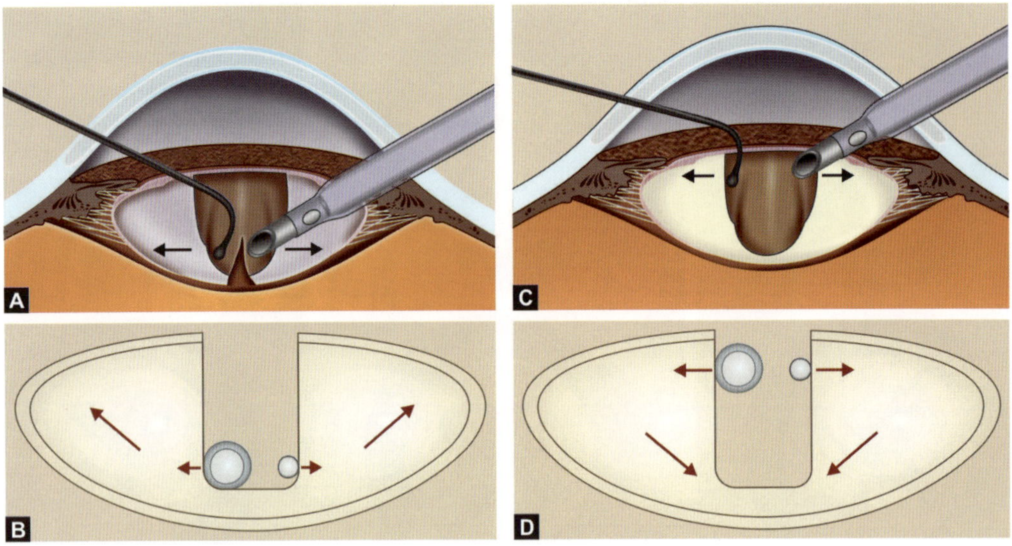

Fig. 15.4.9. ***(A and B)*** *Correct position of two instruments (deep in the trench and at the same level) and direction of forces during nuclear splitting;* ***(C and D)*** *Wrong position of two instruments (superficial in the trench).*

vacuum hold in foot pedal position 2, the piece should be mechanically crushed with the help of second instrument (Sinskey hook or chopper). The crushed pieces should be then aspirated. Phaco power should be used minimal and only when phacoprobe is occluded (judged from the typical sound) and the piece is not getting sucked in. The procedure should be continued till the whole quadrant is phaco-aspirated. Similar manoeuvre should be repeated for removal of other quadrants. While removing the last piece, the vacuum may be decreased and special care should be taken to avoid damage to the posterior capsule.

Crater divide and conquer technique

Crater divide and conquer technique (CDC) was recommended for a harder nucleus, i.e. grade III+.

Salient features of crater divide and conquer (CDC) vis-à-vis trench divide and conquer (TDC) include:

- *Depth of groove is* more in CDC, which is achieved with progressive carving of the central part of the nucleus as far as epinucleus (Fig. 15.4.10A).
- *Width of groove* is made more by peripheral extension to form a crater (Fig. 15.4.10B).
- *Fracture of nuclear rim* is performed using a Sinskey hook and phaco tip into 6–8 pieces (Fig. 15.4.10C).
- *Fragment removal* is then performed as in TDC technique (Fig. 15.4.10D to F).

OTHER TECHNIQUES OF NUCLEOFRACTURE

Other techniques of nucleofracture, which have been described with minor modification, include:

- Shepherd's *in situ* fracture technique,
- Downslope sculpting (DSS) by Gimbel
- Dillman-Maloney's fractional 2/4 phaco-emulsification
- Crater and flip technique (Fine, Maloney, Dillman, 1992).

C. TECHNIQUES OF PHACOEMULSIFICATION WITH PURE NUCLEAR FRACTURE

These techniques include:

- Phaco chop
- Lens quake
- Pre-chop.

PHACO CHOP

Introduced by Nagahara in 1993 the term 'phaco chop' refers to the technique of splitting nucleus into pieces along natural cleavage planes with the help of an instrument called chopper after impaling the nucleus with phacoemulsification

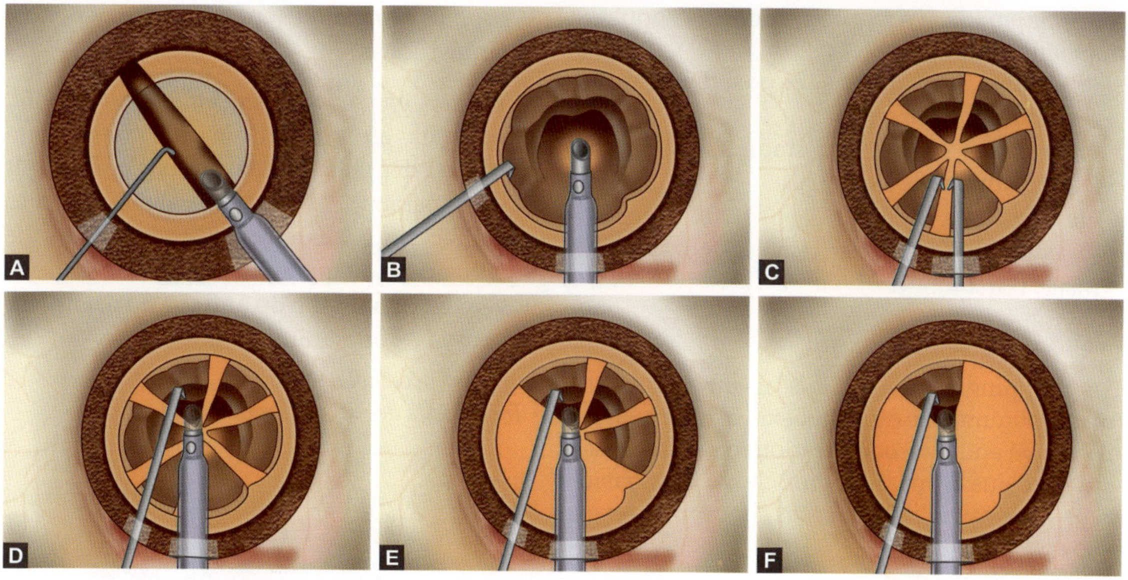

Fig. 15.4.10. *Crater divide and conquer technique:* ***(A and B)*** *Making deep and wide central crater of nucleus by sculpting;* ***(C)*** *Fracture of remaining donut of nucleus into 6–8 pieces using bimanual technique;* ***(D to F)*** *Removal of fragments one-by-one by phacoemulsification.*

tip. Nagahara, who originally described this technique, made an analogy of the technique of chopping to splitting a log of wood with a wedge, taking advantage of the wood's grain or cleavage planes (Fig. 15.4.11).

Since then many modifications have been made in the technique. A few of them will be described briefly:

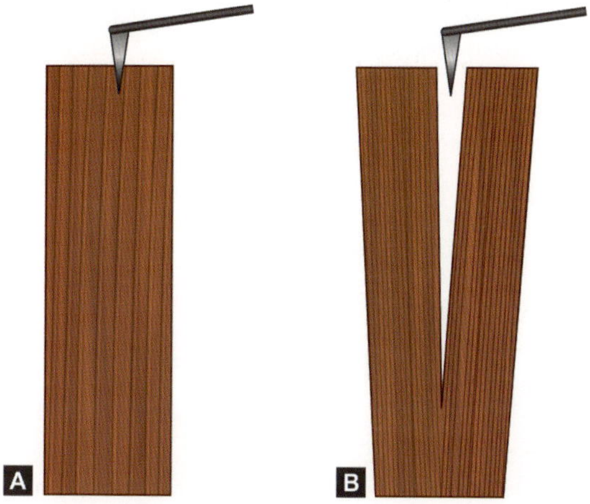

Fig. 15.4.11. *Nagahara's analogy of the technique of nucleus chopping along its natural cleavage planes to the splitting of a log of wood with a wedge along its natural cleavage planes.*

Advantages of phaco chop technique in general over the nucleus cracking technique include:

- Reduction in surgical time
- Reduction in total phaco energy use
- Decreased incidence of posterior capsular tear
- Decreased incidence of corneal complications.

BASIC STEPS OF TECHNIQUE OF PHACO CHOPPING

Before reviewing the various techniques of phaco chop method, it will be worth while to learn about the basic steps of chopping. The chopping manoeuvres known till date, irrespective of the chronology of their discovery, can be grouped as below:

A. *Horizontal chopping*, which can be:
   I. Peripheral chopping
   II. Central chopping
   III. Modified peripheral chopping.

B. *Vertical chopping*

A. Horizontal chopping

In horizontal chopping, the chopping and splitting movements are made in a horizontal plane.

Machine parameters recommended for chopping manoeuvres are:

- *Phaco tip.* Zero degree, exposed more by retracting the sleeve.
- *Vacuum.* For grade I, 80 ; grade II, 100; grade III, 120 and grade IV +, 150.
- *Flow rate.* 24 ± cc/min.
- *Phaco power.* Grade I, 40; II, 50; III, 60; IV ± 70.
- *Mode.* Burst mode.

I. *Peripheral chopping*

For chopping technique, it is essential to have intact optimum size capsulorhexis, a good hydrodissection and hydrodelineation to separate the endonucleus from the epinucleus. The basic steps of peripheral horizontal chopping are as below.

1. *Stabilization of the nucleus.* Stabilization of the nucleus is the key step to success of chopping. Stabilization is done by impaling the tip in the body of nucleus either without a trench, with partial trench or with complete trench (Fig. 15.4.12).

i. *Impaling the phaco tip without trench.* It is preferred to use a zero degree phaco tip. The phaco tip should be implanted with in a position near the proximal margin of the capsulorhexis. The irrigation sleeve should be retracted more than for divide and conquer technique, in order to allow the phaco tip to advance to a depth of midnucleus (1.5–2 mm) while implanting the phaco handpiece should be directed vertically as if aiming towards the optic disc (Fig. 15.4.12A). The phaco tip should be implanted into the centre of the nucleus with short bursts of power by bringing the foot pedal to position 3 for a very short duration.

ii. *Impaling the phaco tip with crater/partial trench.* Making a small partial trench/cratre by sculpting just proximal to the centre and then rotating the nucleus by 180° will provide a better platform for implanting the phaco tip (Fig. 15.4.12B). Further procedure is same as described above.

iii. *Impaling the phaco tip with complete trench.* A complete trench made before chopping will give a full body grip (Fig. 15.4.12C). This is used in 'stop and chop' technique of phacoemulsification.

2. *Creation of vacuum seal and vacuum hold.* Immediately after embedding the phaco tip to a required depth, the pedal should be brought back to position 2, so that the vacuum is build up and a strong vacuum hold is created. If the impalment is adequate, then slight to and fro movement of both the tip and the nuclear piece will move as one unit.

Causes of poor hold include:

- *Inadequate depth,* i.e. superficial grip.

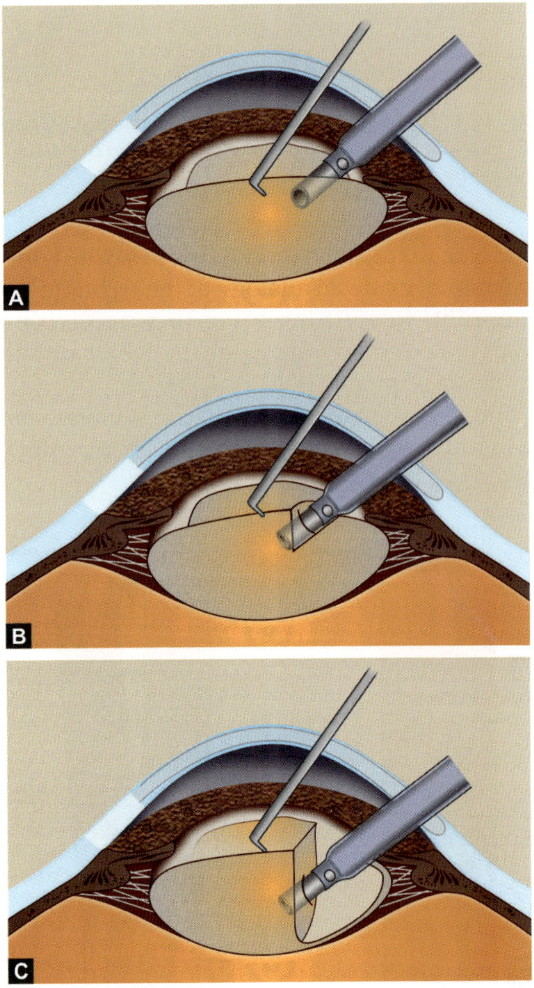

Fig. 15.4.12. *Technique of impaling the phaco tip in the body of nucleus in phaco chop:* ***(A)*** *Impaling without a trench;* ***(B)*** *Impaling with crater/partial trench;* ***(C)*** *Impaling with complete trench.*

- *Keeping foot pedal in position 3 for long* period leads to emulsification of the nucleus material around the tip and loosen the grip.
- *Inadequate vacuum* leads to unstable hold.
- *Soft cataract,* which with high vacuum, gets sucked.

3. ***Peripheral chopping manoeuvres.*** Ideally after pressurizing the eye, the blunt tipped chopper (Fig. 15.4.13A) is passed through a paracentesis, i.e. about one and a half clock hours away from, the main incision, just before the phaco tip. The chopper can assist the proper location of the implanting of the phaco tip by pressing lightly on the nuclear surface and shifting the nucleus gently (about 1 mm) away from the incision. After implanting the phaco tip in nucleus body, the chopper is advanced underneath the CCC margin in horizontal position, and is then turned vertical and positioned around equator of the nucleus, just to the left of the line of the phaco probe at the delineation line and is pulled towards the phaco tip (Fig. 15.4.13B and C). Just before reaching the phaco probe, the chopper is moved laterally (on left side for a right-handed surgeon) to split the nucleus (Fig. 15.4.13D and E).

To make pie-shaped smaller pieces the above procedure should be repeated circumferentially (Fig. 15.4.13F).

Problems with peripheral chopping include:

- *Technically difficult* as complex manoeuvrability is needed while managing the chopper and simultaneously maintaining the nuclear hold.
- *Radial anterior capsular tear* may occur, if accidently the chopper is placed over the anterior capsule rather than beneath it. It may specially occur in a hard cataract with very little cortex.
- *Posterior capsular tear* may occur, especially if a long chopper is used with a soft nucleus in an unstable anterior chamber.

II. Central chopping

- For central chopping, a sharp-pointed chopper (Fig. 15.4.14A) is required in contrast to the blunt-tipped chopper required for peripheral chopping.

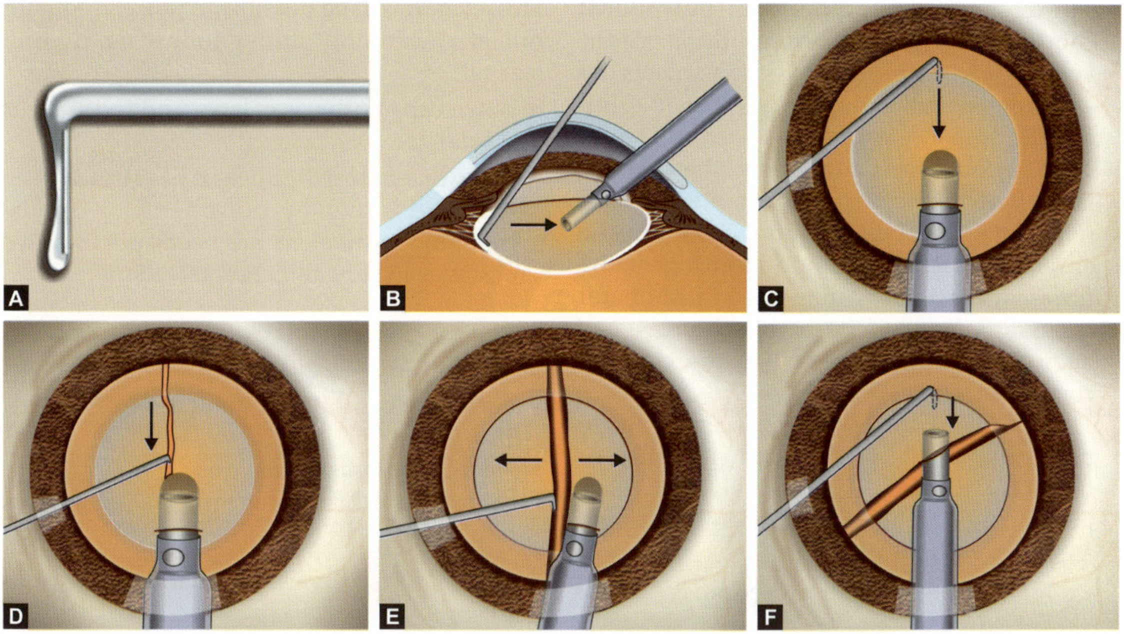

Fig. 15.4.13. *Technique of peripheral chopping without making a trench: **(A)** Blunt tipped chopper; **(B and C)** Implantation of phaco tip in the body of nucleus; and advancing chopper underneath the CCC margin in horizontal position; positioning the chopper around the equator of nucleus after turning it vertically; pulling the chopper towards phaco tip; **(D and E)** Moving the chopper laterally to split the nucleus; **(F)** Further chopping to make pie-shaped pieces.*

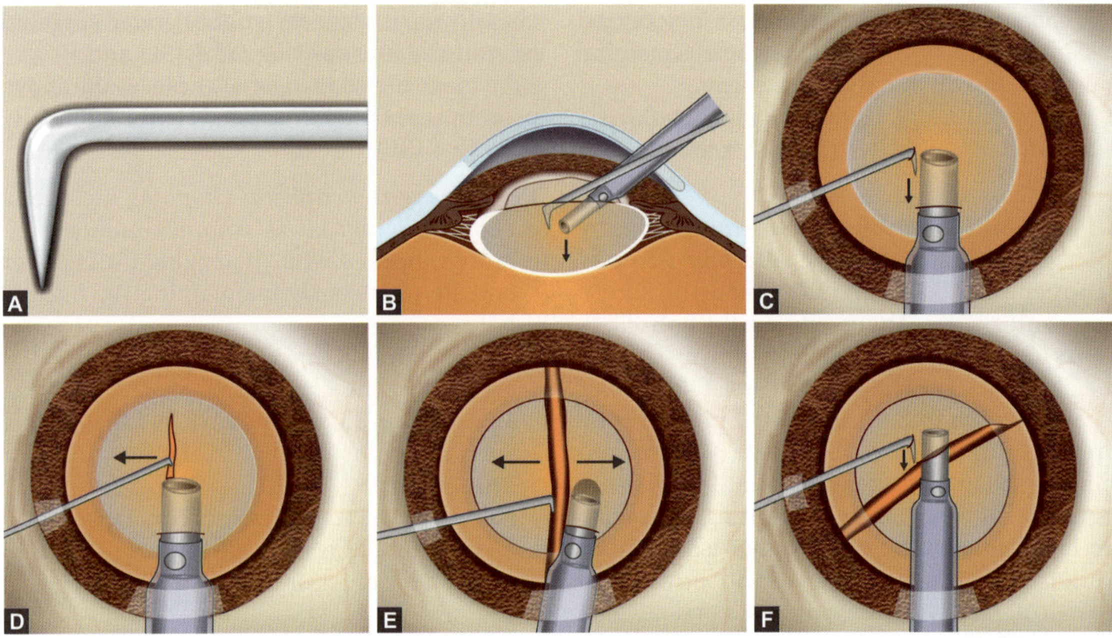

Fig. 15.4.14. *Technique of central chop without making a trench:* ***(A)*** *A sharp chopper;* ***(B and C)*** *Embedding the chopper in the body of nucleus near the phaco tip;* ***(D)*** *Movement of the chopper towards left side to split the nucleus; Splitting of nucleus starts at centre and superficially, and moves deep and towards periphery;* ***(E)*** *Simultaneous movement of phaco tip in opposite direction to complete the split;* ***(F)*** *Further chopping to make pie-shaped pieces.*

- After impaling the phaco tip and stabilizing the nucleus (as described in peripheral chopping), the sharp chopper tip is placed very close to the phaco tip just towards its left and is embedded in the nucleus (Fig. 15.4.14B and C).
- Then, with a steady movement, the chopper is moved to the left to split the nucleus (Fig. 15.4.14D). Thus, in central chopping, the emphasis is essentially on splitting of the fibres rather than cutting (as in peripheral chopping). If required, the phaco probe can be simultaneously moved to the right to complete the split (Fig. 15.4.14E).

  To make pie-shaped smaller pieces the above procedure should be repeated circumferentially (Fig. 15.4.14F). Alternatively the further pieces may be made by peripheral chopping as shown in Fig. 15.4.13F.

III. *Modified peripheral chopping*

In this technique, after impaling the nucleus (Fig. 15.4.15A and B), the equator is pulled out of the rhexis margin (thus avoiding negotiating under the CCC) and then peripheral chopping (Fig. 15.4.15C and D) is done as described above. However, it will be possible to pull the equator out of rhexis only under following circumstances:

- When capsulorhexis is large and the nucleus is small, or
- When one-half of the nucleus has already been removed either by peripheral or central chopping, or nucleus has been split into two pieces as in stop and chop technique.

B. Vertical chopping

- *The concept of vertical forces* to fragment the nucleus was proposed by Vladimir Pfeifer of Slovenia.
- *The technique was developed and taught* by David Dillman and Louis Nichamin as '*Phaco quick chop*'.

Salient points of vertical phaco chop are as below:

- *In vertical phaco chop,* after impaling and vacuum holding the nucleus, the sharp-tipped chopper is embedded in the anterior surface of nucleus just in front and to the left side of

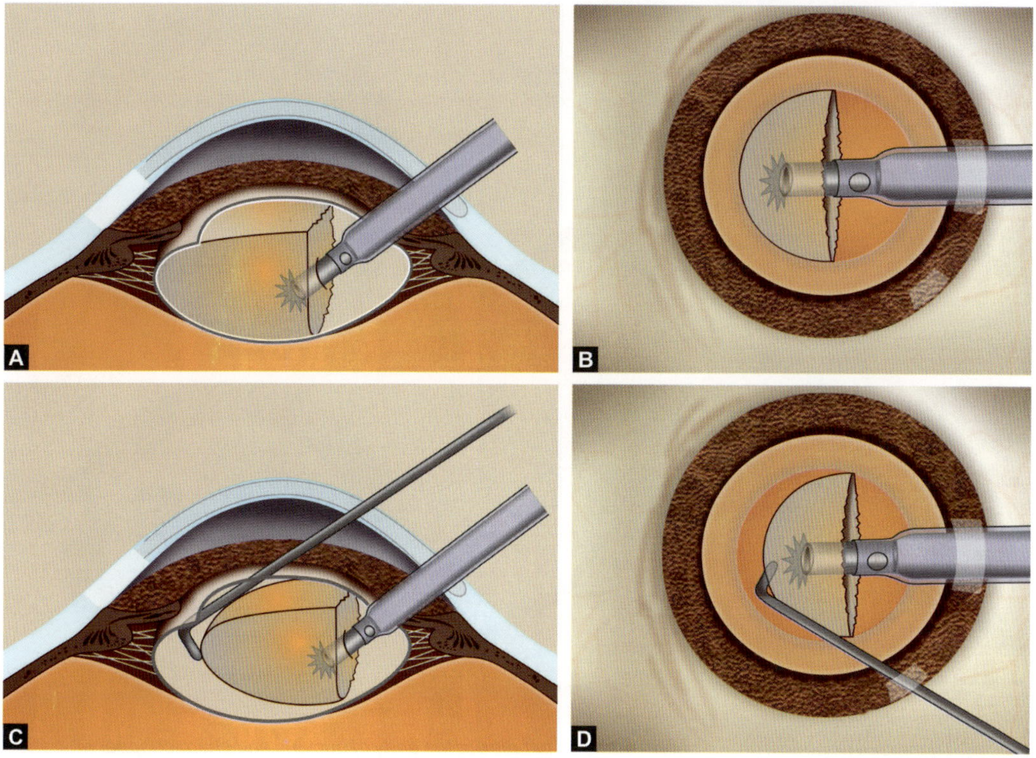

Fig. 15.4.15. *Technique of modified peripheral chop:* ***(A and B)*** *Impaling the phaco tip in the body of nucleus;* ***(C and D)*** *Pulling the fragment out of the bag towards the central safe zone and placing the chopper around the equator and pulling towards phaco tip to split the nucleus.*

the phaco tip (as done for central chopping, pages 265–266) (Fig. 15.4.16A and B).

- *For vertical chopping the chopper is pushed sharply downwards* while the phaco tip is lifted upwards (Fig. 15.4.16A and B). The crisp apposing vertical movements create a split in which left half of nucleus moves down (towards posterior capsule) and right half of the nucleus moves up (towards cornea) (Fig. 15.4.16C). Each instrument moves about one-half of the total amont of vertical separation needed. As soon as the vertical split begins, the two instruments are also moved laterally in the horizontal plane to complete the cleavage of two halves of the nucleus (Fig. 15.4.16D).

Advantages of vertical chopping is that it avoids the need to pass the chopper under the anterior capsule out of the equater and in a quick procedure.

Disadvantages. It wroks only in moderate density cataract. In soft cataract, the chopper and phaco tip pull through the nucleus, and in harder cataract, the higher forces required may threaten the integrity of the posterior capsule and/or zonules.

COMMON HORIZONTAL PHACO CHOPPING TECHNIQUES

After knowing the basic manoeuvres of chopping, it will be appropriate to review the various horizontal phaco chop techniques in Vogue.

1. Nagahara's phaco chop technique

Kunihiro Nagahara (1993), first of all introduced the concept of phaco chop for nuclear disassembly taking advantage of the natural cleavage planes that existed in the nucleus.

Salient points of Nagahara's technique are: Nagahara's phaco chop basically is a peripheral horizontal chopping technique. He first of all described this technique.

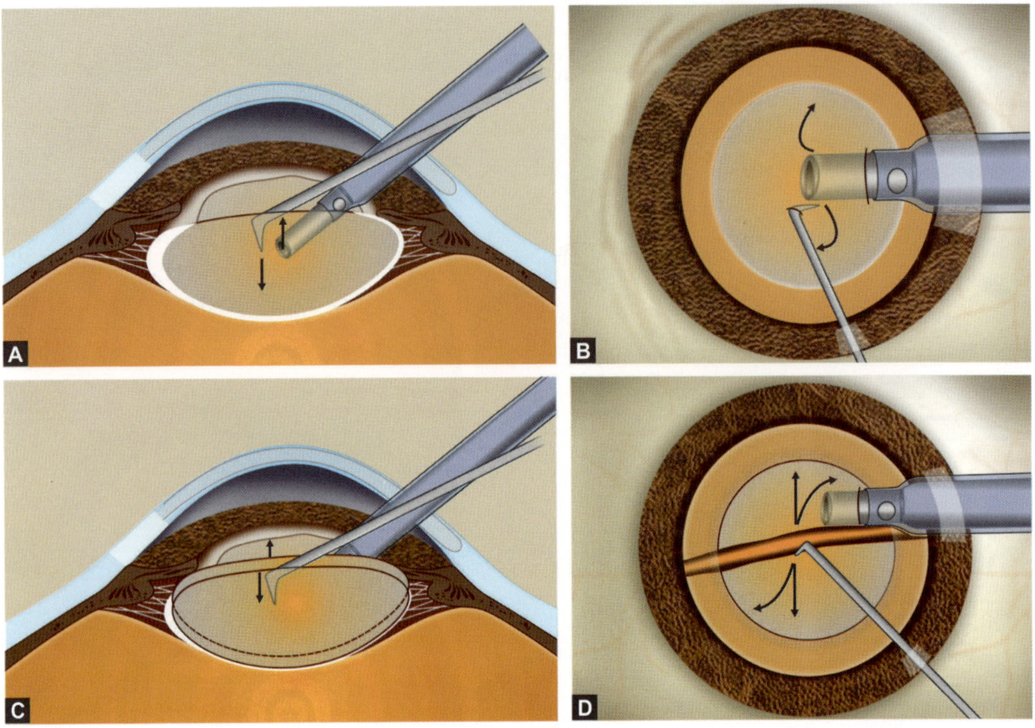

Fig. 15.4.16. *Technique of vertical phaco chop: Phaco tip impaled in the body of nucleus and sharp chopper embedded just in front and to the left side of the phaco tip* ***(A)****. Simultaneous manoeuvre of lifting the phaco tip and pushing down the chopper* ***(B)*** *Creates a split in which left half of nucleus moves down and right half moves up* ***(C)****. At this juncture the two instruments are also moved laterally in the horizontal plane to quickly complete the cleavage between two halves of the nucleus* ***(D)****.*

- *Steps of peripheral horizontal chopping* are described on page 264 (Fig. 15.4.13).
- *Four quadrants* are chopped by repeating the process of peripheral horizontal after rotating the nucleus by 90° three times.
- *Each quadrant* is then phaco aspirated.

2. Stop and chop technique

Paul Koch was stimulated by Nagahara to perform phaco chop. He found that the initial chop intended to bisect the nucleus was most difficult and that there was lack of space in the bag to remove the chopped pieces which adhered to each other. In 1994, he modified Nagahara's technique and named it 'stop and chop' technique.

Salient points of Koch's stop and chop technique are:

- *Deep trench* is sculpted initially (Fig. 15.4.17A).
- *Cracking of nucleus in two halves* is then done using two instruments similar to divide and conquer technique (*see* page 260, Fig. 15.4.17B). At this point, the quadrant cracking technique is stopped and chopping begins, and so the name 'stop and chop' was given to this technique.
- *Horizontal peripheral chopping* (Fig. 15.4.17C) as described by Nagahara is then performed to divide each heminucleus in 2–4 pieces depending upon the hardness of the nucleus.

3. Chop and debulk technique

Steinert (1995) introduced this technique with the idea to create some central space to comfortably perform phacoemulsification in the posterior chamber and iris plane.

Salient points of this technique are:

- *Initial peripheral horizontal chop* similar to Nagahara's technique is performed to bissect the nucleus (Fig. 15.4.13B to D).
- *Sculpting of the central hard nucleus* is then done along the fault line of initial split to create

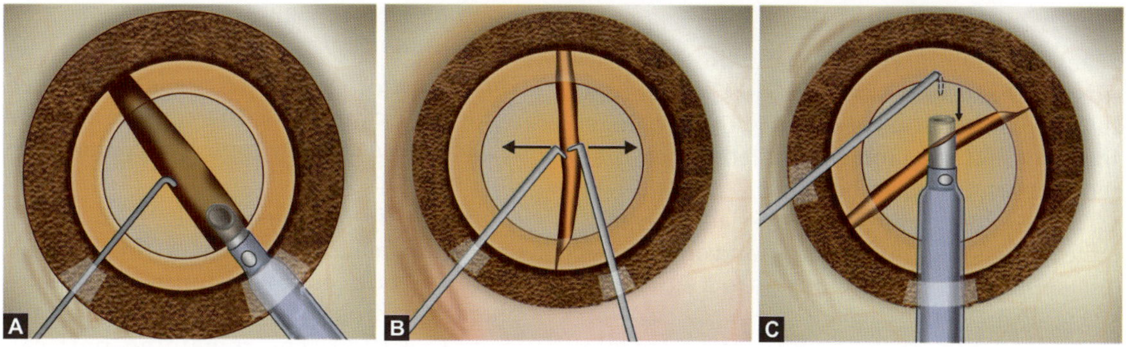

Fig. 15.4.17. *Koch's stop and chop technique of phacoemulsification: **(A)** Sculpting of the central hard nucleus to make a deep trench;**(B)** Splitting (cracking) of nucleus into two halves using two choppers; **(C)** Horizontal peripheral chopping to make multiple pieces of each half of nucleus.*

central space (bigger in the hard cataract than the soft cataract).

- *Horizontal peripheral chopping* is then performed to create multiple pieces, depending upon the hardness of the nucleus.
- *Quadrant removal* is then done by phacoemulsification/aspiration.

4. Choo-choo chop and flip phacoemulsification technique

Introduced by Fine (2001), the technique derives its name from the 'noise created' by phacoemulsification during the burst mode (2 bursts/second), that is used in this technique to create the nucleus lollipop.

Salient features. Peripheral chopping of the endonucleus is performed inside the epinucleus shell. After phacoaspirating the endonucleus, the epinucleus is removed with a flip manoeuvre.

5. Phacodrill technique

Introduced by Choun-ki-Joo (1997), the 'phacodrill' refers to bevel down phaco chop.

Salient features. Central sculpting is done with bevel down 30° phaco tip, followed by standard horizontal phaco chop to remove the remaining nucleus.

6. No vacuum chop technique

It is a modification of, 'phaco drill' technique.

- *Central bowl* is created by sculpting with a 30° bevel down phaco tip, until the red reflex is seen.
- *Chopping of the peripheral nuclear rim* into 6–8 fragments is then made mechanically by apposing movement of chopper and phaco tip without using vacuum.
- *Phacoaspiration* of fragments is then done.

Note. There are various other techniques of horizontal chopping with (Fig. 15.4.13F) minor variations.

TECHNIQUES BASED ON THE VERTICAL PHACO CHOP

Various techniques based on vertical chopping principle (described on page 266, Fig. 15.4.16) were introduced almost at the same time. These include:

- *Phaco crack* by Vladimir Pfiefer
- *Phaco quick chop,* by David Dillman
- *Stop, chop, chop and stuff,* by Abhya Vasavada et al from India (1996)
- *Phaco snap and split ,* by Hidaharu Fukasaku.

LENS QUAKE

Lens quake, also known as *'Auto-crack chop'* introduced by Jack A. Singer, differs completely from the phaco chop technique. The name lens quake is derived from the mechanism of action which resembles an earthquake.

It involves the use of an *auto-crack cobra phaco tip* with 15° bevel and 15° curve upward, modified hexagon external shape with circular lumen and high vacuum to induce stress and strain movement (similar to seismic tremors) near the Y-sutures, resulting in a lens quake that propagates along the natural fault lines in the nucleus.

PRECHOPPING TECHNIQUE

Prechopping, introduced by the Japnese surgeon Takayaki Akahoshi (1993), involves cutting of nucleus into 4 pieces with the help of specially designed forceps (called phaco prechopper) as described below:

- The prechopper forceps is burried deep into the nucleus (Fig. 15.4.18A to C) and on opening it separates the nucleus into two parts (Fig. 15.4.18D).
- Then each heminucleus is further divided into two parts each. The prechopped fragments are then phacoaspirated using high vacuum and flow rate.

EPINUCLEAR PLATE REMOVAL, CORTICAL ASPIRATION AND CAPSULAR POLISHING

EPINUCLEAR PLATE REMOVAL

For removal of epinucleus, principle is to have a moderate flow and moderate vacuum.

Machine parameters include:

- *Flow rate.* 15–20 cc/min
- *Vacuum.* 75–100 mm Hg
- *Power.* Usually not required. Minimum settings (20–30%)
- *Mode.* Pulse or linear

Salient points of technique of epinucleus removal

- ***This is a delicate phase*** and needs to be tackled with great caution, as the capsule is more relaxed and can easily come into contact with the phaco tip.
- ***Chip and flip technique*** can be used for the epinuclear plate. First the size of epinuclear plate is reduced by chipping the peripheral part from under the anterior capsule (Fig. 15.4.19A). The remaining part can then be flipped with the help of second instrument (round iris repositor or rod-shaped iris repositor) and then phaco-aspirated (Fig. 15.4.19B and C).

CORTICAL ASPIRATION

A thorough cortical clean up is essential to prevent postoperative uveitis, glaucoma, and posterior capsular opacification. The cortical aspiration can be done by any of the following methods:

1. Automated irrigation and aspiration
   I. Coaxial irrigation and aspiration
   II. Bimanual irrigation and aspiration
2. Manual irrigation and aspiration

Beginners can even use manual irrigation aspiration technique with Simcoe's two-way

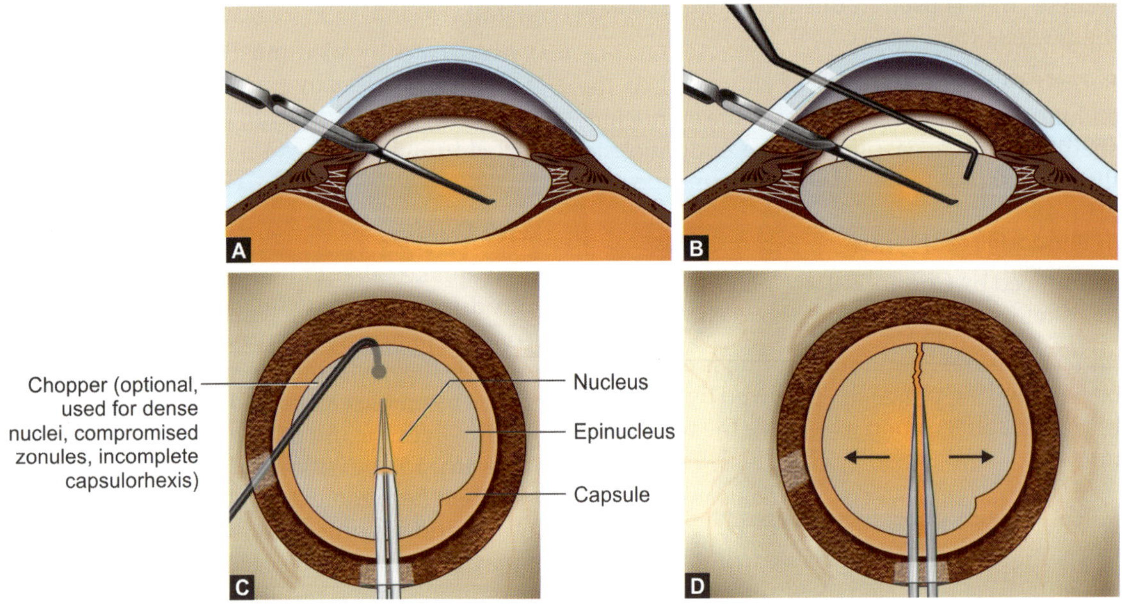

Fig. 15.4.18. *Phaco-prechop: Side view* ***(A and B)****; Top view* ***(C)*** *of phaco-prechop instrument introduced into the nucleus; Nuclear crack produced by the prechopper* ***(D)****.*

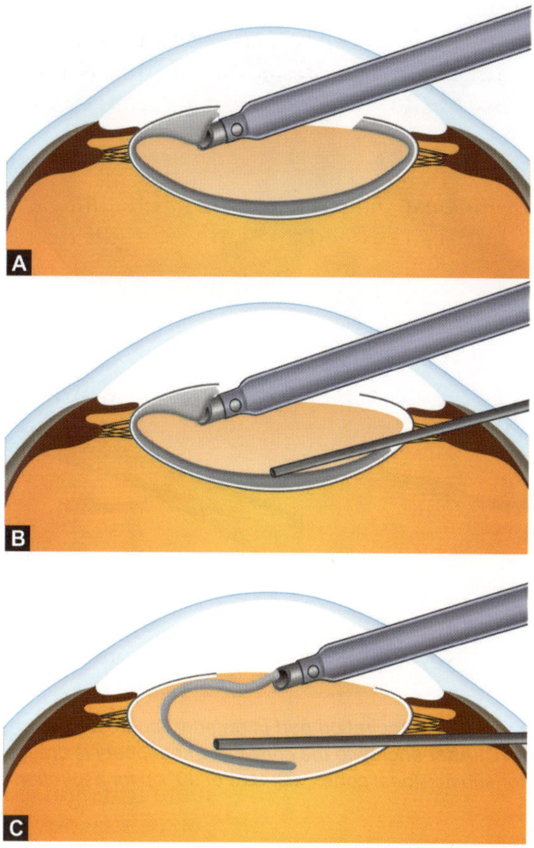

Fig. 15.4.19. *Chip and flip technique for removal of epinuclear plate: **(A)** Chipping of the peripheral part of epinucleus to decrease its size; **(B and C)** Flipping with round repositor and phacoaspiration.*

I/A cannula as in manual small incision cataract surgery (M-SICS), *see* page 214.

Coaxial irrigation and aspiration

The coaxial irrigation and aspiration handpiece is used for this purpose.

Cortical aspiration from the cross-incisional area can be best done with the help of straight I/A handpiece by following manoeuvres:

- *Enter the anterior chamber* after it is partially or fully formed to prevent Descemet's membrane tear.
- *Direction of aspiration port* is kept anterior to engage the cortex from the cross-incisional area (Fig. 15.4.20A).
- *Rotate the aspiration port* of the IA handpiece toward the equator of the lens capsule (Fig. 15.4.20B) for the right- or left-sided cortex and engage the cortical matter with low vacuum and bring the cortical matter in the centre of the bag (Fig. 15.4.20C). Rotate the aspiration port to face anteriorly and increase the vacuum to aspirate the lens matter. Repeat the procedure till all the soft lens matter is aspirated from the cross-incisional area.

Cortical aspiration from the subincisional area is done by rotating aspiration port posteriorly (Fig. 15.4.20D); but may sometimes be difficult with straight I/A cannula. Following measures may be useful:

- *Use of angled tip*—45°, 90° or sharper (180°) aspiration cannula is useful in engaging and aspirating the sub-incisional cortical matter (Fig. 15.4.20E).
- *Cortex resistant to aspiration* can be separated from the capsular bag with OVD (visco-dissection) to allow the I/A cannula to engage it.
- *Aspiration of very resistant cortex* may be tried after IOL implantation. Rotation of IOL in the bag may loosen the cortex and allow aspiration.

Bimanual irrigation and aspiration

Bimanual I/A involves use of two separate cannulas (Fig. 15.2.12). It provides good anterior chamber stability and facilitates removal of the subincisional cortex.

Essential steps are:

- *Two side port incisions* are made approximately 150° apart from each other after inflating the AC with OVD. The incision should be just enough in size to allow smooth fit of the two cannulas (Fig. 15.4.21A). Alternatively, the aspiration cannula may be introduced through the paracentesis while irrigation through the main incision (modified bimanual I/A) (Fig. 15.4.21B).
- *Manoeuvre to aspirate cortex* is same as described above. By interchanging the irrigation and aspiration cannulas, all the cross-incisional as well as subincisional cortices can be removed easily.

Advantages

- Easy removal of subincisional as well as cross-incisional cortices.

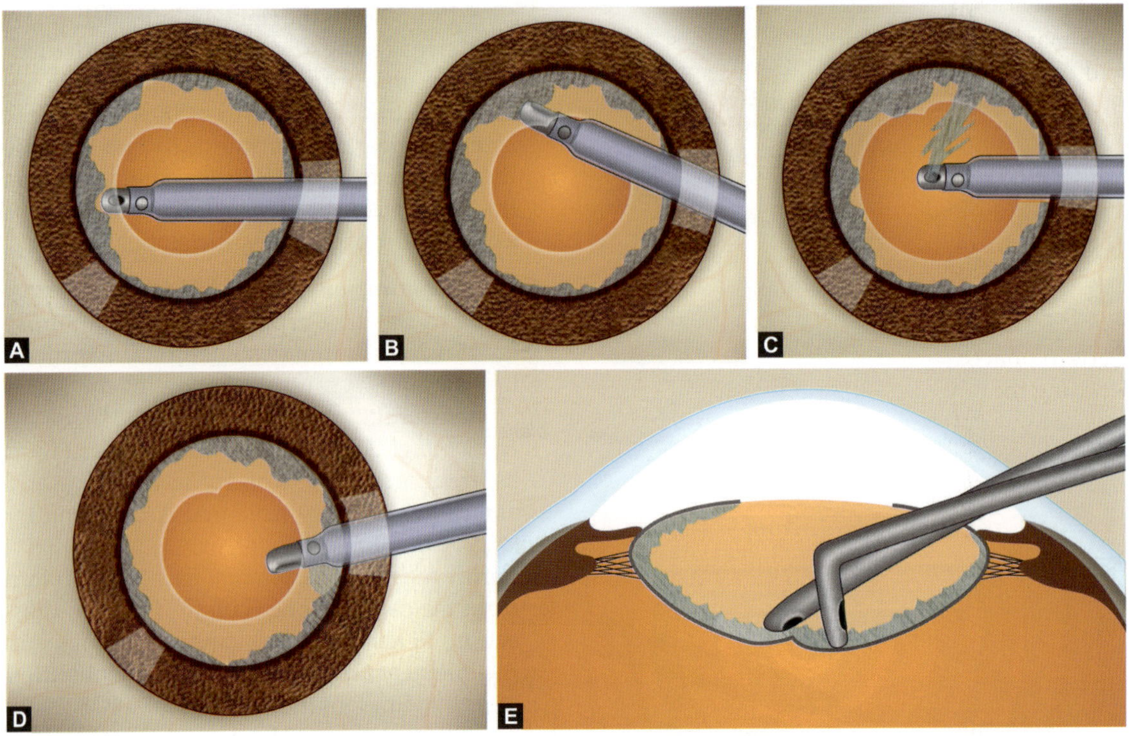

Fig. 15.4.20. *Cortical aspiration with co-axial irrigation and aspiration:* ***(A)*** *Aspiration port is anterior for cross-incisional cortex;* ***(B)*** *Aspiration port is rotated side way for the side cortex;* ***(C)*** *After engaging the cortex from periphery is dragged in the centre and aspirated;* ***(D)*** *Aspiration port turned posterior for subincisional cortex;* ***(E)*** *Use of 90° tip for aspiration of subincisional cortex avoids capsular catch seen with straight tip.*

- Another advantage of bimanual *I/A* is that small nuclear fragments or harder cortical material resistant to aspiration may be crushed between the tip of I/A cannulas.

Disadvantages of bimanual I/A include:

- Need to make two side port incisions, and also
- The surgeon need to be ambidextrous.

CAPSULAR POLISHING

Capsular polishing is required to prevent PCO, specially in the presence of tags of cortex sticking to PC, posterior plaque and vacuolated lens fibres attached to PC in hypermature cataract. Capsular polishing can be done with the help of a polisher or using phaco I/A in cap-vac mode.

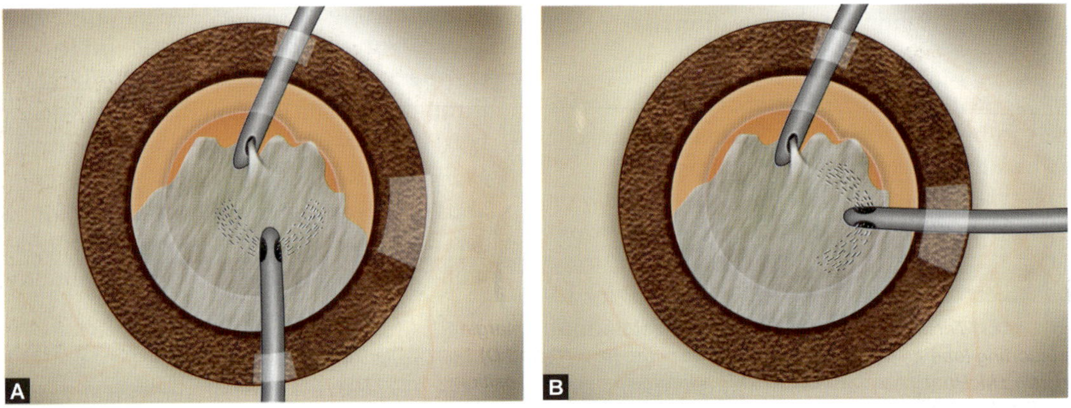

Fig. 15.4.21. *Bimanual irrigation and aspiration:* ***(A)*** *Standard;* ***(B)*** *Modified.*

Use of polisher

Capsular bag should be inflated and pressurized with OVD, and the PC should be gently polished by using any of the following polishers (Fig. 15.4.22):

- Rounded repositor (Fig. 15.4.22A)
- Sand-blasted capsule polisher (Fig. 15.4.22B)
- Ring capsule polisher (Fig. 15.4.22C).

Use of phaco I/A in cap-vac mode

Certain phaco machines have a 'cap-vac mode'. Keeping the machine on this mode, anterior and posterior capsules can be cleaned up very effectively and safely with the help of I/A tip.

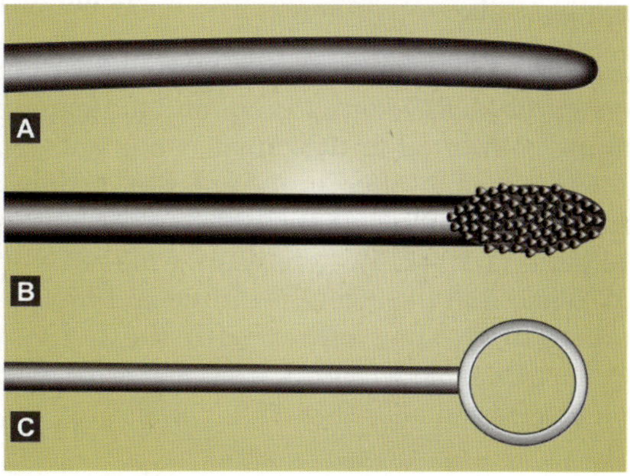

Fig. 15.4.22. *Capsule polishers: **(A)** Round repositor; **(B)** Sand-blasted capsule polisher; **(C)** Ring capsule polisher.*

IOL IMPLANTATION AND COMPLETION STEPS

Foldable IOLs are the choice of most phaco surgeons, however, still phaco profile PMMA IOLs are also used in certain circumstances (mostly economical reasons).

TECHNIQUE OF IMPLANTATION OF PMMA IOL

Enlarging the section

Phaco-profile PMMA IOLs are available in 5, 5.25 and 5.5 mm in size. Accordingly, after pressurizing the eye with OVD, the incision is enlarged to 0.5 mm less than the size of IOLs optic (Fig. 15.4.23A).

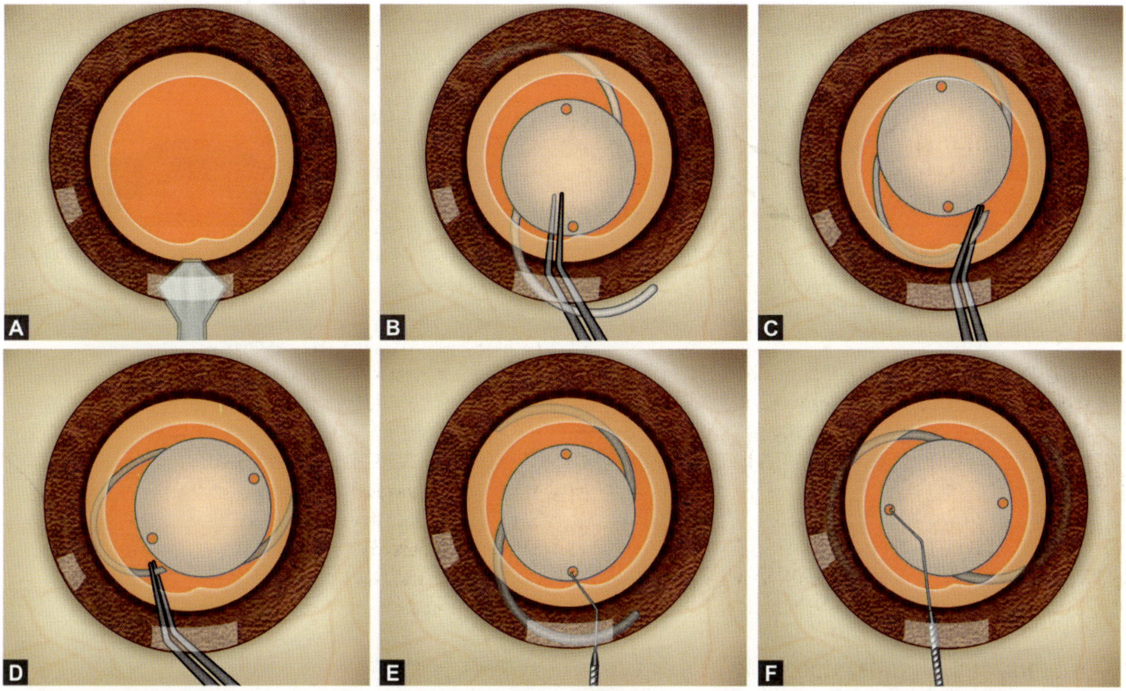

Fig. 15.4.23. *Technique of implantation of a PMMA IOL: **(A)** Enlarging the phacoincision with 5 mm blunt-tipped keratome; **(B)** Inserting leading haptic and part of optic in the bag; **(C and D)** Dialling of the remaining optic and trailing haptic in the bag using McPherson forceps; **(E and F)** Alternate method to position the remaining optic and trailing haptic by dialling with the a Sinskey's hook.*

Insertion of the IOL

The IOL is held either with an IOL holding forceps or McPherson's forceps and the leading haptic is inserted in the capsular bag and the tilted optic is inserted in the anterior chamber in such a way that part of the optic also steps in the bag (Fig. 15.4.23B). Repressurize the eye with OVD and dial the rest of the optic and trailing haptic in the bag either with the help of McPherson forceps (Fig. 15.4.23C and D) or with the help of a dialler (Fig. 15.4.23E and F).

TECHNIQUE OF IMPLANTING FOLDABLE IOL

Enlarging the incision

After pressurizing the eye with OVD, the incision is enlarged to 3.5–4 mm and the foldable IOL can be implanted by any of the following two techniques.

1. IOL implantation with injector system

Nowadays most of the foldable IOLs are available with disposable injector system (Fig. 15.4.24). The IOL is folded in the cartridge with the help of McPherson forceps (Fig. 15.4.25A) which in turn is locked into the injector system (Fig. 15.4.25B) (some IOLs are marketed as pre-loaded in the cartridge with injector system). The injector is then inserted with bevel down up to the centre and up to the level of capsulor-hexis. The IOL is then slowly injected in the capsular bag (Fig. 15.4.25C). The leading haptic is guided under the capsulorhexis margin and slowly the optic is released into the bag where it unfolds and trailing haptic lies outside the bag (Fig. 15.4.25D). Remove the injector and

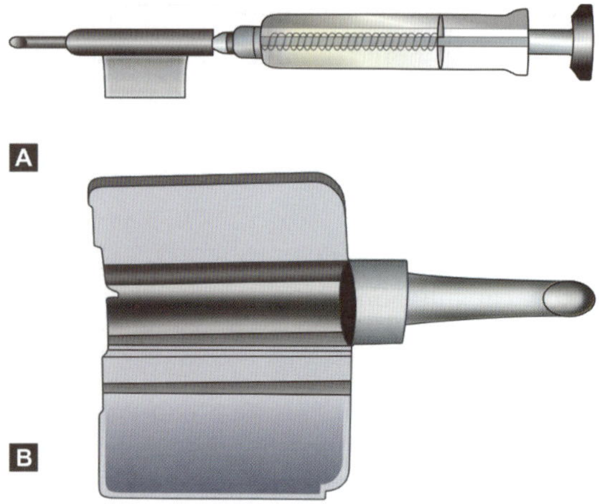

Fig. 15.4.24. *The injector system for foldable IOL* ***(A)*** *with an open cartilage* ***(B)***.

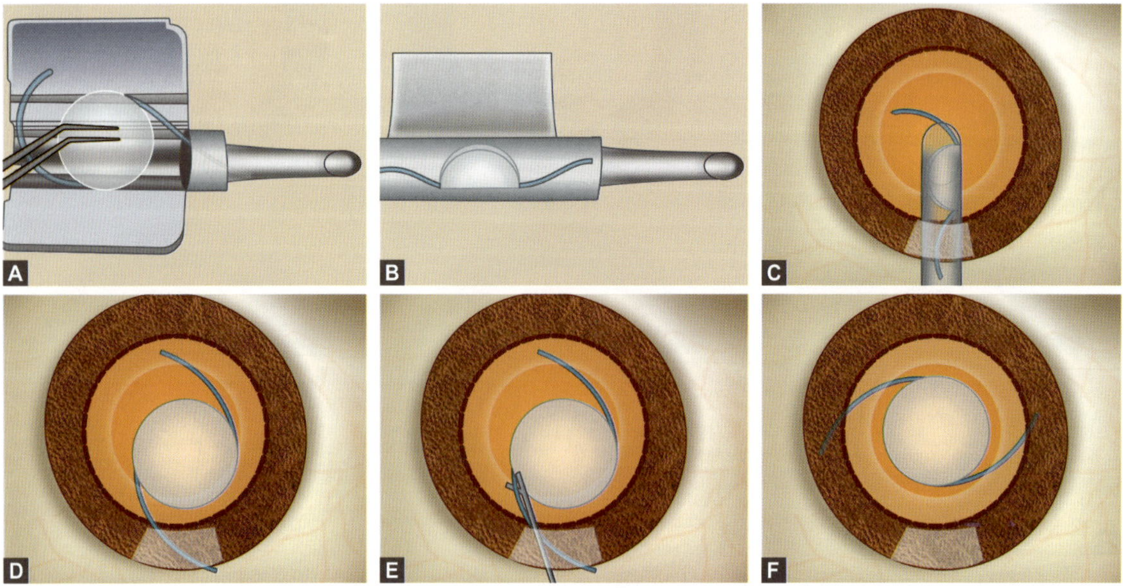

Fig. 15.4.25. *Implantation of foldable IOL with injector system:* ***(A)*** *Folding of IOL in the cartridge;* ***(B)*** *Folded IOL in the closed cartridge;* ***(C)*** *Injection of IOL in the capsular bag with bevel down of the injector tip;* ***(D)*** *Injcted IOL with leading haptic in the bag and trailing haptic out side the bag;* ***(E and F)*** *Dialling of trailing haptic in the bag with Y-dialler.*

again pressurize the eye with OVD. The trailing haptic can be dialled in the bag using a dialler (Fig. 15.4.25E and F).

2. IOL implantation with holder-folder

The holder-folder system comprises two forceps (Fig. 15.4.26A). The grooved forceps folds the IOL (Fig. 15.4.26B) and the other holds the folded IOL (Fig. 15.4.26C). After pressurizing the eye with OVD, insert the folded IOL (Fig. 15.4.26D) in the eye and guide the leading haptic in the capsular bag (Fig. 15.4.26E). Rotate the forceps so the fold of the IOL lies anteriorly and then slowly release it (Fig. 15.4.26F). As the IOL unfolds (Fig. 15.4.26G), insert the dialler in the groove between the haptic and optic and (Fig. 15.4.26H) gently dial the trailing haptic in the bag (Fig. 15.4.26I).

Note. Because of easy availability of injector system and the cumbersome manoeuvring involved with the holder-folder system, the later is sparingly used nowadays.

COMPLETION STEPS

1. ***Aspiration of residual OVD.*** After the IOL is properly implanted and dialled in position, the residual OVD should be thoroughly and meticulously aspirated with automated or manual I/A system.
2. ***Sealing of side port and main incision*** should then be done by hydrating with a jet of BSS, through the hydration cannula.
3. ***Subconjunctival injection*** of antibiotic and steroid should be given.
4. ***Patching*** of the eye should then be done with a self-sticking sterile eye-pad after removing the speculum and drape.

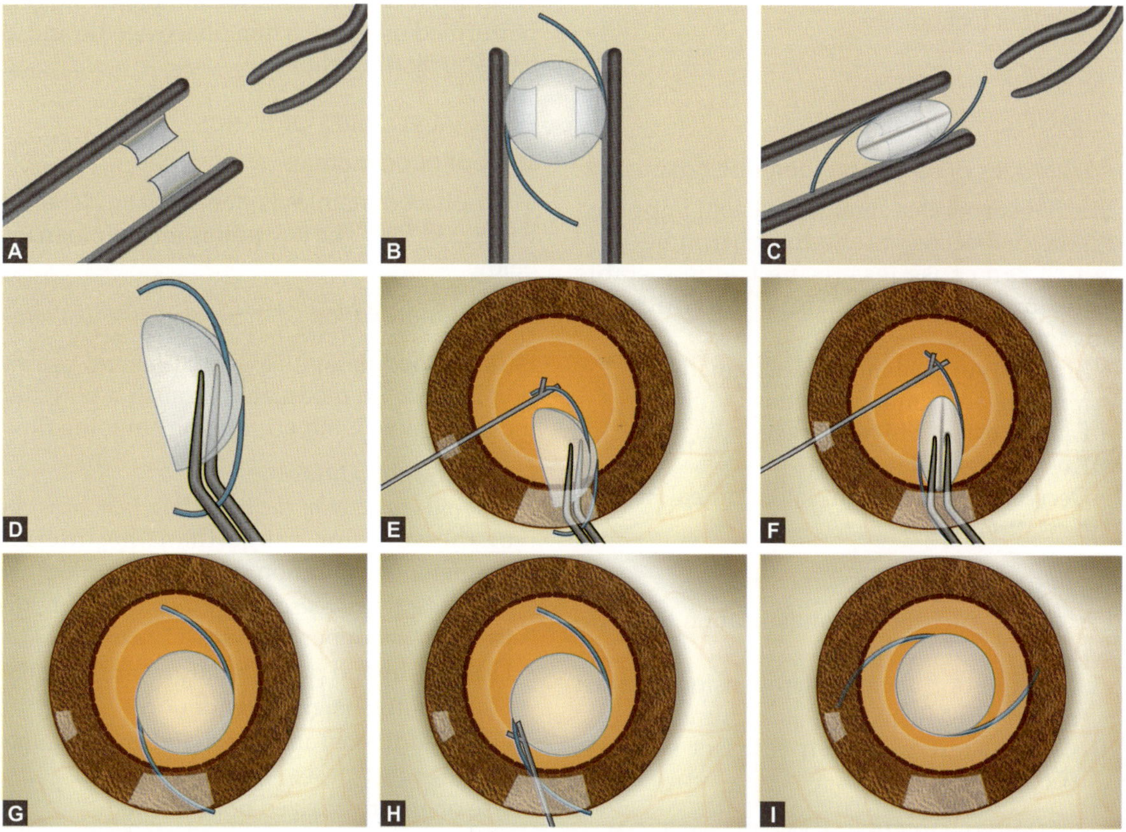

Fig. 15.4.26. *Implantation of foldable IOL using holder-folder system:* ***(A)*** *Holder-folder system comprising two forceps;* ***(B)*** *Grooved forceps folding the IOL;* ***(C)*** *Holding the folded IOL;* ***(D)*** *Folded IOL held by the holding forceps;* ***(E)*** *Inserting the leading haptic and optic of folded IOL in the bag;* ***(G)*** *Released IOL partially in the bag;* ***(H and I)*** *Dialling the trailing haptic in the bag.*

15.5 MICROINCISION CATARACT SURGERY

- Introduction
- Microincision phacoemulsification
- Laser phacolysis
- Aqualase
- High aspiration controlled chop (HACC)

INTRODUCTION

The term 'microincision cataract surgery' (MICS) was coined and patented by Jorge Ilio (Spain) in 2001 to denote all cataract surgical techniques which could be performed through a microincision of 1.5 mm or less. However, presently most MICS are performed through 1.8–2.2 mm incision. The MICS procedures include:

A. Microincision phacoemulsification
B. Laser phacolysis
C. Aqualase
D. High aspiration controlled chop (HACC)
E. Catarex technology.

A. MICROINCISION PHACOEMULSIFICATION

Advantages of microphacoemulsification

MICS incorporates smaller incision, improved fluidics and decreased effective phacotime (EPT) which can cause less tissue trauma, stable anterior chamber and thus, the following advantages:

- Minimal surgical induced astigmatism
- Minimal aberration induction
- Faster postoperative recovery
- Excellent visual recovery
- Decreased incidence of later corneal decompensation.

Types of microphacoemulsification

Essentially microphacoemulsification is of two types:

I. Bimanual or biaxial microincision cataract surgery (BiMICS)
II. Coaxial microincision cataract surgery, (CoMICS)

I. BIMANUAL OR BIAXIAL MICROINCISION CATARACT SURGERY (BiMICS)

BiMICS refers to the surgical technique performed through two microincisions, one for irrigation and the other for aspiration of a reduced size, usually below 1 mm. ***Other terms*** coined for such a technique include the following:

Phakonit is the term used by Prof. Amar Aggarwal from India (1998) for the bimanual *Phaco* done with a *N*eedle *I*ncision *T*echnique through a 1 mm incision. In 2005, the same author performed phakonit through a 0.7 mm incision using a 0.7 mm phaco needle tip and a 0.7 mm irrigating chopper and called it *Microphakonit*.

Microphaco is the term used by Dr. Randall Olsin from USA in 2004 for the phaco surgery performed using a 0.8 mm phaco needle and 21 gauge irrigating chopper.

ESSENTIAL FEATURES OF BiMICS

Microphacodynamics

Microphacodynamics is described in detail on Pages 230–249. The key points are summarized below.

Fluidics modulation

Fluidics modulation, i.e. irrigation and aspiration need to be modulated in such a way that incoming flow is superior to the outgoing flow.

i. *Irrigation modulation*

a. *Internal diameter of the irrigating tube* must be of the superior gauge than the internal diameter of aspiration tube.

b. *Methods to increase irrigation* through the irrigating chopper include:

- Use of fishpond pump to infuse air in the BSS
- Use of bottle height extender
- Use of additional anterior chamber maintainer (ACM)
- Use of air pressurized bottle of BSS
- Mechanized pressure infusion provided in the machines such as Accurus (Alcon) and Millennium (Bausch and Lomb) are very effective

• Use of pressurized plastic bottles using blood pressure apparatus cuff.

ii. *Stable incision* with no leakage plays an important role in providing a stable anterior chamber.

iii. *Flow rate and vacuum* need to be tone down and the whole surgical procedure should be carried out at a slower pace. This allows enough fluid to enter the anterior chamber.

2. *Phaco power modulation in BiMICS*

- *Pulse mode* (3 pulses/second) is recommended over continuous mode.
- *Burst mode* is particularly helpful for hard, brunescent cataracts.
- *Micropulse technology* (e.g. Whitestar), i.e. a cold phaco has added a new impetus and life to the survival and success of microincision phaco.

3. *Surge prevention*

Surge or anterior chamber instability is one of the biggest impediments to the success and further development of microphaco.

Measures to prevent surge include (*see* page 243):

- *Enhanced irrigation* (as discussed above, page 230)
- *Slow pace of surgery* at a low flow rate
- Use of low compliance tubing
- Smaller diameter tube pump
- *Smaller diameter phaco tips.* Flared phaco tips and microflow 2 G phaco tips have an internal bore of 0.6 mm as compared to 0.9 mm in the normal tips (Fig. 15.2.6).

Microphaco technique

Essential features of microphaco technique are summarized:

1. *Incisions.* Two 1–1.5 mm trapezoidal incisions in the clear cornea are made at 10 o' clock and 2 o' clock positions.
2. *Capsulorhexis* can be done with 26 G needle, cystitome or special micro-forceps for capsulorhexis.
3. *Hydrodissection* is performed as for conventional coaxial phaco (*see* pages 203–205).
4. *Nuclear phacoemulsification* is performed bimanually.

Instruments specially needed are:

- *Irrigating chopper*
- *Sleeveless phaco probe,* which is of 2 G and 30° angled
- *Phaco machine* should be high end, e.g. AMO Signature, B and L or Alcon infinity Stellaris.

Nuclear management can be done by divide and conquer or stop and chop or direct chop depending on the surgeon's choice (Fog details *see* pages 256–270).

5. *Cortex removal* is done by using bimanual irrigation and aspiration technique (Fig. 15.4.21, page 271).
6. *IOL insertion.* One of the two microincisions is enlarged to 1.8 mm. The microincision IOLs are inserted through their own dedicated injector by the technique described on page 274, Fig. 15.4.25.

Concluding note. The BiMICS introduced about 25 years ago (Shearing, 1985), has gained some popularity in recent years with the development of advanced high end phaco machines. However, it has still not been widely adopted because of:

- High risk of chamber instability, necessity to decrease fluid parameters, and
- The absence of protective effect of a silicone sleeve introduced between vibrating US needle and the corneal wound.

II. COAXIAL MICROINCISION CATARACT SURGERY

Coaxial microincision cataract surgery (CoMICS) is in fact the conventional phacoemulsification except that it is performed through a microincision (1.8–2.2 mm). This technique was developed after BiMICS to avoid the learning curve and difficulties encountered with BiMICS. It is easier to pass from the conventional phacoemulsification technique to the CoMICS technique as one only needs to change the phaco machine and the machine parameters, as summarized below.

Phaco machine parameters for irrigation and aspiration should be set as below for CoMICS.

- *Phaco sleeve* should be comparatively harder than conventional.
- *Bottle height:* between 80 and 100 cm in order to avoid corneal burns by the phaco tip.

- *For peristaltic pump machine,* parameters when using 21G phaco tip should be:
  - *Flow rate.* 35–60 cc/min, and
  - *Vacuum.* 400 mm Hg (350–500)
- *For Venturi pump machine* when using 21G phaco tip, the parameters should be:
  - *Vacuum:* 350–500 mm Hg

Steps of coaxial micro-phacoemulsification are similar to conventional phacoemulsification except that the main incision is 1.8–2.2 mm. In general, most surgeons prefer phaco chopping techniques.

Phaco machines available for CoMICS and suggested parameters

MICS can be performed with different kinds of aspiration systems. MICS settings with two commonly used phacoemulsification machines are summarized in Tables 15.5.1 and 15.5.2.

Table 15.5.1 *Suggested parameters for CoMICS with Stellaris phaco machine*

Parameter	*Sub-mode 1*	*Sub-mode 2*	*Sub-mode 3*
Suitable grade of lens hardness	+2/+3	+3/+4	+5/+6
Pedal system	Dual foot	Dual foot	Dual foot
Mode	Pulse (80 pulse/sec)	Fix burst (160 milli-sec duration with 320 millisec burst duration)	Multiple Bursts 40 millisec burst duration)
Power	10% US linear	10% US linear	10% US linear
Duty cycle	35%	320 millisec intervals of pulse duration	60%

Table 15.5.2 *Infinity Alcon settings for 19 G MICS*

Step	*Phacoemulsification parameters*	
Chopping	Dynamic rise	0
	Vacuum	150
	Irrigation	110
	Torsional amplitude	Limit 40 On: 20 Off: 40
	Aspiration rate	15
Quadrant removal	Phacoemulsification power	0
	Dynamic rise	2
	Vacuum	500
	Irrigation	110
	Torsional amplitude	Limit 80 On: 20 Off: 40
	Aspiration rate	30
Epinucleus removal	Phacoemulsification power	0
	Vacuum	28
	Irrigation	110
	Torsional amplitude	Limit 30 On: 20 Off: 40
	Aspiration rate	28

TRULY ENDOCAPSULAR MICROINCISION CATARACT SURGERY (TECMIS)

INTRODUCTION

This novel technique described by Dr. AC Cabrera, involves use of 2 corneal incisions of 1.4 mm and 2 micro-capsulorhexes of 1–1.5 mm each. This makes it a minimally invasive technique for faster visual recovery and in the future may help to inject accommodative materials into the capsular bag to provide good vision at all ranges.

Surgical steps

Surgical steps include:

- *Creation of 2 corneal incisions of 1.4 mm each* (Fig. 15.5.1A).
- *2 peripheral small capsulorhexes* (Fig. 15.5.1A). The tiny capsulorhexes are created with a needle cystitome and completed with a 23 G capsulorhexis forceps.
- *Hydrodissections* is performed very gently (Fig. 15.5.1B)
- *Endocapsular phacoemulsification.* Anterior chamber is filled with viscoelastic and endocapsular phacoemulsification is performed using a micro-phaco tip of 0.9 mm and an irrigating chopper introduced into either of the 2 minirhexis openings. The irrigation cannula or chopper and phaco tip should remain in the endocapsular space at all times to prevent PC rupture. Ideally the

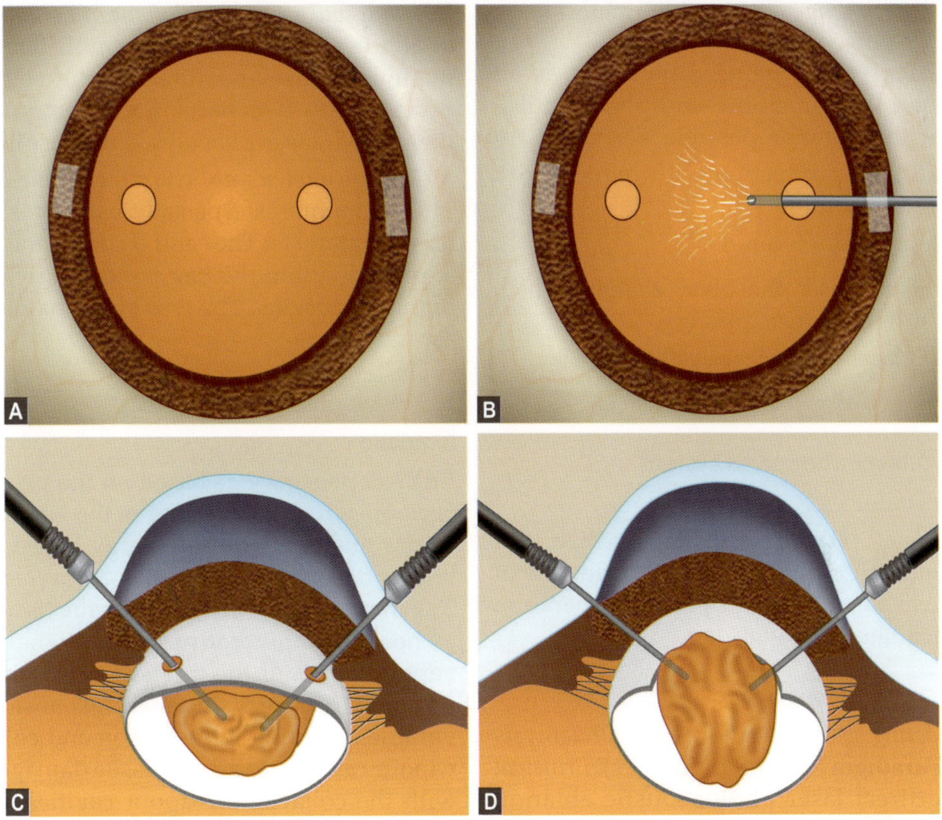

Fig. 15.5.1. *Essential steps of TECMIS vis-à-vis standard MICS:* ***(A)*** *Two tiny capsulorhexes;* ***(B)*** *Hydrodissection;* ***(C)*** *Truly endocapsular bimanual microphacoemulsification;* ***(D)*** *Conventional bimanual micro-phacoemulsification.*

tunnel is created in continuous-burst mode using 10–40% ultrasonic power while emulsification is performed in the pulse mode. Thus, in TECMIS, the entire surgery is completed in the bag minimizing corneal endothelial damage (Fig. 15.5.1C), while in standard micro-phacoemulsification, which is performed partly in the anterior chamber, there occurs anterior chamber tubulence (Fig. 15.5.1D)

- *Bimanual cortical aspiration* and capsular polishing is then performed.
- *The 2 mini-rhexes are then joined* together by giving relaxing incisions.
- *Accommodative IOLs* or injectable gels will be the ideal lens options to maintain capsular elasticity, transparency and accommodation in the future.

Merits

- The entire surgery is completed within the capsular bag minimizing damage to the corneal endothelium because of ultrasonic power and fluid turbulence (Fig. 15.5.1A to C).
- In case of PC rupture, the anterior capsular support may be sufficient for IOL implantation in the sulcus. Further, injectable polymers and accommodative materials of the future could be used in such surgeries.
- The endocapsular irrigation may help to maintain the integrity of the bag in subluxated lenses.

Note. This technique has a steep learning curve and may be challenging to adopt in the beginning but because of the options listed above may become more popular in the coming years.

B. LASER PHACOLYSIS

Laser phacolysis is being developed as an alternative to the microincision phacoemulsification with following possible *advantages*:

- Minimal heat production with reduced risk of corneal burns.
- Smaller and safer wound

The available laser phacolysis systems which work on different principles are:

- Nd:YAG laser phacolysis system, and
- Er:YAG laser phacolase.

1. Nd:YAG laser phacolysis system

Principle

Nd:YAG laser phacolysis systems utilize 1064 nm wavelength and works on the principle of shock wave formation and plasma generation which facilitates removal.

Types of Nd:YAG laser phacolysis systems

i. *Direct acting system* (Photon Laser Phacolysis system, Paradigm Medical Industries). *Principal action* is direct laser photoacoustic ablation under aspiration. With this system, there occurs direct laser disruption of the tissue, which increases efficiency of laser utilization. In these systems, cooling is needed to reduce heat production and prevent tissue damage.

ii. *Indirect acting system* (Dodick Laser Lens Ablation System, ARC Laser, Germany). *Principal action* is indirect: Q switched sonic Laser Transduction. The laser is pulsed (Q-switched) and the probe has an incorporated aspiration function. Inside the tip is present a titanium target towards which laser light (each pulse of 12 mJ energy of 14 nsec duration) is directed. The target acts as a transducer and converts light energy into mechanical shock waves which lyse the nuclear material held at the tip of aspirating port. In this system, there is no need of cooling as heat production is lesser.

Techniques of laser phacolysis

1. ***Pre-slicing and lasing*** *(Dodick technique).* In this technique, the nucleus is pre-sliced into three quadrants. Each quadrant is then lifted, laser phacolysed and aspirated.

2. ***Divide and conquer technique of Zerdab.*** Similar to divide and conquer phacoemulsification, the nucleus is laser-sculpted in the centre and divided into two parts. Each heminucleus is then lifted, laser phacolysed and aspirated.

3. ***Central nucleus ablation technique of Rout.*** This technique is especially useful for grade 4 harder cataracts. The central core of the nucleus is pulsed within the bag, followed by collapse of the epinucleus. The lysed lens matter is then aspirated.

2. Er:YAG phacolase

Principle

Er:YAG phacolase is based on the principle of *photovapourization* of water in the lens and near ocular media. The laser energy in the Er:YAG laser phacolysis system has a wavelength of 2940 nm, which is absorbed by the tissue water as heat. At temperatures greater than 100°C, vapourization of the tissue water occurs. As a result, there occurs a dramatic expansion of the volume, resulting in formation and collapse of vapour cavities leading to tissue damage. Along with the collapse of vapour cavities, acoustic transients (pressure waves) are also produced which cause secondary mechanical damage.

Technique

Pulsed laser energy is used to vapourize and fragment the high water content lens nucleus. The surgical technique is same as for the conventional phacoemulsification except that instead of mechanical ultrasound energy, the laser energy is used. However, with increasing lens hardness, less proteins coagulate, making phacolysis increasingly difficult with Er:YAG laser.

BIMANUAL BI-ENERGY TECHNIQUE FOR CATARACT EXTRACTION

Bimanual Bi-energy (BIMBIE) technique for cataract extraction, still under evaluation involves use of both ultrasonic and laser energy for a faster and better technique:

- *Ultrasonic fragmentation-irrigation* allows efficient fragmentation of the nucleus, and
- *Laser phacolysis-aspiration* allows more efficient aspiration.

C. AQUALASE

In aqualase technology (developed at Alcon Laboratories), instead of mechanical ultrasound energy, small pulses of pre-heated fluid is used to emulsify the nucleus. Nuclei up to grade II are removed with ease while nuclei of grade III or more hardness require slightly larger operating time.

Advantages of aqualase technology over phaco are:

- *Lesser risk of posterior capsular rupture* as this technique avoids the microimplosions and turbulence characteristically seen with phacoemulsification.
- *No corneal wound burns* with aqualase.
- *Less chances of PCO,* as aqualase is more effective in removing lens epithelial cells.
- *Faster technique* than phacoemulsification for soft cataracts.

D. HIGH ASPIRATION CONTROLLED CHOP

High aspiration controlled chop (HACC) is a type of pre-chop technique for microincision cataract surgery (MICS) which is independent of energy-based phacolysis. It does not require phaco handpiece and can be performed just with the help of an automated irrigation-aspiration device. Thus, it is a pre-chop, zero phaco technique which allows easy removal of cataracts up to grade IV nuclear hardness.

Advantages over phacoemulsification

- *Thermal burns,* no risk.
- *Endothelial cell count loss* is less.
- *Posterior capsular tear,* less chances.
- *Universal application,* i.e. even in areas in the developing world where there is limited access to advanced machinery.
- *Low cost MICS,* as compared to other techniques.

E. CATAREX TECHNOLOGY

Catarex technology, also known as vortex phacoemulsicification, is a fundamentally new and different technology which utilises a high speed motor with a 1.5 mm diameter partially shielded impeller probe. This technology utelises a rotation-based vartex flow in the capsular bag through a tiny capsulorhexis.

- Vortex phacoemulsification involves placement of a tiny rotary impeller inside the capsular bag through a tiny capsulorrhexis. The impeller rotates at 60 kHz and causes expansion of the capsular bag with rotation of the nuclear complex, thus allowing extraction of the cataract from a nearly intact lens capsule. Expansion of the capsular bag *minimizes risk* of capsular rupture.

Essential steps of the technique are:

- *Tiny circular capsulorhexis* (1.5 mm) is constructed with a round diathermy instrument, thus reducing the technical demands of such a surgical feat.
- *Hydrodissection* is performed with gentle irrigation by placing the I/A tube containing the rotary impellar over the capsulorhexis.
- *Nuclear material* is removed from the capsular bag with vortex action with no ultrasound at all as described above.
- *Cortex* is then stripped away and aspirated.

Advantages

- This technique is much faster than conventional phacoemulsification.
- Entire capsular bag is left in situ following cataract extraction, as the cataract extraction is done through a very small capsulorhexis. However, this technique like truly endocapsular microincision cataract surgery (TECMIS) will be more useful only when injectable artificial crystalline lenses become available.

15.6 FEMTOSECOND CATARACT SURGERY

- Introduction
- Femtosecond laser
- Steps of femto-cataract surgery
- Advantages and complications
- Limitations of femtosecond cataract surgery

INTRODUCTION

The introduction of the premium IOLs required perfection and precision in cataract surgery as small deviations in surgical technique will have a significant impact on the postoperative vision achieved. For instance, a perfect continuous curvilinear capsulorhexis (CCC) is required to achieve the optimum IOL placement in-the-bag and maintain the correct effective lens position (ELP) to achieve a zero refractive error postoperatively. Similarly surgically induced astigmatism (SIA) should be kept minimal and any pre-existing astigmatism should be further tackled with limbal relaxing incisions (LRI) or opposite-clear corneal incisions (OCCI).

The need for near-perfection is being now achieved with the femtosecond laser cataract surgery which has been introduced in 2010 in the US and in India in 2011.

FEMTOSECOND LASER

MECHANISM OF ACTION OF FEMTOSECOND LASER

A femtosecond laser uses an infrared beam of light to precisely separate the tissues through a process called photo-disruption by generating pulses as short as one-quadrillionth of a second (10^{-15} = femtosecond). It has a wavelength of 1053 nm and is based upon the technology whereby focussed laser pulses divide material at the molecular level without transfer of heat or impact to the surrounding tissue.

The laser beam is focused on a pre-programmed depth and position with each pulse forming a microscopic bubble. As the laser moves painlessly back and forth, the bubbles connect to form a plasma wave which creates a cleavage plane of separation with no trauma to adjacent tissue.

USES OF FEMTOSECOND LASER

So far, the femtosecond laser has been used for the following procedures:

- Creation of a corneal flap for LASIK
- Creation of corneal tunnels for implanting intracorneal ring implants
- Arcuate incisions to correct astigmatism
- Corneal keratoplasty incisions

Femtosecond laser cataract surgery is the latest breakthrough in the use of femtosecond technology, wherein the femtosecond laser is able to create all required surgical incisions with perfect dimensions and architecture, a perfectly centred and sized capsulotomy and help to liquefy and chop the lens. Along with this, precise corneal incisions can be created to treat any pre-existing astigmatism resulting in near perfect outcomes.

The US FDA cleared femtosecond lasers for cataract surgery in 2010 and 3 companies OptiMedica, LensAR (Fig. 15.6.1) and LenSx are developing this technology for widespread use.

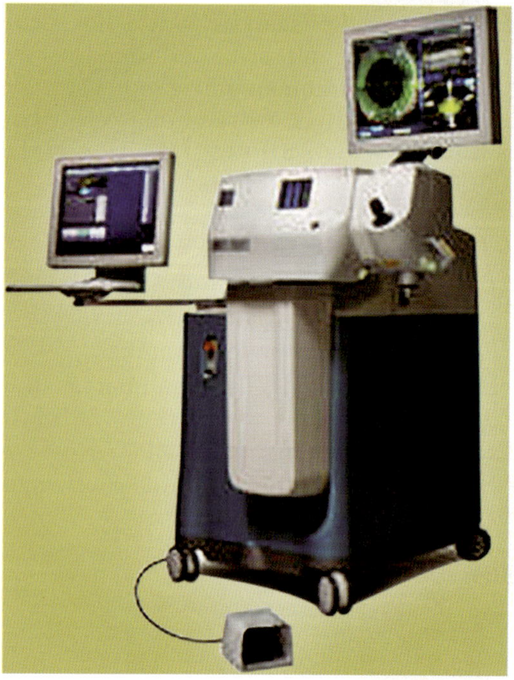

Fig. 15.6.1. *Femtosecond laser cataract surgery system (LenSx; courtesy Alcon).*

The clinical trials of femtosecond cataract surgery in India have been completed and this laser has now become commercially available in India.

The laser causes 43% reduction of phacoemulsification energy and 51% reduction in time which improves the safety profile. In addition, the well-centred, precise continuous capsulorhexis done by the laser is an important consideration for premium IOLs and when combined with limbal relaxing incisions provide a real refractive cataract surgery experience.

STEPS OF FEMTO-CATARACT SURGERY

Steps of femtosecond laser-assisted cataract surgery (FLACS) can be divided into three:

- Pre-femtosecond laser manoeuvres
- Femtosecond laser manoeuvres
- Post-femtosecond laser manoeuvres.

Pre-femtosecond laser manoeuvres

- Pupil is dilated.
- Topical anaesthetic drops are instilled.
- Wire speculum is placed.
- Cornea is applanated with a disposable patient interface cone.
- A high resolution video-microscope combined with a real-time OCT captures images of the anterior segment of the patient's eye (Fig. 15.6.2).
- The images are analyzed and each step is planned and customized according to the patients requirement and surgeons' preference (Fig. 15.6.2)
- Size, shape and location of the incisions is mapped and marked (Fig. 15.6.2).

Femtosecond laser manoeuvres

The laser foot pedal is depressed to begin the laser procedure which includes the following:

Capsulorhexis is created at a depth of 500 microns in the anterior capsule. With FSL, there is a higher degree of circularity, fewer incomplete capsulorhexis-IOL overlap, and better IOL centration. Further, FSL-guided capsulotomy diameter did not show correlation to pupil diameter, eye size, or curvature of the cornea as opposed to manual capsulorhexis. Smooth,

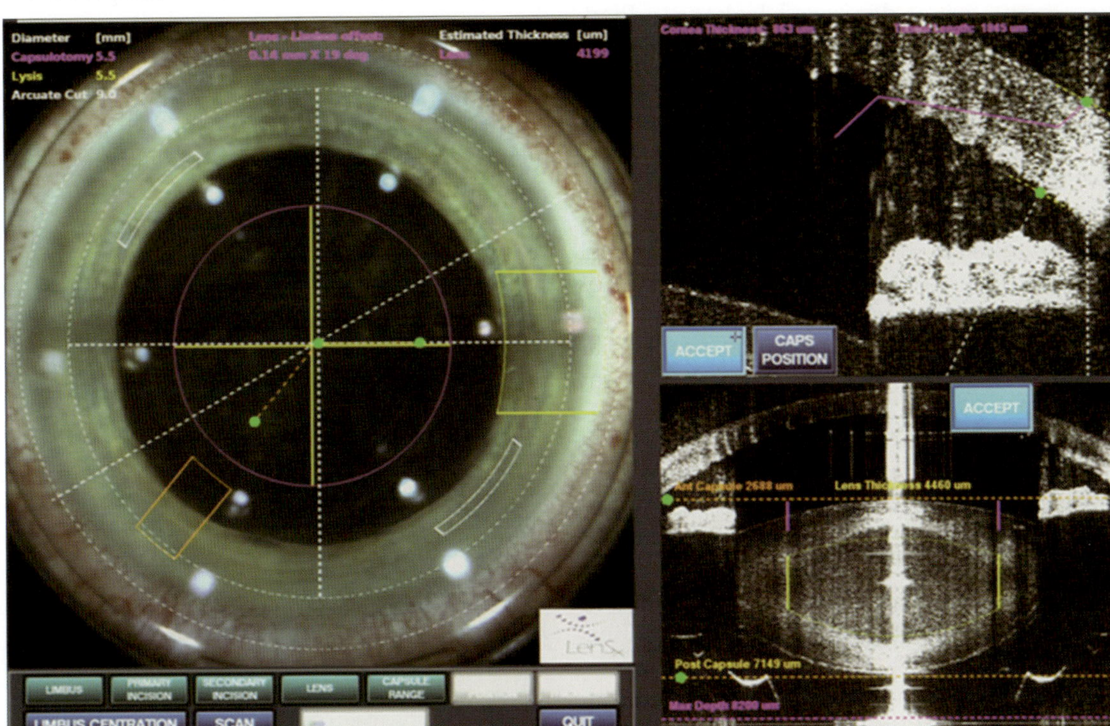

Fig. 15.6.2. *OCT picture of anterior segment and castomized planning for femtosecond cataract surgery.*

regular edges offer superior capsular strength and resistance to capsular tears. Additionally, the unpredictable diameter observed in manual capsulorhexis can have effects on IOL centration, with subsequent poor refractive outcomes, unpredictable anterior chamber depths, and increased rates of posterior capsular opacification.

Lens fragmentation incisions are performed staying 1000 microns above the posterior capsule. Capsulorhexis is done prior to it because lens fragmentation causes release of gas bubbles, which can distort the anatomy and affect capsulotomy planning. The ultrasound phacoemulsification carries the risks of corneal injury because of long duration of ultrasound exposure, damage caused by heat or mechanical manipulation, and injury caused by the fragmenting lens. With prior lens fragmentation with FSL, there occurs reduction in ultrasound energy and instrumentation. Thus, FSLs may show improved safety and decreased complications.

Primary and secondary corneal incisions are carried out. FSL-guided corneal incisions offer the advantages of decreased leakage, added stability, and reproducibility at various IOPs.

Arcuate corneal incisions are created to tackle any co-existing astigmatism.

Post-femtosecond laser manoeuvres

The patient is then wheeled under an operating microscope and the surgery completed with removal of the capsulorhexis flap, phacoaspiration of the lens fragments and cortical clean-up.

The IOL is implanted and the procedure completed.

Primary posterior laser capsulotomy

Steps of performing primary posterior laser capsulotomy (PPLC)

- *Ocular viscous device (OVD) is injected,* in small amount, behind the IOL, after the cataract surgery procedure is complete.
- *Capsulotomy position is confirmed,* then on the live OCT scan.
- *Eye is redocked* to the femtosecond laser system. This is done just like it is at the beginning of laser cataract surgery.
- *Cylindrical treatment zone for anterior capsulotomy is then manually positioned* on the posterior capsule, which is placed in the first inferior third of the treatment zone (diameter 3.5 mm, incision depth 600–800 µm, horizontal spot spacing 5 µm, vertical spot spacing 10 µm, pulse energy 8 µJ). Care is taken to avoid positioning the treatment zone within the IOL optic or the anterior hyaloid.
- *PPLC is then performed* (treatment time about 2.5 seconds). Immediately after treatment, the posterior capsular disc usually starts to contract. There is no need to remove this disc. It curls up, sinks down, disappears, and cannot move into the vitreous because the anterior hyaloid membrane is left intact.[4] It does not cause visual disturbances such as floaters and generally does not bother the patient at all.
- *Eye is undocked*, and the patient is moved back under the operating microscope to confirm whether the posterior capsulotomy is well centered and free-floating for 360°.

ADVANTAGES AND COMPLICATIONS

Advantages. Various studies have shown that *optical coherence tomography (OCT)-guided nuclear fragmentation* improves refractive results, reduces the risk of complications such as posterior capsule rupture, endophthalmitis and endothelial cell density loss. The first clinical results show that femtosecond laser incisions achieved perfect diameter accuracy in 100% of cases, while only 10% of surgeons' manual cuts were within 0.25 mm error. With more than 6000 procedures performed world wide, this is definitely the cataract surgery of the future.

Complications reported so far are *capsular blockage syndrome* (CBS) or *femtocataract intracapsular gass syndrome* in which accumulation of fluid after hydrodissection in the capsular bag led to capsular rupture with nucleus drop. Advanced grade of cataract was the common risk factor along with old age. While only few cases have been published so far, further experience will help to tackle this problem in femto-cataract cases.

LIMITATIONS OF FEMTOSECOND CATARACT SURGERY

Limitations of FLACS are not well-established at this time. Based on relative contraindications to FSL refractive surgery, it is thought that similar contraindications may apply to FLACS.

- ***Patients those who have deep set orbits or those with tremors or dementia*** logistically may do poorly with the initial docking of the lens that requires patient cooperation.
- ***Other exclusions may include*** anterior basement membrane dystrophy, corneal opacities (such as arcus senilis, corneal dystrophies, and trauma- or contact lens-induced scars), ocular surface disease, pannus with encroaching blood vessels, or recurrent epithelial erosion syndrome.
- ***The level of increase in IOP*** induced by the docking device has not been adequately quantified in published studies. This may be a significant contraindication for patients with glaucoma, optic neuropathies, or borderline endothelial pathology.
- ***Diabetics*** may have undiagnosed epithelial disease making them prone to epithelial defects. A foreseeable complication could be persistent epithelial defects from the trauma of docking into an optical system, in an otherwise routine cataract surgery.
- ***Patients with poor dilation would be poor candidates*** because FLACS relies on anterior segment imaging for laser pattern mapping. Such patients would include those with posterior synechiae, intraoperative floppy iris syndrome suspects, or those on chronic miotic medications. High-quality images for mapping of the posterior lens are critical. More studies are needed to assess, if dense posterior subcapsular cataracts, those with vacuoles, anterior subcapsular cataracts, and other types or combinations of cataracts will perform differently with FSL-assisted phacofragmentation.
- ***Patients with phacodonesis and zonular dialysis,*** or even those with risk factors such as pseudoexfoliation syndrome or trauma, may not be ideal candidates since having a stable, stationary lens is needed for precise laser mapping and execution.
- ***Cost*** is the final discussion point for FLACS. Because the size of the laser platforms is quite large, many surgery centres may require an extra step of moving a patient from the preoperative laser suite to the operating room. This will also be an extra cost in both time and efficiency.

BIBLIOGRAPHY

PHACODYNAMICS

1. Fine IH, Packer M, Hoffman RS: Power modulations in new phacoemulsification technology. J Cataract Refract Surg 30:1014–1019,2004.

PHACOEMULSIFICATION

1. Linebarger EJ, Hardten DR, Shah GK, et al. Phacoemulsification and modern cataract surgery. Surv Ophthalmol 44:123–147,1999.
2. Phacoemulsification: Principles and Techniques, Second edition. Lucio Buratto.
3. Shearing SP, Relyca RL, Louiza A et al. Routine phacoemulsification through a one millimetre non sutured incision. Cataract 2:6–11,1985.
4. Unal M, Yücel I, Sarici A et al. Phacoemulsification with topical anesthesia: Resident experience. J Cataract Refract Surg. 32: 1361–1365, 2006.

MICROINCISION CATARACT SURGERY

1. Agarwal A, Agarwal A, Agarwal S, Narang P, Narang S. Phaconit: phacoemulsification through a 0.9 mm corneal incision. J Cataract Refract Surg 27(10):1548–1552,2001 Oct.
2. Alio J, Rodriguez-Prats JL, Galal A, Ramzy M. Outcomes of microincision cataract surgery versus coaxial phacoemulsification. Ophthalmology 112(11):1997–2003,2005 Nov.
3. Allen D; Vasavada, A. "Cataract and surgery for cataract.". *BMJ* 333 (7559): 128–132,Jul 2006. doi:10.1136/bmj.333.7559.128. PMID 16840470.
4. Alió Jorge L; Agdeppa Ma. Cecilia C; Pongo, Vanessa C.; El Kady, Bassam. "Micro-incision cataract surgery with toric intraocular lens implantation for correcting moderate and high astigmatism: Pilot study". *Journal of Cataract & Refractive Surgery* 36, 2010: 44.doi:10.1016/j.jcrs.2009.07.043.
5. Braga-Mele R, Liu E. Feasibility of sleeveness bimanual phacoemulsification with the Millennium microsurgical system. J Cataract Refract Surg 29(11):2199–2203,2003 Nov.
6. Colvard DM. Bimanual technique to manage subincisional cortical material. J Cataract Refract Surg 23(5):707–709,1997 Jun.

8. Duker, Jay S.; Myron Yanoff MD; Yanoff, Myron; Jay S. Duker MD (2009). *Ophthalmology*. St. Louis, Mo: Mosby/Elsevier. ISBN 0-323-04332-1.
9. Fine IH, Hoffman RS, Packer M. Optimizing refractive lens exchange with bimanual micro-incision phacoemulsification. J Cataract Refract Surg 30(3):550–554,2004 Mar.
10. Hoffman RS, Fine IH, Packer M. New phaco-emulsification technology. Curr Opin Ophtalmol 16(1):38–43,2005 Feb.
11. Microincisional cataract surgery: the art and science. Amar Agrawal, Richard Lindstrom.
12. Minimising incisions and maximising outcomes in cataract surgery. Jorge L Aliao, I. Howard Fine.
13. Tsuneoka H, Hayama A, Takahama M. Ultrasmall-incision bimanual phacoemulsification and Acrysof SA30AL implantation through a 2.2 mm incision. J Cataract Refract Surg 29(6):1070–1076, 2003 Jun.

FEMTOSECOND CATARACT SURGERY

1. Batlle JF, Feliz R, Culbertson WW. OCT-guided femtosecond laser cataract & surgery: precision and efficacy. Association for Research in Vision and Ophthalmology Annual Meeting. A4694 Poster #D633. Fort Lauderdale, FL, 2011. www.arvo.org
2. Friedman NJ, Palanker DV, Schuele G, et al. Femtosecond laser capsulotomy. J Cataract Refract Surg 37:1189–1198,2011.
3. Masket S, Sarayba M, Ignacio T, Fram N. Femtosecond laser-assisted cataract incisions: architectural stability and reproducibility. J Cataract Refract Surg 36(6):1048–1049,2010 June.
4. Miháltz K, Knorz MC, Alió JL, et al. Internal aberrations and optical quality after femtosecond laser anterior capsulotomy in cataract surgery. J Refract Surg 27:711–716,2011.
5. Nagy Z, Takacs A, Filkorn T, Sarayba M. Initial clinical evaluation of an intraocular femtosecond laser in cataract surgery. J Refract Surg 25:1053–1060,2009.
6. Palanker DV, Blumenkranz MS, Andersen D, et al. Femtosecond laser-assisted cataract surgery with integrated optical coherence tomography. Sci Transl Med 2:58ra85,2010.
7. Roberts TV, Sutton G, Lawless MA, Jindal-Bali S, Hodge C. Capsular block syndrome associated with femtosecond laser-assisted cataract surgery. J Cataract Refract Surg 37(11):2068–2070,2011 Nov.
8. Steinert R. Presentation. Femtosecond Laser Refractive Cataract Surgery. 63rd Annual Proctor Lecture. Dec 3, 2011 Accessed 6th Junehttp://www.ucsfcme.com/2012/slides/MOP12002/33 Steinert Femto second Laser Cataract Surgery.pdf

CATARACT SURGERY IN SPECIAL SITUATIONS

CHAPTER 16

INTRODUCTION

Through each and every case of cataract surgery is a special situation for the patient as well as the operating surgeon and, so, needs special care on the part of both patient and the surgeon. However, there are certain more special situations, which may be called as difficult situations or challenging situations for the surgeon and require a meticulous planning for:

- Preoperative considerations,
- Peroperative considerations, and
- Postoperative considerations.

Some special situations which are challenging for the surgeons include:

- Small pupil,
- Subluxated cataract,
- Pseudoexfoliation syndrome,
- Cataract in uveitic eye,
- Dense cataract,
- Posterior polar cataract,
- Traumatic cataract,
- Cataract with post-refractive surgery and
- Paediatric cataract (*see* Chapter 17, pages 306–311)

PHACOEMULSIFICATION IN SMALL PUPIL

CAUSES OF SMALL PUPIL

A small non-dilating pupil (4 mm or less after dilation) is one of the common problems in cataract surgery. Common causes of non dilating pupil are:

- Advanced age and arteriosclerosis,
- Post-uveitis (synechiae formation),
- Pseudoexfoliation syndrome,
- Prolonged miotic therapy,
- High hypermetropia,
- Diabetic patients,
- Neurological conditions such as Argyll Robertson pupil

ANTICIPATED RISKS AND COMPLICATIONS

Anticipated risks and complications, in patients with small non-dilating pupil include:
- Difficulty during each step of surgery
- Postoperative inflammation due to excessive iris manipulation
- Iris trauma
- Peroperative and postoperative hyphaema
- Postoperative glaucoma
- Temporary or permanent postoperative mydriasis

MANAGEMENT CONSIDERATIONS FOR NARROW PUPIL

A. Preoperative considerations

Preoperative considerations to decrease complications and maximize outcome of surgery include:

1. ***Educating patients*** about the situation, possible risks and complications and that the patients should have realistic expectations.
2. ***Measures to achieve maximum pupil dilation*** include:
   - *Discontinue miotic agents* at least 3 and preferably 7 days before surgery.
   - *Topical NSAID eyedrops* (flubiprufen 0.03% or ketorolac 0.5%) should be used QID for 3–4 days before surgery and every 15 min 2 hours before surgery.
   - *Topical mydriatics* should include 5–10% phenylephrine, 0.8–1% tropicamide and 0.5–1% cyclopentolate. These should be instilled every 10 min for 2 hours before surgery. Use of cotton wick (soaked in the above drugs) in the inferior fornix may be helpful.
3. ***To prevent hyphaema*** from injury to the iris (due to extensive manipulation), stop aspirin and other anticoagulants 7 days prior to surgery.
4. ***To decrease postoperative inflammation*** (due to extensive iris manipulation):
   - Consider use of topical steroids along with NSAIDs.
   - Oral NSAIDs and/or steroids may also be considered.
   - Consider use of hydrophobic IOLs.

B. Anaesthetic considerations

Always prefer *peribulbar block anaesthesia* rather than topical/intracameral anaesthesia due to anticipated excessive iris manipulation.

C. Peroperative considerations

1. ***Wound considerations***. There are two different recommendations:
   i. *Anterior corneal incision* should be given to prevent higher risk of iris prolapse with posterior corneal incision.
   ii. *Scleral tunnel or limbal approach* should be considered, if there is increased likelihood of conversion to conventional ECCE.
2. ***Viscoelastic considerations***. A high molecular weight viscoelastic agent is recommended to aid in pupillary dilation, synechiolysis and haemostasis.
3. ***Measures to enlarge pupil size*** (when pharmacological dilation is of little help) include:
   i. *Synechiolysis* with viscoelastics and use of spatula to sweep below the iris tissue. At times, cyclitic membrane along the pupillary border can be peeled off to free the pupil.
   ii. *Stretch pupilloplasty* with the use of two y hooks, or Kugler hooks or similar instruments is a simple and effective treatment (Fig. 16.1). Four point pupillary dilation with the use of a microhook and Beechler's pupil dilator is also very effective (Fig. 16.2).
   iii. *Use of iris retractors, and other devices* has also become very popular to sustain the dilation of pharmacologically non-dilating pupil. These include:
   - *Flexible iris retractors or hooks*. These are made of nylon and are applied by making four equidistant paracentesis sites in the peripheral

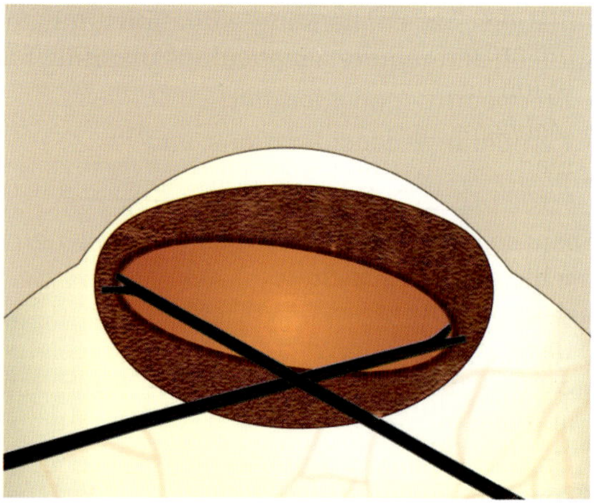

Fig. 16.1. *Stretch pupilloplasty using two hooks.*

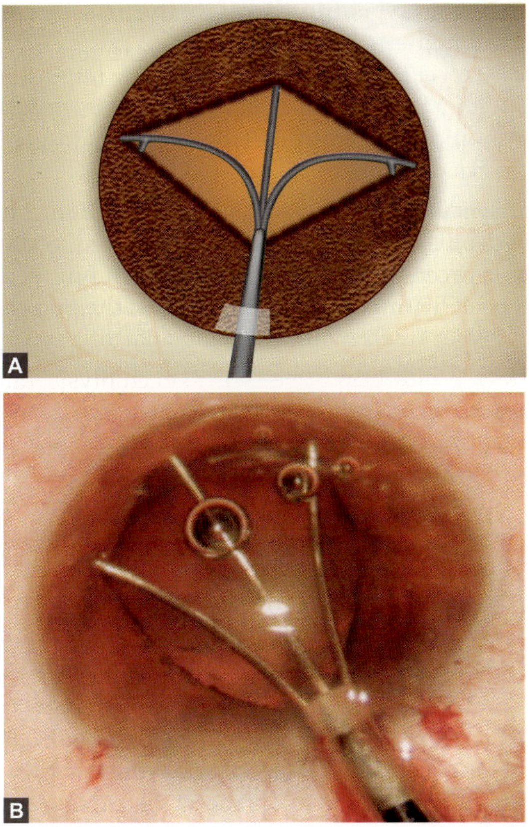

Fig. 16.2. *Stretch pupilloplasty using the Beehler pupil dilator:* **(A)** *Diagrammatic;* **(B)** *Clinical photograph.*

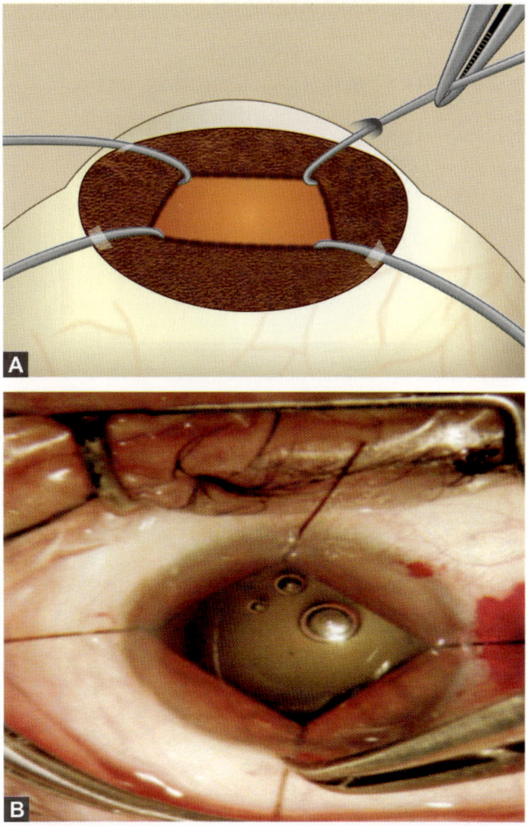

Fig. 16.3. *Pupil stretching using flexible nylon iris retractors equipped with adjustable silicone sleeves:* **(A)** *Diagrammatic;* **(B)** *Clinical photograph.*

cornea. These are anchored with the help of external silicone sleeves (Fig. 16.3).

- *Mackool self-retaining titanium mechanical hooks* can also be used similar to flexible iris hooks, but are much less popular than the disposable nylon hooks.
- *Malyugin ring.* This is a rectangular device made of 5–0 polypropylene which uses the scroll principle to catch the pupillary margin.
- *Hydroview iris protector ring* is a hydrogel ring, which is inserted in the anterior chamber in a dehydrated form (compressed oval). It has flanges on the edge of inner surface that capture the pupil. On hydration, it expands and thus dilates the pupil.
- *Graether pupil expander* system consists of three components: pupil expander, an inserter and an iris glide retractor expander. The pupil expander is a soft silicone ring with a circumferential groove which engages the pupillary margin and allows sustained pupillary dilation.
- *Morcher pupillary dilator* is a semicircular elastic PMMA ring which may be inserted manually or with the help of Geuder dilator injector.

iv. *Surgical measures to enlarge pupil* include:

- *Multiple sphincterotomies* performed at the pupillary border with the help of Vanna's scissors (Fig. 16.4).
- *Radial iridotomy* made through a peripheral iridectomy either at 6 o'clock position or at 12 o'clock position results in keyhole pupil (Fig. 16.5). After completing the surgery, the defect can be closed using McCannel suture.

4. ***Considerations during capsulorhexis.*** It is difficult to perform adequate sized capsulor-

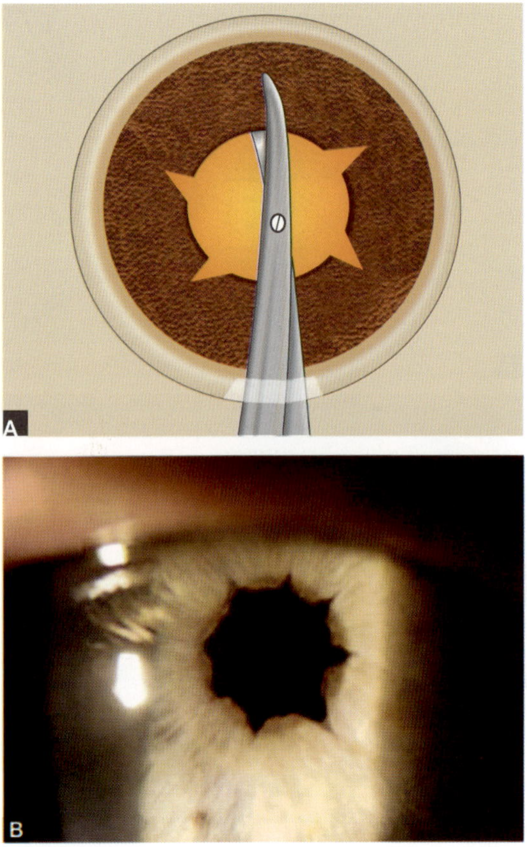

Fig. 16.4. *Multiple sphincterotomies performed at the pupillary border with Vanna's scissors to enlarge the pupil: **(A)** Diagrammatic; **(B)** Clinical photograph.*

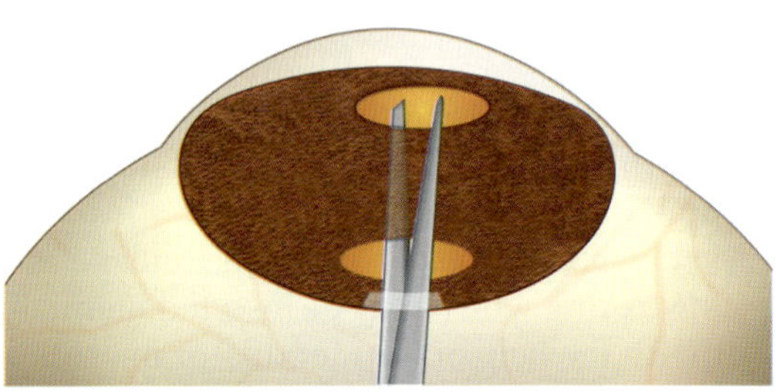

Fig. 16.5. *Radial iridotomy being performed through the peripheral iridectomy.*

hexis with a small pupil. Certain considerations for mid-dilated pupil include:

- *Mechanical retraction of pupil with Sinskey hook* repeatedly in different areas gives a direct view of the running margin of the capsulorhexis.
- *CCC under the iris in an air-filled anterior chamber* is practised by some surgeons. The tearing rhexis is visible through the iris in this technique.
- *Good control of capsulorhexis* is very important with a small pupil. Therefore, the technique should be performed slowly and with great ease.

5. ***Considerations during hydrodissection.*** The hydrodissection should be performed gently but properly with mid-dilated pupil. It is especially important to ensure that the nucleus can spin freely within the capsular bag before proceeding with phacoemulsification.

6. ***Considerations during nuclear emulsification with mid-dilated pupil***
   - *Phaco-chop* should be preferred over the nuclear fractis technique.
   - *Pupillary plane* phacoemulsification should be performed after creating a deep central space.
   - *Phaco parameters* recommended are low aspiration flow rates (AFR) and low vacuum rate to avoid inadvertent aspiration of the iris and posterior capsule.

7. ***Considerations for thorough cortical clean*** include use of a Kuglen hook or y-hook to retract the pupil to allow direct visualization of the remaining cortical matter.

D. Postoperative considerations

1. ***Postoperative inflammation and CME*** are likely to be more severe because in small pupil there is excessive iris manipulation and inadequate cortical clean up. So, intensive topical steroid therapy and topical NSAID therapy are recommended.

2. ***Postoperative glaucoma*** due to debris (blood, pigment and inflammatory cells) is more likely and so needs to be monitored and managed.

PHACOEMULSIFICATION IN SUBLUXATED LENS/ZONULAR DIALYSIS

A. PREOPERATIVE CONSIDERATIONS

A thorough preoperative evaluation should be carried out to:

- *Determine the predisposing conditions* such as trauma, pseudoexfoliation syndrome, high myopia, iris coloboma, hypermaturity, cyclitis and associated systemic conditions such as

Marfan's syndrome or other described in Chapter 6 (pages 83–90).

- *Zonular defect* should be characterized preoperatively in terms of degrees/clock hours of loss.
- *Vitreous loss* is present or absent in the anterior chamber.
- *Phacodonesis* is present or absent.

B. ANAESTHETIC CONSIDERATIONS

- *General anaesthesia* in children and *peribulbar anaesthesia* in adults should be preferred over topical and intracameral anaesthesia.
- *Avoid stress on zonules* in the form of extensive digital massage, Pinky or Honan balloon.

C. PEROPERATIVE CONSIDERATIONS

I. Incision

- *Incision site.* Avoid incision in the zone of subluxation to prevent enlargement of subluxation. Preferable site of incision should be in the zone opposite the subluxation to minimize traction on the zonules. However, if not possible, it may be perfomed 90° to the subluxation.
- *Scleral window* should be precut in the zone of zonular disinsertion, when the need of transscleral suture is anticipated to suture the IOL or capsular ring to the sulcus.

II. Capsulorhexis

- *Highly retentive viscoelastic material* should be used adequately over the area of zonular dialysis so as to tamponade the vitreous and maintain deep non-collapsing anterior chamber.
- *Vitrectomy,* if needed before capsulorhexis, should be performed with two-port system, as co-axial vitrectomy system hydrates the vitreous at the level of zonular dehiscence.
- *Initiation of capsulorhexis* should be done in the area remote from dialysis where the capsule offers sufficient resistance. Initial perforation and creation of flap is most difficult. Effective perforation of the anterior capsule may be achieved by a sharp 15° knife or a diamond blade.
- *Advamcement of capsulorhexis flap* should be in a tangential manner using 26 G bent needle or forceps. Centripetal traction can unzip the remaining zonules.
- *Size of the capsulorhexis* should be relatively large (6 mm) to counteract the tendency for further capsular contraction.

III. Hydrodissection

Gentle but thorough cortical cleavage hydrodissection should be performed carefully so as to free the nucleus maximally and lessen the stress on the zonules during phacoemulsification

IV. Phacoemulsification

Surgical recommendations based on the extent of subluxation

Before commencing nucleus management with phacoemulsification, reassess the zonular dialysis and take following measures:

- *Mild (<3 o'clock hours) zonular dialysis.* In such cases, conventional phacoemulsification can be carried out considering the below mentioned principles.
- *Moderate (3–5 o'clock hours) zonular dialysis.* Capsular tension ring (CTR) is implanted before commencing the phacoemulsification.
- *Severe (up to 7 o'clock hours) zonular dialysis.* Modified CTR (MCTR) or Cionni's CTR is fixed to the sclera with 10–0 prolene before commencing nuclear management.

Capsular tension rings (CTRs)

Types of CTRs

Capsular tension ring (CTR) also known as 'equator ring' or 'endocapsular ring (ECR)' is made of PMMA. Though originally introduced to inhibit the proliferation of equatorial epithelial cells by *Hara et al., the capsular tension rings (CTRs)* are mainly used for zonular dialysis and subluxated lenses. The CTRs work on the principle of traction–expansion and stabilization. These maintain the circular contour of the bag despite zonular dehiscence. Various CTRs available presently are (Fig. 16.6):

- Morcher CTRs
- Cionni CTRs
- Henderson capsular tension ring (HCTR)
- Ahmed capsular tension segment (CTS).

I. ***Morcher capsular tension ring (CTR)***

Morcher CTRs (Fig. 16.6A) are currently most commonly used. These are available in three

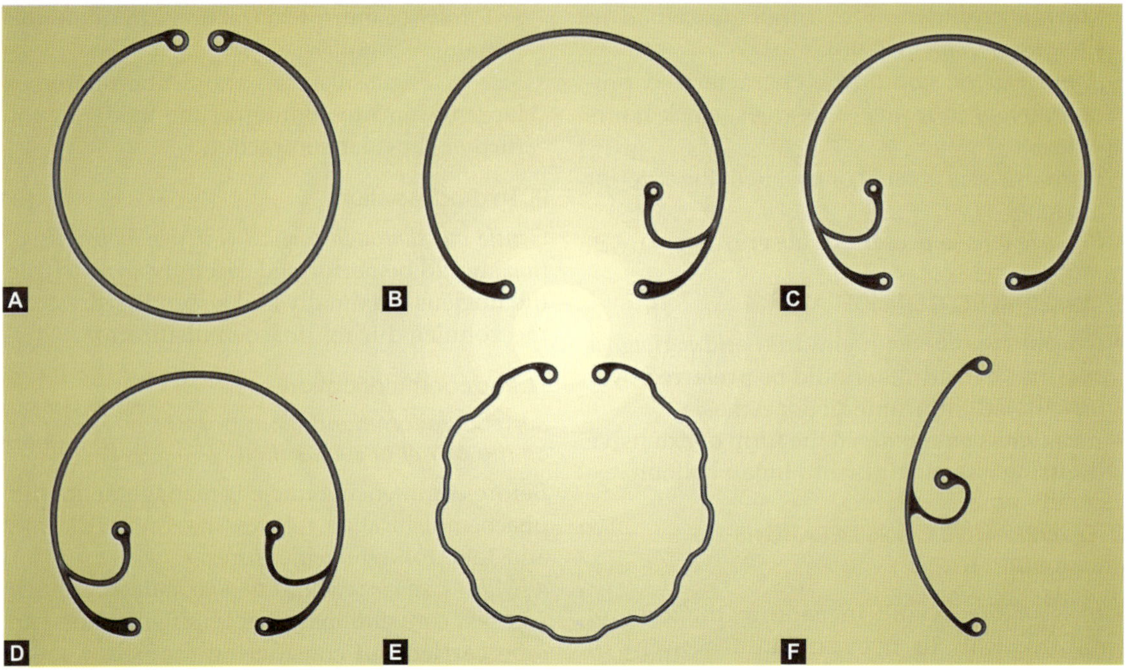

Fig. 16.6. *Various capsular tension rings available:* ***(A)*** *Morcher CTR;* ***(B to D)*** *Cionni's CTR;* ***(E)*** *Henderson CTR;* ***(F)*** *Ahmed CTS.*

types based on their diameters. Their indications are depicted in Table 16.1.

II. ***Cionni's capsular tension ring*** (Fig. 16.6B to D), also called as modified capsular tension ring (MCTR), is specially designed for scleral fixation.

III. ***Henderson capsular tension ring (HCTR)*** is a specially designed open C-shaped loop made of a single piece of PMMA. Its unique design features eight equally spaced indentations spanning the circumference of the ring creating a sinusoidal shape (Fig. 16.6E). The main advantage of the ring is that the new indentations allow for easier nuclear and cortical matter removal while still maintaining the desired stretch of the capsular bag.

IV. ***Ahmed capsular tension segment (CTS)*** is a modified design of Cionni's CTR. It is a partial ring of clear PMMA covering approximately one quadrant with a hole for temporary or permanent fixation (Fig. 16.6F), one or more CTS may be used as necessary to support the area of the capsule with weak or deficient zonules. The CTS can be used even when anterior or posterior capsular tears are present.

Table 16.1 *Three types of Morcher CTR and their indications*

S.no.	*Type*	*Diameter in mm*		*Indications of use based on*		
		Compressed	*Expanded*	*Type of eye*	*axial length*	*Corneal diameter (white to white)*
1.	14	10	12.3	• Paediatric eyes • Microspherophakia	<24 mm	<11 mm
2.	14 C	11	13	• Normal eyes	24–25 mm	11–12.5 mm
3.	14 A	12	14.5	• High myopia	>25 mm	>12.5 mm

Time of insertion of CTR

The CTR can be inserted at variable times as below:

1. ***Before hydrodissection,*** the CTR implantation allows clear visualization of the anterior capsule and the proper placement of the ring. The disadvantage is that it precludes adequate cortical clean up as cortex may remain trapped between the capsule and the CTR.
2. ***After hydrodissection,*** implantation of the CTR keeps the bag stretched and prevents collapse of the capsular fornix during phacoemulsification as well as makes cortex aspiration easier. It also reduces the possibility of vitreous prolapse and provides better capsular bag stability and IOL centration.
3. ***After cortical clean up,*** CTR is implanted, if the zonular dialysis occurs or the initial mild zonular dialysis increases during automated irrigation and aspiration

Technique of insertion of CTR

CTR can be inserted into the bag either manually or with the help of an injector.

1. ***Manual insertion of CTR***

The CTR is inserted with the help of McPherson's forceps through the main incision and its distal end is controlled with a Sinskey hook introduced through the side port incision (Fig. 16.7A). The bent tip of the Sinskey hook is passed in the eyelet (orifice) at the distal end of the CTR. The proximal end of the CTR is released only when it is well below the rhexis margin because if it is lost in the sulcus or the anterior chamber angle, it becomes difficult to retrieve it. The final position of the CTR should be such that the convex part of ring should abut the area of deficient zonules.

2. ***Insertion of CTR with the help of injector.*** The CTR can also be inserted with the help of Gender capsular tension ring injector (Fig. 16.7B).

Technique of Cionni ring fixation

When the zonular dialysis is between 5 and 7 o' clock hours, the Cionni's ring need to be fixed. In such cases, as mentioned earlier, the scleral window is precut in the zone of zonular dehiscence. After hydrodissection, the Cionni's ring is inserted and fixed with the help of trans-scleral 9-0 prolene suture passed through the eyes of the ring and then through the precut scleral window. The eyelets of the Cionni's ring are at a higher plane protruding about 0.25 mm forward from the main CTR body hence lie over the anterior capsule.

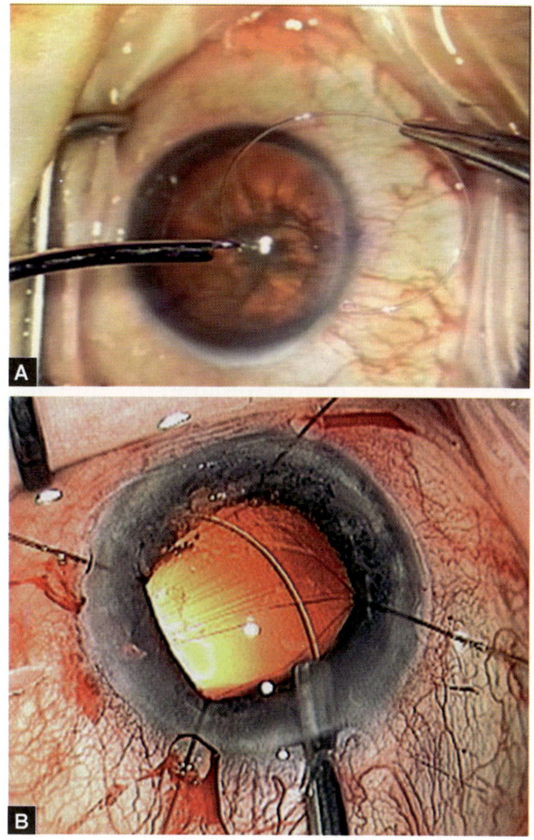

Fig. 16.7. *Techniques of insertion of CTR: **(A)** Manual with the help of a McPherson's forceps; **(B)** With the help of an injector.*

Contraindications of CTR and MCTR

- Anterior capsular tear
- Posterior capsular tear
- Incomplete capsulorhexis
- Severly subluxated lens (>7 o' clock hours). In such cases, it is often prudent to plan ICCE, followed by anterior vitrectomy and implantation of ACIOL or a scleral fixated PCIOL (preferably).

V. Nucleus management, cortical aspiration and IOL implantation

Nuclear phacoemulsification can be performed in the bag after implantation of the CTR or outside the bag depending upon the surgeon's choice. With the latter, it is necessary to have carried out an extensive capsulorhexis, which enables nuclear prolapse either by hydrodissection or viscoexpression.

Special points to be considered are:

- *Slow motion phaco* is recommended, i.e. vacuum, flow rate and bottle height should be kept at low to minimize the turbulence. Phaco power should be appropriate for grade of cataract.
- *For soft nuclei,* phacoaspiration or 'chip and flip' technique is recommended.
- *For moderate to hard nuclei,* phaco chop technique is performed by many surgeons. Some surgeons recommend V-Kelman technique of nucleus cracking as it limits the need for rotating the nucleus and thus may prove useful.
- *Two-port anterior chamber viterctomy* is recommended, if vitreous is detected in the AC at any stage.

Cortical aspiration. Some recommendations are:

- *Viscodissection* of cortical matter reduces stress on the zonules.
- *Manual cortical aspiration* is more controllable.
- *Bimanual technique* is considered better than the co-axial technique of automated aspiration.
- *Tangential traction movements* are advised when performing automated aspiration. The radial movements increase risk of traction on the ring and capsular bag.

IOL implantation. Considerations are:

- *Large diameter lens (>6 mm)* is advised to minimize the symptoms, if lens decentration occurs in the future.
- *CTR ring,* if not used earlier, may be implanted before the IOL is implanted.
- *Orientation of the haptics* parallel to the dialysis, while implanting in the bag, provides optimal zonular support. Most surgeons prefer in the bag implantation.
- *Dialling movement* should be kept to minimum.
- *Implantation on the sulcus,* where zonular support still exists along with the capturing of the optic in the capsulorhexis is recommended by some surgeons.

PHACOEMULSIFICATION IN PSEUDOEXFOLIATION SYNDROME

ANTICIPATED AND/OR EXISTING PROBLEMS

Patients with pseudoexfoliation syndrome may have associated or develop any of the following problems:

- Zonular breaks or zonulolysis
- Subluxation of the lens
- Poor pupillary dilation
- Secondary glaucoma

CONSIDERATIONS DURING PHACOEMULSIFICATION

- *Exfoliative glaucoma,* if associated should be managed first.
- *Poor pupillary dilation,* considerations are the same as described for miotic pupil (page 288)
- *Zonular weakness/subluxated lens,* considerations are described on page 290–299.

PHACOEMULSIFICATION IN UVEITIC EYE

A. PREOPERATIVE CONSIDERATIONS

1. ***Appropriate work-up:***
   - Find out the cause of uveitis.
   - Evaluate status of corneal endothelium.
   - Look for pupillary fibrosis, synechiae and membrane formation which would help to plan surgery.
   - Record IOP for evaluation of glaucoma and to keep it under control.
   - Evaluate posterior segment.
2. ***Practice zero tolerance for inflammation,*** i.e. must ensure that inflammation is totally controlled for at least 2 months before surgery.
3. ***Visual prognosis should always be guarded,*** so that patients have realistic expectations because of potential postoperative complications.
4. ***Preoperative treatment*** should include:
   - Steroid cover (topical as well as oral) is must for three days before surgery.
   - Continue preoperative immunosuppressive agents.
   - Ensure control of IOP.

- Topical antibiotics and NSAID drops, 3 days before surgery
- Two hours before surgery, instill phenylephrine 5–10%, tropicamide 1%, cyclopentolate 0.5–1% and flubiprufen 0.03% or ketorolac trimethamine 0.5% every 15 minutes.

B. OPERATIVE CONSIDERATIONS

1. ***Anaesthesia*** should be peribulbar block and not topical or intracameral.

2. ***Viscoelastics*** should be used copiously to:
   - Protect corneal endothelium, and
   - Minimize trauma to the iris.

3. ***Narrow pupil*** should be managed by following measures, i.e. iris retractors, multiple sphincterotomies, synechiolysis, viscodialators (For details *see* pages 288–290).

4. ***Capsulorhexis*** should always be large (6 mm) and well centred to prevent problems from the potential risks of capsular contraction syndrome.

   Note. Capsular fibrotic bands or calcific plaques in the anterior capsule may cause difficulties. Use of capsulotomy scissors may be helpful.

5. ***Phacoemulsification*** should preferably be done by phaco chop technique.

6. ***Cortical aspiration*** should be thorough to prevent occurrence of severe postoperative inflammation.

7. ***Capsular polishing*** should be done to remove residual epithelium from the under surface of the anterior capsular rim and the residual cortical strands from the posterior capsule.

8. ***IOL considerations*** include:
   - In the bag implantation is always best.
   - *Avoid: ACIOLs, and IOLs with polypropylene haptics.*
   - Heparin surface modified (HSM) PMMA IOL induces comparatively less inflammation.
   - Foldable IOLs of hydrogel and acrylic also induce less inflammation. Avoid silicone foldable IOLs. Hydrophobic IOLs should be preferred.
   - Avoid using IOLs in patients with systemic diseases characterized by chronic inflammation, e.g. juvenile rheumatoid arthritis (JRA), as formation of fibrotic bands causes distortion of pupil and marked displacement of IOL.

9. ***Intracameral wysolone*** is recommended by many surgeons after completion of the surgery.

10. ***Posterior sub-Tenon injection*** of triamcinolone 40 mg will reduce postoperative inflammation.

C. POSTOPERATIVE CONSIDERATIONS

1. ***Aggressive postoperative treatment (to control inflammation)*** by:
   - Topical prednisolone for 3–4 months
   - Topical NSAIDs for at least 1 month
   - Oral NSAIDs and steroids for 4–6 weeks
   - Short acting cycloplegics instilled at night for 4–6 weeks
   - Systemic immunosuppressants may be continued.

2. ***Frequent postoperative follow-up*** to monitor inflammation, CME and IOP.

3. ***Special watch is required*** for pigment deposits on the IOL surface and opacification of the posterior capsule.

PHACOEMULSIFICATION IN DENSE CATARACT

ANTICIPATED DIFFICULTIES AND RISKS

A dense or brunescent cataract is a challenge for emulsification because of:

- Hard and sticky leathery nucleus fibres
- Thin capsules and less epinuclear cushion
- Weak zonules
- Large mass of the nucleus
- Poor flowability and greater chatter due to poor moulding of the nucleus pieces to the phaco tip during phacoemulsification.

Anticipated or potential risks and complications include:

- Inability to complete an anterior capsulorhexis
- Corneal or scleral incision burns
- Endothelial damage and corneal oedema due to a reduced safety zone between the phaco probe and endothelium, as well as prolonged phaco time
- Capsular rupture, capsular rent or vitreous loss
- Drops of nucleus or nuclear fragments.
- Iris trauma
- Postoperative inflammation and CME.

SPECIAL CONSIDERATIONS TO MAXIMIZE OUTCOME

A. Preoperative considerations

1. ***Thorough clinical evaluation*** especially to note corneal status, pupillary dilation, anterior chamber depth, pseudoexfoliation syndrome and grade of nuclear hardness.
2. ***Information to the patient*** about potential risks of hard cataract.
3. ***Pupillary dilation and its maintenance*** should be ensured by sufficient use of mydriatic-cycloplegic and topical NSAIDs, to prevent miosis during prolonged phaco procedure.
4. ***Local anaesthetics (peribulbar block)*** should be preferred over topical anaesthesia in view of the prolonged surgical time and greater risk of intraoperative complications.

B. Operative considerations

1. ***Wound considerations.*** A short scleral tunnel incision may be preferred over the clear corneal incision to prevent thermal burns. Temporal incision may be more comfortable than the superior incision.
2. ***Viscoelastic considerations.*** The 'soft shell technique' should be preferred, i.e. first inject a small amount of viscodispersive viscoelastic to coat the endothelium, and then inject a second high molecular weight highly cohesive viscoelastic just above the lens capsule to push the first viscoelastic against the endothelium and maintain the anterior chamber.
3. ***Capsulorhexis*** should neither be large nor small. A size between 5.5 and 6 mm may be preferred, especially if conversion to SICS or ECCE is required.
4. ***Hydrodissection*** should be performed very gently, low volume but adequate to ensure mobility. Avoid hydrodelineation because the lens fibres do not clear well and because the increased intracapsular volume can rupture the bag.
5. ***Nuclear emulsification considerations*** need special attention:

Phaco probe and parameter considerations include:

- *With standard phacoemulsification*, a 45° bevel tip provides better cutting for denser nuclei.
- *Special facilities in the handpiece* of high end phaco machines have been provided for hard cataracts, e.g.:
  - Mackool system offered by Alcon provides protection against thermal burns.
  - Kelman flared Mackool ABS tip allows efficient nuclear sculpting.
  - Transverse ultrasound and rotational Ozil technology facilitate easier emulsification.
- *Parameters recommended* include: a higher flow rate and high phaco power (100%). Pulse and burst mode, if available, should be preferred.

Technique recommendations include:

- Phaco chop should be preferred over nucleofracture methods.
- Sculpting a deep central zone is essential in either technique.
- Vertical chop should be preferred over horizontal chop.
- Bevel down phaco (phaco drill technique) further reduces energy transfer to the corneal endothelium.
- Chopping nucleus into multiple quadrants before emulsifying is a good option.
- Some recommend a technique called 'transverse cracking and serial chopping'.

6. ***Cortical aspiration.*** Though minimal cortical matter is left after emulsification of hard cataracts, but a thorough clean-up is essential to prevent postoperative inflammation.

C. Postoperative considerations

Postoperative considerations are based on the postoperative complications noted as below:

1. ***Prolonged corneal oedema*** may occur due to reduced safety zone between the phaco probe and endothelium, as well as prolonged phaco time. Postoperative considerations for corneal oedema include:
   - Intensive topical steroid therapy.
   - Use of topical hypertonic saline eyedrops and eye ointment.

2. ***Excessive inflammation*** may occur due to increased phaco energy and iris trauma. Special treatment considerations include:
   - Intensive topical steroid therapy
   - Use of cycloplegic drugs
   - Use of oral steroids.

3. ***Wound burns*** may occur due to thermal damage and may be even associated with wound leak.

Wound leak may be treated with:
- Aqueous suppressants,
- Pressure patching,
- Bandage contact lens, and
- Wound revision, if necessary.

4. ***Cystoid macular oedema*** may occur due to prolonged phaco time and postoperative inflammation. Additional postoperative considerations include:
- Topical NSAIDs, preferably nepafenac eyedrops QID for about a month.
- Oral NSAIDs may also be considered.
- Sub-Tenon steroid injection may be needed.
- Acetazolamide 500 mg orally may be considered, if no response is achieved after one month of above therapy.

D. Considerations for alternative procedures

Phacoemulsification should be deferred and ECCE or SICS may be considered under following situations:
- Preoperative poor endothelium
- Weak zonules
- One-eyed patients
- Previous vitrectomy
- Advanced cataracta brunescence or nigra.

POSTERIOR POLAR CATARACT

Posterior polar cataract typically presents as dense white opacities in the centre of posterior capsule with a characteristic concentric 'whorl like' pattern and central thickening (Fig. 16.8). These may be associated with remnants of hyaloid system. About 26–36% of cases of posterior polar cataract are associated with dehiscence of the posterior capsule. Special considerations in the management of posterior polar cataracts are summarized below.

A. PREOPERATIVE CONSIDERATIONS

1. ***Meticulous slit-lamp examination*** with dilated pupil should be carried out. Look for the details of posterior polar cataract and associated anomalies, if any.

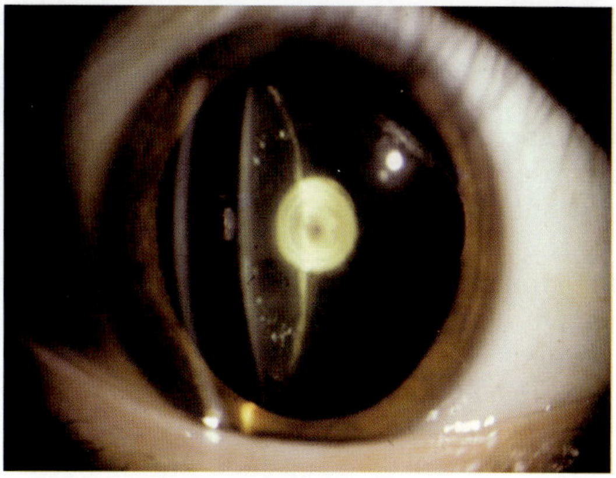

Fig. 16.8. *A typical posterior polar cataract.*

2. ***Defer cataract surgery*** until the patient's visual complaints are truly troublesome.
3. ***Proper information and counselling*** of the patient should be done about the risks of the surgery such as nucleus drop, vitreous loss and longer surgical time.
4. ***Preparation for anterior vitrectomy*** should be done preoperatively, i.e. the case should be scheduled for cataract extraction with anterior vitrectomy.
5. ***Pupillary dilatation and its maintenance*** should be ensured by sufficient use of mydriatic-cycloplegics and topical NSAIDs to prevent miosis during prolonged surgery. A well-dilated pupil is important in order to optimize visualization of the polar cataract and to evaluate the behaviour when the capsule is manipulated.
6. ***Local anaesthetic (peribulbar block)*** should be preferred over topical anaesthesia in order to minimize ocular movements with concomitant positive pressure on the vitreous and forward movement of the posterior capsule. Further it will be also useful for prolonged surgery, especially if vitrectomy is required for the posterior capsular tear.

B. OPERATIVE CONSIDERATIONS

1. ***Wound construction.*** A short scleral tunnel incision may be preferred over the clear corneal incision in view of the high risk of capsular complications and the possible need for conversion to ECCE.
2. ***Capsulorhexis.*** Both too large and too short capsulorhexis should be avoided. Just adequate

anterior capsulorhexis of 4–5 mm should be performed, so as to ensure enough anterior capsular support for a sulcus-fixated IOL, if necessary. Too small a capsulorhexis may increase hydrostatic pressure on the bag during hydrodelineation, predisposing to capsular rupture.

3. ***Hydrodissection*** is contraindicated in such cases to avoid hydraulic rupture of the posterior capsule at the point of adhesion.

4. ***Hydrodelineation*** should be performed to separate the endonucleus from the epinucleus bowl which will act as cushion during nuclear emulsification.

5. ***Nuclear rotation*** should preferably be avoided in order to minimize tractional forces between the polar cataract and the posterior capsule.

6. ***Nuclear phacoemulsification*** considerations are:

- *Anterior chamber fluctuation* should be minimized by:
  - Generous use of viscoelastic material
  - Infusion bottle height should be low to prevent over distension of the posterior capsule
- *Technique of nuclear emulsification.* Most of the time nucleus is soft and should be managed by central sculpting with low vacuum and low aspiration flow rate, taking care to keep the epinuclear layer intact. A moderately hard nucleus (rare finding) should be managed by the chopping technique rather than nuclear fractis technique to avoid stress on the posterior capsule.

7. ***Epinucleus and cortex*** should first be removed from the periphery, leaving the central area for the last. Avoid performing capsular polishing or capsular vacuuming (cap-vac) and attempt to remove the posterior plaque. This can be managed with Nd:YAG laser at a later date.

Management of posterior capsular tear

- *If posterior capsular tear occurs in early stages,* hail out to ECCE may be required
- *If posterior capsular tear occurs* during advanced stage of nuclear phacoemulsification, efforts should be made to remove the remaining lens matter gently without disturbing the vitreous by *dry aspiration* after plugging the tear area with high density viscoelastics.
- *Two port anterior vitrectomy* is, however, recommended to manage capsular rupture with vitreous prolapsed into the anterior chamber.

8. ***IOL implantation***

i. *In the absence of capsular tear,* the foldable IOL should be implanted in the capsular bag.

ii. *In the presence of capsular tear, without vitreous prolapse* also the foldable IOL can be gently implanted in the capsular bag.

iii. *In the presence of capsular tear with vitreous prolapse,* after meticulous two port vitrectomy, depending upon the circumstances IOL may be implanted as below:

- *In the capsular bag,* foldable IOL can be implanted, if the tear is small.
- *In the sulcus,* foldable IOL can be implanted when the anterior capsular support is sufficient but posterior capsular support is deficient.
- *Sclera-fixated (or suture) PCIOL* can be placed when the anterior capsular support is deficient.
- *Anterior chamber Kelman-Multiflex IOL* can be implanted as an alternative to sutured posterior chamber IOL.

C. POSTOPERATIVE CONSIDERATIONS

Special postoperative considerations are required for the complications as below:

1. *Residual posterior capsular plaque* may require Nd:YAG capsulotomy at later date.

2. *Dropped nucleus or lens fragments* need management by pars-plana vitrectomy.

3. *Postoperative IOP elevation* is mainly caused by retained viscoelastic material, lens particles and inflammation. Consider postoperative use of:

- *Acetazolamide* orally 250 mg TDS
- *Topical aqueous suppressants* such as 2% timolol maleate
- *Mannitol i/v* may be needed, if IOP is very high.

4. *Postoperative inflammation* can be treated by:

- Intensive topical steroids therapy
- Use of cycloplegics
- Oral steroids may be required in moderate to severe cases.

5. *Postoperative CME* should be treated by:

- Intensive topical NSAIDs therapy.
- Acetazolamide 500 mg orally may be considered in non-responsive cases.

FEMTODELINEATION IN POSTERIOR POLAR CATARACTS

Femtolaser-assisted cataract surgery (FLACS) can enhance safety and reduce PCR rates in surgery for posterior polar cataracts.

Advantages of femtolaser-assisted cataract surgery (FLACS):

- *Femtodelineation creates multiple nuclear layers or zones that act as shock absorbers* during surgery. These shock absorbers prevent the transmission of mechanical forces and fluidic turbulence to the weakest part of the posterior capsule until the end of surgery.
- *Risk for buildup of hydraulic pressure within the bag is eliminated*, since no hydro-based procedures are involved.
- Produces extremely well-demarcated and predictable walls of division, this is the biggest advantages of using the laser to create nuclear delineation. These sharp vertical walls separating the layers from each other make removal easy, requiring minimal mechanical manoeuvring with the second instrument. When the last layer of epinucleus is finally removed, gently stripping it off the fornices around 180° creates a plane of separation between the lens material and the posterior capsule.
- *Even if there is a preexisting or intraoperative PCR, there is no or minimal enlargement of this rupture*, because a cleavage is created between the epinucleus and the posterior capsule and passage of fluid into this space will not lead to buildup of hydraulic pressure. If there is a PCR, the final goal of being able to implant an IOL in the capsular bag can be achieved by converting this small rupture into a continuous posterior capsulorhexis.
- *Size, number, and depth of the delineated cylinders can be customized* by the surgeon depending on the size of the pupil, the size of the capsulorhexis, or surgeon's preference. This is not possible with manual techniques.
- *Femtodelineation is also useful in posterior polar cataracts with an associated dense nucleus.* As the nucleus is already predivided by the laser, it is easily debulked without the need for any mechanical division techniques, which could otherwise cause stress on the capsular-zonular complex.

Procedure

- *Docking of eye and programing of laser.* Once the laser interface is docked onto the patient's eye, (Fig. 16.9) the cylindrical pattern of lens division is selected. The laser is programmed to create three cylinders within the nucleus, with the diameter of the outermost cylinder generally set at 5.5–6 mm. The number, depth, and width of the cylinders can be customized depending on the characteristics of each eye. Safety margin of at least 500 μm from the posterior capsule, guided by the live anterior segment optical coherence tomography incorporated in the laser is preferred.
- *Creation of anterior capsulotomy and laser delineation of nucleus.* As the laser fires, it first creates the capsulotomy, followed by the generation of the three cylinders within the lens, from inside out. This produces three distinct zones of demarcation within the nucleus, surrounded by a peripheral fourth zone of epinucleus (Fig. 16.10).
- *Phacoemulsification.* Once the laser part of the surgery is completed, the phacoemulsification portion is begun. Immediately after the capsulotomy is removed, lens emulsification can start; no hydrodissection or hydro-delineation procedure is performed. Starting from the innermost layer, each of the sharply laser-demarcated zones is emulsified from inside out, within the cushion of the outer zones (Fig. 16.11). Minimal ultrasound energy

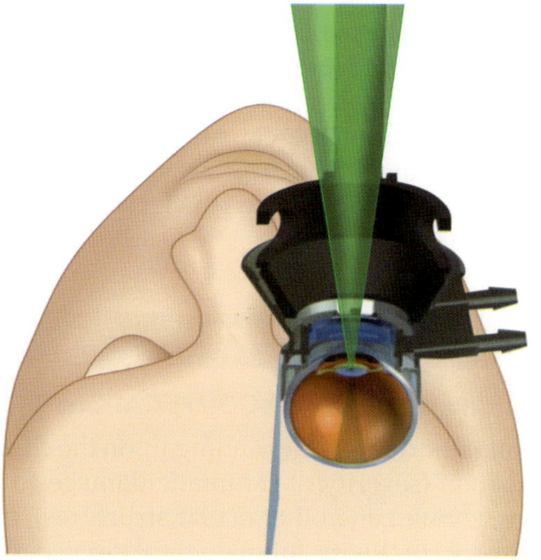

Fig. 16.9: Docking the laser interface on to the patient's eye

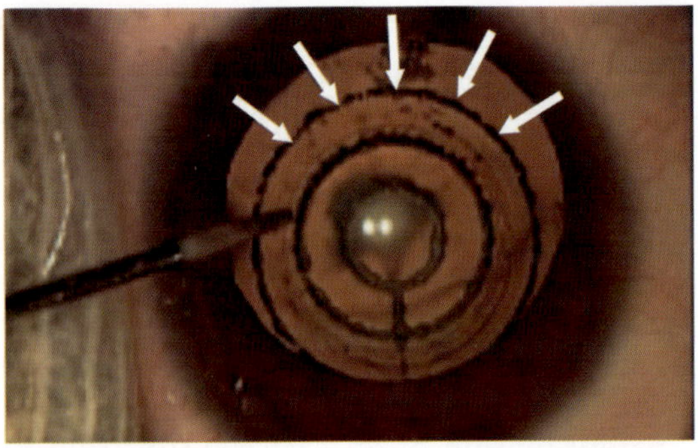

Fig. 16.10: Laser delineation of the nucleus. Note: Small air bubbles generated by firing of the femtosecond laser, which may not drastically increase intracapsular pressure

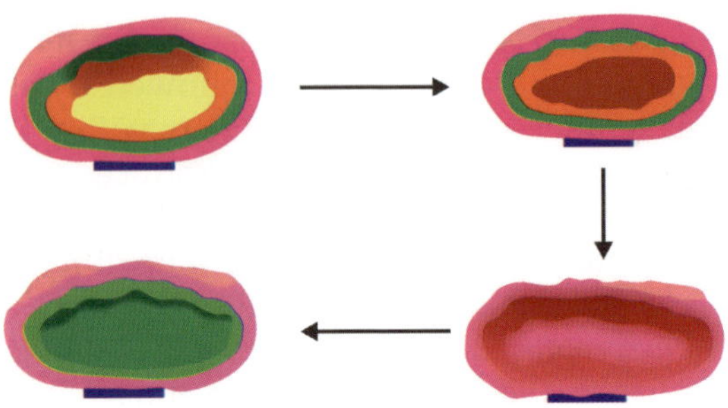

Fig. 16.11: How, as each nuclear layer is removed sequentially, the epinuclear cushion remains, guarding the potentially dehiscent or weak posterior capsule

can be used, with an aspiration flow rate of 14–16 ml/min and a modest bottle height of 60–70 cm. When all three zones have been removed, a thick and uniform epinuclear cushion remains. At the end of this surgical phase, owing to the sharp vertical wall created by the laser circumferentially, removal of this epinuclear cushion is easy. It can be gently stripped from the capsular bag. Once the epinucleus is detached circumferentially, it can be aspirated with irrigation and aspiration.

TRAUMATIC CATARACT

ANTICIPATED RISKS AND COMPLICATIONS

Traumatic cataract, depending upon the clinical situation (severity of traumatic damage to the lens, zonules and other ocular structures), may be associated with following anticipated risks and complications.

A. Preoperatively anticipated risks and complications

1. *Calculation of IOL power* may be difficult due to irregular corneal astigmatism.
2. *Surgical procedure* may be difficult and may require vitrectomy.

B. Peroperatively anticipated risks and complications

1. *Anterior capsulorhexis* may be difficult or not possible.
2. *Posterior capsular rupture (PCR)* incidence and the incidence of associated complications may be more.
3. *Nuclear fragment loss* may occur through the PCR and/or zonular dehiscence.
4. *Vitreous loss* may occur depending upon the extent of PCR and/or zonular dehiscence.
5. *Positioning of IOL* may be difficult.

C. Anticipated postoperative risks and complications

1. *Exuberant postoperative inflammation* may be expected because of lens matter or vitreous present in the anterior chamber or injury to the iris.
2. *Prolonged postoperative increase in IOP* may be expected due to multiple factors in ocular trauma.
3. *Prolonged postoperative corneal oedema* may be expected due to associated damage to the corneal endothelium, glaucoma or hyphaema.
4. *Cystoids macular oedema (CME)* may be severe and prolonged.
5. *Postoperative refractory error* due to inaccurate biometry and IOL malposition.

MANAGEMENT CONSIDERATIONS

- Preoperative considerations
- Operative considerations
- Postoperative considerations

A. Preoperative considerations

Preoperative considerations should include:

I. *Meticulous preoperative evaluation*

- Decision and planning for surgery
- IOL consideration
- *Meticulous preoperative evaluation*

A thorough preoperative evaluation should be carried out to:

- *Examine for RAPD* to assess for traumatic optic neuropathy
- *Corneal evaluation* for oedema, scarring, astigmatism, status of endothelium
- *Pupillary dilatation* should be assessed
- *Examination of lens* with slit-lamp to note for:
  - Signs of capsular rupture
  - Presence of a fibrotic anterior capsular plaque
  - Phacodonesis is present or absent
  - Zonular defects, when present, should be characterised preoperatively in terms of degree/clock hours of loss
  - Subluxation or dislocation of the lens
  - Vitreous prolapse is present or absent in the anterior chamber
- *Indirect ophthalmoscopy* to evaluate the posterior segment
- *B-scan ultrasonography* should be performed to evaluate the posterior segment when visualisation is not possible due to opaque media. Efforts should also be made to discover any retained intraocular foreign body.
- *Biometry and keratometry* should be carried out to calculate IOL power. Many a times it may be erroneous due to difficulty obtaining axial length and keratometry measurements. Biometry of other eye should be performed to compare for accuracy.

II. *Decision and planning for surgical management*

Depending on the clinical situation, the following decision and planning should be done:

- Time of surgery
- Surgical approach
- Special arrangements

Time of surgery

The indications for removal of traumatic cataract can be acute (immediate), subacute (early) or elective (delayed).

Immediate (acute) removal of traumatic cataract is required only when there is:

- Risk of worsening of the lens-related inflammation (phacoanaphylactic uveitis)
- Loss of lens fragments in the posterior segment
- Significant risk of lens particle glaucoma from a highly disrupted lens capsule.

Early (subacute) removal of traumatic cataract is indicated during conservative management in post-traumatic period patient develops:

- Persistent inflammation
- Phacogenic uveitis
- Lens particle glaucoma

Delayed (elective) extraction of traumatic cataract should be preferred, as it permits:

- Proper management of traumatic inflammation.
- Proper decision in small traumatic cataracts which may not progress to visual axis and thus may not need extraction.
- Proper healing and stability of open globe wounds.
- More accurate measurement of IOL power calculation and planning of cataract surgery.

Surgical approaches

Once decision to operate is made, depending on the clinical situation, the surgical management of a traumatic cataract is performed using either a standard anterior limbal or posterior pars plana approach.

- ***Anterior approach*** is best for a traumatic cataract unless there is complete lens dislocation or capsular rupture with significant lens material incarcerated in the vitreous. The surgeon should perform a standard phacoemulsification cataract extraction using a large capsulorhexis and initiated at the site of greatest zonular stability.
- ***Posterior approach*** with vitrectomy and lensectomy is reserved for cases of posterior capsular rupture with vitreous prolapse or a posteriorly dislocated lens.

III. *IOL consideration*

- *Power of IOL, when not possible to measure accurately, take fellow eye values. Further, plan to balance the refraction in the fellow eye to within 2 to 3 D. Always err on the myopic side.*
- *Size of IOL.* Large diameter IOL (>6 mm optic size) should be preferred to minimize the symptoms, if lens decentration occurs in the future. An IOL with over all diameter 13 mm (never less than 12 mm) should be preferred.

- *IOL with PMMA haptics* should be preferred, since they are stiffer and may help to prevent capsular contraction and IOL decentration. Recommended IOLs are:
  - Foldable acrylic with PMMA haptics,
  - One piece PMMA,
  - Foldable one piece acrylic
- *Heparin surface modified and acrylic IOLs* are reported to produce minimal corneal oedema, anterior chamber reaction, formation of synechiae, and deposits on IOL.

B. Anaesthesia considerations

General anaesthesia is required in children and un-cooperative adults.

Local anaesthesia is recommended for adult patients.

- Always prefer peribulbar block anaesthesia than topical or intracameral anaesthesia.
- Avoid stressing of the zonules by overpressing the eye during local anaesthesia (i.e. avoid digital massage, Honon balloon and Super-Pinky after administration of anaesthetic solution).

C. Peroperative considerations

1. *Incision considerations*

- *In the presence of narrow pupil,* the incision considerations are as given on page 288
- *In the presence of subluxated lens/zonular dehiscence,* follow the incision considerations given on page 291.

2. *Viscoelastic considerations*

- *In the presence of zonular dehiscence,* avoid hyperinflation of the anterior chamber.
- *In the presence of small pupil,* a high molecular weight viscoelastic agent is recommended to aid in pupillary dilation, synechiolysis and haemostasis. A soft shell technique should be preferred.

3. *Pupil and iris considerations*

- *Measures to enlarge pupil,* when pharmacological dilation is of little help are described on page 291.
- *Iridodialysis,* when present may need repair after removal of the cataract and placement of IOL.

4. *Considerations during capsulorhexis*

- *Staining the capsule with trypan blue dye is recommended in all complicated and white cataracts.*
- *In the presence of narrow of pupil,* follow the considerations described on page 289.
- *In the presence of zonular dehiscence,* follow the considerations described on page 291.
- *In the presence of dense fibrotic subcapsular plaque,* start away from the plaque and tear completely around the plaque, if possible. Avoid tearing through the plaque.

5. *Hydrodissection and hydrodelineation*

Gentle but thorough cortical cleavage hydrodissection should be performed carefully so as to free the nucleus maximally and lessen the stress on the zonules during phacoemulsification. Aggressive hydrodissection may cause a hydraulic rupture at the point of capsular compromise.

Hydrodelineation may be preferred in the absence of zonular dehiscence and phacodonesis. This technique creates a small endonucleus that can be phacoemulsified more easily.

6. *Phacoemulsification, nucleus management, cortical aspiration and IOL implantation*

- *In the presence of subluxation,* the degree of zonular dehiscence dictates the management approach (For details *see* pages 291–295).
- *In the absence of subluxation but presence of a narrow pupil,* the management considerations are described on pages 288–290.
- *Traumatic cataract* without any associated complication should be managed in standard way but with more gentle and careful approach.

Note. In cases of an unsalvageable capsular bag, other IOL options include ciliary sulcus-fixated IOLs, trans-sclerally sutured PCIOLs, and ACIOLs. Although the ACIOLs have been advocated in special circumstances (elderly patient, good iris support, no evidence of glaucoma, no vitreous in anterior chamber), they should not be used in younger patients because of the increased risk of corneal endothelial injury and glaucoma from further angle injury.

- *Ciliary sulcus-fixated IOLs* in children following traumatic cataract removal are reported to result in visual outcomes similar to those for capsular bag IOLs but with more complications, in particular uveitis and pupillary capture.
- *Sclerally sutured PCIOLs* are also reported to produce good postoperative visual results.
- The use of *multifocal capsular bag IOLs* following removal of a traumatic cataract has also been explored. In comparison with standard, mono-focal, capsular bag IOLs, the multifocal lenses resulted in improved uncorrected near visual acuity and stereopsis, as well as decreased spectacle dependency.

7. Wound closure

Since complicated traumatic cataract patients often require additional surgical procedures, so preferably the tunnel wound should be closed with at least one suture.

Consideration for alternative surgical procedures

- *Combined phaco with trabeculectomy* or other glaucoma procedures need to be considered in the presence of intractable glaucoma.
- *Postponement of cataract surgery* needs to be considered in patients with uncontrolled inflammation, except in case of phacogenic uveitis.
- *ICCE* may need to be considered in markedly subluxated lens.
- *Pars plana approach* may be needed in patients with posterior capsular rupture associated with lens matter in the vitreous and in completely posteriorly dislocated lens.
- *Consider deferring surgery* in the presence of associated traumatic optic neuropathy.

D. Postoperative considerations

1. *Postoperative inflammation and CME* are likely to be more severe in patients with traumatic cataract. So, intensive topical steroid and NSAID therapy and frequent follow-up examination is recommended.
2. *Postoperative glaucoma* due to debris, (blood, pigment and inflammatory cells) is more likely to occur, and so needs to be monitored and managed efficiently.
3. *Malpositions of IOL* are frequent postoperatively and may need repositioning in patients with selective complaints or persistent intraocular inflammation.
4. *Posterior dislocation of IOL*, which may occur postoperatively, requires removal by a retina surgeon via a pars plana approach.
5. *Retinal detachment* and other posterior segment complications which are comparatively more common after traumatic cataract surgery need timely detection and management.

CATARACT SURGERY IN A POST-REFRACTIVE SURGERY PATIENT

ANTICIPATED RISKS AND COMPLICATIONS

Likely complications during cataract surgery in a post-refractive surgery patient include:

- *True corneal power* is difficult to assess. Therefore, standard IOL power formulas using routine keratometry yield significant under correction with postoperative hyperopic surprises in patients who have undergone LASIK, PRK or RK.
- *Dehiscence of refractive keratotomy* incisions may occur in patients with RK.
- *Transient refractive shifts* may occur in radial keratotomy patients after surgery, which may last for weeks with wide fluctuations.
- Risks of developing *bullous keratopathy* after cataract surgery are more in patients who had RK.
- Increased risk of *retinal hole, tear or detachment* in the pseudophakic state is expected in post-myopic refractive surgery eyes especially those having long axial lengths. Such patients should be advised and warned for the early warning signs and urgent nature thereof.

MANAGEMENT CONSIDERATIONS

A. Preoperative considerations

Steps that can be taken to reduce the operative risks are:

- Counsel the patient about increased likelihood of a lens power calculation error.
- Counsel post-radial keratotomy patients about diurnal fluctuations.

- Calculate effective corneal power by different methods.
- For details of IOL power calculation after keratorefractive surgery *see* page 128. Some key points to be considered are:
  - Corneal topography is must in each case to evaluate asphericity and irregular astigmatism.
  - Always use flattest k-reading for myopes and steepest k-reading for hypermetropes.
  - For myopes, use multiple third-generation formulas for IOL power calculation and choose the highest calculated power. The opposite is true for hyperopes.

B. Operative considerations

- Avoid cutting into or across radial and arcuate keratotomy incisions to avoid dehiscence.
- Consider sclera tunnel incision, if radial incisions of radial keratotomy are too close together to avoid.
- Avoid crossing interface of LASIK flap with the keratome incision.
- Consider combined corneal transplant and cataract surgery in patients with markedly abnormal corneal endothelium.

C. Postoperative considerations

1. ***Unexpected refractory error*** may occur even after best possible measures. Review pre-operative data and wait till stabilisation of refraction:.
   - An eye with history of incisional keratotomy may take weeks to several months to obtain refractive stability.
   - If a lens exchange is necessary, it should be performed only after refractive stability has been achieved.
2. ***Bullous keratopathy,*** when occurs should be managed effectively.

BIBLIOGRAPHY

PHACOEMULSIFICATION IN SMALL PUPIL

1. Centrion VC, Fine IH, Lu LW. Management of the small pupil in phacoemulsification. In: Lu LW, Fine IH, (eds). Phacoemulsification in difficult and challenging cases. New York: Thieme, 62–64,1999.
2. Dinsmore SC. Modified stretch technique for small pupil phacoemulsification with topical anesthesia. J Cataract Refract Surg 22:27–30,1996.
3. Fine IH. Phacoemulsification in the presence of a small pupil. In: Steinert RF, ed. Cataract surgery: technique, complications and management. Philadelphia: Saunders; 199–208, 1995.
4. Gimbel HV. Nucleofractis phacoemulsification through a small pupil. Can J Ophthalmol 27: 115–119,1992.
5. Oetting TA, Omphroy LC. Modified technique using flexible iris retractors in clear corneal surgery. J Cataract Refract Surg 28:596–598,2002.

PHACOEMUSIFICATION IN PSEUDOEXFOLIATION SYNDROME

1. Akman A, Yilmaz G, Oto S, Akove Y. Comparison of various pupil dilatation methods for phacoemulsification in eyes with small pupil secondary to pseudoexfolication. Ophtalmology 111:1693–1698,2004.
2. Fine IH, Hoffman RS. Phacoemulsification in the presence of pseudoexfoliation: challenges and options. J Cataract Refract Surg 23:160–165, 1997.
3. Osher RH, Icon RJ, Gimbel HV, Crandall AS. Cataract surgery in patients with pseudo-exfoliation syndrome. Eur J Implant Refract Surg 5:46–50,1993.

PHACOEMUSIFICATION IN UVEITIC EYE

1. Jalali S, Das T, Gupta S. Presumed non-infectious endophthalmitis after cataract surgery. J Cataract Refract Surg 22:1492–1497,1996.
2. Jehan FS, Mamalis N, Spencer TS, Fry LL, Kerstine RS, Olson RJ. Postoperative sterile endophthalmitis (TASS) associated with the memorylens. J Cataract Refract Surg 26:1773–1777, 2000.
3. John CC, Mili R. Epidemic bacillus endo-phthalmitis after cataract surgery II. Chronic and recurrent presentation and outcome. Ophthalmology 107:1038–1041,2000.
4. Madhavan HN, Sara R. Effects of viscoelastic ophthalmic solution on cell cultures. Indian J Opthalmology 46:37–40, 1998.
5. Schmitz K. Postsurgery Intraocular inflamma-tion. BenEzra. D, editor. Uveitis Update. Dev Ophthalmol. Basel: Karger. Vol 31, 175–191, 1999.
6. Wenkel H, Rummelt V, Knorr H, Naumann GO. Chronic postoperative endophthalmitis following cataract extraction and intraocular lens implantation. Report on nine patients. Ger J Ophthalmol 2: 419–425, 1993.

PHACOEMUSIFICATION IN DENSE CATARACT

1. Vasavada A, Singh R. Step-by-step chop in situ and separation of very dense cataracts. J Cataract Refract Surg 24:156–159, 1998.

PHACOEMUSIFICATION IN POSTERIOR POLAR CATARACT

1. Anon. Consultation section: Cataract surgical problem. J Cataract Refract Surg 23:819–822, 1997.
2. Luntz MH. Clinical types of cataracts. Duane's Ophthalmology; CD ROM, 1996.
3. Osher RH, Yu BC, Koch DD. Posterior polar cataracts: a predisposition to intraoperative posterior capsular rupture. J Cataract Refract Surg 16:157–162,1990.
4. Vasavada A, Singh R. Phacoemulsification in eyes with posterior polar cataract. J Cataract Refract Surg 25:238–245,1999.
5. Vasavada A, Singh R. Surgical techniques for difficult cataracts. Curr Opin Ophthalmol 10:46–52,1999.

SURGERY IN TRAUMATIC CATARACT

1. Bienfait MF, Pameijer JH, Wildervanck de Biecourt-Devilee M. Intraocular lens implantation in children with unilateral traumatic cataract. Int Ophthalmol 14:271–276, 1990.
2. Binkhorst CD, Gobin MH. Treatment of congenital and juvenile cataract with intraocular lens implants (pseudophakoi). Br J Ophthalmol 54:759–765,1970.
3. Blumenthal M, Yalon M, Triester G. Intraocular lens implantation in traumatic cataract in children. Am Intraocular Implant Soc J 9:40–41, 1983.
4. Gupta AK, Grover AK, Gurha N. Traumatic cataract surgery with intraocular lens implantation in children. J Pediatr Ophthalmol Strabismus 29:73–78,1992.
5. Hemo U, Benezra D. Traumatic cataracts in young children (correction of aphakia by intraocular lens implantation). Ophthalmic Paediatr Genet 8:203–207,1987.
6. Juler F. Amblyopia from disuse: visual acuity after traumatic cataract in children. Trans Ophthalmol Soc UK 41:129–139,1921.
7. Kozer Bilgin L, Pakter S, Sezen F, Tugal Tutkun I. Binocular vision regained after monocular traumatic aphakia by wearing contact lenses. Eur J Ophthalmol 2:86–90,1992.
8. McKinna AJ. Results of treatment of traumatic cataract in children. Am J Ophthalmol 52:43–53,1961.
9. Morgan KS, Arffa RC, Marvelli TL, Verity SM. Five year follow-up of epikeratophakia in children. Ophthalmology 93:423–432,1986.
10. Morgan KS, et al. The nationwide study of epikeratophakia for aphakia in older children. Ophthalmology 95:526–532,1988.
11. Morgan KS, Stephenson GS. Epikeratophakia in children with corneal lacerations. J Pediatr Ophthalmol Strabismus 22:105–108,1985.

CATARACT SURGERY IN A POST-REFRACTIVE SURGERY

1. Awwad ST, et al. Intraocular lens power calculation after radial keratotomy: estimating the refractive corneal power. J Cataract Refract Surg, 33(6):1045–1050,2007.
2. Holladay JT, Consultations in refractive surgery. Refract Corneal Surg, 5:203,1989.
3. Holladay JT, WE Hill, A. Steinmueller, Corneal power measurements using scheimp-flug imaging in eyes with prior corneal refractive surgery. J Refract Surg, 25(10):862–868, 2009.
4. Koch DL Wang. Calculating IOL power in eyes that have had refractive surgery. J Cataract Refract Surg, 2003;29:2039–2042.
5. Qazi MA, et al. Determining corneal power using Orbscan II videokeratography for intraocular lens calculation after excimer laser surgery for myopia. J Cataract Refract Surg, 33(1):21–30,2007.
6. Ridley F. Development in contact lens theory-moulding, computation, and veiling. Trans Ophthalmol Soc, 68:385–401,1948.
7. Shammas HJ, et al. Correcting the corneal power measurements for intraocular lens power calculations after myopic laser in situ kerato-mileusis. Am J Ophthalmol, 136(3):426–432, 2003.

CHAPTER 17

PAEDIATRIC CATARACT SURGERY

SPECIAL PREOPERATIVE CONSIDERATIONS

Before attempting surgery for paediatric cataracts, one must be aware about some special preoperative considerations:

Considerations for paediatric eyeball

- *Co-existing ocular defects* such as a small or micro-ophthalmic eye or any other ocular defect which may complicate the situation, e.g. presence of persistent pupillary membrane or synechiae or an atonic pupil can result in inadequate pupillary dilation.
- *Low ocular rigidity* present in children may cause the eye to collapse in cases of poor controlled ocular hydrodynamics. Further, sutureless self-sealing wound may not be successful due to low ocular rigidity.
- *Elasticity of anterior capsule* is comparatively more in infants and young children and is thus prone to radial extension during capsulorhexis. Use of high density viscoelastic may help.
- *Maintenance of anterior chamber* is of major concern during surgery, as children tend to have shallow anterior chamber.
- *Increased intravitreal pressure* owing to scleral collapse and/or due to variation in the intraocular pressure under general anaesthesia predisposes to vitreous loss. Therefore, lowering of IOP by IV mannitol is recommended.

Considerations for IOL power

IOL power is calculated under general anaesthesia just before surgery. No satisfactory answer is still available for the power of IOL to be implanted. Till date best option is based on the axial length as described by Dahan et al. For details *see* page 57.

Some surgeons (Vasada AR) prefer following approach for better outcome.

Age	*Under correction*
0–3 months	35%
3–6 months	30%
6–12 months	25%

1–2 years	20%
2–4 years	15%
4–6 years	10%
>6 years	5%

Considerations for general anaesthesia

General anaesthesia should be administered by an anaesthesiologist skilled for young patients. For important points to be considered during various steps of anaesthesia, *see* page 105.

TECHNIQUES OF SURGERY FOR CHILDHOOD CATARACT

Surgical techniques employed for childhood cataract are essentially of two types:
- Lens aspiration
- Lensectomy.

1. LENS ASPIRATION

Lens aspiration can be performed by:
- Conventional ECCE technique
- Manual SICS technique
- Phaco-aspiration technique.

The corneoscleral tunnel techniques (closed chamber surgery), i.e. manual SICS or phaco-aspiration is preferred over the conventional ECCE technique (open chamber surgery which is obsolute and not practiced nowadays).

SURGICAL STEPS OF LENS ASPIRATION BY CORNEOSCLERAL TUNNEL INCISION TECHNIQUES

1. ***Exposing the eye***
2. ***Bridle suture and conjunctival flap***
3. ***Sclerocorneal tunnel incision***
4. ***Injection of viscoelastic device in the anterior chamber***
5. ***Side port incision***

Note. 1–5 initial steps up to making of side port entry are similar to as described for manual SICS in adults (*see* pages 194–198) *except that*:
- *Size of the sclerocorneal incision* is 3 mm (for foldable IOL) and the preferred site is superior.
- *Bridle suture* should preferably be avoided as it may cause traction on the soft sclera and may mask extraocular contractions, if anaesthesia becomes light.
- *Cohesive viscoelastic* should always be preferred to facilitate easy removal and prevention of postoperative IOP spikes.

6. ***Anterior capsulorhexis*** of about 5 mm in size is made as described on page 201–203 (Figs 14.10 and 14.12). As mentioned above, in children, the anterior capsule is more elastic than in adults and, therefore, the capsulorhexis may be difficult due to tendency to run outwards. Use of high density viscoelsatic and Utrata's capsulorhexis forceps are helpful in having a controlled capsulorhexis. Tractional forces must be directed centripetally at all times, rather than circumferentially in order to avoid extension of the CCC out to the equator.

- *Radiofrequency thermal cautery capsulotomy.* In cases with intense capsular fibrosis, use of radiofrequency diathermy to perform CCC gives good results. It involves coagulation and cutting of the capsule using a high frequency probe providing a safe, regular and predictable capsulorhexis. The capsulotomy size and shape are controlled by the surgeon, as the tip is moved along a circular path. This procedure is also useful in cases with total white cataracts in which there is no red reflex, in eyes with small pupil and especially for surgeons with less experience with CCC. Use of tryphan blue dye is also helpful under such situations.
- *Vitrectorhexis,* i.e. anterior capsulotomy with vitrectomy probe can also be done as alternative to the radiofrequency thermal cautery capsulotomy.

7. ***Irrigation and aspiration of lens matter*** (which is soft in children) can be done by any of the following methods:

- *Manual irrigation and aspiration* with the help of two-way Simcoe's cannula.
- *Automated irrigation and aspiration* with a phaco I/A handle, is being preferred by most of the surgeons. A well-performed hydrodissection will not only loosen the lens matter and assist in its aspiration but also dislodge the equatorial cells responsible for posterior capsular opacification thus decreasing the incidence of PCO. It is best to have a linear control of the suction pressure while using I/A tip. A meticulous removal of lens matter as

much as possible from the fornices of the capsular bag will markedly reduce the post-operative inflammation. A bimanual approach (Fig. 17.1) minimizes anterior chamber fluctuations and aids in thorough removal of the cortex especially in the subincisional area. In cases of posterior capsular rupture with efflux of lens material into the vitreous, pars plana vitrectomy should be performed, ideally at the same setting.

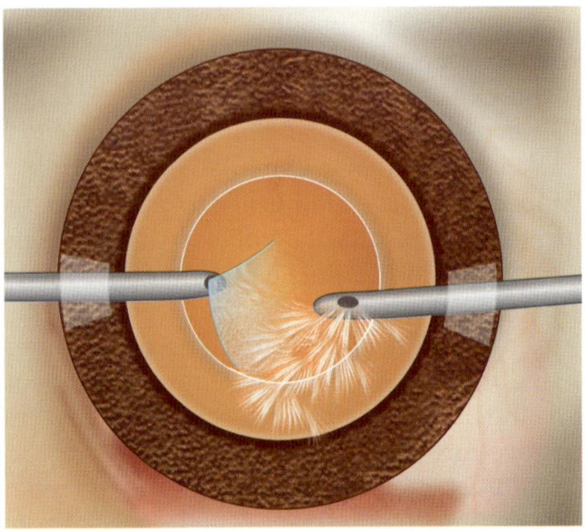

Fig. 17.1. *Technique of manual/irrigation and aspiration*

- *Membranectomy* along with anterior vitrectomy may be required in patients with membranous or calcified cataracts, where anterior and posterior capsules are fused to form a membrane.

Note.

Some surgeons recommend using a permanent anterior chamber maintainer (ACM) throughout the case to maintain inflation of the soft eye and to provide more room to manoeuvre within the deep anterior chamber.

- Heparin in the irrigation solution is recommended by some research to reduce incidence of postoperative inflammation and posterior capsular opacification.

8. ***Posterior capsulorhexis*** of about 3–4 mm size (Fig. 17.2) performed by a technique similar to anterior CCC is recomnended in children under the age of 6 years to avoid the problem of posterior capsule opacification.

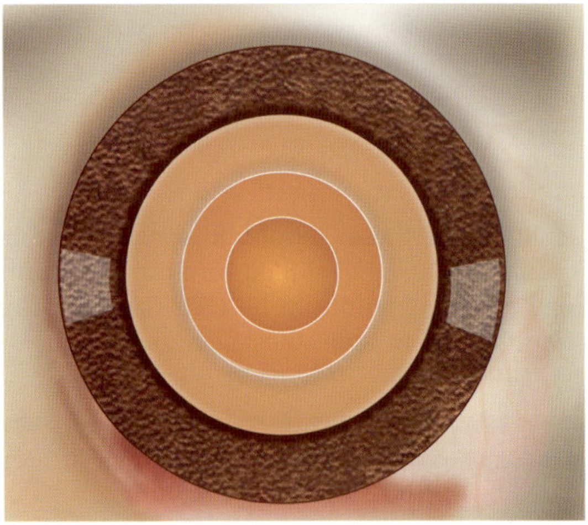

Fig. 17.2. *Depicting posterior central carvilinear capsulorhexis (PCCC) along with anterior central curvilinear capsulorhexis (ACCC)*

- *Posterior vitrectorhexis.* Alternatively many surgeons perform posterior capsulotomy with posterior vitrectorhexis. The initial capsule puncture can be carried out with a cystitome. The resultant flap is engaged with the vitrector, and the desired capsulotomy is then sculpted.
- *With automated vitrector,* there is no need to initiate flap with the cystitome. The anterior capsule is directly engaged by the automated vitrector at a low cut rate and the desired capsulotomy size is vitrected. A venturi pump vitrector is used for capsulotomy.
- *YAG laser posterior capsulotomy* may also be performed at the conclusion of surgery, if a ceiling mount YAG laser is available.

9. ***Anterior vitrectomy*** of limited amount should be performed with a vitrector. Primary anterior vitrectomy is necessary along with posterior capsulorhexis in children <2 years, because posterior capsulotomy without a central vitrectomy would unlikely prevent the development of secondary membrane. It is reported that opacification rate is not significantly decreased by posterior capsulotomy alone. The reasons supporting anterior vitrectomy are:

- Anterior vitrectomy places the vitreous face posterior to the plane of iris, thus reducing posterior synechiae formation.

- Anterior vitreous face is more reactive in infants and young children.
- Inflammatory response in small children is severe and fibrous membrane may form on an intact vitreous face.
- Intact vitreous face acts as scaffold for lens epithelial cell migration and proliferation and also for proliferation of metaplastic epithelial cells.

Note. Advent of primary posterior capsulorhexis and primary vitrectomy in young children has dramatically increased the success rate and minimized the complications and the need for secondary surgery.

10. ***Implantation of IOL*** is done in the capsular bag after inflating it with viscoelastic substance. Heparin or fluorine coated PMMA IOLs were earlier preferred in children. However, presently most surgeons prefer foldable IOLs made of hydrophobic acrylic material, e.g. Acrysof IOL, Alcon labs USA. In general, implantation of IOL in the capsular bag has its own advantages.

Optic capture through the posterior capsulorhexis has been recommended to reduce after cataract formation (Fig. 17.3A). Most surgeons now recommend implantation in the bag and pushing the optic of the lens anterior to the anterior capsulorhexis (Fig. 17.3B). As a result of this manoeuvre, the capsular bag remains closed and there is less opportunity for the remaining cells to migrate and create secondary cataract. The IOL remains stable and well centred. The vitreous body stays behind the IOL and the capsular bag. With this method of IOL implantation, there occurs less inflammation and less synechiae formation between the IOL and the iris.

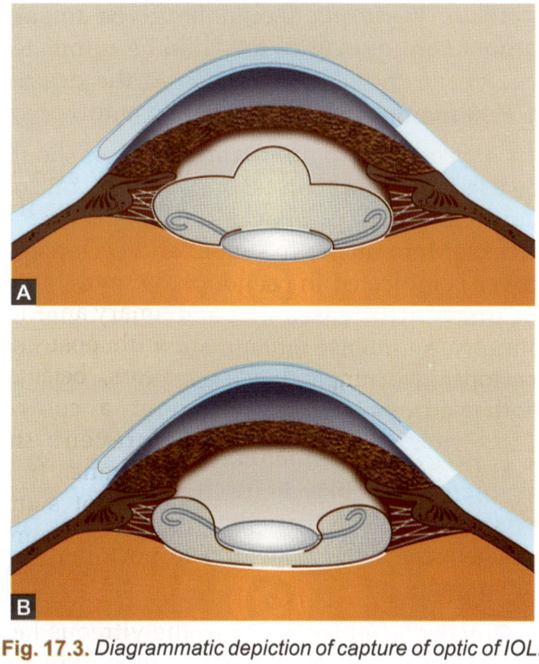

Fig. 17.3. *Diagrammatic depiction of capture of optic of IOL: **(A)** Posterior to posterior capsulorhexis; **(B)** Anterior to anterior capsulorhexis*

- *Bag-in-the-lens implantation* has been recomended recently. In this technique, anterior and posterior CCC one made of same size and the margins of both the capsulorhexis are placed in the groove of a specially designed IOL having groove at the periphery of optic (Fig. 17.4).

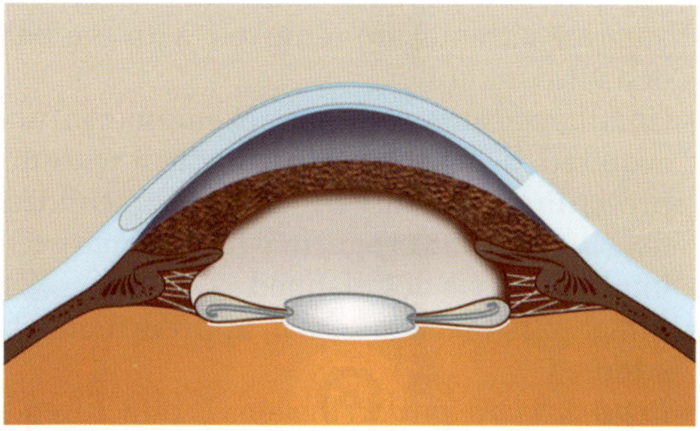

Fig. 17.4. *Diagrammatic depiction of bag-in-the-lens implantation*

Note. Steps 8 and 9, and optic capture as described in step 10 are measures to prevent formation of thick after cataract, the incidence of which is very high in young children.

11. ***Removal of viscoelastic substance*** is carried out with the help of two-way cannula or I/A phaco probe.

12. ***Wound closure.*** A well-constructed corneoscleral tunnel often does not require a suture in adults. However, it is mandatory to close the wound in children to ensure wound stability and reduce postoperative astigmatism. The water-tight closure with multiple interrupted absorbable sutures (10-0 vicryl) is adequate for closure of the wound as there occurs rapid healing. Further, it avoids the problem of suture

removal (under general anaesthesia) as is required with non-absorbable sutures.

13. ***Posterior sub-tenon injection of long acting steroid*** (triamcinolone), in addition to routine subconjunctival injection of gentamicin and dexamethasone, is useful in reducing post-operative inflammation.

Microphakonit in paediatric cataract

Many ophthalmologists are preferring micro-incision lens aspiration for paediatric cataract. With MICS, the anterior chamber is much more stable than in coaxial phaco with much less turbulence, endothelial cells trauma and less spend of BSS. For details of technique of micro-phakonit, *see* pages 276–281.

2. LENSECTOMY

- In this operation, most of the lens including anterior and posterior capsules along with anterior vitreous are removed with the help of a vitreous cutter.
- Childhood cataracts, both developmental and acquired, being soft are easily dealt with this procedure especially in very young children (less than 1 years of age) in which primary IOL implantation is not planned.
- Either pars plana or limbal approach may be adopted.
- *In pars plana approach,* the lens is punctured at its equator and stirred with the help of a Ziegler's or any other needle-knife introduced through the sclera and ciliary body, from a point about 2.5–3 mm behind the limbus.
- The cutter (ocutome) of the vitrectomy machine is introduced after enlarging the sclerotomy and lensectomy along with anterior vitrectomy is completed using cutting, irrigation and aspiration mechanisms. The aim of modern lensectomy is to leave in situ a peripheral rim of the capsule as an alternative to complete lensectomy.
- *In the limbal approach,* the steps are similar to phacoaspiration of lens as described above except that all the steps, i.e. anterior capsulorhexis, lens matter removal, posterior capsulorhexis and anterior vitrectomy are all performed with vitrectomy probe.
- Secondary IOL implantation can be planned at a later date.

Merits and demerits of lensectomy

Advantages of lensectomy include:
- Least postoperative inflammation,
- No posterior capsular opacification, and
- Early postoperative rehabilitation with aphakia.

Disadvantages of lensectomy:
- Child is made aphakic, and
- There is increased risk of retinal detachment.

Epilenticular IOL with lensectomy

This technique has the obvious advantages of an IOL but there is a high rate of IOL related complications as the lens is not in the capsular bag.

Note. With the advances in microsurgical technique in cataract surgery, the phaco *lens aspiration* is being preferred over lensectomy and thus have become the procedure of choice.

POSTOPERATIVE MANAGEMENT

I. Follow-up and advice to parents

Regular follow-up to look for any postoperative complication.

Advice to parents should be given to take proper care of eyes of the child.

II. Postoperative medications

1. ***Corticosteroid and antibiotic eyedrops*** should be used one hourly on 1st day, 2 hourly on 2nd day, 3 hourly on 3rd day and then QID for 6–8 weeks. More intensive steroid and cycloplegic cover is indicated in pseudophakic eyes. Even in uneventful cases of paediatric cataract surgery, an intense inflammation is a common postoperative complication. Therefore, compliance with eyedrops is essential.

2. ***Topical antiglaucoma drugs* and *oral acetazolamide*** may be used, if one suspects postoperative IOP spikes due to left out viscoelastic material or due to postoperative inflammation.

3. ***Oral prednisolone*** in a dose of 1.5 mg/kg body weight should also be given to decrease fibrous inflammatory reaction in the anterior chamber.

III. Spectacle correction and amblyopia therapy

1. ***Postoperative spectacle correction*** should be given within 2 weeks to correct an ametropia exceeding 1 D of hyperopia or 4 D of myopia in pseudophakic cases.

2. ***Amblyopia therapy by occlusion*** is the most critical part of postoperative care especially in unilateral and asymmetrical bilateral cataract surgeries and should be started one week post-operatively.

COMPLICATIONS OF PAEDIATRIC CATARACT SURGERY

Complications of cataract surgery and their mangement is described in detail in Chapter 20. However, a few important complications of paediatric cataract surgery are mentioned here.

I. ***Intraoperative complications*** include:

- Small pupil,
- Hyphaema,
- Iris damage, and
- Anterior chamber collapse.

II. ***Immediate postoperative complications***

1. *Wound leak* usually occurs when the corneo-scleral tunnel is not proper and/or when the wound is not secured with sutures.
2. *Anterior plastic uveitis,* i.e. intense inflammatory reaction may be seen in the early post-operative period.
3. *Increased intraocular pressure* may occur due to inflammation and left out viscoelastic material.
4. *Incarceration of iris* in the wound may sometimes occur when it is not secured with sutures.
5. *Haemorrhagic retinopathy, i.e.* occurrence of flame-shaped retinal haemorrhages with or without vitreous haemorrhage has been reported to occur rarely during first 24 hours of surgery.
6. *Postoperative endophthalmitis,* incidence is same as for adult cataract surgery.

III. ***Late postoperative complications***

1. *Secondary membrane formation* may occur in cases with intense inflammatory reaction. Use of intracameral tissue plasminogen activator (TPA) is recommended in such cases.
2. *Chronic smoldering uveitis* may occur in cases with left out lens matter.
3. *IOL decentration* is quite common in children. However, with in-the-bag placement and use of optic capture, the incidence is reduced.
4. *Secondary glaucoma.* Late glaucoma usually occurs due to post-inflammatory scarring in the trabecular meshwork or annular synechiae formation.
5. *Posterior capsular opacification* is the most common complication with the reported incidence varying from 51–100%. However, with use of optic capture and anterior vitrectomy, the incidence is reduced.
6. *Late endophthalmitis* may occur due to *Propionobacterium acnes* or fungal infection.
7. *Cystoid macular oedema.* Exact incidence is not known, however, the younger eyes are thought to be more resistant to develop CME.
8. *Corneal oedema and bullous keratopathy* may occur due to endothelial damage. Exact incidence is not known as long-term follow-up is not available.
9. *Retinal detachment* is reported to occur in 2–25% of cases. Mean interval after surgery is 23–43 years.

BIBLIOGRAPHY

1. Aasuri MK, Fernandes M, Pathan PP. Comparison of acrylic and polymethylmethacrylate lenses in a pediatric population. Indian J Ophthalmol 54:105–109,2006.
2. Ahmadieh H, Javadi MA. Intraocular lens implantation in children. Curr Opin Ophthalmol 12:30–34,2001.
3. Dahan E. Intraocular lens implantation in children. Curr Opin Ophthalmol 11:51–55,2000.
4. Faramarzi A, Javadi MA. Comparison of 2 techniques of intraocular lens implantation in pediatric cataract surgery. J Cataract Refract Surg 35:1040–1045,2009.
5. Javadi MA, Ahmadieh H. Opacification of the ocular media. In: Wilson ME, editor; Trivedi RH, editor; Pandey SK, editor. Pediatric cataract surgery techniques; complications, and management. Philadelphia: Lippincott Williams & Wilkins 236–243,2005.

CHAPTER 18

ASTIGMATISM CONTROL IN CATARACT SURGERY

ASTIGMATISM IN CATARACT SURGERY

The present day cataract surgery aims at not only removal of cataract but also correction of pre-existing spherical as well as cylindrical component of the refraction, and so is rightly called as *'refractive cataract surgery'*. Infact, the term 'refractive cataract surgery' no longer simply engenders a shift in philosophy, rather has come to represent a reality for our cataract patients. The spherical refractive error can be eliminated through a meticulously performed accurate IOL power calculation, while control of final postoperative astigmatism during cataract surgery involves management of:

- Pre-existing astigmatism (PEA)
- Surgically induced astigmatism

PRE-EXISTING ASTIGMATISM

Pre-existing astigmatism (PEA) is quite commonly encountered. Variable prevalence is reported in the literature. In a study conducted by us (unpublished data) in consecutive 3000 patients undergoing cataract surgery (from 2005 to 2011), of the total patients, the results are as below:

- 73% of patients were having astigmatism, out of which:
  - 70% had 0.25–1 D
  - 20% had 1–2 D
  - 10% had >2 D of astigmatism
- 31% of patients had with-the-rule (WTR) astigmatism
- 69% had against-the-rule (ATR) astigmatism.

The PEA may be corneal and/or lenticular. Only corneal astigmatism (identified by keratometry or topography) need to be corrected.

Factors about PEA, which need to be considered for the management of final postoperative astigmatism, include:

- Amount of astigmatism
- Axis of the cylinder
- Age of the patient
- Status of the fellow eye.

* *Courtesy:* Dr. Saurabh Sawhney and Dr. Aashima Aggarwal, Insite Eye Clinic, New Delhi

SURGICALLY INDUCED ASTIGMATISM

Astigmatic change introduced because of surgical treatment of the cornea is referred to as surgically induced astigmatism (SIA). This change may be intended or incidental. Technically, SIA = Postoperative astigmatism–Preoperative astigmatism. It is important to note that only corneal astigmatism is being considered.

Surgically induced astigmatism (SIA), depends upon the incision characteristics such as: its length, location, shape and direction.

Observations about SIA vis-à-vis incision characteristics reported in the literature are as follows:

- *Concept of astigmatically neutral funnel of Koch* is described on page 196 and Fig. 14.2. Incision placed in this funnel induces minimal astigmatism.
- *Clear corneal tunnel incision* induces more astigmatism than the sclerocorneal tunnel incision.
- *Location.* Farther the incision from the centre of cornea, lesser is the SIA.
- *Size.* Smaller the incision, lesser the SIA.
- *Direction.* Incision placed in the temporal quadrant induces less astigmatism than placed in the superior quadrant.
- *Shape.* Straight sclerocorneal tunnel incision is reported to induce more astigmatism than the frown and v-shaped (Chaveron incision).
- *Superior incision* induces against the rule astigmatism and thus neutralizes pre-existing with-the-rule (WTR) astigmatism.
- *Temporal incision* induces WTR and this neutralizes the pre-existing ATR.
- *Corneal relaxing incision* (CRI), limbal relaxing incision (LRI) and clear corneal incision (CCI), when placed along and at 180° to the main cataract incision enhance the flattening produced by the main cataract incision; and when placed at 90° to the main cataract incision try to neutralize the flattening produced by the main cataract incision.

METHODS TO EVALUATE SIA

SIMPLE SUBTRACTION AND ALGEBRAIC METHODS

In the past, a number of strategies have been adopted to estimate SIA. However, since astigmatism is a vector quantity, i.e. it possesses both magnitude and direction, the simplistic methods used earlier do not provide accurate results, and are often misleading, in fact.

Among the methods that mislead are the simple subtraction method, which entails subtracting the preoperative astigmatic magnitude from the postoperative magnitude, ignoring the axis altogether. This is obviously incorrect. Another method that may mislead is the ***algebraic subtraction method,*** in which the investigator assigns a plus or minus sign to the astigmatic magnitude, to roughly account for with or against the rule astigmatism. This begins to approach the problem of considering the axis, but is just a rudimentary first step, and hence, inaccurate.

VECTOR ANALYSIS METHODS

Accurate analysis of astigmatic changes requires that the rules of vector transformation be followed. This can be done by means of actual drawing of vectors, or by using trigonometric functions to obtain the same results. This latter approach is recommended as it is easier to extrapolate it to aggregate analysis. Technically, it is possible to perform aggregate analysis using traditional vector analysis, but observer errors inherent in the process of physically drawing and measuring vectors makes it less accurate.

The proper methods for evaluating vector changes were elucidated more than a century ago. The milestone in aggregate data analysis was the paper in 1998, by Holladay et al, that laid down the methodology for calculating mean astigmatic vectors.

By convention, astigmatic analysis is performed using vectors in the plus-cylinder form. This is calculated by taking the difference of the keratometric values in the two meridians as the magnitude of astigmatism, and the axis of the steeper meridian as the axis of astigmatism, as depicted by example below.

EXAMPLE 1 OF VECTOR ANALYSIS METHOD

Consider the following values:

Kh = 44.50 D @ 165°

Kv = 43.75 D @ 75°

The plus-cylinder format would then be 0.75 D @ 165°.

This is the form in which calculations are performed and results presented. Since the value has both direction and magnitude, it is called an 'astigmatic vector'.

Calculating SIA using trigonometric functions

As we know, SIA = Postoperative astigmatism – Preoperative astigmatism..........(1)

The first problem encountered in using trigonometric functions for astigmatic data analysis is the fact that whilst astigmatic direction repeats after 180°, geometrical angles repeat after 360°. In the field of directional statistics, the two types of data are termed 'orientational' and 'directional' data, respectively.

This difficulty is tackled by doubling the angle of astigmatism prior to calculations, and halving it at the end of the procedure, thereby adapting the 180° refractive scheme to the 360° geometrical one. Once this is done, the rest of the procedure follows standard trigonometric strategies.

The preoperative astigmatic vector is transformed to a point on a Cartesian grid using the following equations.

X_{preop} = a cos 2p................(2a)

Y_{preop} = a sin 2p.................(2b)

where 'a' is the magnitude of the astigmatic vector and 'p' is the axis which is doubled to '2p' for the calculations.

The location of the point is now represented as (X_{preop}, Y_{preop}) (Fig. 18.1).

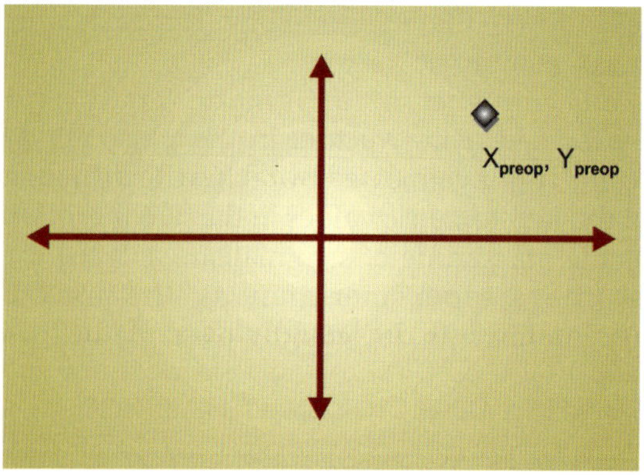

Fig. 18.1. *A representation of preoperative astigmatism on the Cartesian system.*

A similar transformation is carried out for the postoperative vector, producing (X_{postop}, Y_{postop}) (Fig. 18.2).

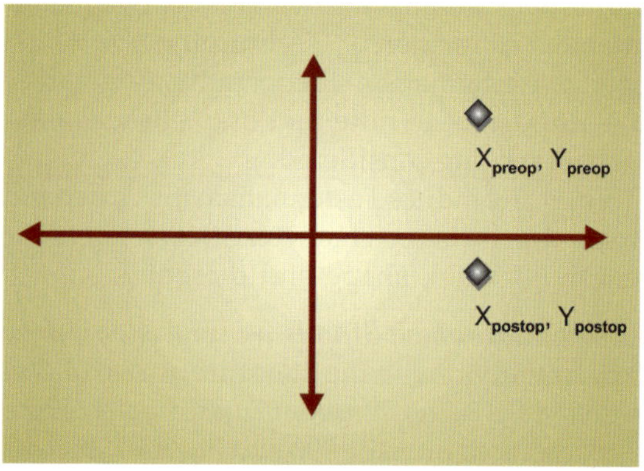

Fig. 18.2. *Both preoperative and postoperative vectors are now represented. From this point, connecting the two dots would produce the resultant SIA vector, as classically done by the vector calculation method. This illustrates how cartesian coordinates and vector analysis are essentially identical.*

The SIA coordinates are calculated by simply subtracting the preoperative values from the postoperative values, independently for 'X' and 'Y'

Thus,

$X_{SIA} = X_{postop} - X_{preop}$..........(3a)

$Y_{SIA} = Y_{postop} - Y_{preop}$..........(3b)

The SIA Cartesian values now need to be converted back into the vector form that can be understood clinically. The magnitude of SIA (M_{SIA}) and its axis (A_{SIA}) are calculated separately, as follows:

Magnitude of SIA (M_{SIA}) = $\sqrt{X_{SIA}^2 + Y_{SIA}^2}$ ...(4a)

Angle of SIA (θ) = ½ arctan $\frac{Y_{SIA}}{X_{SIA}}$ ...(4b)

Note that the angle has been halved to revert back to the orientational (refractive) scheme from the directional scheme.

The angle of SIA thus obtained is not the final axis. It needs further refinement as follows. The rules are valid for general conversion of (X,Y) values to the vector form.

If $X_{SIA} > 0$ and $Y_{SIA} \geq 0$, then axis = θ...(5a)

If $X_{SIA} > 0$ and $Y_{SIA} < 0$, then axis = θ + 180°...(5b)

If $X_{SIA} < 0$, then axis = θ + 90°...(5c)

If $X_{SIA} = 0$ and $Y_{SIA} > 0$, then axis = 45°...(5d)

If $X_{SIA} = 0$ and $Y_{SIA} < 0$, then axis = 135°...(5e)

The last two caveats (5d and 5e) are specifically added to avoid the problem of dividing by zero.

In this manner, the SIA vector is obtained and represented as M_{SIA} Diopters @ A_{SIA} degrees.

Let us see the process at work using hypothetical data.

EXAMPLE 2 OF VECTOR ANALYSIS

Preoperative astigmatic vector = 1.5 D @ 65°
Postoperative astigmatic vector = 1.0 D @ 35°
Then,

$X_{preop} = 1.5 * \cos 2*65 = 1.5*\cos 130 = -0.964181$
$Y_{preop} = 1.5 * \sin 2*65 = 1.5*\sin 130 = 1.149067$

$X_{postop} = 1.0 * \cos 2*35 = 1.0*\cos 70 = 0.342020$
$Y_{postop} = 1.0 * \sin 2*35 = 1.0*\sin 70 = 0.939693$

From the above values, it is fairly straightforward to calculate SIA (X, Y) values.

$X_{SIA} = X_{postop} - X_{preop} = 1.306201$
$Y_{SIA} = Y_{postop} - Y_{preop} = -0.20937$

Applying equations 4 and 5

Magnitude of astigmatism, M_{SIA}=

$$\sqrt{(1.306201)^2 + (-0.20937)^2} = 1.322875 \text{ Diopters}$$

$$\text{Angle of SIA } (\theta) = \tfrac{1}{2} * \arctan \frac{-0.20937}{1.306201} = -4.5533°$$

Applying qualifiers as per equation 5

Since X > 0 and Y < 0, the final axis =

$$\theta + 180° = 175.4467°$$

Therefore, SIA is 1.32 D @ 175°

A WORD ABOUT PRESENTING DATA

Notice that the use of mathematical functions allows calculations up to as many decimal places but the final results must be rounded off to clinically relevant decimal places for the evaluation to be meaningful. It is all too easy to present diopteric values going to five or six decimal places, creating a false impression of great accuracy. The same holds true for the direction data as well, where we recommend no decimal places at all, just whole numbers.

AGGREGATE DATA ANALYSIS

The elegance of the Cartesian system is truly appreciated when analyzing aggregate data. The preoperative data is converted to (x,y) format using equations (2a and 2b) above. For instance, if evaluating the outcome of 20 cases, one obtains a set of 20 preoperative 'x' values, 20 preoperative 'y' values, and similar sets of postoperative (x,y) values. From these, SIA (x,y) values can be generated (equations 3a and 3b).

Next, each of the x and y values are averaged to determine mean values. This is done by simply adding up all x values (in our example, 20 values each for preop, postop and SIA data), mindful of the sign, and then dividing by the total number of cases (20, in our example).

$$\bar{X} = \frac{\sum_{(i)}^{n} xi}{n} \quad \text{..} (6)$$

Here, $\bar{X}$ is the mean value, x_i is the individual value, and n is the total number of cases.

Now, the mean (x,y) values thus obtained are converted to the vector form using the set of equations 4 and 5.

The mean vector thus obtained is called the ***centroid.***

Further descriptions of standard deviations for x,y values in each set have been quoted in the literature, but are erroneous in concept and value of interpretation, and will not be discussed.

Automated computer software is available that can help with the calculations. One such free software is the SIA Calculator Version 2.1, which can be downloaded from http://www.insighteyeclinic.in

How to interpret the data?

The centroid yields the mean astigmatic vector for a group of data points. It should be plotted on a double-angled plot (DAP), which is essentially a modification of the rose diagram. The DAP is drawn in the form of concentric rings, each representing an incremental step in the magnitude of astigmatism. Thus, the innermost point is zero, the first ring represents one diopter of astigmatism, the second ring represents two diopters, and so on and so forth. Typically, three to four rings would suffice for all depictions.

The axis on the DAP is marked at twice the standard notation for circles. Thus, the 0° and 180° marks coincide. This is intended to allow visualization of clusters without splitting the points around the 0° mark into a fallacious, bimodal-appearing pattern. The vectors are plotted as points on the DAP, and the centroid can be plotted as a point of a different colour or shape to highlight it.

When interpreting data on a DAP, one should look for clustering of points. A good, tight cluster means that the data is composed of similar vectors and has low variability, factors which make the set more useful clinically.

For example, look at the sample DAP below (Fig. 18.3). This represents the SIA vectors from a group of 20 cases.

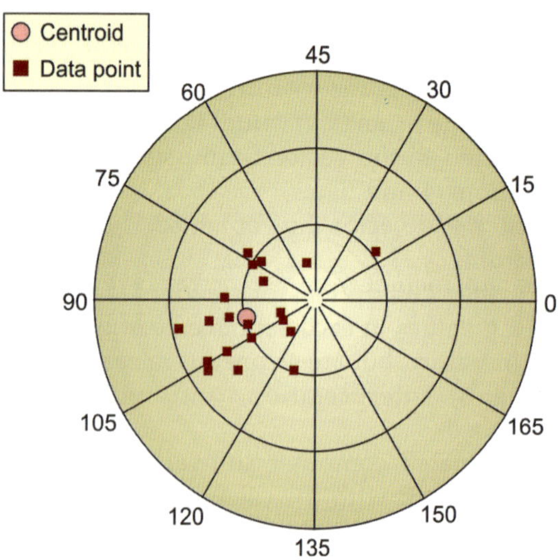

Fig. 18.3. *Clustered data as represented on a doubled-angle plot.*

The vectors are clustered around the 90° mark, and the centroid occupies a position that instinctively appears to represent the mean. This is a tight data set, and can be used to make reasonably accurate predictions.

Now look at this DAP (Fig. 18.4).

The points are spread out, creating no specific patterns. In such a case, the opposing astigmatic vectors tend to neutralize each other, resulting in a lower mean value. The centroid is, therefore, placed closer to the centre of the DAP, and is not truly representative of the data. Therefore,

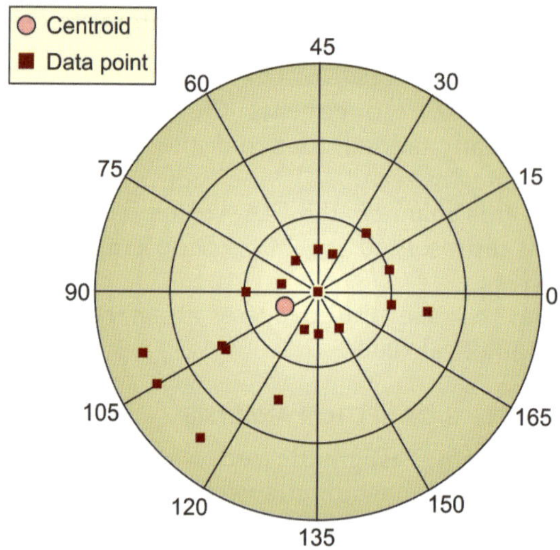

Fig. 18.4. *Scattered data as represented on a doubled-angle plot.*

the clinical utility of a data set with well-spread vectors showing poor clustering is rather limited.

THE SIA CALCULATORS—CALCULATING SURGICALLY INDUCED ASTIGMATISM USING MS EXCEL

The SIA calculators are a series of computer programmes of increasing complexity that are based on the principles of vector transformation using trigonometric functions. There are three current versions, namely 1.1, 2.1 and 3.1. All these versions can be run using MS Excel 2007 or higher. An earlier SIA Calculator 1.0 is now obsolete and has been withdrawn.

SIA CALCULATOR VERSION 1.1

SIA Calc v 1.1 is a basic calculator that allows the user to enter data for one single patient at a time. This data is entered in the form of preoperative and postoperative keratometric readings. The calculator first generates the amount of astigmatism from these values, then converts them into Cartesian coordinates using well-defined functions. These coordinates (x,y values) are displayed by the calculator screen. A complete calculation and the resultant SIA vector are also displayed. There is also an option for entering any coordinates you desire, and the programme will tell you what the corresponding vector would be. The primary utility of this version of the calculator is to gain acquaintance with the way the system works. It allows you to *see* the processes at work.

SIA CALCULATOR VERSION 2.1

The SIA calculator version 2.1 takes data from multiple patients simultaneously. It then does all the number crunching automatically, and the final results are available instantly. The method used is scientifically ratified and was published first by Jaffe and associates, with later refinements added by Jack Holladay and coworkers to allow aggregate data analysis.[2–4]

The SIA calculator version 2.1 consists of a protected MS Excel document, with three sheets. Since the document is protected, you cannot inadvertently harm it, making it secure to use. The three sheets that comprise the calculator are:

- User manual
- The calc 2.1
- Detailed report

User manual

This contains a brief description of the procedure for entering data into the calculator, and a theoretical segment that explains in detail on the methodology used in calculating SIA, including all formulae used.

The calc 2.1

This is the actual calculator sheet, containing segmented columns where one can enter the patients' identification data, clinical data, as well as postoperative data. Data for a single patient is to be entered in a single row. After this is done, a comments column will notify you on the suitability of the data. For example, if you have accidentally typed in 100° in the horizontal axis space, the comments column will report this. If all data entered is consistent and ready for analysis, the comments column will indicate this.

Once a complete entry has been made, the SIA calc 2.1 will do two things. One, it will instantly display the induced astigmatism in that particular case. Secondly, it will store the x,y values generated and use them for aggregate analysis, so that when a second case is entered, it will generate not only the individual SIA for the two cases, but also the combined, average SIA of the two cases together. In this manner, it will add the third case, the fourth case, and so on and so forth. It can handle up to 200 cases at a time in this manner.

Any incomplete entries will not be analyzed till complete information is available. This allows you to enter partial data without worrying about its impact on the calculations. For example, preoperative data might be entered on the day of surgery, but postoperative data can be put on hold till the final refraction is carried out, at which point of time it may be entered to make the entry complete and eligible for analysis.

The following screen shot (Fig. 18.5) gives an idea of how the blank calculator appears, and Fig. 18.6 shows the sheet with four cases entered.

Exclusions

There may be occasions when you feel a particular case is behaving abnormally in terms of induced astigmatism. In such a situation, you might wish to exclude that particular case from overall analysis and see the effect of that exclusion. One way to do that would be to delete the entry entirely. However, in case you wish to include that data again, you would then need to type all the details again.

The SIA Calc 2.1 provides a simple way out of this by providing a special exclusion column. This column is placed just before the comments column on the right side of the sheet (Fig. 18.7). By typing 'yes' in this column, you may exclude the entry temporarily. To reverse this and reconsider the entry, simply delete the 'yes'. Notice that the reports bar (top rows) now indicates that only three cases are being considered for evaluation. Compare this with Fig. 18.6, where the number of cases is 4.

Results

The results are displayed in the top rows, which are protected against scrolling, so even if you scroll down to enter more cases, the results bar stays in place. You may view the centroid here, which consists of the magnitude of aggregate SIA, its axis, and the 'coherence' value. The coherence value is indicative of the 'tightness' of the data. The higher the coherence, the more aligned are the astigmatic vectors.

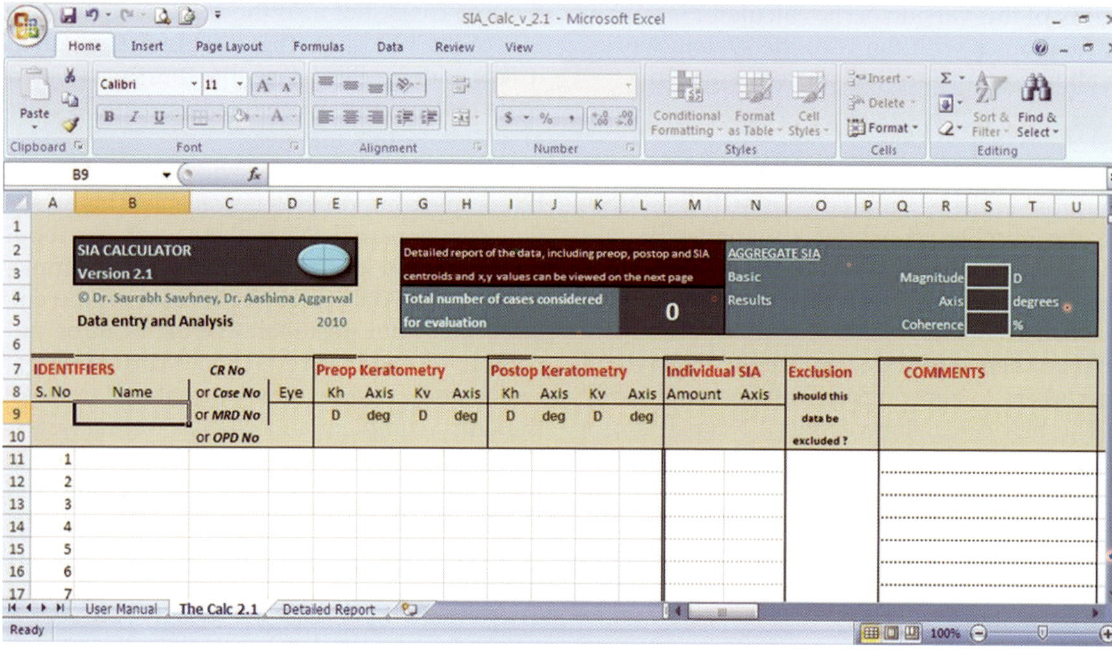

Fig. 18.5. *The empty calculator screen.*

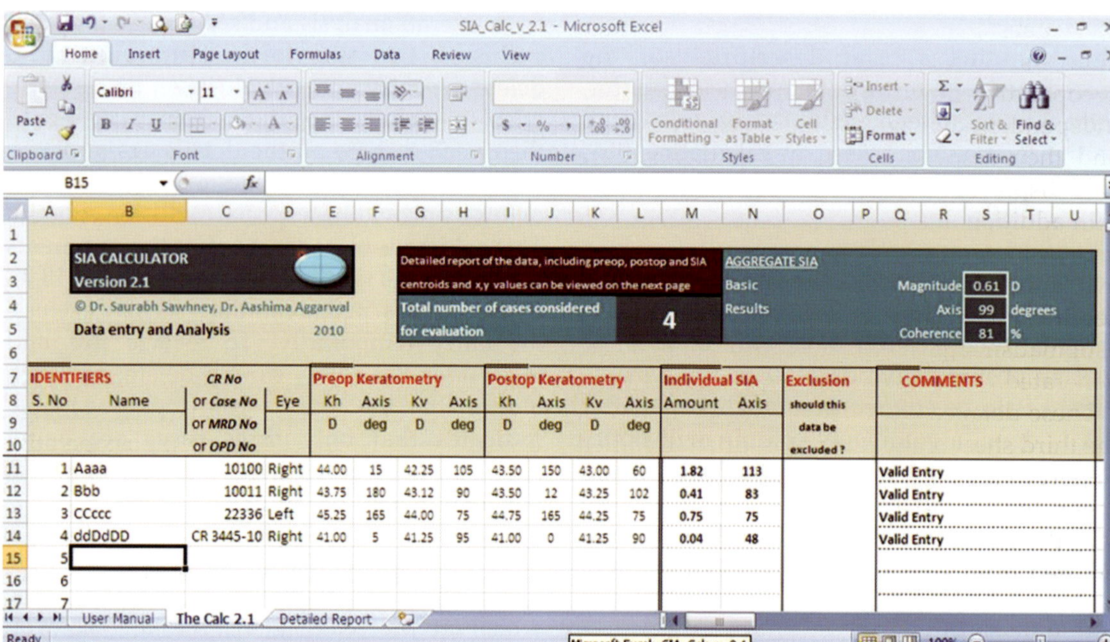

Fig. 18.6. *Four complete entries have been made. The individual SIA is noted against each entry, while the centroid or aggregate SIA is displayed in the top right corner.*

Thus, a higher coherence means a more reliable centroid, having a greater predictive value for future predictions.

Detailed analysis

The SIA calculator 2.1 is also a research tool. For all cases analyzed, it generates and stores

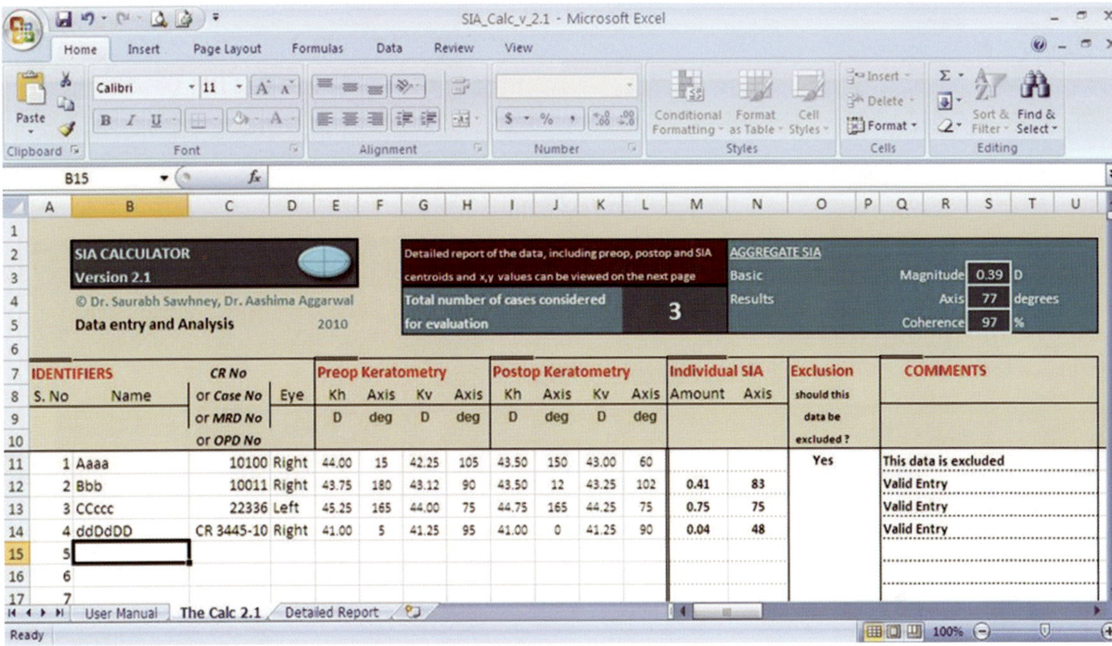

Fig. 18.7. *Notice that the first entry is excluded by typing yes in the 'Exclusion' column. The comment identifies it as such.*

x,y values that are useful in aggregate data analysis. These values are generated for preoperative, SIA, and postoperative data. The independent average of these x and y values, and their respective standard deviations are also displayed.

In addition, the aggregate preoperative, SIA and postoperative astigmatic vectors are also available, along with their coherence values. A separate analysis of mean amplitude of astigmatism and its standard deviation is also generated.

These detailed parameters can be viewed in the third sheet of the calculator, titled 'Detailed Report'. Figure 18.8 gives a screenshot of the report for the cases as entered in Figure 3. Note that the temporarily excluded entry has been omitted from analysis.

Tips to maximize the utility of the SIA calculator 2.1

1. Make multiple copies of the programme and rename them to reflect the type of data. For example, one file could be renamed 'Temporal 2.8 mm' to indicate that only surgeries with 2.8 mm incisions and temporal wounds will be entered. This makes the analysis more focused and useful. Since the software is free to use, any number of copies can be made at no cost whatsoever.
2. The quality of data entered determines the quality of analysis. Good, accurately centred keratometric readings taken on the same keratometer consistently will produce high-worth results.
3. If you are using a manual keratometer, take the time to record the axis of astigmatism correctly.
4. Avoid using a hand-held keratometer as the axis can vary significantly between readings.
5. Be consistent in the timing of the postoperative readings, since astigmatism may shift over time. As a rule of thumb, instruct your staff to record the keratometry on the day that final postoperative refraction is done.
6. Your data is precious. Always save a backup copy.

THE SIA CALCULATOR VERSION 3.1– THE WAY AHEAD

The final utility of calculating SIA lies in being able to predict what would happen in a given case. For instance, if a patient has a pre-existing corneal astigmatism of 1.25 D @ 165°, a surgeon

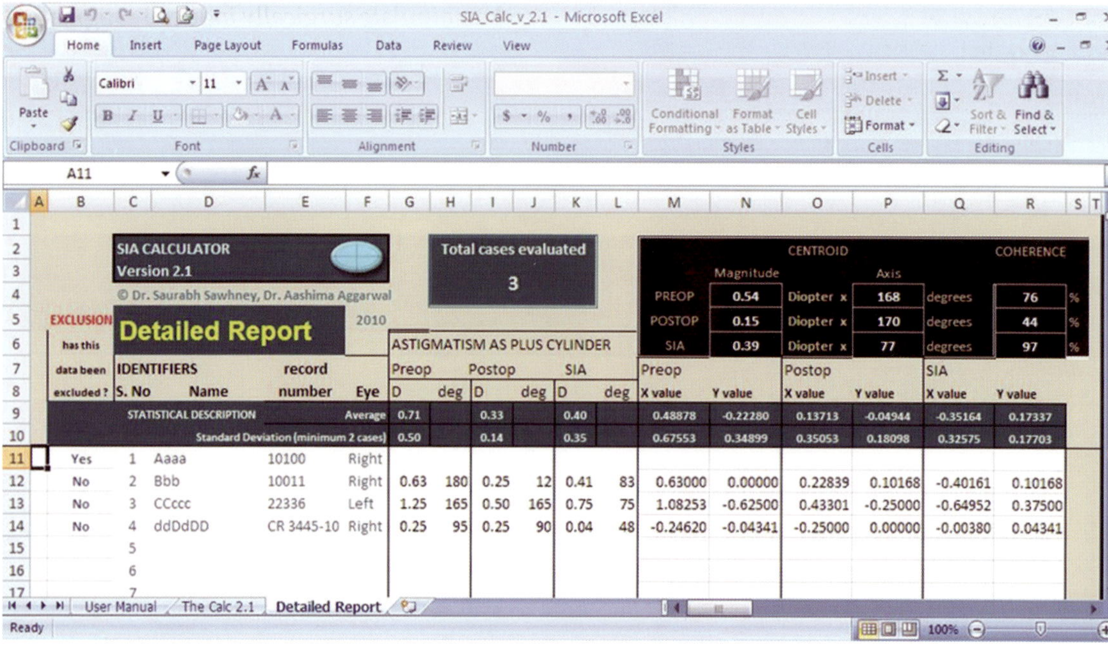

Fig. 18.8. *Detailed report.*

would want to know whether his/her standard incision at 15° would be sufficient to take care of this. *Interestingly, we found that for this particular example, if we went ahead and made an incision at 15°, it was surprisingly ineffective at reducing the astigmatism. We had to shift closer to the axis to have any measurable impact.*

Merely calculating the SIA leaves us halfway; we need to know how to incorporate this data for making predictions. Since vector analysis works both ways, the solution is obvious. We just take the preoperative astigmatic vector, add the SIA vector, and the resultant is our expected postoperative vector.

So, preoperative astigmatism + SIA = postoperative astigmatism

Once again, the catch is that adding vector quantities is easier said than done.

The SIA calculator version 3.1 is designed to take this last step. Like the previous two versions, it is a fully automated programme. The basic design involves taking in a lot more data, so that targeted SIA results can be generated, which will have actual, real-life clinical value.

The process begins by creating a database of surgeries. Once this is available, it functions a sort of analytical pool. Whenever a prediction is required, specific preoperative information is fed into the predictions page of the calculator. The calculator then scans its database for matching entries within a narrow bandwidth. For example, if the preoperative astigmatism is 0.5 D @ 90°, the calculator will automatically reject all database entries that have a preoperative astigmatism of, say, 2.5 or 2.75 D. It will also reject preoperative data that is steep at 180°. The 'tightness' of this fit is adjustable by the user, with tight fits being more likely to produce accurate predictions.

After the analytical pool, data has been selected to match the user-entered data, the calculator performs a selective SIA analysis on the chosen data. The 'non-matched' data is not considered for evaluation, unlike the version 2.1 where all valid entries were evaluated. In this manner, a specific SIA value is generated, which is then vector-added to the specific preoperative data fed by the user. This produces the predicted postoperative astigmatism.

The SIA calculator 3.1 is an extensive tool, and its detailed functions require a lot of space to explain, so we will not discuss it further here, but the online user guide covers it comprehensively. With this tool, we finally hope to provide users with a complete grip over astigmatism analysis and predictions.

WEB RESOURCES AND SYSTEM REQUIREMENTS

Web Resources

All SIA Calculator versions are available for free download from the webpage www.insighteyeclinic.in, by accessing the physician resources. Alternatively, just type the following URL into your internet browser window. http://www.insighteyeclinic.in/SIA_calculator.php. Any updates will also be available at the same site in the future. The site features on the useful links panel of the AIOS webpage, as well as the online toolbox of the Premier Surgeon web magazine, and can be accessed from any of these routes.

Dr. Saurabh Sawhney can also be personally contacted for any clarifications or assistance (saurabhsawhney@rediffmail.com).

System requirements

Any computer with MS Windows and Office 2007 or Office 2010 installed will support the software. The programme occupies a miniscule space on the hard-drive, so even older computers can run it quite comfortably. It can be easily run on a laptop or netbook, or even a cellphone with the requisite software support. The programme is well-protected against inadvertent data-entry errors. As of today, there are no known software bugs.

SUMMARY

Analysis of astigmatism is a difficult proposition for those of us not comfortable with mathematics. However, there is no solution that is simple yet accurate. Older methods like simple or algebraic subtraction are fallacious, whilst vector analysis is tedious. Of the more advanced methods, the Cartesian coordinates based system is the simplest to understand, and has the added advantage of being freely available as a programmed calculator. It is worthwhile to remember, however, that no matter how accurate your data collection and analysis, prediction of postoperative astigmatism is an exercise that can often surprise you.

As cataract surgeons set their sights on postoperative emmetropia, the need to calculate and manipulate surgically induced astigmatism is increasing. Using software to do this task makes it fast, accurate and hassle-free.

CLINICAL APPLICATIONS OF SIA ANALYSIS

Not only should the surgeon not add to the burden of astigmatism, but every effort must be made to reduce it as a part and parcel of surgery. Only meticulous observation and accurate of interpretation of results can show the way forward.

The results of your own SIA analysis are relevant for all patients, but especially for the use of toric IOLs. The website for Alcon has a calculator that lets the surgeon calculate the toric IOL specifications, and one of the data that needs to be input is the surgeon's SIA. Obviously, if the surgeon has diligently calculated mean SIA using his past surgical records, the output of the toric IOL calculator would be much more reliable than if mere guesswork is used.

In some cases, you might actually want to leave a small amount of residual cylindrical error, e.g. in an effort to match the other eye. Once again, only sound previous analysis can guide you on the best way to achieve your target.

A word of caution

A number of factors influence postoperative astigmatism.

One source of error is the simplistic view of the whole cornea being defined by just two variables. This presupposes a uniform corneal contour when this is clearly not the case. In an uncomplicated situation, this view might suffice, but irregular preoperative astigmatism, or in the presence of an off-visual axis corneal opacity, the whole analysis may go haywire.

Another point of concern is that till now, we have only considered anterior corneal astigmatism. Various researchers have indicated the contribution of posterior corneal curvature towards the overall astigmatism. In addition, there is the variation in individual incisions, even if the same surgeon makes them in ostensibly the same manner. The response of the individual cornea to incisions is also not cut and dried, and there may be significant variations.

Surprisingly, IOL tilting does not seem to add too much to astigmatism.

Because of these influences, the end-result of a cataract surgery in terms of astigmatism lies in a zone, rather than being a specific figure, and this should be kept in mind at all times.

MODALITIES OF CORRECTING ASTIGMATISM

Peroperatively, the astigmatism in cataract surgery can be controlled by using any of the following described modalities alone or in combination:

- ***On axis cataract incision*** with manipulation of its characteristic shape, size and type, i.e. unipolar/bipolar/tripolar/hinged.
- ***Corneal relaxing incision*** (CRI), limbal relaxing incision/opposite clear corneal incision (OCCI)
- ***Toric IOLs***
- ***Postoperative*** by the residual astigmatism can be corrected by laser ablative procedures (e.g. astigmatic LASIK).

MANAGEMENT OF ASTIGMATISM IN PHACOEMULSIFICATION

RELAXING INCISIONS

ON-AXIS CATARACT INCISION

On-axis cataract incision alone can correct the PEA as below:

- *3.2 mm phacoincision* placed on the steep axis is reported to correct up to 0.5 D of pre-existing astigmatism (PEA) (Fig. 18.9A).
- *Enlarging the phacoincision* at the end of surgery to 4.5 and 5.5 mm can approximately correct up to 1.00 and 1.50 D of PEA, respectively (Fig. 18.9B).

CORNEAL AND LIMBAL RELAXING INCISIONS

Limbal relaxing incisions (LRIs), placed in the periphery, are less powerful than their shorter, more central counterparts, the so-called corneal relaxing incisions (CRIs) (Fig. 18.10), but are preferred because of certain advantages given as follows:

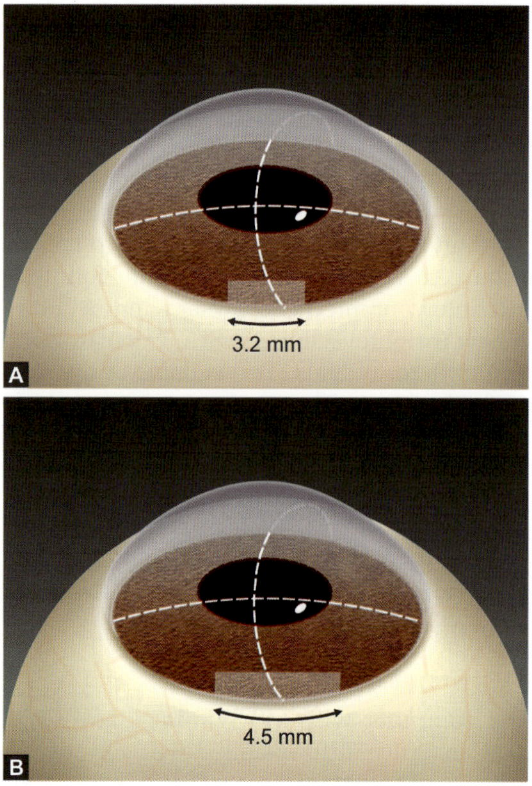

Fig. 18.9. *On-axis cataract incision:* ***(A)*** *3.2 mm phacoincision;* ***(B)*** *Phacoincision enlarged after completion of the procedure to correct astigmatism.*

ADVANTAGES, DISADVANTAGES, AND CONTRA-INDICATIONS

Advantages of LRIs

- *Overcorrection* is a less likely complication.
- *Stabilization* of the refractive effect is quicker as compared to the CRI, because the incisions made close to the limbus heal faster.
- *Complications* like irregular astigmatism, glare and foreign body sensation are less likely with LRIs as compared to CRIs.

Disadvantages of LRIs

- *Regression.* The higher the astigmatism, the greater is the regression. Most regression occurs in eyes with more than 3.5D of astigmatism.
- *Mechanical instability.* LRIs may lead to weakening of the globe, which is prone to rupture or trauma.
- *Ocular surface discomfort* may occur due to postoperative tear film irritability.

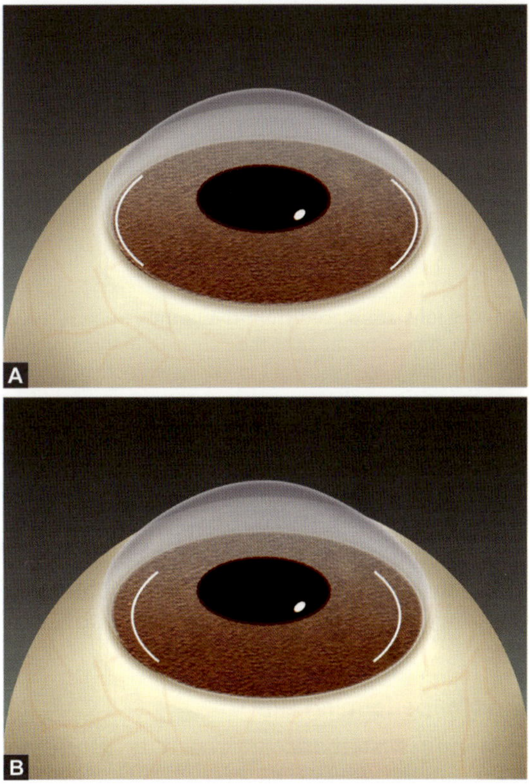

Fig. 18.10. *Limbal relaxing incisions (LRIs) and corneal relaxing incisions (CRIs) at steep axis.*

Contraindications to LRIs

- *Radial keratoplasty* (RK), performed earlier, is a contraindication for LRI.
- *Irregular astigmatism,* e.g. patients with keratoconus, other topographic abnormalities and those with peripheral corneal diseases are also contraindications for LRIs.
- *Advanced autoimmune rheumatoid disease* that might predispose to healing problems after peripheral corneal incisions, should also be considered a contraindication.

Amount of astigmatism correction with LRIs

LRIs along with cataract incision can correct up to 3 D of astigmatism. The amount of correction of course depends upon the:

- *Length of incision* (4–8 mm)
- *Number of incisions* (single, double, paired doubled)
- *Depth of incision* (about 600 microns depth gives good results)
- *Age of the patient* (more the age, greater the effect)
- *Amount of pre-existing astigmatism.*

LRI with a toric IOL or excimer laser ablation can correct up to 6.0 D of astigmatism.

LRI with toric IOL and excimer laser ablation, i.e. by using all three modalities, one can correct even up to 9.0 D of astigmatism.

Nomograms for LRIs

Various nomograms have been evolved as guides for making LRIs, a few are:

1. *Wang et al's nomogram* is depicted in Table 18.1.
2. *Gill's nomogram* is shown in Table 18.2.
3. *The NAPA nomogram* is summarized in Table 18.3.
4. *Donnenfeld nomogram (DONO)* is depicted in Table 18.4.
5. *Kevin Miller nomogram.* In this nomogram, one clock hour paired LRIs are given on the steep axis for each dioptre, i.e.

- 1 D=1 clock hour (30° = 3 mm),
- 2 D = 2 clock hours (60° = 6 mm) and so on.

Coupling effect

Cravy has described Gauss's law of elastic domes."

Table 18.1 *Wang et al's*[Δ] *nomogram for peripheral corneal incisions combined with cataract incision (Temporal 3.2–3.5 mm clear corneal incision)*

Preop astigmatism (D)	*Age (Y)*	*Number*	*Length (degrees)*
WTR*			
0.75–1.00 D	< 65	2	45
	≥ 65	1	45
1.0–1.50 D	< 65	2	60
	≥ 65	2	45 (or 1 × 60)
>1.50 D	< 65	2	80
	≥ 65	2	60
ATR/oblique*			
1.00–1.25 D#	—	1	35
1.26–2.00 D	—	2	45
> 2.0 D	—	2	45

(1 mm incision = 10° of arc and 1 o'clock incision = 30° of arc = 3 mm)

ΔWang L, Misra M, Koch DD. Peripheral corneal incisions combined with cataract surgey. J Cataract and Refractive Surgery

* WTR = with the-rule; ATR = against-the-rule

#especially if cataract incision is not directly centred on steep meridian.

Table 18.2 *Gill's nomogram*

Amount of astigmatism	*Number of incisions*	*Length of incisions*
1 D	1	6
2 D	2	6
3 D	2	7
4 D	2	8
> 4 D	2	10

Table 18.3 *The NAPA nomogram (Nichamin Age and Pach adjusted Intralimbal Arcuate Astigmatic Nomogram) with the rule astigmatism (10° arc = 1 mm)*

Preop Cyl (diopters)	*Paired incision in degrees of arc 50–60 yrs of age*
0.75	30
1.00	35
1.25	40
1.50	45
1.75	50
2.00	55
2.25	60
2.50	65
2.75	70
3.00	80

Against-the-rule astigmatism (10° arc = 1 mm)

Preop Cyl (diopters)	*Paired incision in degrees of arc 50–60 yrs of age*
0.75	35
1.00	40
1.25	45
1.50	50
1.75	55
2.00	60
2.25	65
2.50	70
2.75	75
3.00	80

For every change in curvature in one meridian, there is equal and opposite change 90° away". This phenomenon of corneal behaviour is known as coupling effect. Corneal room coupling is ratio of magnitude of corneal flattening or steepening in the axis of surgery divided by magnitude of flattening or steepening 90° away. LRIs have a coupling of ratio of 1, i.e. they result in one-to-one steepening-flattening effect. Because of the coupling effect, LRIs do not influence the IOL power and thus there is no need to change the IOL power when giving LRIs.

Table 18.4 *Donnenfeld nomogram (1 clock hour = 30 degrees)*

Preoperative astigmatism	*Number of incisions**	*Length of incisions, clock hours#*
0.50 D	1	1.5
0.75 D	2	1
1.50 D	2	2
300 D#	2	3

* All incisions are placed from the limbus in correct axis

\# Patients who have against-the-rule astigmatism or who are less than 45 years old may benefit from slightly longer incisions. Shorter incisions may be indicated for patients older than 65 years.

Note. Longer incisions might induce the RK effect, and there may be a need to increase the IOL power in order to achieve a good spherical effect.

Steps for performing LRIs

Following systematic approach is useful for effectively performing LRIs.

1. *Determination of pre-existing astigmatism*

Determination of pre-existing astigmatism is the important first step. Unfortunately, preoperative measurements—keratometry, refraction and topography—do not always agree. Lenticular astigmatism may account for some disparity. Only corneal astigmatism should be corrected. It has been reported that *preoperative corneal topography* gives compatively accurate measurement of the amount and axis of the astigmatism and also helps to rule out conditions like mild keratoconus and pellucid degeneration.

In the operating room, the topography map should be placed in front of the surgeon in such a way that its orientation should coincide with that of the patient's eye in surface position. The surgeon should triple check the orientation of incision. The worst common mistake is to place the incisions on the flat meridian, i.e. 90° away from the correct orientation.

2. Plan of surgery

Plan of surgery is most important and should include the following:

Nomogram should be chosen, once the amount of astigmatism to be corrected has been determined. Always choose a nomogram that includes *age as a variable* in addition to the amount of astigmatism. Age has a large impact on the cornea's response to incisions: An 80-year-old responds twice as much as a 40-year-old to the same incision.

Cataract incision induced astigmatism should be exactly known to the surgeon and this should be factored in the surgical plan.

Paired incision should be planned to optimize symmetric corneal flattening.

Express incision in degrees of arc rather than millimetres, since corneal diameter may significantly impact the relative length of the arcuate incision and its resultant effect.

Plan of placement *of LRIs* may be as below:

- *Negligible pre-existing astigmatism:* Single plane temporal phacoincision alone may be emoployed.
- *Against-the-rule astigmatism:* Along with temporal phacoincision either single (nasal) or double (nasal and temporal) LRIs may be planned depending upon the degree of PEA. The temporal LRI, when required, the cataract incision should be created within it.
- *With-the-rule astigmatism.* Some surgeons prefer a superior cataract incision alone, or with single LRI (superior or inferior) or double LRIs (superior and inferior), depending upon the amount of WTR astigmatism. However, the superior cataract incision drifts against the wound more than the temporal incision. Therefore, many surgeons prefer a temporal cataract incision 3.5 mm or less in size and apply LRIs over the steep vertical axis.

3. Surgical technique of LRIs

Surgical technique of LRIs includes the following essential steps:

Identification and marking of the axis. Proper centration of the LRI over the steep meridian (plus cylinder axis) is the final key to success and this step starts with a reliable orientation mark. Before beginning the case, i.e. even before anaesthesia, it is advisable to place orientation marks with a surgical marking pen while the patient is upright (Fig. 18.11). Most surgeons do well with marks at 3 and 9 o'clock positions. Vertical marks at the 6 and 12 o'clock positions pose difficulty in many patients due to coverage of limbus by the lids. Some surgeons prefer to use multiple radial lines with markers, e.g. by a modified four-ray marker made by Master Precision Inc. It does not require ink for marking.

The steep meridian during placing the LRIs may be identified by aligning a Mendez ring (Fig. 18.12) or similar degree gauge with the previously placed limbal orientation marks. Alternatively, a simple hand-held device such as the Maloney works well.

Making the LR incisions. Intraoperatively, the LRIs should preferably *be created prior to cataract surgery* incision on a dry cornea. If the cataract incision is placed first, the subsequent LRIs may intersect and cause major problems with the wound sealing. The LRIs should be approximately 90% corneal depth and should be placed at the most peripheral extent of clear

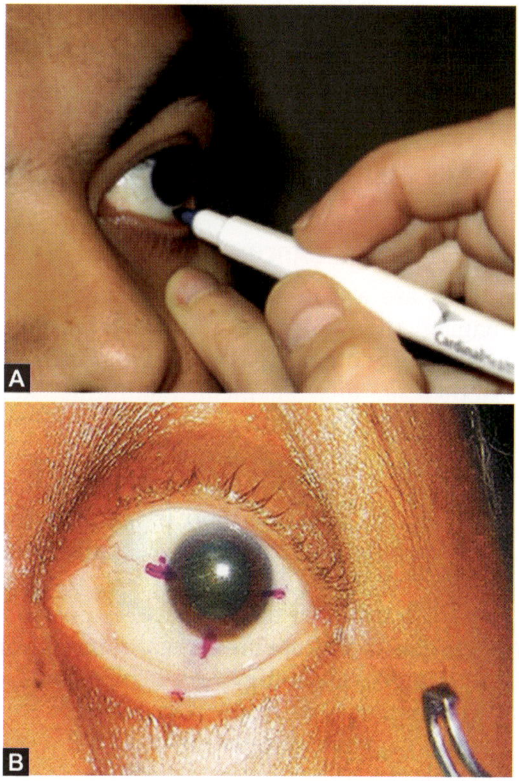

Fig. 18.11. *Marking the axis of astigmatism in sitting position.*

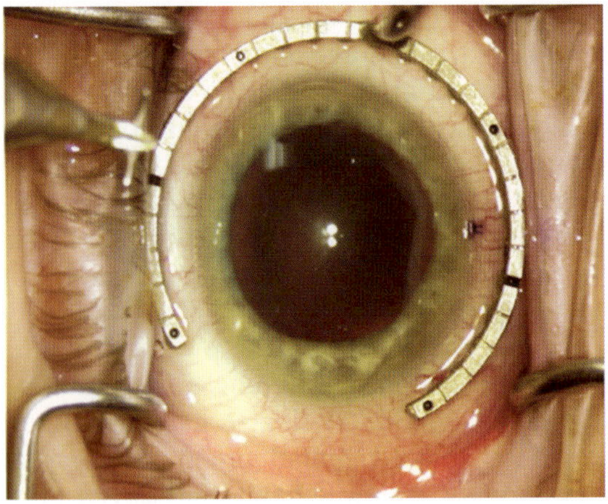

Fig. 18.12. *Marking the axis of astigmatism in supine position using Mendez ring.*

corneal tisuue, just inside the true surgical limbus. If the main cataract incision coincides with the LRI, it should be created within the LRI and when the LRI coincides with the paracentesis the later should be placed just central to the location of LRI.

It is advisable to use a diamond knife preset at 550 or 600 µm for making LRIs, but this setting potentially increases the risk of perforation, if there is peripheral thinning of cornea. It is important to hold the knife perpendicular to the corneal surface in order to achieve a consistent depth and effect to avoid gaping the incision.

POTENTIAL COMPLICATIONS OF LRIs

The LRIs are a safe and effective method of managing astigmatism as compared to more central placed corneal relaxing incisions (CRIs). Nonetheless, any surgical technique has potential complications. A few reported complications are listed below:

- *Placement of incision on the wrong axis,* i.e. at 90° upon the opposite flat meridians is the most common error reported. This error almost doubles the pre-existing astigmatism.
- *Corneal perforation,* though rare, is possible either due to peripheral corneal thinning or due to improper setting of depth of the blade.
- Misalignment/axis shift
- Wound gape and discomfort
- Infection
- Decreased corneal sensations
- Weakening of the globe
- Induced irregular astigmatism

OPPOSITE CLEAR CORNEAL INCISION

Opposite clear corneal incision (OCCI) refers to an identical penetrating CCI placed opposite, i.e. at 180° to the main cataract incision on steep axis. The OCCI enhances the flattening effect of on-axis cataract incision.

Manipulation of paired CCIs for correcting variable amount of PEA

The paired opposite CCIs are placed on the steepest meridian axis to flatten it. One CCI is used to perform cataract surgery and OCCI is made to enhance the flattening effect.

It is possible to correct up to 4 D of PEA with this method by simple manipulation of the *incision characteristics* as below:

- *Size of incision.* Larger the incision, more the flattening effect.
- *Location of incision.* Farther the incision from the centre of cornea, lesser is flattening.
- *Type of incision,* i.e. unipolar/bipolar/tripolar/hinged (Fig. 18.13). As one progresses from unipolar to hinged incision, the amount of astigmatism corrected can be doubled.
- *Direction of incision.* Superior incision gives more correction than the superonasal and temporal incisions.

Nomograms for CCI

The nomogram which can be used as a guideline for giving CCIs is shown in Table 18.5.

Advantages and disadvantages of CCI

Advantages of CCI

- *No special training and instruments* are required, as all surgeons are familiar with the creation of cataract incision.
- *Stability of cornea,* which is achieved in 2 weeks' time, is the biggest advantage of this technique. Therefore, postoperatively there are minimum fluctuations in vision and there is minimal regression.
- *No change in IOL power (calculated)* is required due to the *coupling effect,* that for every change in curvature in one meridian there is an equal and opposite change 90° away (Gauss's law

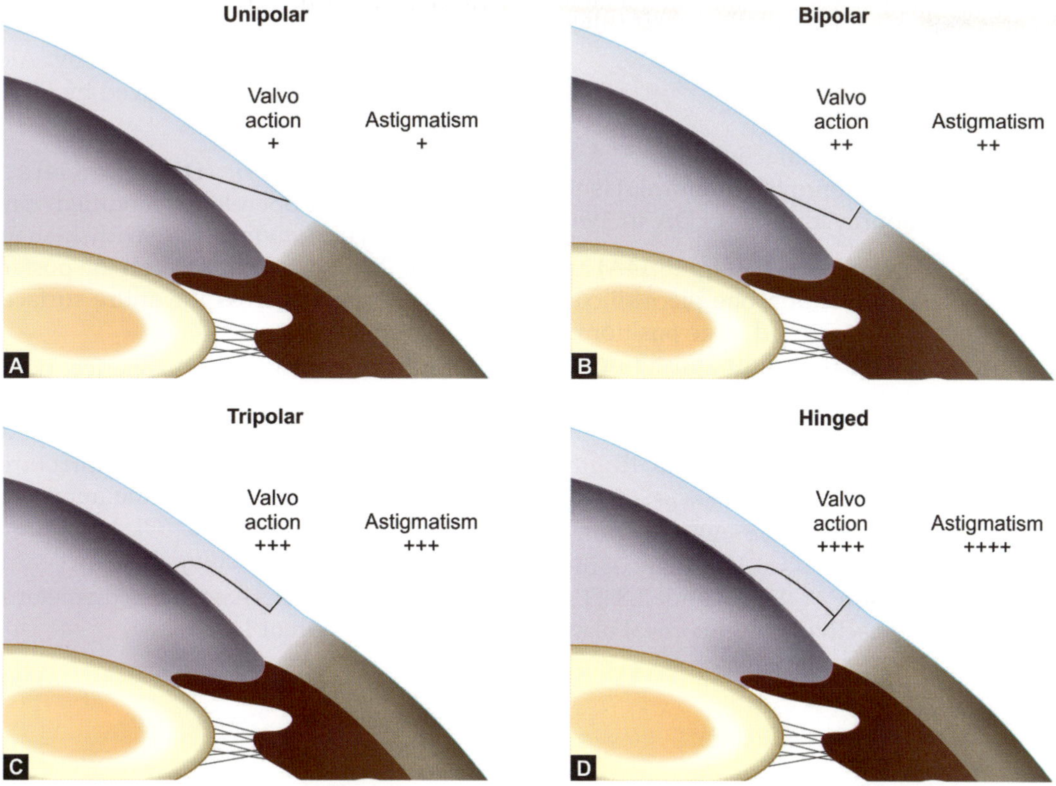

Fig. 18.13. *Types of clear corneal incisions: **(A)** Uniplanar; **(B)** Biplanar; **(C)** Triplanar; **(D)** Hinged triplanar.*

Table 18.5 *Lal et al.'s nomogram for CCI**

Type of incision	*Amount of astigmatism corrected*
Single steep axis, 3.2 mm	<0.5 D
OCCI (uniplanar) and 3.2 mm cataract incision	0.5–1 D
OCCI (biplanar, triplanar, hinged) and 3.2 mm incision	1–1.5 D
OCCI (biplanar, triplanar, hinged) and 3.2 mm incision	1.5–2 D (if incision placed superiorly)
OCCI (biplanar, triplanar, hinged) 4.0 mm incision	1.5–2 D (if incision placed temporally)
OCCI (biplanar, triplanar, hinged) 4.5 mm incision	2.0–2.5 D
OCCI (biplanar, triplanar, hinged) 5.0 mm incision	2.5–3.0 D
OCCI (biplanar, triplanar, hinged) 5.5 mm incision	3.0–4.0 D

*North Zone Journal of Ophthalmology, Vol 17. No. 1, June 2010, p. 26–31.

of elastic domes). This flattening produced by CCI is associated with steepening of the axis at 90°. Because of this, spherical equivalent is unchanged.

Disadvantages of CCI include:

- *Limited amount* of correction produced.
- *Large wounds* made to correct astigmatism may be leaky and not self-sealing, and thus may even require sutures. Once the sutures are removed or dissolve, the amount of astigmatism may change.
- *Technically awkward location* of the wound may be required, depending upon the meridian of steeper axis.

TORIC INTRAOCULAR LENSES FOR CONTROL OF ASTIGMATISM DURING CATARACT SURGERY

PRESENTLY AVAILABLE TORIC INTRAOCULAR LENSES

The toric IOLs, designed to correct astigmatism were first introduced in 1994 by Shimizu et al.

presently available toric IOLs and their salient features are as below.

STAAR toric IOL

STAAR Toric IOL (manufactured by STAAR Surgical company, Monrovia, California) is the first toric IOL approved by the FDA in 1998.

Features of STAAR toric IOL (Fig. 18.14A) are:

- *Design.* It is a plate haptic, one-piece silicone lens with an axis mark and large positioning holes on each plate that allows posterior and anterior capsules to fuse within the hole, reducing rotation of the lens.
- *Length.* Available in 10.8 and 11.2 mm lengths.
- *Power.* It is available in a full range of spherical powers but with only two cylinder power options: 2.0 D and 3.5 D at IOL plane which achieve reduction of 1.4 D and 2.3 D of astigmatism respectively at the corneal plane.

AcrySof toric IOL

AcrySof toric IOL (manufactured by Alcon Laboratories, Texas) was approved by FDA in September 2005.

Features of acrySof toric IOL (Fig. 18.14B) are:

- *Design.* It is an open-loop, modified, single piece, acrylic polymer IOL with L-shaped haptics. Toric power, placed on the posterior surface, extends across the entire surface of the spherical optic.
- *Power.* It is available in all spherical powers from 0 D to 30 D with 7 cylinder power options as 7 models. Table 18.6 depicts the 7 models of the IOLs along with the manufacturer's information for selection of the appropriate model and power of toric IOL based on the pre-existing corneal astigmatism.
- *Dimensions.* The lens has a 6 mm diameter and an overall length of 13.0 mm.

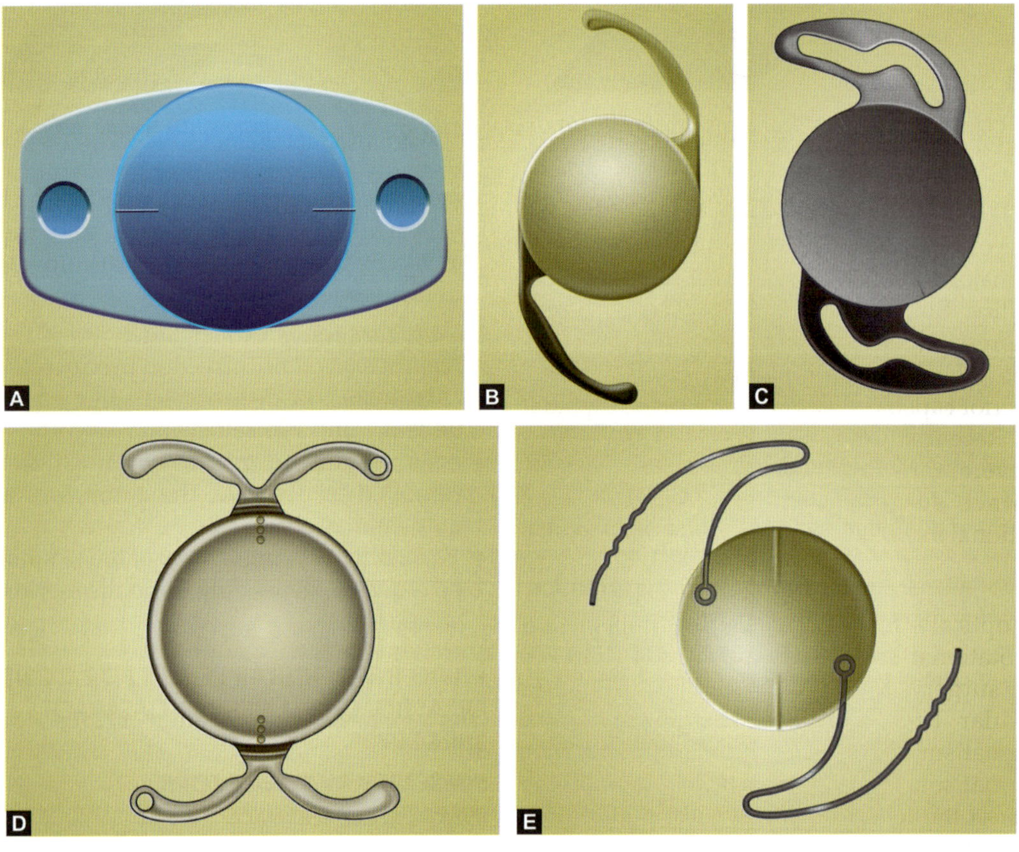

Fig. 18.14. *Toric IOLs:* ***(A)*** *STAAR toric IOL;* ***(B)*** *AcrySof toric IOL;* ***(C)*** *Raynor toric IOL,* ***(D)*** *Ankosis toric IOL;* ***(E)*** *Leis toric IOL.*

Table 18.6 *Acrysof toric IOL: models, power and selection based on the pre-existing corneal astigmatism*

Toric IOL model	*Power (diopters)*		*Range of pre-existing astigmatism*
	At IOL plane	*At corneal plane*	
SN60T3	1.50	1.03	0.75 D–1.50 D
SN60T4	2.25	1.55	1.50 D–2.25 D
SN60T5	3.00	2.06	2.25 D–3.00 D
SN60T6	3.75	2.57	3.00 D–3.75 D
SN60T7	4.50	3.08	3.75 D–4.50 D
SN60T8	5.25	3.60	4.50 D–5.25 D
SN60T9	6.00	4.11	5.25 D–6.00 D

- *Lens stability and lack of rotation* are crucial for the effectiveness of toric IOL. Its biomaterial adheres to the capsular bag using a single layer of lens epithelial cells. As a result, there is a lack of space for nutrients to pass, which leads to cell death. The lens then adheres directly to the lens capsule, which also minimizes the lens rotation.

Other toric IOLs

Some other toric IOLs available include Raynor toric IOL (Fig. 18.14C), Ankosis toric IOL (Fig. 18.14D) and Leis toric IOL (Fig. 18.14E).

TORIC IOLs: SOME PERSPECTIVES

Toric IOL–rotational stability

The major requirement for toric IOL is rotational stability. Rotation is mainly caused by haptic compression resulting from capsule contraction. Until IOLs form a bioadhesive bond with the posterior capsule, they can rotate in the capsular bag. Recent studies have analyzed the results of several toric IOL models' implantation after cataract surgery and have shown good rotational stability and good functional results.

Optical effect of the toric IOLs

The optical effect of the toric IOL depends on its rotational stability in the capsular bag. If, after surgery, the toric IOL rotates 30° in the capsular bag, there will be an increased astigmatism compared with the preoperative astigmatism. If the toric IOL rotates 15°, the effect of the IOL will be halved. If the rotation is 10°, one-third of the toric effect of the IOL will be lost. If a toric IOL that fully corrects the astigmatism is rotated by as little as 3°, there will be a 10% loss in the compensatory antiastigmatic effect. Additionally, because axial alignment of a toric IOL determines the efficacy of astigmatic correction, accurate surgical placement is important.

Optical and visual quality with toric IOL

Mendicute et al. in a study of toric intraocular lens versus opposite clear corneal incisions to correct astigmatism in eyes having cataract surgery compared higher order aberrations in both groups. No statistically significant differences were found between the toric IOL group and OCCI group in spherical aberration, coma-like aberration or higher order corneal or ocular aberrations. In the same study, contrast sensitivity in both groups was also studied and found that under photopic and mesopic conditions performance was similar between groups. At 18 cycles per degree (cpd), log10 CS was significantly better in the toric IOL group.

Toric IOL versus opposite clear corneal incision

Toric IOL implantation has been reported to achieved a slight enhanced effect over opposite clear corneal incisions in treating pre-existing astigmatism. Toric IOL implantation has advantages over corneal procedures including the potential to decrease induced irregular astigmatism from corneal manipulation and to provide the option of irreversibility.

POSTOPERATIVE CORNEAL LASER ABLATION PROCEDURES

Postoperative corneal laser ablation procedures such as phacorefractive keratomy (PRK), and LASIK are very useful in correcting the residual astigmatism in pseudophakic patients.

MANAGEMENT OF ASTIGMATISM IN SICS

Though phacoemulsification is presently the ideal cataract surgery, but is still beyond the reach of majority of patients from developing countries. Manual small incision cataract surgery (SICS) is, therefore, being practised abundantly and has emerged as a useful alternative to phacoemulsification. The uncorrected visual acuity (UCVA) can be markedly improved by becoming astigmatism conscious during SICS.

BASIC PRINCIPLES AND MODALITIES

Basic principles of managing astigmatism are similar to phacoemulsification technique (*see* page 322).

Modalities for control of astigmatism in SICS are similar to that for phacoemulsification and include:

- *Cataract incision* on the steep axis.
- *Relaxing incisions* such as corneal relaxing incisions (CRI), limbal relaxing incisions (LRIs) and opposite clear corneal incisions (OCCI) (For details *see* pages 322–327).
- *Toric IOL,* is usually not considered an option in SICS, because of financial reasons and comparatively unpredicted surgically induced astigmatism in SICS.
- *Postoperative corneal laser ablation procedures* to manage pseudophakic astigmatism include PRK and LASIK.

CATARACT INCISION AND OCCI: PROTOCOLS FOR MANAGEMENT OF ASTIGMATISM IN SICS

Based on the pre-existing astigmatism (PEA) and expected surgically induced astigmatism (SIA), the author has evolved a standard protocol (unpublished data), which provides a reasonably good control of astigmatism in SICS. The protocol is as below:

A. Nil pre-existing astigmatism

1. ***Cataract incision*** in patients with nil pre-existing astigmatism may be either temporal or superior.
   - *A 6 mm corneoscleral* tunnel incision on an average produces SIA varying from 1.25 to 1.75 D.
   - *Superior incision* will induce against-the-rule astigmatism (ATR).
   - *Temporal incision* will induce with-the-rule astigmatism (WTR).
2. ***Opposite clear corneal incisions (OCCIs)*** are preferred as relaxing incisions to neutralise the SIA as given:
   - *On horizontal axis,* two OCCIs (temporal and nasal) of 3 mm each are made when cataract incision is made superiorly (Fig. 18.15A).
   - *On vertical axis,* two OCCIs (superior and inferior) of 2 mm each are made when cataract incision is made temporally (Fig. 18.15B).

B. Against-the-rule pre-existing astigmatism

1. ***Temporal cataract incision*** of 6 mm is given in all patients with PEA up to 2 D.
2. ***OCCIs*** are made depending upon the amount of pre-existing ATR astigmatism as below:
   - *For 0 to 0.5 D of PEA,* a 2 mm clear corneal incision (CCI) is made on vertical axis (superiorly in left eye and inferiorly in right eye) (Fig. 18.16A).
   - *For 0.5 to 1.25 D of PEA,* no CCI is made (Fig. 18.16B).

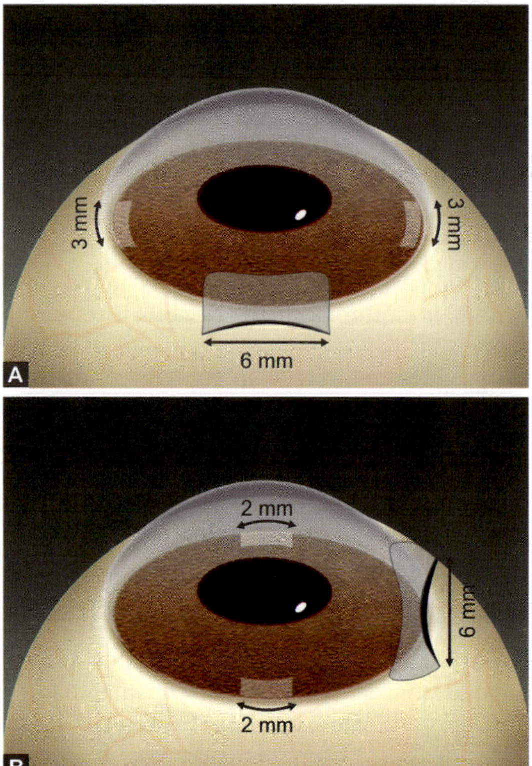

Fig. 18.15. *Sclerocorneal tunnel (SCT) cataract incision and OCCI for managing final astigmatism after SICS in patients with nil pre-existing astigmatism: **(A)** OCCIs on horizontal axis with superior cataract incision; **(B)** OCCIs on vertical axis with temporal cataract incision.*

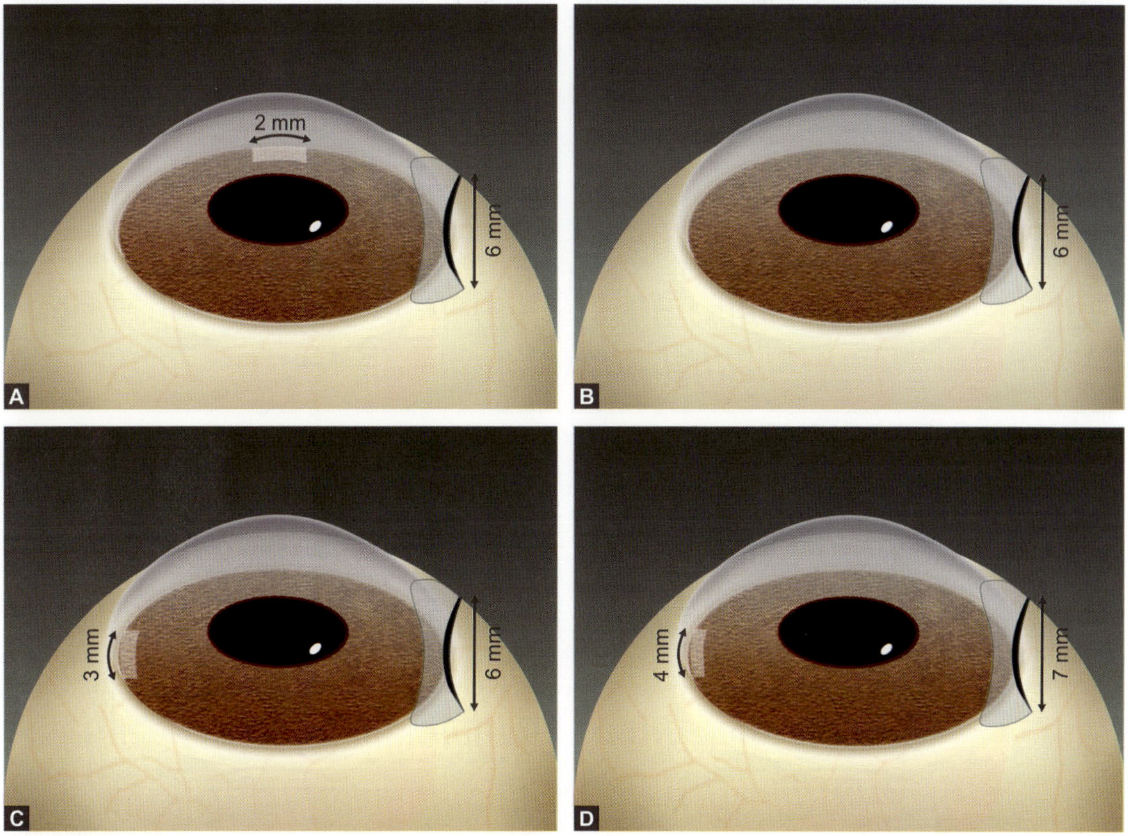

Fig. 18.16. *Sclerocorneal tunnel (SCT), cataract incision and OCCI for managing final astigmatism after SICS in patients with against-the-rule (ATR) pre-existing astigmatism (PEA):* ***(A)*** *For 0.5 DPEA;* ***(B)*** *For 0.5–1.25D PEA;* ***(C)*** *For 1.25–2 D PEA; and* ***(D)*** *For >2 D PEA (for explanation see text).*

- *For 1.25 to 2 D of PEA,* a 3 mm OCCI is made nasally on the horizontal axis (Fig. 18.16C).
- *For >2 D of PEA,* the cataract incision of 7 mm temporally and 4 mm OCCI is made nasally on the horizontal axis (Fig. 18.16D).

C. With-the-rule pre-existing astigmatism

1. ***Superior cataract incision*** of 6 mm is made in all patients with PEA of up to 2 D.

2. ***Clear corneal incisions (CCIs)*** are made depending upon the amount of PEA as below:

- *For 0 to 0.75 D of WTR PEA,* a 3 mm CCI is made temporally (horizontal axis) (Fig. 18.17A).
- *For 0.75 to 1.5 D of WTR PEA,* no CCI is required (Fig. 18.17B).
- *For 1.5 to 2 D, of WTR PEA,* an OCCI of 3 mm is made inferiorly (Fig. 18.17C).
- *For > 2 D, of WTR PEA,* a 7 mm cataract incision is made superiorly and OCCI of 4 mm is made inferiorly (Fig. 18.17D).

BIBLIOGRAPHY

1. Carvalho MJ, Suzuki SH, Freitas LL, et al. Limbal relaxing incisions to correct corneal astigmatism during phacoemulsification. J Refract Surg 23:499–504,2007.
2. Eydelman MB, Drum B, Holladay J, Hilmantel G, Kezirian G, Durrie D, Stulting RD, Sanders D, Wong B. Standardized analyses of correction of astigmatism by laser systems that reshape the cornea. J Refract Surg. 22(1):81–95,2006 Jan-Feb.
3. Frranks JB, Binder PS: Keratotomy procedure for the correction of astigmatism. J. Refract Surg 1:11–17,1985.
4. Holladay JT, Dudeja DR, Koch DD. Evaluating and reporting astigmatism for individual and

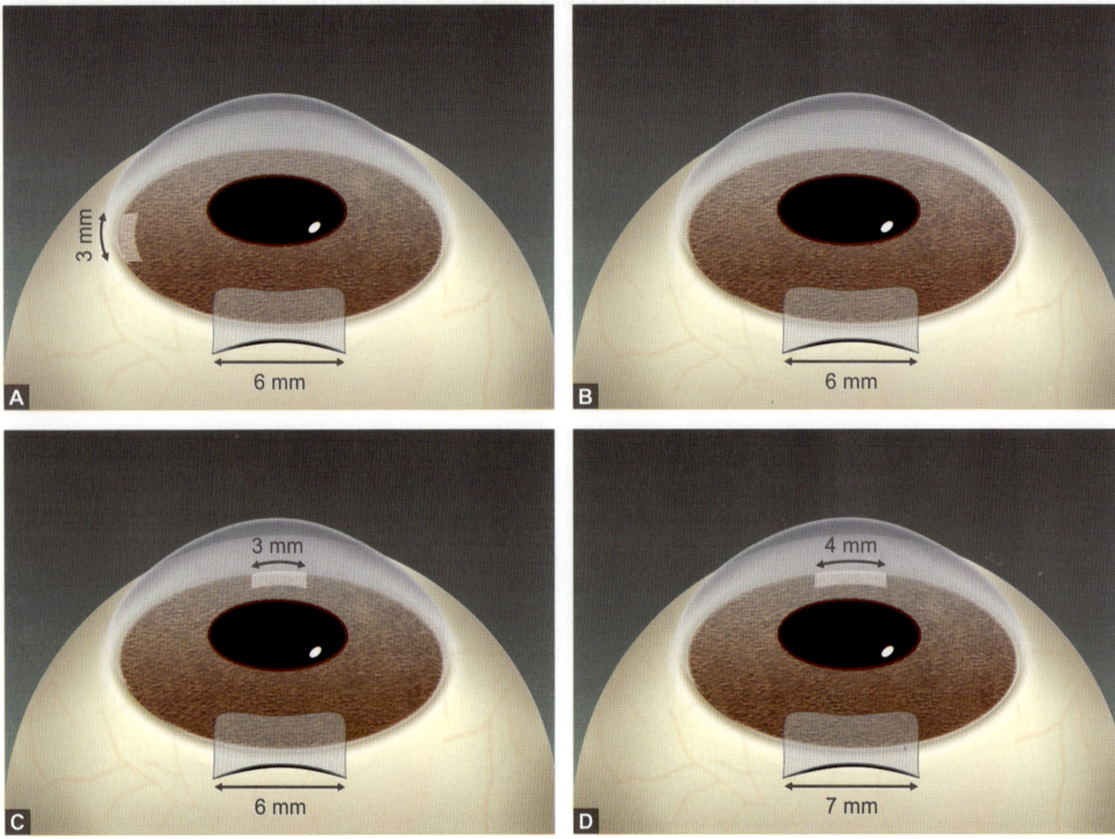

Fig. 18.17. *Sclerocorneal tunnel (SCT), cataract incision and OCCI for managing final astigmatism after SICS in patients having with-the-rule (WTR) pre-existing astigmatism (PEA):* ***(A)*** *For up to 0.75 D PEA;* ***(B)*** *For 0.75–1.5 D PEA;* ***(C)*** *For 1.5–2 D PEA; and* ***(D)*** *For >2 D, PEA (for explanation see text).*

aggregate data. J Cataract Refract Surg 24(1):57–65,1998 Jan.

5. Holladay JT, Moran JR, Kezirian GM. Analysis of aggregate surgically induced refractive change, prediction error, and intraocular astigmatism. J Cataract Refract Surg 27(1):61–79,2001 Jan.
6. Koch DD, Lindstrom RL: Controlling astigmatism in cataract surgery Semin Ophthalmol 7:214–223, 1992.
7. Muller-Jensen K, Fischer P, Siepe U: Limbal relaxing incisions to correct astigmatism in clear corneal cataract surgery. J Refract Surg 15:506–509,1999.
8. Sawhney S. Theoretical validity of vector analysis for aggregate astigmatic data. J Cataract Refract Surg 28(3):385–386,2002 Mar.
9. Shepherd JR: Induced astigmatism in small incision surgery. J Cataract Refract Surg 15:85–88,1989.
10. Shimizu K, Misawa A, Suzauki Y. Toric intraocular lenses: Correcting astigmatism while controlling axis shift. J Cataract Refract Surg 20:523–526,1994.
11. Wang L, Missa M, Koch DD. Peripheral corneal relaxing incisions combined with cataract surgery. J Cataract refract Surg 29:712–722,2003.

INTRAOCULAR LENS IMPLANTATION IN THE ABSENCE OF POSTERIOR CAPSULAR SUPPORT

CHAPTER 19

GENERAL CONSIDERATIONS

Implantation of an intraocular lens (IOL) in the capsular bag is the most ideal choice available at present following successful cataract extraction with intact capsulorhexis. In the absence of intact capsular bag, but sufficient posterior capsule, the option is implantation in the ciliary sulcus. However, inspite of best efforts, many a times posterior capsular support is not available for implantation of posterior chamber IOL in the bag or even in the ciliary sulcus. Such a situation comprises aphakia without capsular support.

IOL implantation in aphakia without capsular support

Primary IOL implantation in the absence of posterior capsular support is required in cases with:

- Large posterior capsular tear in the absence of intact anterior capsulorhexis.
- Accidental intracapsular cataract extraction.
- Accidental aspiration of the whole capsular bag.
- After explantation of markedly subluxated in-the-bag IOL.
- Zonular dehiscence of more than 3/4th area following trauma or due to other causes such as Marfan's syndrome.
- IOL exchange in patients with pseudophakic bullous keratopathy with ACIOL.

Secondary IOL implantation for the pre-existing aphakia without posterior capsule is required in following cases:

- Planned intracapsular cataract extraction (in the past)
- Accidental intracapsular cataract extraction (in the past)
- Posterior dislocation of IOL-capsule complex
- Posterior dislocation of the crystalline lens.

Options available

Options available for primary or secondary IOL implantation in the absence of posterior capsular support include:

Anterior chamber IOLs
- Angle-supported ACIOLs
- Iris-supported ACIOLs

Posterior chamber IOLs
- Iris-fixated PCIOLs
  - Retroiris-fixated PCIOLs
  - Sutureless iris-fixated Binderflex PCIOLs
- Transscleral-fixated PCIOLs
  - Transscleral suture-fixated PCIOLs
  - Sutureless transscleral-fixated PCIOLs

ANTERIOR CHAMBER IOLs

ANGLE-SUPPORTED ANTERIOR CHAMBER (AC) IOLs

The angle-supported ACIOLs in use are modern 4-point fixation flexible open-loop type (e.g. Kelman-multiflex, Fig. 19.1).

Technique

Technique of implantation of angle-supported ACIOLs is described on page 188, Fig. 13.1. Salient points of the technique are as below:

1. *Anterior vitrectomy* is performed to thoroughly clear the vitreous from the anterior chamber either by pars plana approach or limbal approach.
2. *Pupil is constricted* with the help of preservative free intracameral pilocarpine or acetylcholine.
3. *Peripheral iridectomy,* one or two are performed with the help of vitrector or Vanas scissors to avoid pupillary block.

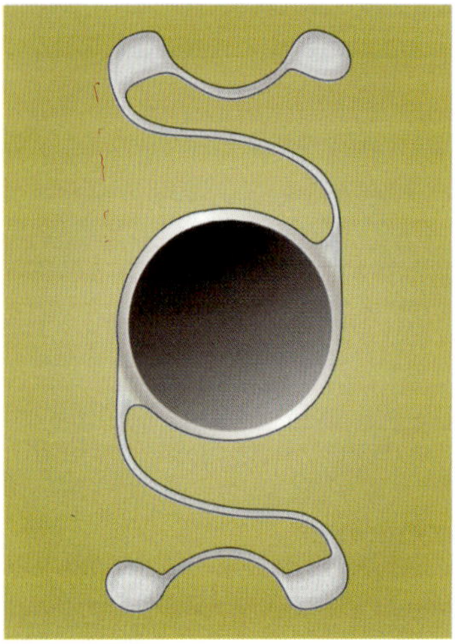

Fig. 19.1. *Kelman multiflex angle-supported ACIOL.*

4. *Viscoelastic material* is injected to stabilize the anterior chamber and to protect the endothelium
5. *Valvular sclerocorneal incision* of 5.5 mm size is made superiorly when secondary IOL implantation is being done or the phaco-incision is enlarged with 5.5 mm keratome in cases with primary IOL implantation during complicated phaco surgery.
6. *Lens glide* may be inserted across the anterior chamber into the distal angle. However, the use of lens glide is not must.
7. *IOL is inserted* in the anterior chamber by pushing the leading haptic into the distal angle. The lens glide when placed will protect the iris from the advancing IOL haptic. At this juncture, the lens glide is removed and the trailing haptic is flexed and gently pushed after retracting the posterior lip of the incision.
8. *Removal of OVD* is done by aspirating it and the anterior chamber is maintained with BSS.
9. *Incision* is checked for valvular stability. If required 10-0 nylon suture may be applied for wound stability.

Advantages

- ACIOLs are easy to implant.
- In an older patient with no history of glaucoma who had a normal anterior segment with a healthy endothelium, an ACIOL might be best.
- These are useful in those with bleeding disorders or severe conjunctival scarring who would benefit from minimal uveal manipulation and conjunctival dissection.

Limitations

- Shallow anterior chamber
- Structural abnormality of anterior chamber or angle
- Decompensated cornea

Features of modern day ACIOLs

1. *Vaulting.* In contrast to a closed-loop anterior chamber IOL, the vault engineered into a well-designed open-loop lens is maintained even under high compression. This minimizes IOL touch against the cornea or posterior touch against the iris.
2. *Sizing* is less critical with flexible open-loop designs.

3. *Haptic* or footplate fixation elements designed by Choyce is tissue friendly; a protective fibrosis occurs around the footplate which helps minimize erosion and/or chafing.
4. *Point-fixation* is possible since haptics subtend only small areas of the angle outflow structures.
5. *Finishing.* Most present-day lenses now have an excellent finish with highly polished smooth surfaces and rounded edges. Tissue contact by any component of the IOL (optic or haptic) is much gentler with less possibility of chafing damage.
6. *Easy to remove.* Most of these open-loop IOL designs are much easier to remove, if necessary, especially those with Choyce style haptic or footplate designs. The well-polished surfaces are usually not completely surrounded by goniosynechias or "cocoon" membranes and will usually slide out without undue difficulty to excessive tissue damage.

Complications

Earlier rigid, closed-loop ACIOLs were associated with an unacceptable rate of complications:

- Irreversible endothelial loss leading to pseudophakic bullous keratopathy, intractable inflammation
- Cystoid macular oedema (CME)
- Structural change to the angle leading to glaucoma, and hyphaema.

In modern ACIOLs, the optic is anteriorly vaulted just enough to minimize IOL-iris touch and iris chafing while the flexible open-loop haptics resist increased vaulting under high compression, which prevents endothelial damage. Rounded, highly polished edges, particularly at the optic-haptic junction, minimize trauma to the iris, if the IOL inadvertently contacts the iris. The haptics are designed to provide three- or four-point fixation, instead of continuous apposition, that minimizes the area of contact with the outflow structures within the angle. Each point of fixation features a highly polished footplate that prevents erosion into the angle structures and minimizes fibrous overgrowth of the haptic.

However, even with a perfectly implanted ACIOL, *subclinical uveitis* secondary to lens-tissue contact creates inflammatory products that could be directly toxic to the endothelium and angle and could also result in CME. The rate of CME associated with ACIOL implantation has been reported at 1–10%. *Other complications* include corneal decompensation, glaucoma, retinal detachment and endophthalmitis.

IRIS-SUPPORTED ACIOLs

Out of the various iris-supported ACIOLs, *Worst iris claw lens* and its modified version (Singh's modified iris claw lens) have been widely used and are still used by some surgeons. The iris claw lens (Fig. 19.2) used presently is plano-convex lens with optic size of 4.25 mm and overall size of 7.25 mm.

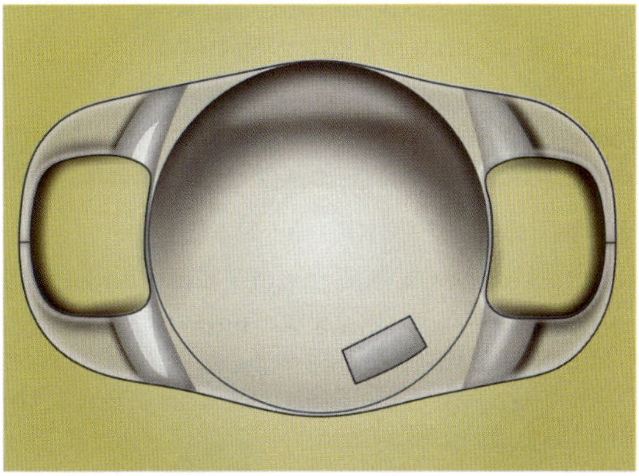

Fig. 19.2. *Iris claw lens.*

Technique

1. to 5. *Initial steps* are same as described above for angle supported ACIOL (*see* page 334).
6. *Fixation of iris claw lens.* The lens is introduced into the anterior chamber with convexity upward and fixed to the anterior surface of the iris with the claw mechanism using a lens stabilisation forceps and an enclavation needle or a forceps to tuck the iris into the claw (Fig. 19.3). A sufficient fold of iris must be tucked into the claw for it to hold securely to this iris and to prevent shacking of the lens.

Disadvantages and complications

- *Progressive loss of endothelial cells* is the major problem which has made this lens very unpopular or almost obsolete presently.

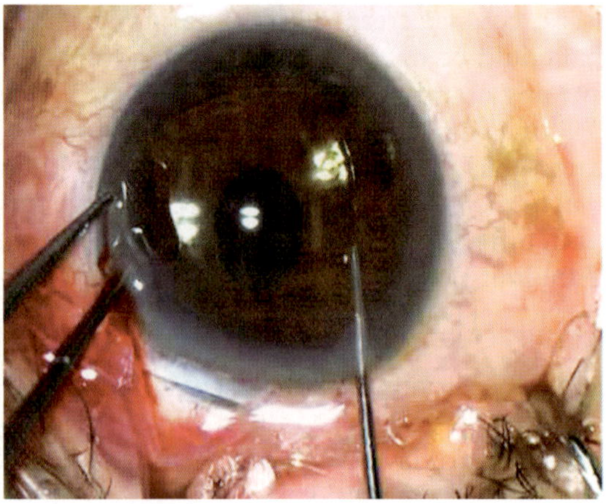

Fig. 19.3. *Technique of fixation of iris claw lens on the anterior iris surface.*

- *Other complications* are similar to angle-supported ACIOLs and include anterior uveitis, hyphaema and glaucoma.

POSTERIOR CHAMBER IOLs

ADVANTAGES OF PCIOLs OVER ACIOLs

- These lenses are closer to the anatomical position and nodal point of eye.
- They place the IOL in a position furthest from the corneal endothelium and avoid the trabecular meshwork.
- They may provide a mechanical barrier against vitreous movement or diffusion of vasoactive substances that could lead to retinal detachment or cystoid macular oedema.
- They can be put in cases of shallow anterior chamber or in cases of structural abnormality of anterior chamber.

IRIS-SUPPORTED PCIOLs

Retroiris-fixated iris claw lens

- Iris-supported PCIOL is basically retroiris fixation of the iris claw lens and is nowadays the preferred method of fixation of iris claw lens.
- Retroiris fixation markedly decreases the endothelial cell loss associated with fixation on the anterior surface of iris.
- IOL power for retrofixation is +1 D more than for the anterior fixation.

Technique

1 to 5 *initial steps* are similar to implantation of angle-supported ACIOL (*see* page 334).

6. *Fixation of the IOL.* Retroiris fixation is achieved with the help of specially designed right and left forceps (one for either side of the lens) and a 27 gauge cannula (3/4th of an inch long and bent at 45° in the middle) mounted on a 1 ml syringe (used for enclavation of the iris tissue into the claw mechanism) (Fig. 19.4).

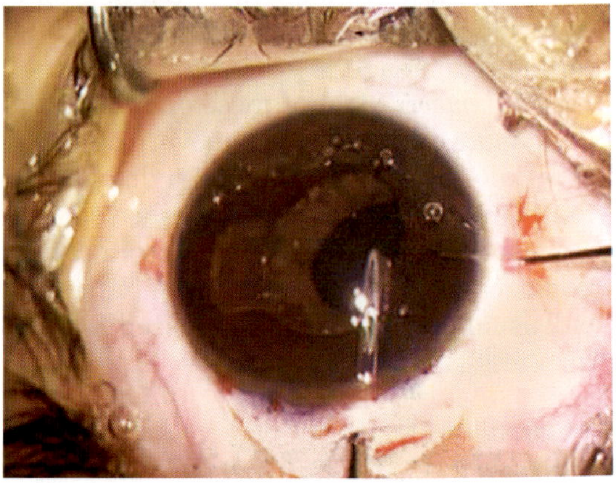

Fig. 19.4. *Technique of fixation of iris claw lens on the posterior iris surface.*

Sutureless iris-fixated Binderflex PCIOL

Features of Binderflex PCIOL

Binderflex PCIOL (named after the designer H. Binder) is a new PCIOL which can be fixed to the peripheral iris in aphakic patients. Its features are (Fig. 19.5):

- Optic diameter is 6 mm.
- Overall diameter is 15 mm.
- Haptics are long, C-shaped, and only 0.4 mm thick (very flexible) with 12° angulation from the optic plane.
- T-shaped anchor is mounted at each end of the haptic.
- PMMA (non-foldable) as well as foldable (hydrophilic acrylic) models of Binderflex lens are available.

Technique

1 to 5 *initial steps* are similar to as described on page 334.

6. *Paracentesis,* two in number at 3 and 9 o'clock, are made in the peripheral cornea with the help of 15° MVR blade.

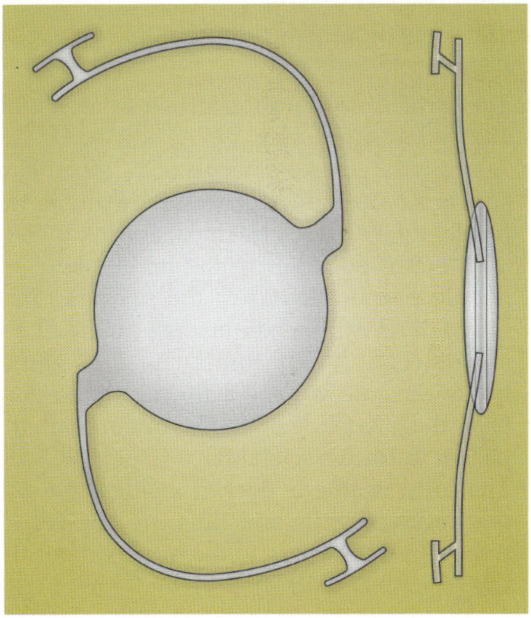

Fig. 19.5. *Binderflex PCIOL.*

7. ***Sclerocorneal*** *(6 mm for non-foldable lens)* ***or clear corneal tunnel incision*** (4 mm for foldable lens) is made superiorly.

8. ***Iridotomies,*** two in number at 3 and 9 o'clock are made in dry modes with the vitrectomy machine, using smallest diameter.

9. ***Implantation of Binderflex IOL.*** After filling the AC with viscoelastic material, the Binderflex lens (available in pre-folded cartridge) is held in folded form with forceps and is inserted into the AC through the tunnel incision one haptic with anchor is allowed to go behind the iris towards periphery and the IOL is allowed to get unfolded in the AC. The IOL is then rotated towards 3 and 9 o'clock positions. Then holding the optic securely the second haptic is also allowed to go behind the iris. At this juncture, a haptic forceps is used through the paracentesis or tunnel incision to grasp and position the haptic ends (anchors) through the iridotomies. After both anchors are securely placed in the iridotomies, the optic of IOL is exactly centred (Fig. 19.6).

10. ***Removal of OVD*** is done by aspirating it and the anterior chamber is maintained with BSS.

Advantages of Binder's lens

- Sutureless technique
- Stable and well-centred IOL. Stability is provided by following three features of Binder's lens:
  - Long C-haptics which abut in the sulcus
  - Necks of the anchors which extend through iridotomies
  - Head (T) of anchor which lie on the anterior surface of iris.
- Well-known optical properties of standard PCIOL implanted in the sulcus.

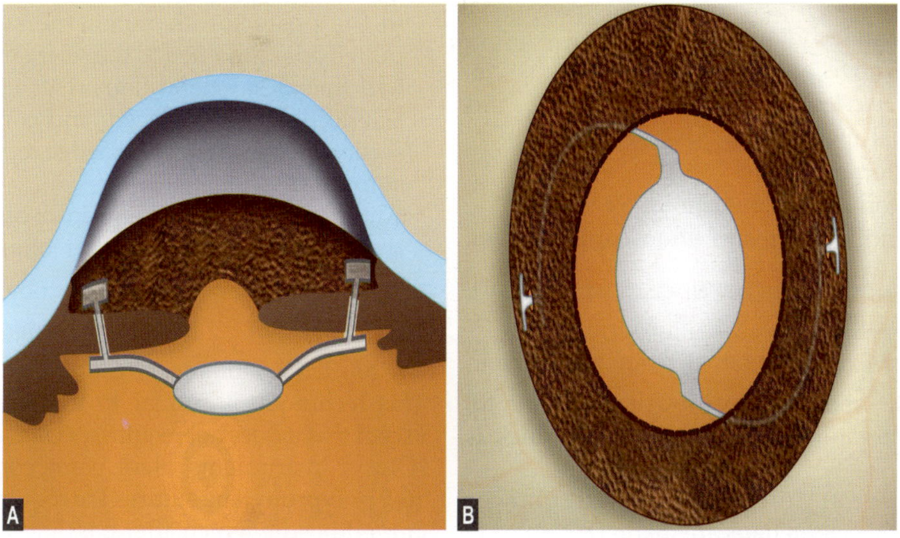

Fig. 19.6. *Diagrammatic depiction of fixation of Binderflex PCIOLs seen in:* ***(A)*** *Cut section;* ***(B)*** *Anterior view.*

- Technique is simple and less cumbersome than the scleral suture fixation.

TRANS-SCLERAL-FIXATED PCIOLs

A. TRANS-SCLERAL SUTURE FIXATION OF PCIOLs

Since the introduction of trans-scleral suture fixation of PCIOL by Malbran (1986), several techniques have been described. Variations in the techniques of several trans-scleral suture fixation of PCIOL include:

- *Ab interno versus ab externo* suturing technique. The former is technically easier, whereas the latter facilitates the increased accuracy of suture placement.
- *Variations in the method of securing the haptic with fixation suture* and the number of points of PCIOL fixation. It can be two point or four point fixation. Four point fixation provides better stability.
- *Variations in the method to avoid erosion of suture knot* (the most significant complication in late postoperative period).

TECHNIQUES OF TRANS-SCLERAL SUTURE FIXATION OF PCIOL

Presently available techniques can be divided into two groups:

I. *Conventional (non-endoscopic) techniques,* which include:

- Ab interno techniques
- Ab externo techniques.

II. *Endoscopic techniques,* which include:

1. Bimanual methods of
   - Ab externo fixation
   - Ab interno fixation techniques.
2. One hand technique of endoscopic fixation.

I. CONVENTIONAL (NON-ENDOSCOPIC) TECHNIQUES

1. Ab externo (external to internal) techniques

- Low IOP is achieved by intravenous mannitol and super pinkie ball, peribulbar block is given.
- Two partial thickness, rectangular or triangular scleral flaps are made 180° apart in horizontal meridian after the conjunctival flap dissection (Fig. 19.7A).
- The crystalline lens/IOL is removed, when present.
- The corneoscleral section is then secured with 10-0 nylon suture (Fig. 19.7A).
- A long, straight, solid needle of a 10-0 prolene suture is passed through the sclera (under the partial thickness scleral flaps) approximately 0.75–1 mm posterior to the limbus keeping needle perpendicular to the sclera so that inside the eye the needle emerges in the ciliary sulcus (Fig. 19.7B). Similarly, a 27 gauge hollow needle is passed through the sclera from the other side of the eye underneath the partial thickness scleral flaps (Fig. 19.7C).
- The solid needle is docked inside the tip of the hollow needle and thus prolene suture passes from one side to the other side of the eye (Fig. 19.7C and D).
- The suture is then pulled out of the eye with the help of a hook or McPherson's forceps from the corneoscleral section (Fig. 19.7D) and cut into two, each end of the suture is tied to the haptic of the IOL which has got eyelet near the tip of the haptic (Fig. 19.7E). Thus, in all cases, a specially designed IOL having eyelet near the tip of haptics to thread the prolene suture is used. Its optic diameter is 6.5 mm, and overall length is 13–13.5 mm. This is available in the market from Domilens (model PERLENS-2), and Aurolab (model SF 6530).
- This sutured IOL is then placed behind the iris in the posterior chamber; the sutures are pulled apart and tied to the sclera beneath the half thickness scleral flaps (Fig. 19.7F to H). Scleral flaps are replaced, and corneoscleral section is closed, the conjunctiva reposited and sutured (Fig. 19.7I).
- Anterior vitrectomy is done in all cases to clear the vitreous from anterior chamber and around the lens.

Modifications of ab externo technique

i. ***Modified technique of Shapirno and Leen.*** This technique is similar to the previous one except that it does not require specialized sutures, IOLs or instruments. Here, same conventional 10-0 polypropylene sutures are required having curved needle which after passing through the sclera is pulled out of the eye with the help of a McPherson forceps.

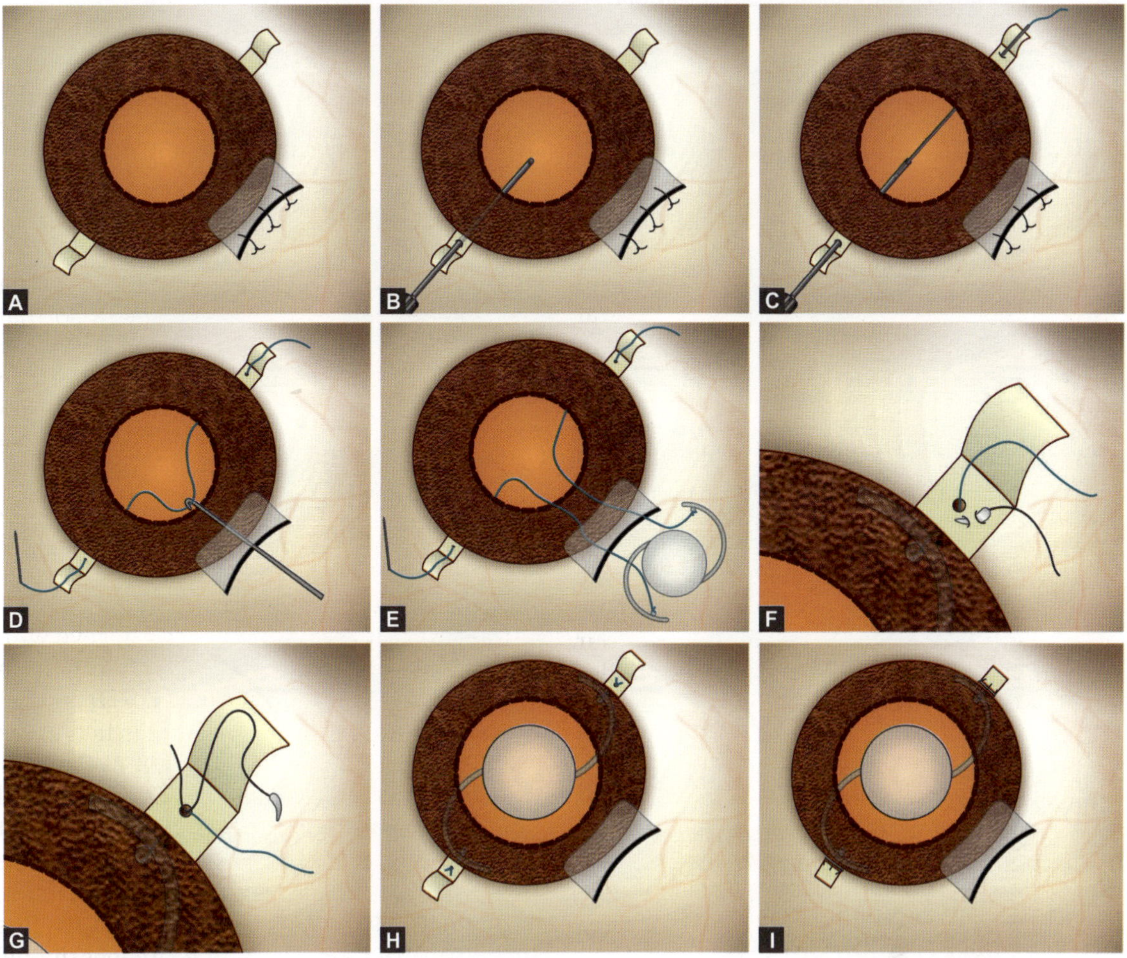

Fig. 19.7. *Ab externo technique of trans-scleral suture fixation of PCIOL. For explanation see text.*

ii. ***Four-point suture fixation technique.*** The technique is similar to the external to internal approach using long straight needle, but here IOL is fixed at 4 points, 2 placed on each haptic. As in this technique, two 10-0 polypropylene sutures are passed, at two places, this will avoid tilt or decentration of IOL.

2. Ab interno (internal to external) technique

In this technique, the curved needle is passed from inside the eye under the iris through the corneoscleral section aiming for the ciliary sulcus out under the scleral flaps (Fig. 19.8A and B). The same is repeated on the other side. The two ends of the suture are tied to the IOL haptic (Fig. 19.8C) and the two external ends with needle are tied to the sclera securing the IOL into position (Fig. 19.8D).

Advantages

- Quicker than outside to inside technique
- Easier with PKP

Disadvantages

- Blind procedure of passing needle into ciliary sulcus from behind the iris.
- More chance of intraocular bleeding and damage to corneal endothelium.

Intraoperative problems

- Difficulty in handling prolene suture
- Lens rotation/instability during passage of suture through it
- Iris distortion
- Iris/ciliary body bleeding obscuring visibility

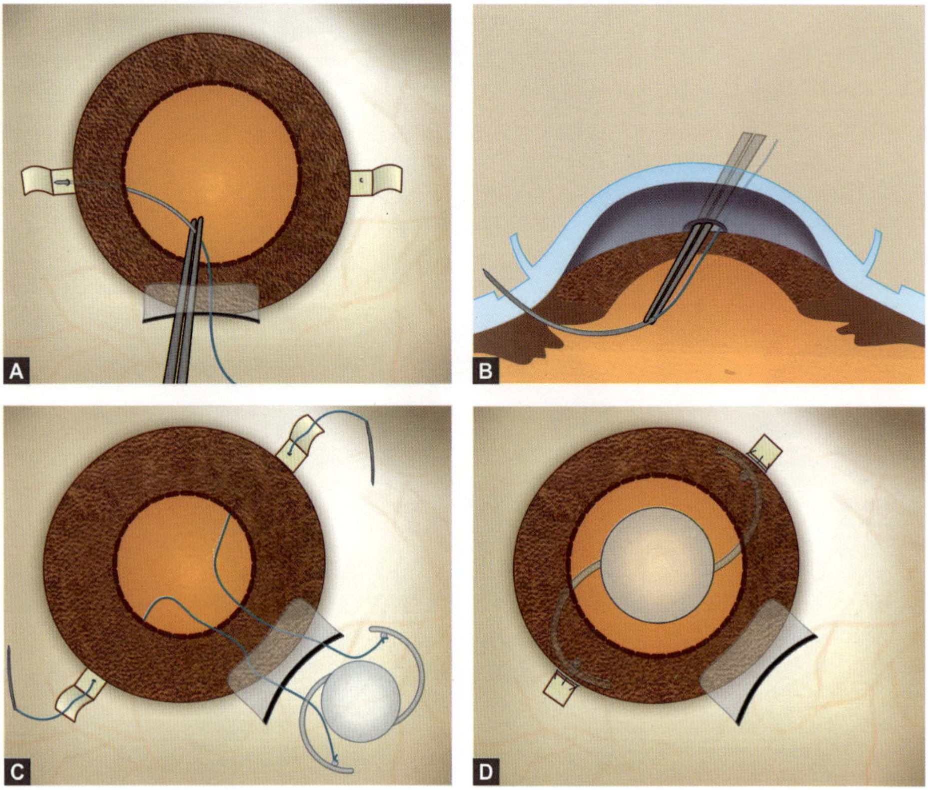

Fig. 19.8. *Ab interno technique of trans-scleral suture fixation of PCIOL. For explanation see text.*

II. ENDOSCOPIC TECHNIQUES OF TRANS-SCLERAL SUTURE FIXATION OF PCIOL

Endoscopic techniques of trans-scleral suture fixation of PCIOL was first described by Eguchi and Araie (1990). For direct visualisation of the ciliary sulcus, endoscope can be introduced either through the limbal or pars plana approach.

Methods

Two methods have been described for endoscopic technique of suture fixation:

1. ***Bimanual method.*** In this method, with one hand the surgeon holds the endoscope and with second hand introduces the needle. There are two variants of bimanual method:

i. *Ab externo technique.* In this technique, the bent 27 gauge needle is passed through the outer wall of the sclera (under the partial thickness flap) and is directly observed at the sulcus. Further procedure is same as described for conventional (non-endoscopic) ab externo technique (*see* page 338).

ii. *Ab interno technique.* In this technique, the surgeon observes the sulcus through the endoscope and with other hand passes the suture from inside of the eye to outside by a technique similar to as described above for the conventional ab interno technique (Fig. 19.8).

Disadvantage of bimanual methods. It is very difficult to coordinate the both hand movements.

2. ***One-hand method.*** One-hand method of endoscopic technique (Fig. 19.9) has been described by Boris Malyugin from Russia in 2005. Basically it is an ab interno technique in which after tying the suture to the IOL haptics, the needle is attached by a silicone sleeve to the endoscopic probe (Fig. 19.9A). The latter is then passed through the surgical incision, and via pupil behind the iris (Fig. 19.9B and C). In this way, needle penetrates in the sulcus region under direct visualization (Fig. 19.9C). Needle holder is used to catch the needle which penetrates through the sclera posterior to the

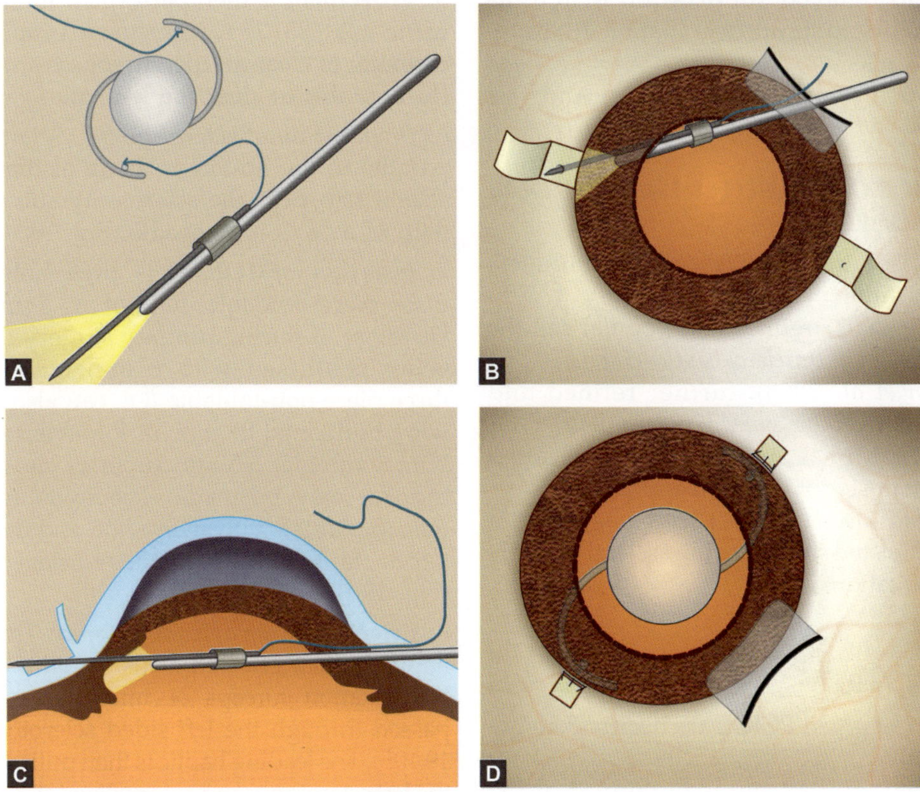

Fig. 19.9. *One hand method of endoscopic technique of trans-scleral suture fixation of PCIOL. For explanation see text.*

corneoscleral limbus under the partial thickness scleral flap. Further steps are similar as described above for conventional ab interno technique (Figs 19.8C and D and 19.9D).

COMPLICATIONS OF SUTURE FIXATION TECHNIQUES

- ***Problems related to prolene suture,*** like suture loosening or exposure (most frequently observed problem). This may produce scleral and conjunctival erosion causing foreign body sensation or they may act as a nidus for endophthalmitis. To avoid this, one should always bury the sutures underneath the scleral flaps. The exposed Prolene suture should ideally be trimmed or reburied but if this happens late (after 12–24 months) then it can be removed, if it is creating trouble even after reburying it.

- ***IOL tilt/decentration*** is seen when sutures are tied loose or IOL diameter is less than 6.5 mm or when pupil is large and distorted. To avoid this, pass the suture from slightly below the horizontal line, secondly optic size of IOL should be 6.5 mm or more.
- Pupillary distortion
- Episcleritis
- Trans-scleral haptic erosion through sclera
- Corneal decompensation
- Secondary glaucoma
- Intraocular haemorrhage through iris or ciliary body

B. SUTURELESS TRANS-SCLERAL FIXATION OF PCIOL

Techniques of sutureless trans-scleral fixation of PCIOL have been developed to achieve the following:

- To avoid suture-related problems.
- To use a foldable IOL through a small self-sealing wound.
- To achieve better centration and stabilization of IOL.

- To avoid delayed subluxation of IOL as reported due to suture degradation in suture-fixated IOLs.
- To reduce uveal tissue contact and iris changes.

TECHNIQUES OF SUTURELESS TRANS-SCLERAL FIXATION OF PCIOL

- *Maggi* (1997), introduced the idea of sutureless scleral fixation of PCIOL.
- *Scharioth* (2002), refined and popularised the technique as *'intrascleral haptic fixation'.*
- *Agarwal et al* (2008), further refined and revolutionized the *'glued IOL technique'.*
- *Prenna* (2012) has suggested a modification from the posterior segment approach.
- *Yotan and Keradag* (2012) have suggested a Trocar-assisted sutureless intrascleral foldable PCIOL fixation.

GLUED IOL

Surgical technique

Basic steps of glued PCIOL are decribed below (Fig. 19.10):

1. ***Conjunctival peritomy*** is performed at the sites of planned scleral flaps creation.
   - *Horizontal flaps.* When horizontal white-to-white (WTW) measurement is 11 mm then IOL can be fixed horizontally and flaps should be made at 3 and 9 o'clock position (Fig. 19.10A).
   - *Vertical flaps.* When WTW is more than 11 mm it would be better to fix the IOL vertically and so flaps should be made at 6 and 12 o'clock positions.

2. ***Intraocular infusion.*** After peritomy, the eyeball should be stabilised by either pars plana infusion (i.e. 25 G) or by an anterior chamber maintainer (Fig. 19.10A).

3. ***Preparation of scleral flaps.*** Two partial thickness limbal based scleral flaps about 2.5 mm × 2.5 mm are created exactly 180° from each other at the planned site (Fig. 19.10A).

4. ***Creation of sclerotomies under the scleral flaps.*** Two straight sclerotomies ab externo are prepared with a sharp 20–22 G needle about 1.5 mm from the limbus under the scleral flaps exactly 180° from each other and directed towards the centre of globe (Fig. 19.10B).

5. ***Vitrectomy*** is then performed meticulously using a 20/23/25 G vitrectomy probe. This is essential to clear all the vitreous from AC and PC and also to clear the lenticular remnants.

6. ***Preparation of scleral tunnel.*** Scleral tunnel parallel to the limbus is made at the edge of scleral flap near the sclerotomy site with the help of a 26 G bent needle (Fig. 19.10C).

7. ***Insertion of IOL.*** It is preferable to use three-piece foldable IOL of 13.5 mm size. However, if during primary surgery SICS was being performed with 6 mm incision, then three piece non-foldable IOL can also be used. For a horizontal fixation of foldable secondary IOL, a valvular 3.5 mm superior clear corneal incision may be made. The foldable IOL is then implanted with an injector, and the trailing haptic is kept out of the corneal incision (Fig. 19.10D and E).

8. ***Externalization of leading haptic.*** The leading haptic is then grasped at its tip with a special IOL fixation forceps or microrhexis forceps) passed through the left sided sclerotomy (Fig. 19.10F). The leading haptic is then pulled through the left sclerotomy and externalized (Fig. 19.10G).

9. ***Externalization of trailing haptic.*** The trailing haptic is flexed in the anterior chamber by grasping the tip with a McPherson forceps and transferred to a microrhexis forceps held in left hand by hand-shake technique. With the right hand, another special IOL fixation is then passed through right-sided (or superior) sclerotomy and the tip of haptic is transferred to this right-handed forceps again by the hand-shake technique (Fig. 19.10H). The trailing haptic is then pulled through the sclerotomy and externalized (Fig. 19.10I).

10. ***Vitrectomy around the sclerotomy*** should then be performed to remove tucked vitreous.

11. ***Tucking of the haptic ends in the scleral tunnel*** is then done by flexing the haptic with the help of McPherson forceps and then pushing inside the scleral tunnel (Fig. 19.10J and K).

12. ***Application of fibrin glue.*** Fibrin glue works in a dry area. So at this juncture, the infusion cannula is turned off and air is injected in the AC to have a firm globe. Then the reconstituted fibrin glue is prepared and injected through

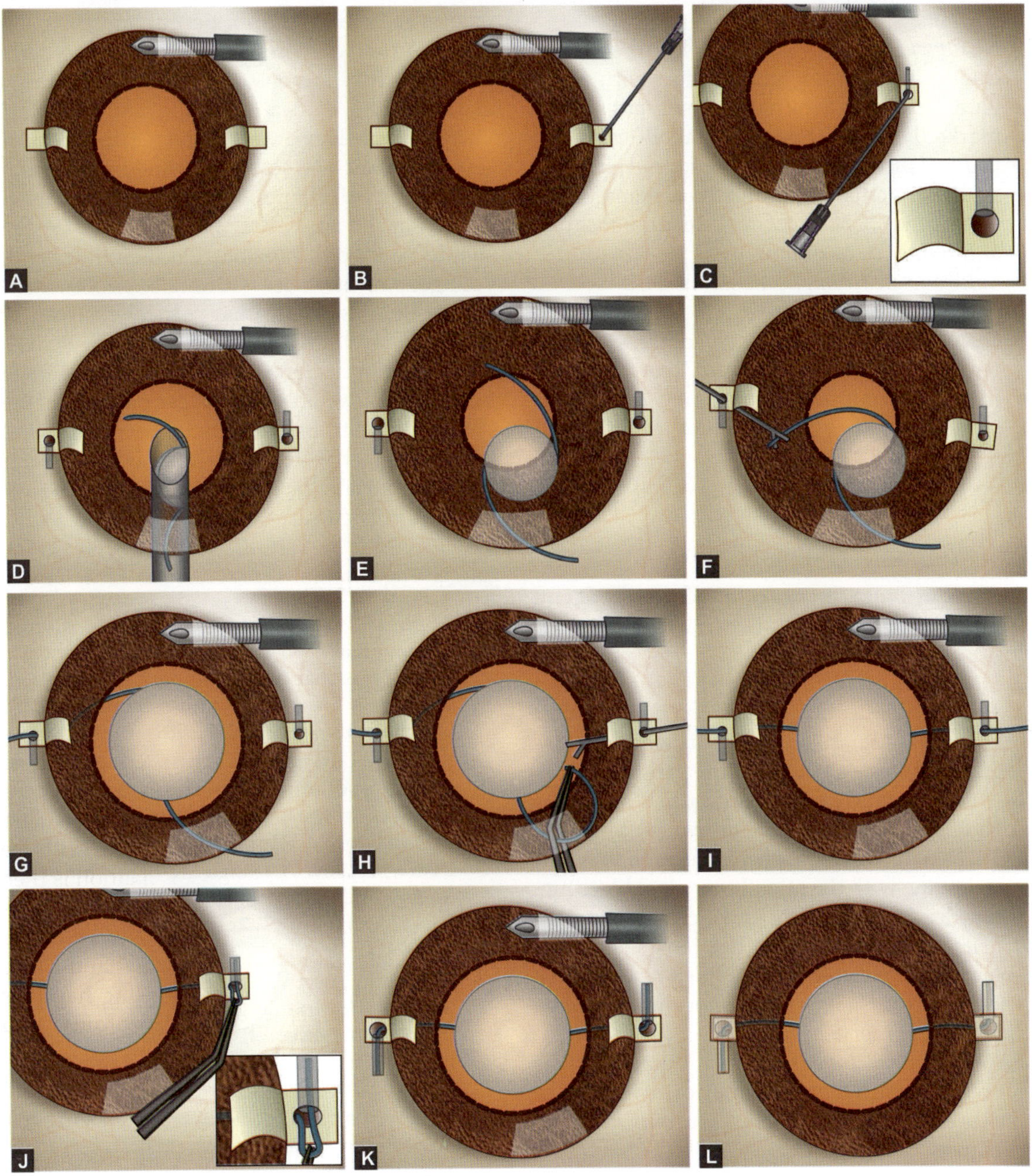

Fig. 19.10. *Technique of glued PCIOL. For explanation see text.*

the cannula under the scleral flaps after thoroughly dry mapping the area. The scleral flaps are reposited and gentle pressure is applied for 10 to 20 seconds for the formation of fibrin polypeptides. The infusion cannula or anterior chamber maintainer (whichever is used) is then removed and after drying the surface the fibrin glue can be used over the conjunctiva and clear corneal incision to seal them too (Fig. 19.10L).

Advantages of glued IOL technique

- *No need for special IOLs with eyelets,* as the standard three-piece IOLs, routinely available are used. Thus, there is no need for maintaining a special inventory.

- *No tilt and better stabilization of IOL* is obtained due to haptic tuck and fixation with fibrin glue. This leads to minimum astigmatism and markedly reduced pseudophakodonesis.
- *Reduced incidence of postoperative complications* such as uveitis, glaucoma, hyphaema (UGH syndrome), CME, corneal decompensation and retinal detachment.
- *Suture-related complications* (as described on page 341) are not there.
- *Fast and easy technique.* The glued IOL technique once learnt is faster and easier than the suture fixation technique.

Disadvantages of glued IOLs

- Needs an end opening glued IOL forceps.
- Has a longer learning curve.

COMPLICATIONS OF PCIOLs

1. ***Cystoid macular oedema.*** Most important cause of its occurrence after SFIOL is vitreous loss.
2. ***Endophthalmitis.*** Endophthalmitis is a dreaded complication, which can happen after any intraocular procedure. Its chances are increased in cases where suture erosion occurs due to improperly covered or buried knot.
3. ***Hyphaema/vitreous haemorrhage.*** Suturing PCIOLs require needle passes through vascular uveal tissue with the attendant risk of bleeding. It may lead to red cell or ghost cell glaucoma.
4. ***Lens tilt/decentration.*** The lens stability is solely due to sutures and not due to any fibrous encapsulation, so lens may dislocate at any time following surgery.
5. ***Retinal detachment.*** Retinal detachment is more common when the anterior hyaloid face has been disturbed with or without vitreous prolapse.
6. ***Suprachoroidal haemorrhage.*** This is a rare complication considering the uveal manipulation that occurs during scleral fixation of a PCIOL.

CONCLUSION

Thus, considering the advantages and disadvantages of various techniques, it is clear that PCIOLs have a better prognosis than ACIOLs, but wherever facilities do not permit and there are less chances of complications as in elderly patients where there is a normal angle with no glaucoma, no corneal disorder, and an intact vitreous face. Those with bleeding disorders or severe conjunctival scarring would benefit from minimal uveal manipulation and conjunctival dissection and an ACIOL with improved design should be used, if possible. On the other hand, younger patients, those with angle abnormalities, iris tissue loss, glaucoma, corneal disease, or simultaneous PKP should have a PCIOL implanatation. Scleral flaps for knot coverage may not be advisable in younger patients as the flap tends to atrophy with time. For these cases, it may be better to use a method involving rotation/burying of the knot or fibrin glue may be used in such cases.

BIBLIOGRAPHY

1. Apple DJ, Price FW, Gwin T, et al. Sutured retropupillary posterior chamber intraocular lenses for exchange or secondary implantation. The 12th annual Binkhorstlecture, 1988. Ophthalmology 96:1241–7,1989.
2. Bas AM, Bulacio JL, Carrizo R. Monoscleral xation forposterior chamber intraocular lenses in cases of posteriorcapsule rupture. Ann Ophthalmol 22:341–345,1990.
3. Basti S, Tejaswi PC, Singh SK, et al. Outside-in trans-scleral fixation for ciliary sulcus intraocular lens placement. J Cataract Refract Surg 20:89–92,1994.
4. Bellucci R, Pucci V, Morselli S, et al. Secondary implantation of angle-supported anterior chamber and scleral-fixated posterior chamber intraocular lenses. J Cataract Refract Surg 22:247–252,1996.
5. Hu BV, Shin DH, Gibbs KA, et al. Implantation of posterior chamber lens in the absence of capsular and zonular support. Arch Ophthalmol 106:416–420,1988.
6. Jaffe NS, Horwitz J. Anterior chamber lenses and secondarylens implantation, in Podos SM, Yanoff M (eds): Textbook of Ophthalmology: Lens and Cataract. New York: Gower Medical Publishing 11.81–90,1992.
7. Ju¨rgens I, Lillo J, Buil JA, et al. Endoscope-assisted trans scleral suture fixation of intraocular lenses. J Cataract Refract Surg 22:879–881,1996.

COMPLICATIONS OF CATARACT SURGERY AND THEIR MANAGEMENT

20 CHAPTER

INTRODUCTION
PREOPERATIVE COMPLICATIONS
OPERATIVE COMPLICATIONS
- Superior rectus muscle laceration
- Excessive bleeding
- Incision-related complications
- Injury to cornea, iris and lens
- Iris injuries and iridodialysis
- Complications related to anterior capsulorhexis
- Complications during hydrodissection
- Posterior capsular rupture (PCR)
- Zonular dehiscence
- Nucleus drop into the vitreous cavity
- Suprachoroidal effusion or haemorrhage
- Expulsive choroidal haemorrhage

POSTOPERATIVE COMPLICATIONS
- Hyphaema
- Iris prolapse
- Flat anterior chamber
- Corneal oedema
- Postoperative anterior uveitis
- Toxic anterior segment syndrome
- Bacterial endophthalmitis
- Delayed chronic postoperative endophthalmitis
- Cystoid macular oedema (CME)
- Retinal detachment (RD)
- Epithelial ingrowth
- Fibrous downgrowth
- After cataract
- Postoperative glaucoma
- IOL-related complications

INTRODUCTION

Nowadays cataract surgery is being performed largely by extracapsular cataract extraction techniques. Therefore, complications encountered during these techniques are described in general. Wherever necessary a specific reference of the technique, viz. conventional ECCE, manual SICS and phacoemulsification in relation to the particular complication is highlighted.

Complications encountered during surgical management of cataract can be enumerated under the following heads:

A. Preoperative complications
B. Operative complications
C. Postoperative complications

A. PREOPERATIVE COMPLICATIONS

1. Anxiety. Some patients may develop anxiety, on the eve of operation due to fear and apprehension of operation.

Treatment. Anxiolytic drugs such as diazepam 2–5 mg at bedtime usually alleviate such symptoms.

2. Nausea and gastritis. A few patients may develop nausea and gastritis due to preoperative medicines such as acetazolamide and/or glycerol.

Treatment. Oral antacids and omission of further dose of such medicines usually relieve the symptoms.

3. Irritative or allergic conjunctivitis may occur in some patients due to preoperative topical antibiotic drops.

Treatment. Postponing the operation for a few days along with withdrawal of such drugs is required.

4. Corneal abrasion may develop due to inadvertent injury during tonometry especially Schiotz tonometry.

Treatment. Patching with antibiotic ointment for a day and postponement of operation for a few days is required.

5. Complications due to local anaesthesia

i. *Retrobulbar haemorrhage* may occur due to retrobulbar block.

Treatment. Immediate pressure bandage after instilling one drop of 2% pilocarpine and postponement of operation for a week is advised.

ii. *Oculocardiac reflex,* which manifests as bradycardia and/or cardiac arrhythmia, has also been observed due to retrobulbar block. *Prevention and treatment.* An intravenous injection of atropine is helpful.

iii. *Perforation of globe* may also occur sometimes. To prevent such catastrophy, gentle injection with blunt-tipped needle is recommended. Further, peribulbar anaesthesia should be preferred over retrobulbar block.

iv. *Subconjunctival haemorrhage* is a minor complication observed frequently, and does not need much attention.

v. *Spontaneous dislocation of lens* in the vitreous has also been reported (in patients with weak and degenerated zonules especially with hypermature cataract) during vigorous ocular massage after retrobulbar block.

Treatment. The operation should be postponed and further management is on the lines of posterior dislocation of nucleus (*see* page 351).

Note. For complications due to anaesthesia also *see* page 104.

B. OPERATIVE COMPLICATIONS

1. Superior rectus muscle laceration and/or haematoma, may occur while applying the bridle suture in patients being operated by ECCE or SICS. In phacoemulsification, bridle suture is generally not required.

Treatment. Usually, no treatment is required for such an injury.

2. Excessive bleeding may be encountered during the preparation of conjunctival flap in ECCE or SICS. A few surgeons prepare conjunctival flap for sclerocorneal tunnel incision in phacoemulsification also.

Treatment. Bleeding vessels may be gently cauterized with wet field cautery.

3. Incision-related complications depend upon the type of cataract surgery being performed.

a. *In conventional ECCE,* there may occur *irregular incision.* Irregular incision leading to defective coaptation of wound may occur due to blunt cutting instruments.

b. *In sclerocorneal tunnel incision, during manual SICS or phacoemulsification,* following complications may occur as compared to a normal self-sealing tunnel incision (Fig. 20.1A):

i. ***Thin flap and/or button holing of anterior wall of tunnel*** (Fig. 20.1B) can occur because of superficial dissection of the scleral and/or corneal flap. A shallow initial groove is the commonest cause. Other causes are a too sharp or too blunt knife. The thin flaps are predisposed to develop a torn edge and are also liable to develop corneal burns leading to a leaking wound with unstable chamber and unsafe surgery.

Treatment. As a remedy, abandon this dissection and re-enter at a deeper plane from the other side of the external incision.

ii. ***Premature entry into the anterior chamber*** (Fig. 20.1C) can occur because of deep dissection following deep initial groove. Most common cause of premature entry is the failure to move the knife in accordance with the curvature of corneal dome. The smaller corneal lip thus produced will not have an efficient valvular function resulting in an unstable chamber and repeated iris prolapse.

Treatment. Once this is detected initially, dissection in that area should be stopped and a new dissection started at a lesser depth at the other end of the tunnel.

iii. ***Scleral disinsertion*** can occur due to very deep groove incision. In it, there occurs complete separation of inferior sclera from the sclera superior to the incision (Fig. 20.1D). Scleral disinsertion needs to be managed by radial sutures.

Prevention. Sclera disinsertion can be prevented by making the groove incision of partial thickness only, either by judicious use of free hand incision or with a guarded blade designed for this purpose.

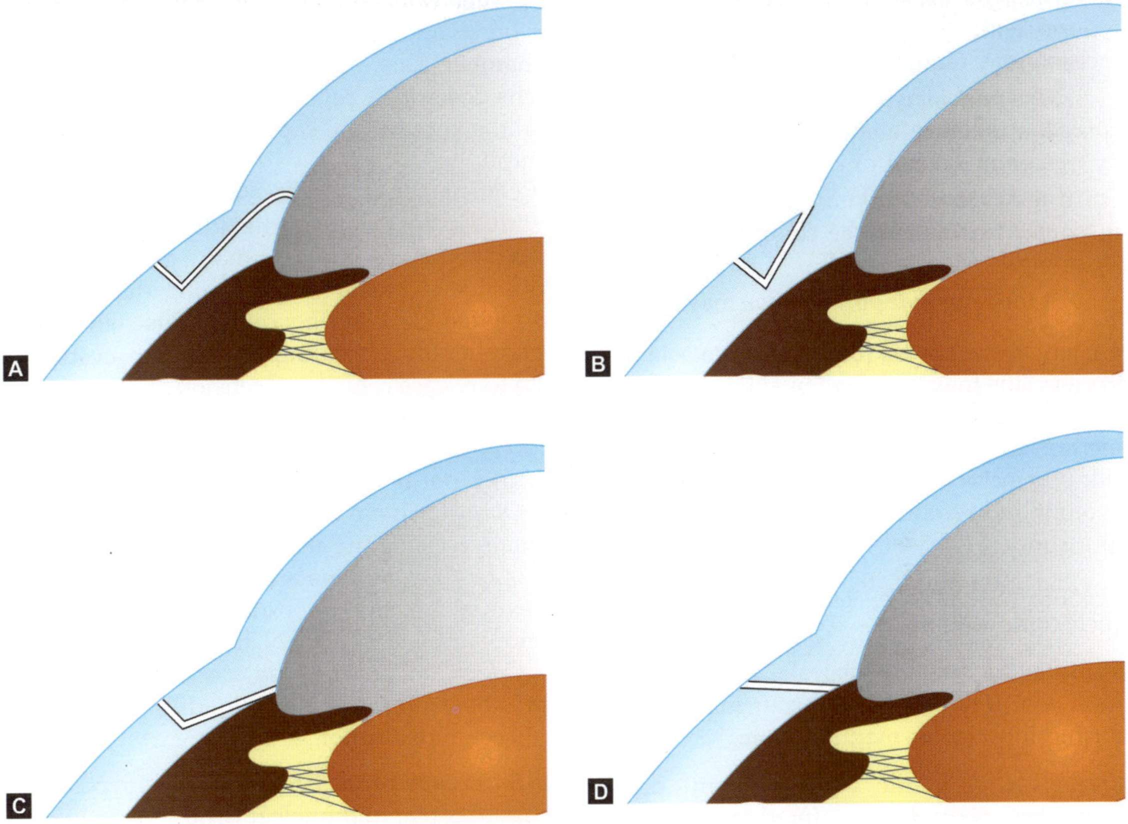

Fig. 20.1. *Tunnel incision-related complications:* ***(A)*** *Normal tunnel;* ***(B)*** *Button holing of anterior wall of the tunnel;* ***(C)*** *Premature entry into the anterior chamber;* ***(D)*** *Scleral disinsertion.*

c. *Complications with clear corneal incision:* Presently 2–4 mm clear corneal tunnel incision is preferred to sclerocorneal tunnel incision for phacoemulsification, when implanting foldable IOLs, as there is no need to further enlarge the incision. Complications encountered include:

i. *Thin flap and button holing of anterior wall of corneal tunnel* may occur as described for sclerocorneal tunnel incision.

ii. *Premature entry* may occur due to similar causes as described for sclerocorneal tunnel incision. Premature entry in clear corneal incisions occurs more commonly with uniplanar incision especially with a very sharp knife.

iii. *Torn edges* are not uncommon especially with beginners. The edges are cut by the shoulder of the knife due to inadvertent lifting of the anterior flap while entry the anterior chamber.

- *Prevention.* One should understand the configuration of curvature of the cornea and should press the shoulder of knife down while entering the anterior chamber.
- *Management.* A small tear may be ignored. Large tear of the edge of the flap which causes a leaking wound should be sutured with 10-0 nylon suture.

iv. *Long tunnel* may be inadvertently formed sometimes especially in myopes and soft eyes where anterior chamber is not firm enough to facilitate the smooth movement of the knife. A long tunnel makes the surgery uncomfortable because of the poor visibility occurring due to distortion of the cornea. To prevent long tunnel, always construct the tunnel in a tense eyeball and tend to perforate the cornea a little early in myopes.

d. *Complications during side port incision*

i. *Too far peripheral paracentesis incision* accidently made in the sclera causes bleeding, increases the incidence of iris prolapse and wound leak. A leaky non-sealing side port incision may require to be sutured in the end.

ii. ***Side port incision too far central into the cornea,*** accidently made, may be complicated by Descemet's membrane stripping.

iii. ***Side port incision too small for the instrument entry*** may be complicated by DM stripping.

iv. ***A too large side port incision*** may be leaky.

4. Injury to the cornea (Descemet's detachment), iris and lens may occur when anterior chamber is entered with a keratome. During the main incision or with the paracentesis knife, during side port incision, especially when the instrument is blunt and requires excess force which leads to a sudden entry.

Prevention. Always use a sharp knife to prevent such complications.

5. Iris injury and iridodialysis, i.e. tear of iris from root (Fig. 20.2) may occur inadvertently during intraocular manipulation.

Prevention. A gentle handling with proper hypotony reduces the incidence of such inadvertent injuries.

6. Complications related to anterior capsulorhexis. Continuous curvilinear capsulorhexis (CCC) is the preferred technique for opening the anterior capsule for SICS and phacoemulsification. Following complications may occur:

i. *Escaping capsulorhexis*, i.e. capsulorhexis moves peripherally and may extend to the equator (Fig. 20.3A) or posterior capsule.

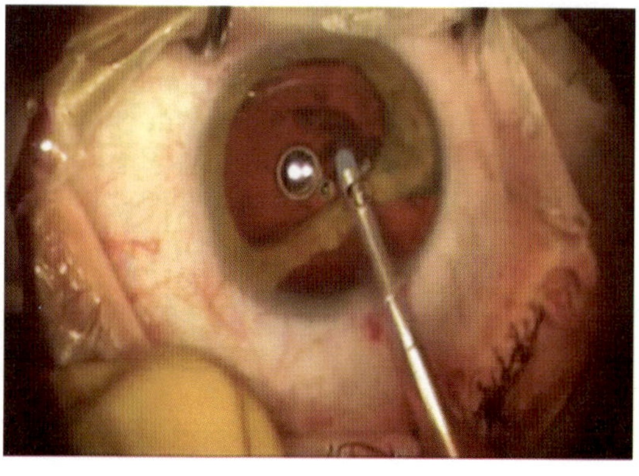

Fig. 20.2. *Iridodialysis due to preoperative trauma.*

Management. Take following measures:

- *Inject viscoelastic* to pressurize the anterior chamber. This will deepen the AC, displace the lens posteriorly relieving the centrifugal stress on the zonules and capsule and also widen the pupil.
- *Option 1: Catch the capsular flap* (preferably with forceps) close to the advancing tear and pull the flap centrally. In many cases, it will be possible to recover the escaping rhexis.
- *Option 2: Cut the capsule* just ahead of peripherally extending rhexis with cystitome tip to release centrifugal tension on the capsule and then pull the flap centrally with capsular forceps. Option 2 should be opted when option 1 does not help.
- *Option 3: Raise the opposite flap* by making a small incision in the capsule with Vanna's scissors or cystitome and start a new capsulorhexis in direction opposite to the previous one and complete it (Fig. 20.3B to D).
- *Option 4: Convert to can-opener capsulotomy,* if the above options fail and modify technique of phacoemulsification.

ii. *Small capsulorhexis.* It predisposes to posterior capsular tear and nuclear drop during hydrodissection. It also predisposes to occurrence of zonular dehiscence. Therefore, a small-sized capsulorhexis should always be enlarged by taking following steps:

- *Inject viscoelastic* (preferably cohesive) to pressurize the AC, deepen it, and widen the pupil.
- *Make an oblique cut in the rim of capsulorhexis* with the help of Vanna's microscissors to create a flap of the capsule.
- *Catch the flap with rhexis forceps* and tear it with a wider required diameter until the circle is completed. If required, the procedure can be repeated.

iii. *Very large capsulorhexis* may cause problems for phacoemulsification. Following measures may be used:

- *Limit hydrodissection* to minimum without mobilizing the nucleus.
- *Use dispersive viscoelastic* to keep the nucleus in the bag.
- Phacoemulsification should be done either by *emulsifying the nucleus* tilted as described by

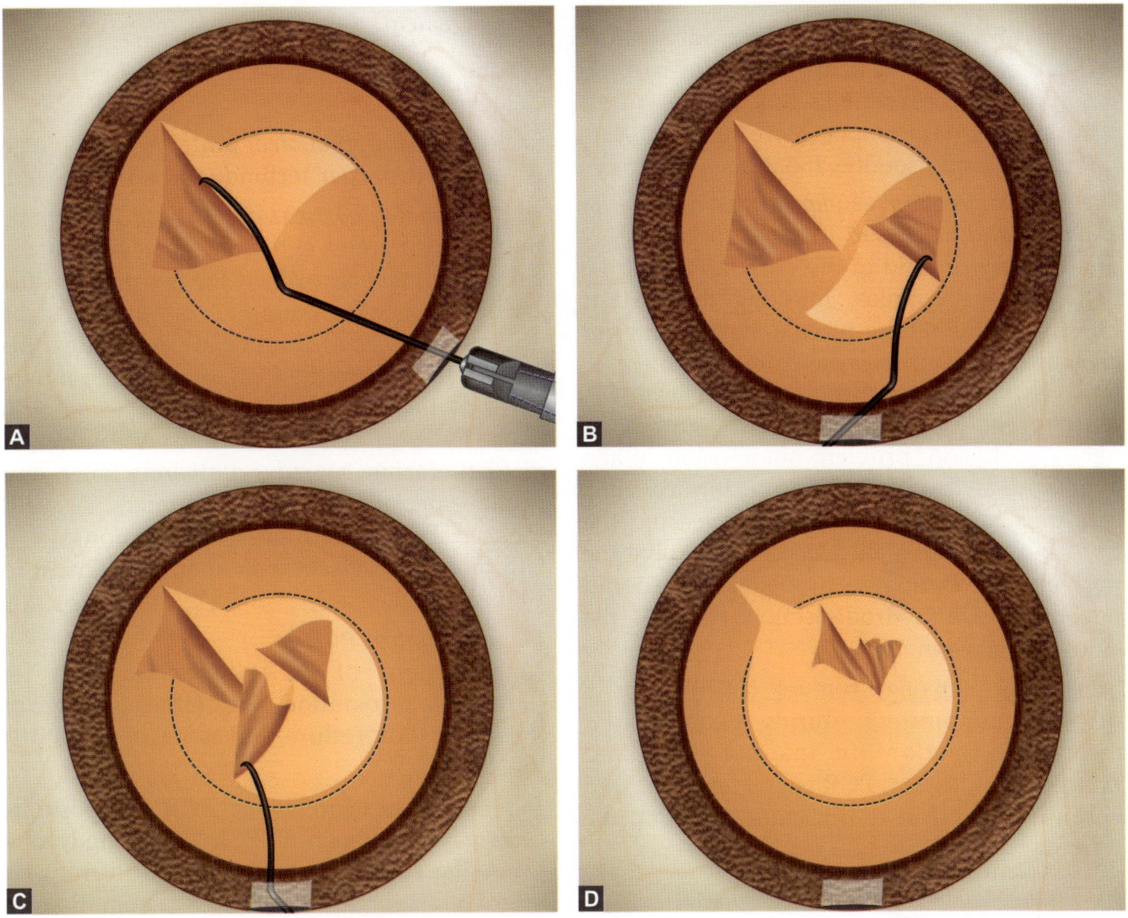

Fig. 20.3. *Peripheral extension of anterior capsulorhexis **(A)** and its management by starting a new capsulorhexis in the opposite direction and completing it **(B to D)**.*

Brown or by the quick chop, i.e. Pfeiffer-Maloney technique. This technique gives the best control with a mobile nucleus.

iv. ***Eccentric capsulorhexis*** can lead to IOL decentration at a later stage.

7. Complications during hydrodissection

i. ***Insufficient hydrodissection*** will make all successive manoeuvres difficult and may cause further complication such as zonular dialysis, PCR and nucleus drop. Suspect insufficient hydrodissection, if difficulty is encountered during nucleus rotation and so repeat hydrodissection gently.

ii. ***Posterior capsular rupture (PCR)*** with or without nuclear drop may occur during hydrodissection. First tell-tale sign of PCR occurring during hydrodissection is *pupil snap sign*. PCR may occur under following situations:

- *Forcefully performed hydrodissection* with injection of too much fluid can lead to PCR.
- *Block to outflow, e.g.* when the capsulorhexis is of small size, the excess of fluid will lift the nucleus, block the capsulorhexis margin and capsule will be burst. This condition is known as *'capsular block syndrome'*. Increased resistance offered by too much viscoelastic in the anterior chamber can also cause block to fluid outflow and PCR.
- *Inherent weakness of posterior capsule,* e.g. posterior polar cataracts are associated with dehiscence of the posterior capsule in 20–25% cases. Even a normal hydrodissection in these cases can cause PCR and may lead to nucleus drop. In such cases, hydrodelineation should

be performed rather than hydrodissection. Inherent weakness of the posterior capsule may also be present in the high myopes, traumatic cataracts, post-vitrectomy cataractous eyes and pseudoexfoliation syndrome.

iii. ***Fluid misdirection resulting in shallow anterior chamber and increased IOP*** may occur rarely due to entry of fluid in the vitreous through a defect in the zonules. Injecting too fast or injecting in the wrong place (over the anterior capsule) may be the cause of this problem.

iv. ***Over inflated eye leading to increased IOP, tense eyeball,*** patient discomfort, and optic nerve perfusion problem may occur when aggressive hydrodissection is performed via a side port incision. Immediately releasing the fluid through the main incision will solve the problem. To avoid the problem, one should never perform hydrodissection through the side port incision.

8. Posterior capsular rupture (PCR). It is a dreaded complication during extracapsular cataract extraction. In manual SICS and phacoemulsification, PCR is even more feared because it can lead to nucleous drop into the vitreous.

PCR can occur in following situations:

i. ***During hydrodissection*** (as described above).

ii. ***By direct injury*** with some instrument such as Sinskey's hook, chopper or phaco tip.

iii. ***PCR during nucleotomy*** may occur at any stage but is more common in the end, since at this stage capsule can move forward particularly in hypermature cataract and may strike the phaco tip or tip of the chopper. To prevent this, one should reduce vacuum settings and perform phaco more anteriorly under the visco cover.

Cardinal signs of PCR during phacoemulsification (nucleotomy) are:

- Sudden deepening of anterior chamber
- Momentary pupillary dilatation
- Non-flowability of nuclear fragments towards phaco tip
- Movements of nuclear fragments away from the phaco tip.

Posterior loss of lens fragments into the vitreous cavity may occur after PCR or zonular dehiscence during phacoemulsification. It is potentially serious because it may result in glaucoma, chronic uveitis, chronic CME and even retinal detachment.

iv. ***PCR during epinuclear plate removal*** is also common, if proper technique is not followed.

v. ***PCR during cortical aspiration,*** is perhaps the most common situation, especially in the sub-incisional area. When PC is caught in the suction probe/cannula, a star-shaped area appears (Fig. 20.4). Immediate release at this stage will prevent the PCR, but sudden movement of the probe/cannula at this stage will cause PCR.

vi. ***PCR during capsular polishing*** may also occur especially with the beginners. A well-focused PC under high magnification and a bag filled with viscoelastic material is must to prevent PCR.

Management of PCR

Management of PCR depends upon its immediate recognition, size of the tear, stage of the surgical procedure, and associated vitreous loss, etc.

Immediate recognition of PCR is of prime importance; as soon as PCR is detected, take following steps:

- Stop working
- Maintain a closed chamber
- Preserve as much of the posterior capsule as possible.

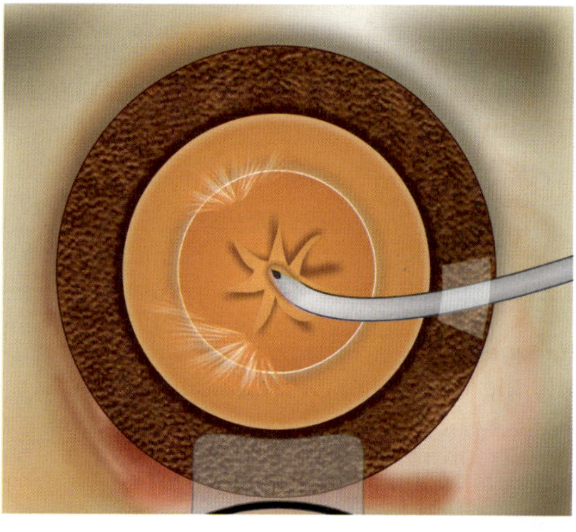

Fig. 20.4. *Star sign of posterior capsular catch during cortical aspiration.*

Management of PCR is as below:

i. *PCR occurring in initial stage.* When PCR occurs early, i.e. during capsulorhexis, hydrodissection or early sculpting, then the procedure should be converted to an ECCE.

ii. *PCR in late stage with intact hyloid phase.* Immediately inject highly dispersive viscoelastic under the lens fragments to plug the PCR and proceed as below:

- *In case of small nuclear fragments left,* move the lens fragment in anterior chamber with spatula and emulsify with short bursts.
- *In case of large nuclear material,* enlarge the incision and extract the fragments using Sheet's glide loop or by 'chopstick technique'. *Cortex and epinuclear plate* should be removed by manual dry aspiration using Simcoe's cannula, taking care not to extend the PCR and not to rupture the hyaloid face.

iii. *PCR with vitreous loss without luxation of nuclear material into vitreous.* Lens matter remnants should be managed as above. Depending upon the size of PCR and amount of vitreous loss, a vitrectomy should be performed using an anterior or posterior approach.

iv. *PCR with vitreous loss with dislocation of nuclear material into the vitreous.* The management is similar to nuclear drop, as described below.

9. Zonular dehiscence may occur in all techniques of ECCE but is especially common during nucleus prolapse into the anterior chamber in manual SICS.

10. Nucleus drop into the vitreous cavity. It occurs more frequently with phacoemulsification, less frequently with manual SICS and sparingly with conventional ECCE. It is a dreadful complication which occurs due to sudden and large PCR. PCR with nucleus drop can occur at any stage of phacoemulsification, i.e. during hydrodissection, rotation, sculpting, cracking or chopping and emulsification of the nuclear quadrants.

Management. Once the nucleus has dropped into the vitreous cavity, no attempt should be made to fish it out. The case must be referred to vitreoretinal surgeon after a thorough anterior vitrectomy and cortical clean up and proper wound closure.

Management by vitreoretinal surgeon

Three-port vitrectomy is performed after control of intraocular inflammation and raised IOP. After vitrectomy, depending upon the amount and hardness of the lens, following measures may be taken:

- *Removal by limbal route* is recommended for hard almost complete nucleus. PFCL should be injected to raise the nucleus up to just beneath the iris. Then a light pipe or any other soft tipped cannula can be used to manipulate the lens into AC, after which it can be removed by limbal incision.
- *Removal by phacofragmentation* is good for soft and small dropped in lens matter. Small amount of PFCL is injected behind the lens fragment to raise it in the midvitreous. Then keeping the power at 5–10% and aspiration at 150–200 mmHg, the lens fragments are aspirated by a phacofragmentome.
- *Favit* is a newer technique of removal of dislocated lens. In this technique, a vitrectomy probe connected to a peristaltic pump is used from the initial corneal incision. Endoilluminator is passed through a side port and adequate vitrectomy is done. Then a phaco probe is passed via the corneal incision and lens matter is removed using 50% power, 50 mm Hg suction and 18 cc/min flow rate.

11. Suprachoroidal effusion or haemorrhage. Suprachoroidal effusion refers to sudden exudation of fluid from choroidal vasculature occurring during any decompression procedure performed in the eye. Suprachoroidal haemorhage may follow suprachoroidal effusion or may occur de novo under similar circumstances.

Etiopathogenesis. Suprachoroidal effusion and/or haemorrhage can occur as a complication during any intraocular surgery. Their incidence was high in ICCE and conventional ECCE. Fortunately, both complications are much less likely with modern phacoemulsification because of the relatively closed system formed by the architecture of the small self-sealing incision and the relative tight fit of the phaco tip incision. Both complications occur more commonly in people who are elderly or have arteriosclerosis, hypertension, diabetes mellitus, blood dyscrasias, obesity, high myopia, glaucoma, chronic ocular inflammation.

Clinical features. Clinically, it may be difficult to differentiate between suprachoroidal effusion and haemorrhage. Both are characterized by a forward prolapse of posterior ocular structures including iris and vitreous accompanied by shallowing of anterior chamber and change in the red reflex. Typically, such a situation is referred to *'operative hard eye'*. Patient agitation and pain followed by an extremely firm globe suggest suprachoroidal haemorrhage.

Management.

- *Closure of the wound* should be done rapidly.
- *Hyperosmotic agents* such as 20% mannitol should be administered intravenously.
- *Posterior sclerotomy* may be performed to drain the suprachoroidal fluid and/or haemorrhage. If required sclerotomy may be repeated after 7–10 days to drain the residual suprachoroidal blood detected on B-scan USG.
- *Topical antiglaucoma drugs and steroids* help maintaining the IOP and reducing the inflammation.

12. Expulsive choroidal haemorrhage. It is one of the most dramatic and serious complication of cataract surgery. It usually occurs in hypertensives and patients with arteriosclerotic changes.

Etiopathogenesis. It is an exaggerated, acute and severe form of suprachoroidal haemorrhage. Therefore, etiopathogenesis, and predisposing factors are same as described above.

Characteristic features. It is characterized by spontaneous gaping of the wound followed by expulsion of the lens, vitreous, retina, uvea and finally a gush of bright red blood.

Management. Principles of management are same as described above for choroidal effusion. Although treatment is unsatisfactory, the surgeon should attempt to:

- Rapidly close the incision
- Drain subchoroidal blood by performing an equatorial sclerotomy
- Most of the times eye is lost and so evisceration operation has to be performed.

C. POSTOPERATIVE COMPLICATIONS

1. Hyphaema. Collection of blood in the anterior chamber may occur from conjunctival or scleral vessels due to minor ocular trauma or otherwise. Hyphaema from the wound may follow ECCE, SICS and in phacoemulsification with sclerocorneal tunnel incision. Inadvertent trauma to the iris especially iris root may also result in hyphaema.

Treatment. Most hyphaemas absorb spontaneously and thus need no treatment. Sometimes hyphaema may be large and associated with rise in IOP. In such cases, IOP should be lowered by acetazolamide and hyperosmotic agents. If the blood does not get absorbed in a week's time, then a paracentesis should be performed to drain the blood.

2. Iris prolapse. It is usually caused by inadequate suturing of the incision after ICCE and conventional ECCE and occurs during first or second postoperative day. This complication is almost not known with manual SICS and phacoemulsification technique, except in cases where incision is not valvular.

Management. A small prolapse of less than 24 hours duration may be reposited back and wound sutured. A large prolapse of long duration needs abscission and suturing of wound.

3. Flat (shallow or non-formed) anterior chamber. It has become a relatively rare complication due to improved wound closure. It may be due to wound leak, ciliochoroidal detachment or pupil block.

i. *Flat anterior chamber with wound leak* is associated with hypotony. It is diagnosed by Seidel's test. In this test, a drop of fluorescein is instilled into the lower fornix and patient is asked to blink to spread the dye evenly. The incision is then examined with slit-lamp using cobalt-blue filter. At the site of leakage, fluorescein will be diluted by aqueous. In most cases, wound leak is cured within 4 days with pressure bandage and oral acetazolamide. If the condition persists, injection of air in the anterior chamber and resuturing of the leaking wound should be carried out.

ii. *Ciliochoroidal detachment.* It may or may not be associated with wound leak. Detached ciliochoroid presents as a convex brownish mass in the involved quadrant with shallow anterior chamber. In most cases, choroidal detachment is cured within 4 days with pressure bandage and use of oral acetazolamide. If the condition persists, suprachoroidal drainage with injection of air in the anterior chamber is indicated.

iii. *Pupil block* leads to formation of iris bombe and shallowing of peripheral anterior chamber. If the condition persists for 5–7 days, permanent peripheral anterior synechiae (PAS) may be formed leading to secondary angle closure glaucoma.

Causes. Common causes of postoperative pupil block are vitreous bulge following PCR, ACIOL without PI and air entrapment.

Management. Pupil block is managed initially with mydriasis, hyperosmotic agents (e.g. 20% mannitol) and acetazolamide. If not relieved, then laser or surgical peripheral iridectomy should be performed to bypass the pupillary block.

4. Corneal oedema

Causes. Corneal oedema may occur due to damage (mechanical, chemical or thermal) to endothelium, intraocular inflammation or raised IOP. One or more factors may be responsible for the corneal oedema. Incidence of corneal oedema is higher in eyes with pre-existing corneal endothelial dysfunction such as Fuch's dystrophy.

i. *Damage to endothelium*

- *Mechanical damage to the endothelium* may be caused by instruments, lens matter or shock waves due to fluid turbulence. Rubbing of a hard nuclear fragment against the endothelium is often responsible for endothelial damage. Small nuclear fragments retained in the anterior chamber angle may contribute to persistent focal corneal oedema. *Note.* Corneal oedema from surgical trauma generally resolves completely within 4–6 weeks of surgery.
- *Chemical damage to the endothelium* may be caused by irrigating solution, viscoelastic and drugs such as adrenaline, xylocard and pilocarpine. Certain toxic substances inadvertently introduced into the anterior chamber can also cause endothelial dysfunction.
- *Thermal damage to endothelium* occurs due to excessive use of phaco power.

ii. *Intraocular inflammation,* *i.e.* uveitis with associated endothelitis also causes corneal oedema.

iii. *Postoperative raised IOP* may result in acute endothelial decompensation with an increase in the corneal thickness. When epithelial oedema is present in the face of compact stroma immediately after surgery, it is likely due to elevated IOP with an intact endothelium. Decreasing IOP, via aqueous release from the paracentesis site after results in immediate resolution of epithelial oedema in these cases.

Some facts about postoperative corneal oedema

- *When corneal periphery is clear,* the corneal oedema usually resolves with time.
- *Corneal oedema persisting after 3 months* usually does not clear.
- *Chronic corneal oedema* from significant loss of endothelial cells results in bullous keratopathy which is associated with reduced visual acuity, irritation, foreign body sensation and watering.
- *Striate keratopathy,* characterized by mild corneal oedema with Descemet's folds is a common complication observed during immediate postoperative period. This occurs due to endothelial damage during surgery. Mild striate keratopathy usually disappears spontaneously within a week. Moderate to severe keratopathy may be treated as described below.
- *Brown–McLean syndrome* refers to a condition of peripheral corneal oedema with a clear central cornea occurring after cataract surgery. Punctate brown pigment often underlies the oedematous area.
- *Irvine–Gass syndrome* refers to a condition of vitreocorneal adherence, persistent corneal oedema and cystoid macular oedema following ICCE or complicated ECCE or phacoemulsification. A vitrectomy is needed for treatment.
- *Pseudophakic bullous keratopathy (PBK)* is usually a continuation of postoperative corneal oedema produced by surgical or

chemical insult to a healthy or compromised corneal endothelium. PBK is becoming a common indication for penetrating keratoplasty (PK).

Treatment of corneal oedema

- *Topical hyperosmotic agents along with topical steroids* (5% NaCl) may be useful in early cases.
- *Bandage contact lenses (BCL)* may be required in persistent cases with bullae formation.
- *Penetrating or endothelial keratoplasty* may be required in bullous keratopathy not responding to conservative treatment.
- *Gunderson conjunctival flap or amniotic membrane transplantation (AMT)* may help in alleviating pain due to recurrent rupture of bullae in patients with little visual potential.

5. Postoperative anterior uveitis can be induced by instrumental trauma, undue handling of uveal tissue, reaction to residual cortex or chemical reaction induced by viscoelastics, pilocarpine, etc.

Management includes more aggressive use of topical steroids, cycloplegics and NSAIDs. Rarely systemic steroids may be required in cases with severe fibrinous reaction.

6. Toxic anterior segment syndrome (TASS) is an acute severe intraocular inflammation accompanied by diffuse corneal oedema which is most commonly associated with cataract surgery. TASS presents within 12–48 hours after surgery where infectious endophthalmitis typically develops 2–7 days after surgery.

Etiology. TASS has numerous causes, and most cases are attributed to:

- Bacterial endotoxins or particulate contamination of balanced salt solutions.
- Intraocular irrigating solutions with abnormal pH, osmolarity or ionic composition.
- Denatured ophthalmic viscosurgical devices (OVD).
- Intraocular medications (antibiotics in the irrigation solutions or intracameral antibiotics)
- Inadequate sterilization of surgical instruments and tubing.
- Inadequate flushing of instruments between cases resulting in build-up of ophthalmic viscosurgical devices (OVD).
- Preservative
- Metallic precipitate
- Other substances that enter the eye during or after surgery, such as topical ointments or talc from surgical gloves.

Clinical features. Clinical features of TASS typically appear within 12–48 hours after surgery and include the following:

Symptoms reported usually are:

- Vision loss or blurry vision
- Pain ranging from mild to severe
- Photophobia.

Signs noted are:

- *Corneal oedema* typically extending from limbus to limbus
- *Pupil* is dilated or irregular
- *Intraocular pressure* may be increased
- *Anterior chamber* shows severe inflammation appearing within 12–48 hours postoperative period. Hypopyon may be present occasionally.

Diagnosis is made as below:

- *Clinical diagnosis* is made from the typical clinical features mentioned above. All patients must have a slit-lamp examination, measurement of IOP and dilated fundus examination.
- *Ultrasound B-scan,* to rule out any posterior segment reaction, is required in the presence of hazy media due to severe anterior chamber reaction.
- *Aqueous and vitreous taps* should be taken and sent for bacterial culture (both aerobic and anaerobic) and fungal culture to investigate for an infectious process.

Management. Management of TASS includes its differential diagnosis, prevention and treatment.

Differential diagnosis should be made from

- Infectious endophthalmitis
- Retained lens material
- Uveitis

Prevention of TASS includes:

- *Use of proper balance salt solution* (BSS) with the correct pH, osmolarity, and ionic composition.
- *Good filtration of the BSS* at the manufacturing site to eliminate particulate contamination and endotoxins.

- *Avoid any kind of preservatives* in the intraocular solutions, intracameral medications and irrigating solutions.
- *Use of fresh ophthalmic viscosurgical devices.*
- *Adequate sterilization* of instruments and tubing according to the manufacturer's protocol. Standard and clear operative and instrument processing procedures (SOP) need to be implemented.
- *The staff and surgeon should be well aware* of the SOPs.

Treatment. Treatment is mainly medical, rarely surgical intervention may be required.

Medical treatment consists of:

- *Topical steroids*—most patients do well with medical management using topical steroids only.
- *Systemic steroid* treatment may be needed in rare cases, depending on the severity.

Note. The patient should be followed closely and needs to be evaluated by a retina specialist to rule out infectious causes.

Surgical treatment. Rarely in severe cases, there may occur need for surgical intervention in the form of cornea transplant, glaucoma surgery or both.

7. Bacterial endophthalmitis. This is one of the most dreaded complication with an incidence of 0.2–0.5%. The principal sources of infection are contaminated solutions, instruments, surgeon's hands, patient's own flora from conjunctiva, eyelids and air-borne bacteria.

Symptoms and signs of bacterial endophthalmitis are generally present between 48 and 72 hours after surgery and include: ocular pain, diminshed vision, lid oedema, conjunctival chemosis and marked circumciliary congestion, corneal oedema, exudates in the pupillary area, hypopyon and diminished or absent red pupillary glow (Fig. 20.5).

Management. It is an emergency and should be managed energetically.

i. *Microbiological diagnosis.* As soon as the diagnosis of endophthalmitis is suspected, the first step is to obtain a vitreous sample in order to find the causal microorganism. A sample of aqueous humour may be useful also but the probability to find a microorganism by direct examination or by culture is higher in the vitreous (40–69% of the cases) than in the aqueous humour (22–30%). The micro organisms found are Gram-positive bacteria in 85–94% of the cases: *Staphylococcus epidermidis* is the most common (45–50%), followed by *Streptococcus* species (24–38%) and *Staphylococcus aureus* (7–11%).

ii. *Intravitreal antibiotics*

- *When a bacterial endophthalmitis is suspected*, in order to cover all the germs that can be responsible for the endophthalmitis, two combinations of two antibiotics are to be recommended.
  - The first one is vancomycin 1 mg/0.1 ml + ceftazidine 2.25 mg/0.1 ml, and
  - The second one is vancomycin 1 mg/0.1 ml + amikacin 0.4 mg/0.1 ml. Vancomycin is

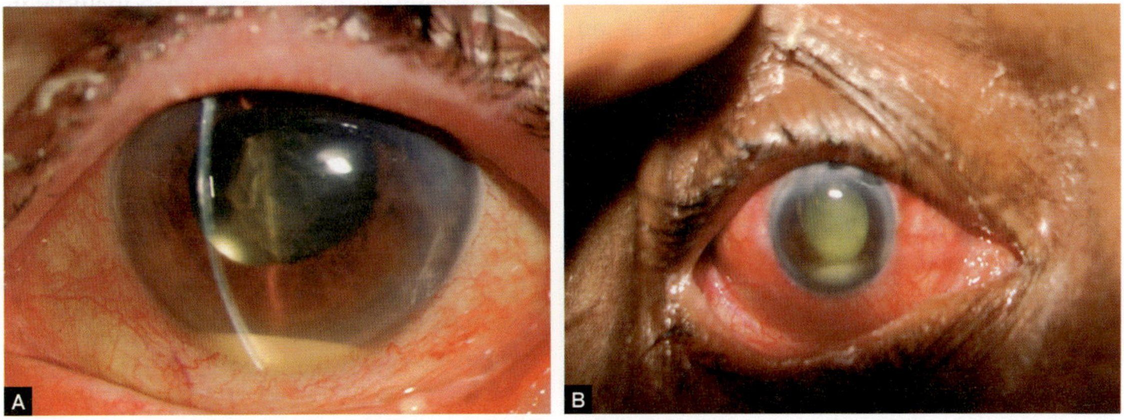

Fig. 20.5. *Postoperative endophthalmitis.*

useful to cover the Gram-positive organisms and particularly *Staphylococcus epidermidis*. Either ceftazidine or amikacin may be efficient against Gram-negative organisms. However, both have a drawback. When used together with vancomycin, ceftazidine may precipitate and become less bio-available. Amikacin has the advantage to have a synergistic activity with vancomycin against Gram-positive organisms, but may cause macular infarction in up to 0.5% of the cases.

- *When a fungal endophthalmitis is suspected or proved*, intravitred injection of amphotericin 5 μg is the treatment of choice. If the organism is resistant, voriconazole 100 μg might be useful.

iii. ***Systemic antibiotics.*** So far, there has been no definitive study to prove that the endophthalmitis patient is better managed with than without systemic antibiotic therapy along with intravitreal antibiotics. In daily clinical practice, systemic antibiotics are usually prescribed, and the drug of choice for this purpose is a quinolone. This family of antibiotics is characterized by a good bioavailability, a long half-life, and a good penetration in the vitreous cavity. The quinolones are quickly bactericidal. Ciprofloxacine has been the first one to be used, but several cases of bacterial resistance have emerged. So third generation quinolones such as moxifloxacine and gatifloxacine are now being used.

iv. ***Vitrectomy.*** Immediate vitrectomy is recommended when the initial visual acuity is reduced to light perception only, and delayed vitrectomy is recommended, if there is no clinical improvement 48 hours after intravitreal antibiotic injection. Once the infection is well controlled, a functional vitrectomy may also be necessary in order to improve the final visual acuity, should the vitreous remains opaque.

v. ***Corticosteroids.*** The use of corticosteroids in the treatment of endophthalmitis is still a matter of debate. There is not a single prospective randomized study which could have proved the efficacy of corticosteroids in this situation. The rationale for the use of corticosteroids is that the ocular inflammation that occurs during endophthalmitis may become the main cause of irreversible complications. Corticosteroid therapy may probably be started as soon as 48 hours after the beginning of the antibiotherapy, if a fungal infection is not suspected. Dexamethasone may be injected in the vitreous cavity. The recommended dose is 400 μg. Systemic corticosteroids are not advised because of the many general contraindications and side effects. Most often steroid drops and sub-conjunctival injections are used, but their action is mainly directed toward the anterior segment.

8. Delayed chronic postoperative endophthalmitis is caused when an organism of low virulence (*Propionibacterium acnes* or *Staph epidermidis*) becomes trapped within the capsular bag. It has an onset ranging from 4 weeks to years (mean 9 months) postoperatively and typically follows an uneventful cataract extraction with a PCIOL in the bag.

9. Cystoid macular oedema (CME). Collection of fluid in the form of cystic loculi in the Henle's layer of macula is a frequent complication of cataract surgery. However, in most cases, it is clinically insignificant, does not produce any visual problem and undergoes spontaneous regression. In few cases, clinically significant CME typically produces visual diminution one to three months after cataract extraction. On fundoscopy, it gives *honeycomb appearance*. On fluorescein angiography, it depicts typical *flower petal pattern* due to leakage of dye from perifoveal capillaries. In most cases, it is associated with vitreous incarceration in the wound and mild iritis.

Prevention. Role of some prostaglandins is being widely considered in its etiopathogenesis. Therefore, immediate preoperative and post-operative use of antiprostaglandins (indomethacin or flurbiprofen or ketorolac) eyedrops is re-commended as prophylaxis of CME.

Management. In cases of CME with vitreous incarceration, anterior vitrectomy along with steroids and antiprostaglandins may improve visual acuity and decrease the amount of discomfort.

10. Retinal detachment (RD). Incidence of retinal detachment is higher in aphakic and pseudo-phakic patients as compared to phakics. It has been noted that retinal detachment is more common after ICCE than after ECCE. Incidence is lower with phacoemulsification as compared to ECCE and SICS. Other risk factors for retinal detachment include vitreous loss during operation, associated myopia and lattice degeneration of the retina.

11. Epithelial ingrowth. Rarely conjunctival epithelial cells may invade the anterior chamber through a defect in the incision. This abnormal epithelial membrane slowly grows and lines the back of cornea and trabecular meshwork leading to intractable glaucoma. In late stages, the epithelial membrane extends on the iris and anterior part of the vitreous.

12. Fibrous downgrowth into the anterior chamber may occur very rarely when the cataract wound apposition is not perfect. It may cause secondary glaucoma, disorganisation of anterior segment and ultimately phthisis bulbi.

13. After cataract. It is also known as 'secondary cataract'. It is the opacity which persists or develops after any technique of extracapsular lens extraction.

Causes. (i) *Residual opaque lens matter* may persist as after cataract when it is imprisoned between the remains of the anterior and posterior capsules, surrounded by fibrin (following iritis) or blood (following hyphaema). (ii) *Proliferative type* of after cataract may develop from the left-out anterior epithelial cells. The proliferative hyaline bands may sweep across the whole posterior capsule.

Clinical types. After cataract may present as:

- *Thickened posterior capsule*, or dense membranous after cataract (Fig. 20.6A),
- *Soemmering's ring* which refers to a thick ring of after cataract formed behind the iris, enclosed between the two layers of capsule (Fig. 20.6B),

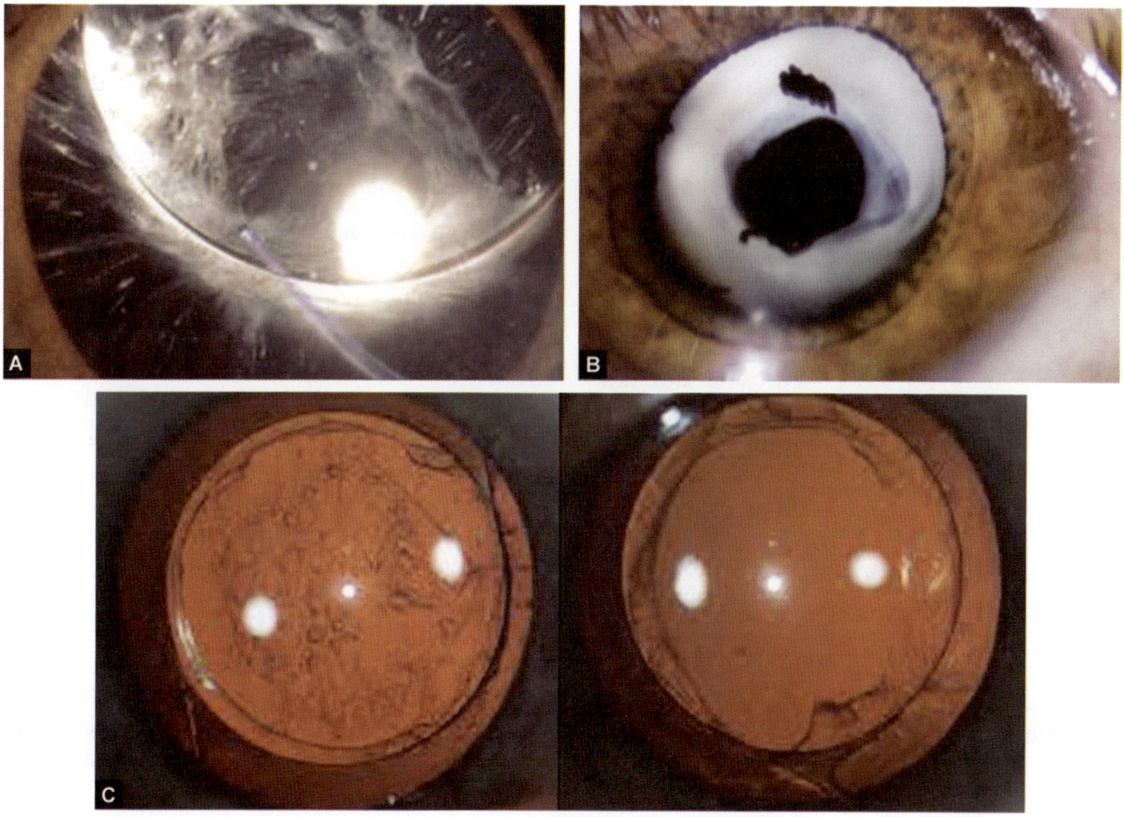

Fig. 20.6. *Types of after cataract: **(A)** Membranous posterior capsule opacification (PCO); **(B)** Soemmering's ring; **(C)** Elschnig's pearls.*

- *Elschnig's pearls* in which the vacuolated subcapsular epithelial cells are clustered like soap bubbles along the posterior capsule (Fig. 20.6C).

Treatment is as follows:

i. Thin membranous after cataract and thickened posterior capsule are best treated by YAG-laser capsulotomy. Alternatively discission with cystitome or Ziegler's knife can be done.
ii. Dense membranous after cataract needs surgical membranectomy.
iii. Soemmering's ring after cataract with clear central posterior capsule needs no treatment.
v. Elschnig's pearls involving the central part of the posterior capsule can be treated by YAG-laser capsulotomy or discission with cystitome.

14. Postoperative glaucoma

Causes. Postoperative glaucoma includes following conditions:

i. *Raised IOP with deep anterior chamber in early postoperative period.* It may be due to hyphaema, inflammation, retained cortical matter or vitreous filling the anterior chamber.

ii. *Secondary angle-closure glaucoma due to flat anterior chamber.* It may occur following long-standing wound leak.

iii. *Secondary angle-closure glaucoma due to pupil block.* It may occur following formation of annular synechiae or vitreous herniation.

iv. *Undiagnosed pre-existing primary open-angle glaucoma* may be associated with aphakia/ pseudophakia.

v. *Steroid-induced glaucoma.* It may develop in patients operated for cataract due to postoperative treatment with steroids.

vi. *Epithelial ingrowth* may cause an intractable glaucoma in late postoperative period by invading the trabeculum and the anterior segment structures.

vii. *Aphakic/pseudophakic malignant glaucoma* first described by von Graefe in 1869, is also known as aqueous misdirection, ciliary block glaucoma and lens block angle closure. It is characterized by elevated IOP with a shallow or flat anterior chamber, and it occurs following intraocular surgery, usually in patients having or prone to angle closure glaucoma.

Malignant glaucoma is one of the most complex and difficult of all the glaucomas to treat, and it can progress to permanent blindness without prompt intervention.

Etiopathogenesis

Risk factors. Malignant glaucoma occurs in 2–4% of eyes undergoing surgery for angle-closure glaucoma, and though it may occur at any time during the postoperative period, most cases occur shortly after incisional surgery. It may also occur within hours to days or years after cataract extraction with or without IOL implantation. Risk factors include:

- Hyperopia
- Chronic angle closure with plateau iris configuration
- Nanophthalmos
- History of malignant glaucoma in the fellow eye
- Women are three times more likely than men to develop malignant glaucoma, possibly because they have a smaller mean axial length than men, their ocular volume is 10% less and they have shallower anterior chambers.

Note. Preoperative IOP is not a good indicator of the likelihood of developing malignant glaucoma postsurgically.

Pathogenesis. The mechanism of this disorder remains unclear. Following theories have been proposed:

- *Shaffer* proposed posterior segment pooling of aqueous due to a blockage of the normal anterior aqueous flow by an abnormal vitreociliary relationship. He coined the term *ciliary block glaucoma.*
- Another theory by *Epstein* and colleagues proposed anterior displacement of the vitreous due to posterior diversion of aqueous. They also proposed that there may be associated thickening of the anterior hyaloid. According to this theory, the accumulation of aqueous within the posterior segment forces the ciliary body and the anterior hyaloid face forward, shallowing the anterior chamber and causing secondary angle closure.
- *Quigley* and colleagues implicated the poor conductivity of fluid through the vitreous and stated that past theories proposing misdirected

aqueous violate the laws of physics. Dr. Quigley believes that the inciting event for malignant glaucoma is more likely to be the inability to generate sufficient fluid flow across the vitreous to compensate for aqueous outflow anteriorly under the higher pressure conditions generated by choroidal expansion. With such choroidal expansion, the pressure within the corneoscleral shell increases and anterior outflow increases.

Whatever the underlying pathophysiology may be, it is clear that the iris, ciliary processes, lens and vitreous are intimately involved in the development of malignant glaucoma.

Diagnosis

- Malignant glaucoma presents difficult diagnostic and treatment challenges. Slit-lamp examination reveals anterior displacement of the IOL-iris diaphragm in pseudophakic patients and of the anterior hyaloid face in aphakic patients, shallowing of both the central and peripheral anterior chamber and elevated IOP. Physical findings include unequal anterior chamber depths, increasing myopia and progressive shallowing of the anterior chamber.
- If there is no iridotomy or if patency is in doubt, an iridotomy must be created to rule out pupillary block.
- If there is a patent iridotomy and the IOP remains high, choroidal detachment and suprachoroidal haemorrhage must be excluded clinically or by ultrasound biomicroscopy (UBM).

Imaging

i. *UBM* has documented swelling or anterior rotation of the ciliary body with forward rotation of the IOL-iris diaphragm and relaxation of the zonular apparatus, causing anterior IOL displacement and direct angle closure by physically pushing the iris against the trabecular meshwork. In some eyes, a shallow supraciliary detachment, which is not evident on routine B-scan examination, is responsible for anterior rotation of the ciliary body. Consequently, there is diffuse shallowing of the anterior chamber. In ciliary block, a pressure differential is created between the vitreous and aqueous compartments, a situation analogous to pupillary block, in which the angle becomes occluded by the iris because of a pressure differential between the posterior and anterior chambers.

ii. *Anterior segment optical coherence tomography (AS-OCT)* is a new imaging method that allows for objective and quantitative imaging of the anterior segment. AS-OCT is similar to UBM in its ability to determine angle parameters quantitatively. Although the resolution is lower and details behind the iris are not reliably seen, AS-OCT has the benefit of being easier to use and does not require a coupling agent.

Management

I. *Medical management.* Initial medical therapy includes:

- *Aqueous suppressants* to lower the IOP.
- *Hyperosmotic agents* to shrink the vitreous.
- *Cycloplegic*, such as atropine, for an attempt to posteriorly displace the IOL-iris diaphragm.

The effect of medical therapy is often not immediate, but approximately 50% of cases will be relieved within five days.

II. *Laser therapy* may be useful in following forms:

- *Laser iridotomy* must be performed, if one is not present or if patency of a previous iridotomy cannot be established.
- *Nd:YAG laser therapy* may be attempted to disrupt the posterior capsule and anterior hyaloid face, if medical management is unsuccessful, or if lens-cornea touch occurs.
- *Argon laser* through a peripheral iridectomy may also be used in an attempt to shrink the ciliary processes and relieve ciliolenticular blockage of the anterior flow of aqueous.

III. *Posterior vitrectomy* should be performed with disruption of the anterior hyaloid face when laser therapy is not possible or is unsuccessful.

Note. Once the anterior chamber deepens and the IOP has been normalized, medical treatment can be withdrawn gradually. The patient may require indefinite treatment with cycloplegics to prevent recurrence, if vitrectomy was not performed.

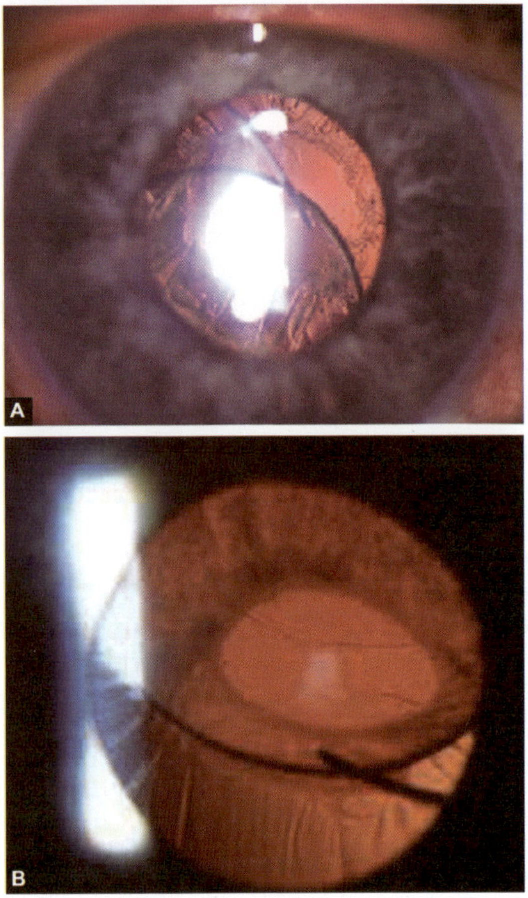

Fig. 20.7. *Decentration of posterior chamber IOL: **(A)** Inferior subluxation; **(B)** Superior subluxation.*

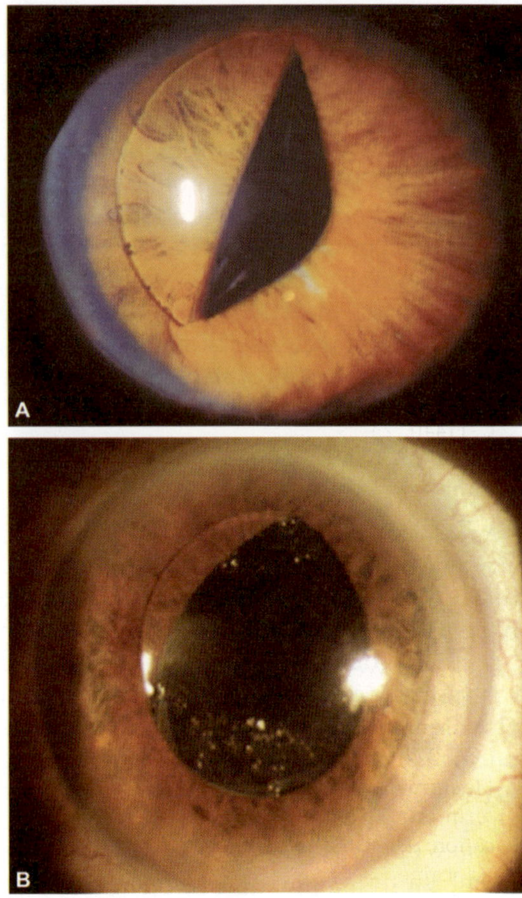

Fig. 20.8. *Pupillary capture of posterior chamber IOL.*

15. IOL-related complications. In addition to the complications of cataract surgery, following IOL-related complications may be seen:

a. ***Complications like cystoid macular oedema, corneal endothelial damage, uveitis and secondary glaucoma*** are seen more frequently with IOL implantation, especially with anterior chamber and iris-supported IOLs.

- *UGH syndrome* refers to concurrent occurrence of uveitis, glaucoma and hyphaema. It used to occur with rigid anterior chamber IOLs, which are not used now.

b. ***Malpositions of IOL.*** These may be in the form of decentration, subluxation and dislocation. The fancy names attached to various malpositions of IOL are:

- *Sunset syndrome,* i.e. inferior subluxation of IOL (Fig. 20.7A).
- *Sunrise syndrome* superior subluxation of IOL (Fig. 20.7B).
- *Windshield wiper syndrome.* It results when a very small IOL is placed vertically in the sulcus. In it, the superior loop moves to the left and right, with movements of the head.
- *Lost lens syndrome* refers to complete dislocation of an IOL into the vitreous cavity.

c. ***Pupillary capture of the IOL*** (Fig. 20.8) may occur following postoperative iritis or proliferation of the remains of the lens fibres.

BIBLIOGRAPHY

COMPLICATION ASSOCIATED WITH CATARACT SURGERY

1. Chang DF, Masket S, Miller KM, Braga-Mele R, Little BC, Mamalis N, et al. Complications of

sulcus placement of single-piece acrylic intraocular lenses: recommendations for backup IOL implantation following posterior capsule rupture. J Cataract Refract Surg 35(8):1445–1458,2009 Aug.
2. Kuchle M, Schonherr U, Dieckmann U. Risk factors for capsular rupture and vitreous loss in extracapsular cataract extraction. The Erlangen Ophthalmology Group. Fortschr Ophthalmol 86(5):417–421,1989.
3. Stainer L. Cataract surgery complications. Intra-operative complications. Continuing education and training. On line publication; course code C-11440. 23–29,2009.
4. Zare M, Javadi M-A, Einollahi B, Baradaran-Rafii A-R, Feizi S, Kiavash V. Risk factors for posterior capsule rupture and vitreous loss during phacoermulsification. J Ophthalmic Vis *Res* 4(4):208–212,2009.

TOXIC ANTERIOR

1. Avisar R, Weinberger D. (2010). Corneal endothelial morphologic features in toxic anterior segment syndrome. Cornea 29:251–3,2010. ISSN: 0277-3740.
2. Heuermann T, Hartman C, Anders N. Long-term endothelial cell loss after phacoemulsification; peribulbar anesthesia versus intracameral lidocaine 1%; prospective, randomized clinical trial. J Cataract Refract Surg, 28:639–643;2002. ISSN: 0886-3350.
3. Holland SP, Lee TL, Morck DW (2007). Update on toxic anterior segment syndrome. Curr Opin Ophthalmol 18:4–8, 2007. ISSN: 1040–8738.

MACULAR OEDEMA

1. Ah-Fat FG, Sharma MK, Majid MA, Yang YC. Vitreous loss during conversion from conventional extracapsular cataract extraction to phacoemulsification. J Cataract Refract Surg, Vol. 24: (801–805),1998.
2. Chan E, Mahroon OAR, Spalton DJ. Complications of cataract surgery. Clin Exp Optom Vol. 93; No. 6: (379–389), 2010.
3. Ferrari MT, Cavallo M, Minnino L, Cardascia N. Macular edema induced by phacoemulsification. Doc Ophthalmol, Vol. 97:(325–7),1999.
4. Irvine AR. Cystoid maculopathy. Surv Ophthalmol Vol. 21:(1–17),1976.
5. Irvine SR. A newly defined vitreous syndrome following cataract surgery. Am J Ophthalmol, Vol. 36; No. 5: (499–619),1953.

INTRAOCULAR FLOPPY

1. Blouin MC, Blouin J, Perreault S, Lapointe A, Dragomir A: Intraoperative floppy-iris syndrome associated with alpha1-adrenoreceptors: comparison of tamsulosin and alfuzosin. J Cataract Refract Surg 33:1227–1234,2007.
2. Chang DF, Campbell JR. Intraoperative floppy iris syndrome associated with tamsulosin. J Cataract Refract Surg 31:664–673,2005.
3. Edelhauser HF, Hyndiuk RA, Zeeb A, Schultz RO: Corneal edema and the intraocular use of epinephrine. Am J Ophthalmol 93:327–333,1982.

ENDOPHTHALMITIS

1. Aaberg TM Jr., Flynn HW Jr., Schiffman J, Newton J. Nosocomial acute-onset postoperative endophthalmitis surgery: a ten-year review of incidence and outcomes. Ophthalmology 105: 1004–1010,1998.
2. Aaberg TM Jr, Rubsamen PE, Joondeph BC, Flynn HW Jr. Chronic postoperative Gram-negative endophthalmitis. Retina. 17:260–262, 1997.
3. Allen HF, Mangiaracine AB. Bacterial endophthalmitis after cataract extraction: a study of 22 infections in 20,000 operations. Arch. Ophthalmol. 72:454–462, 1964.

Index

D

E

P

R